Lecture Notes in Artificial Intelligence 7867

Subseries of Lecture Notes in Computer Science

LNAI Series Editors

Randy Goebel
University of Alberta, Edmonton, Canada

Yuzuru Tanaka
Hokkaido University, Sapporo, Japan

Wolfgang Wahlster
DFKI and Saarland University, Saarbrücken, Germany

LNAI Founding Series Editor

Joerg Siekmann
DFKI and Saarland University, Saarbrücken, Germany

Jiuyong Li   Longbing Cao
Can Wang   Kay Chen Tan   Bo Liu
Jian Pei   Vincent S. Tseng (Eds.)

Trends and Applications in Knowledge Discovery and Data Mining

PAKDD 2013 International Workshops:
DMApps, DANTH, QIMIE, BDM, CDA, CloudSD
Gold Coast, QLD, Australia, April 14-17, 2013
Revised Selected Papers

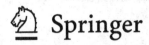 Springer

Volume Editors

Jiuyong Li
University of South Australia, Adelaide, SA, Australia
E-mail: jiuyong.li@unisa.edu.au

Longbing Cao
Can Wang
University of Technology, Sydney, NSW, Australia
E-mail: longbing.cao@uts.edu.au; canwang613@gmail.com

Kay Chen Tan
National University of Singapore, Singapore
E-mail: eletankc@nus.edu.sg

Bo Liu
Guangdong University of Technology, Guangzhou, China
E-mail: csbliu@gmail.com

Jian Pei
Simon Fraser University, Burnaby, BC, Canada
E-mail: jpei@cs.sfu.ca

Vincent S. Tseng
National Cheng Kung University, Tainan, Taiwan
E-mail: tsengsm@mail.ncku.edu.tw

ISSN 0302-9743   e-ISSN 1611-3349
ISBN 978-3-642-40318-7   e-ISBN 978-3-642-40319-4
DOI 10.1007/978-3-642-40319-4
Springer Heidelberg Dordrecht London New York

Library of Congress Control Number: 2013944975

CR Subject Classification (1998): H.2.8, I.2, H.3, H.5, H.4, I.5

LNCS Sublibrary: SL 7 – Artificial Intelligence

Typesetting: Camera-ready by author, data conversion by Scientific Publishing Services, Chennai, India

Printed on acid-free paper

Springer is part of Springer Science+Business Media (www.springer.com)

Preface

This volume contains papers presented at PAKDD Workshops 2013, affiliated with the 17th Pacific-Asia Conference on Knowledge Discovery and Data Mining (PAKDD) held on April 14, 2013 on the Gold Coast, Australia. PAKDD has established itself as the premier event for data mining researchers in the Pacific-Asia region. The workshops affiliated with PAKDD 2013 were: Data Mining Applications in Industry and Government (DMApps), Data Analytics for Targeted Healthcare (DANTH), Quality Issues, Measures of Interestingness and Evaluation of Data Mining Models (QIMIE), Biologically Inspired Techniques for Data Mining (BDM), Constraint Discovery and Application (CDA), Cloud Service Discovery (CloudSD), and Behavior Informatics (BI). This volume collects the revised papers from the first six workshops. The papers of BI will appear in a separate volume.

The first six workshops received 92 submissions. All papers were reviewed by at least two reviewers. In all, 47 papers were accepted for presentation, and their revised versions are collected in this volume. These papers mainly cover the applications of data mining in industry, government, and health care. The papers also cover some fundamental issues in data mining such as interestingness measures and result evaluation, biologically inspired design, constraint and cloud service discovery.

These workshops featured five invited speeches by distinguished researchers: Geoffrey I. Webb (Monash University, Australia), Osmar R. Zaïane (University of Albert, Canada), Jian Pei (Simon Fraser University, Canada), Ning Zhong (Maebashi Institute of Technology, Japan), and Longbing Cao (University of Technology Sydney, Australia). Their talks cover current challenging issues and advanced applications in data mining.

The workshops would not be successful without the support of the authors, reviewers, and organizers. We thank the many authors for submitting their research papers to the PAKDD workshops. We thank the successful authors whose papers are published in this volume for their collaboration in the paper revision and final submission. We appreciate all PC members for their timely reviews working to a tight schedule. We also thank members of the Organizing Committees for organizing the paper submission, reviews, discussion, feedback and the final submission. We appreciate the professional service provided by the Springer LNCS editorial teams, and Mr. Zhong She's assistance in formatting.

June 2013

Jiuyong Li
Longbing Cao
Can Wang
Kay Chen Tan
Bo Liu

Organization

PAKDD Conference Chairs

Hiroshi Motoda   Osaka University, Japan
Longbing Cao   University of Technology, Sydney, Australia

Workshop Chairs

Jiuyong Li   University of South Australia, Australia
Kay Chen Tan   National University of Singapore, Singapore
Bo Liu   Guangdong University of Technology, China

Workshop Proceedings Chair

Can Wang   University of Technology, Sydney, Australia

Organizing Chair

Xinhua Zhu   University of Technology, Sydney, Australia

DMApps Chairs

Warwick Graco   Australian Taxation Office, Australia
Yanchang Zhao   Department of Immigration and Citizenship, Australia
Inna Kolyshkina   Institute of Analytics Professionals of Australia
Clifton Phua   SAS Institute Pte Ltd, Singapore

DANTH Chairs

Yanchun Zhang   Victoria University, Australia
Michael Ng   Hong Kong Baptist University, Hong Kong
Xiaohui Tao   University of Southern Queensland, Australia
Guandong Xu   University of Technology, Sydney, Australia
Yidong Li   Beijing Jiaotong University, China
Hongmin Cai   South China University of Technology, China
Prasanna Desikan   Allina Health, USA
Harleen Kaur   United Nations University, International Institute for Global Health, Malaysia

QIMIE Chairs

Stéphane Lallich   ERIC, Université Lyon 2, France
Philippe Lenca   Lab-STICC, Telecom Bretagne, France

BDM Chairs

Mengjie Zhang   Victoria University of Wellington, New Zealand
Shafiq Alam Burki   University of Auckland, New Zealand
Gillian Dobbie   University of Auckland, New Zealand

CDA Chairs

Chengfei Liu   Swinburne University of Technology, Australia
Jixue Liu   University of South Australia, Australia

CloudSD Chairs

Michael R. Lyu   The Chinese University of Hong Kong, China
Jian Yang   Macquarie University, Australia
Jian Wu   Zhejiang University, China
Zibin Zheng   The Chinese University of Hong Kong, China

Combined Program Committee

Aiello Marco   University of Groningen, The Netherlands
Alípio Jorge   University of Porto, Portugal
Amadeo Napoli   Lorraine Research Laboratory in Computer
                                      Science and Its Applications, France
Arturas Mazeika   Max Planck Institute for Informatics, Germany
Asifullah Khan   PIEAS, Pakistan
Bagheri Ebrahim   Ryerson University, Canada
Blanca Vargas-Govea   Monterrey Institute of Technology
                                      and Higher Education, Mexico
Bo Yang   University of Electronic Science and
                                      Technology of China
Bouguettaya Athman   RMIT, Australia
Bruno Crémilleux   Université de Caen, France
Chaoyi Pang   CSIRO, Australia
David Taniar   Monash University, Australia
Dianhui Wang   La Trobe University, Australia
Emilio Corchado   University of Burgos, Spain
Eng-Yeow Cheu   Institute for Infocomm Research, Singapore

Evan Stubbs	SAS, Australia
Fabien Rico	Université Lyon 2, France
Fabrice Guillet	Université de Nantes, France
Fatos Xhafa	Universitat Politècnica de Catalunya, Barcelona, Spain
Fedja Hadzic	Curtin University, Australia
Feiyue Ye	Jiangsu Teachers University of Technology, China
Ganesh Kumar Venayagamoorthy	Missouri University of Science and Technology, USA
Gang Li	Deakin University, Australia
Gary Weiss	Fordham University, USA
Graham Williams	ATO, Australia
Guangfei Yang	Dalian University of Technology, China
Guoyin Wang	Chongqing University of Posts and Telecommunications, China
Hai Jin	Huazhong University of Science and Technology, China
Hangwei Qian	VMware Inc., USA
Hidenao Abe	Shimane University, Japan
Hong Cheu Liu	University of South Australia, Australia
Ismail Khalil Johannes	Kepler University, Austria
Izabela Szczech	Poznan University of Technology, Poland
Jan Rauch	University of Economics, Prague, Czech Republic
Jérôme Azé	Université Paris-Sud, France
Jean Diatta	Université de la Réunion, France
Jean-Charles Lamirel	LORIA, France
Jeff Tian	Southern Methodist University, USA
Jeffrey Soar	University of Southern Queensland, Australia
Jerzy Stefanowski	Poznan University of Technology, Poland
Ji Wang	National University of Defense Technology, China
Ji Zhang	University of Southern Queensland, Australia
Jianwen Su	UC Santa Barbara, USA
Jianxin Li	Swinburne University of Technology, Australia
Jie Wan	University College Dublin, Ireland
Jierui Xie	Oracle, USA
Jogesh K. Muppala	University of Science and Technology of Hong Kong, Hong Kong
Joo-Chuan Tong	SAP Research, Singapore
José L. Balcázar	Universitat Politècnica de Catalunya, Spain
Julia Belford	University of California, Berkeley, USA
Jun Ma	University of Wollongong, Australia
Junhu Wang	Griffith University, Australia
Kamran Shafi	University of New South Wales, Australia

Robert Stahlbock	University of Hamburg, Germany
Rohan Baxter	Australian Taxation Office, Australia
Ross Gayler	La Trobe University, Australia
Rui Zhou	Swinburne University of Technology, Australia
Sami Bhiri	National University of Ireland, Ireland
Sanjay Chawla	University of Sydney, Australia
Shangguang Wang	Beijing University of Posts and Telecommunications, China
Shanmugasundaram Hariharan	Abdur Rahman University, India
Shusaku Tsumoto	Shimane University, Japan
Sorin Moga	Telecom Bretagne, France
Stéphane Lallich	Université Lyon 2, France
Stephen Chen	York University, Canada
Sy-Yen Kuo	National Taiwan University, Taiwan
Tadashi Dohi	Hiroshima University, Japan
Thanh-Nghi Do	Can Tho University, Vietnam
Ting Yu	University of Sydney, Australia
Tom Osborn	Brandscreen, Australia
Vladimir Estivill-Castro	Griffith University, Australia
Wei Luo	The University of Queensland, Australia
Weifeng Su	United International College, Hong Kong
Xiaobo Zhou	The Methodist Hospital, USA
Xiaoyin Xu	Brigham and Women's Hospital, USA
Xin Wang	University of Calgary, Canada
Xue Li	University of Queensland, Australia
Yan Li	University of Southern Queensland, Australia
Yanchang Zhao	Department of Immigration and Citizenship, Australia
Yanjun Yan	ARCON Corporation, USA
Yin Shan	Department of Human Services, Australian
Yue Xu	Queensland University of Technology, Australia
Yun Sing Koh	University of Auckland, New Zealand
Zbigniew Ras	University of North Carolina at Charlotte, USA
Zhenglu Yang	University of Tokyo, Japan
Zhiang Wu	Nanjing University of Finance and Economics, China
Zhiquan George Zhou	University of Wollongong, Australia
Zhiyong Lu	National Institutes of Health, USA
Zongda Wu	Wenzhou University, China

Table of Contents

Data Mining Applications in Industry and Government

Data Analytics for Targeted Healthcare

Quality Issues, Measures of Interestingness and Evaluation of Data Mining Models

Biological Inspired Techniques for Data Mining

Constraint Discovery and Cloud Service Discovery

Using Scan-Statistical Correlations
for Network Change Analysis

Adriel Cheng and Peter Dickinson

Command, Control, Communications and Intelligence Division
Defence Science and Technology Organisation, Department of Defence, Australia
{adriel.cheng,peter.dickinson}@dsto.defence.gov.au

Abstract. Network change detection is a common prerequisite for identifying anomalous behaviours in computer, telecommunication, enterprise and social networks. Data mining of such networks often focus on the most significant change only. However, inspecting large deviations in isolation can lead to other important and associated network behaviours to be overlooked. This paper proposes that changes within the network graph be examined in conjunction with one another, by employing correlation analysis to supplement network-wide change information. Amongst other use-cases for mining network graph data, the analysis examines if multiple regions of the network graph exhibit similar degrees of change, or is it considered anomalous for a local network change to occur independently. Building upon Scan-Statistics network change detection, we extend the change detection technique to correlate localised network changes. Our correlation inspired techniques have been deployed for use on various networks internally. Using real-world datasets, we demonstrate the benefits of our correlation change analysis.

Keywords: Mining graph data, statistical methods for data mining, anomaly detection.

1   Introduction

Detecting changes in computer, telecommunication, enterprise or social networks is often the first step towards identifying anomalous activity or suspicious participants within such networks. In recent times, it has become increasingly common for a changing network to be sampled at various intervals and represented naturally as a time-series of graphs [1,2]. In order to uncover network anomalies within these graphs, the challenge in network change detection lies not only with the type of network graph changes to observe and how to measure such variations, but also the subsequent change analysis that is to be conducted.

Scan-statistics [3] is a change detection technique that employs statistical methods to measure variations in network graph vertices and surrounding vertex neighbourhood regions. The technique uncovers large localised deviations in behaviours exhibited by subgraph regions of the network. Traditionally, the subsequent change analysis focuses solely on local regions with largest deviations.

J. Li et al. (Eds.): PAKDD 2013 Workshops, LNAI 7867, pp. 1–13, 2013.

Despite usefulness in tracking such network change to potentially anomalous subgraphs, simply distinguishing which subgraph vertices contributed most to the network deviation is insufficient.

In many instances, the cause of significant network changes may not be restricted to a single vertex or subgraph region only, but multiple vertices or subgraphs may also experience similar degrees of deviations. Such vertex deviations could be interrelated, acting collectively with other vertices as the primary cause of the overall network change. Concentrating solely on the most significantly changed vertex or subgraph, other localised change behaviours would be hidden from examination. The dominant change centric analysis may in fact hinder evaluation of the actual change scenario experienced by the network.

To examine the network more conclusively, rather than inspect the most deviated vertex or subgraph, scan-statistic change analysis should characterise the types of localised changes and their relationships with one another across the entire network.

With this in mind, we extend scan-statistics with correlation based computations and change analysis. Using our approach, correlations between the edge-connectivity changes experienced by each pair of network graph vertices (or subgraphs) are examined. Correlation measurements are also aggregated to describe the correlation of each vertex (or subgraph) change with all other graph variations, and to assess the overall correlation of changes experienced by the network as a whole.

The goal in supporting scan-statistical change detections with our correlations-based analysis is to seek-out and characterise any relational patterns in the localised change behaviours exhibited by vertices and subgraphs. For instance, if a significant network change is detected and attributed to a particular vertex, do any other vertices in the network show similar deviation in behaviours? If so, how many vertices are considered similar? Do the majority of the vertices experience similar changes, or are these localised changes independent and not related to other regions of the network.

Accounting for correlations between localised vertex or subgraph variations provides further context into the possible scenarios triggering such network deviations. For example, if localised changes in the majority of vertices are highly correlated with one another, this could imply a scenario whereby a network-wide initialisation or re-configuration took place. In a social network, such high correlations of increased edge-linkages may correspond to some common holiday festive event, whereby individuals send/receive greetings to everyone on the network collectively within the same time period. Or if the communication links (and traffic) of a monitored network of terrorist suspects intensifies as a group, this could signal an impending attack.

On the other hand, a localised vertex or subgraph change which is uncorrelated to other members of the graph may indicate a command-control network scenario, In this case, any excessive change in network edge-connectivity would be largely localised to the single command vertex. Another example could involve the failure of a domain name system (DNS) server or a server under a denial-of-service attack. In this scenario, re-routing of traffic from the failed server to an alternative server would take place. The activity changes at these two server vertices would be highly localised and not correlated to the remainder of the network.

To the best of our knowledge, examining scan-statistical correlations of network graphs in support of further change analysis has not been previously explored. Hence, the contributions of this paper are two-fold. First, to extend scan-statistics network change detection with correlations analysis at multiple levels of the network graphs. And second, to facilitate visualisation of vertex clusters and reveal interrelated groups of vertices whose collective behaviour requires further investigation.

The remainder of this paper is as follows. Related work is discussed next. Section 3 gives a brief overview of scan-statistics. Sections 4 to 6 describe the correlation extensions and correlation inspired change analysis. This is followed by experiments demonstrating the practicality of our methods before the paper concludes in Section 8.

2   Related Work

The correlations based change analysis bears closest resemblance to the anomaly event detection work of Akoglu and Faloutsos [4]. Both our technique and that of Akoglu and Faloutsos employ 'Pearson ρ' correlation matrix manipulations. The aggregation methods to compute vertex and graph level correlation values are also similar. However, only correlations between vertices in/out degrees are considered by Akoglu and Faloutsos, whereas our method can be adapted to examine other vertex-induced k hop subgraph correlations as well – e.g. diameter, number of triangles, centrality, or other traffic distribution subgraph metrics [2,9]. The other key difference between our methods lies with their intended application usages.

Whilst their method exposes significant graph-wide deviations, employing correlation solely for change detection suffers from some shortcomings. Besides detecting change from the majority of network nodes, we are also interested in other types of network changes, such as anomalous deviations in behaviours from a few (or single) dominant vertices. In this sense, our approach is not to deploy correlations for network change detection directly, but to aid existing change detection methods and extend subsequent change analysis.

In another related paper from Akoglu and Dalvi [5], anomaly and change detection using similar correlation methods from [4] is described. However, their technique is formalised and designated for detecting 'Eigenbehavior' based changes only. In comparison, our methods are general in nature and not restricted to any particular type of network change or correlation outcome.

Another relevant paper from Ide and Kashima [6] is their Eigenspace inspired anomaly detection work for web-based computer systems. Both our approach and [6] follow similar procedural steps. But whilst our correlation method involves a graph adjacency matrix populated and aggregated with simplistic correlation computations, the technique in [6] employs graph dependency matrix values directly and consists of complex Eigenvector manipulations.

Other areas of research related to our work arise from Ahmed and Clark [7], and Fukuda et. al. [8]. These papers describe change detections and correlations that share similar philosophy with our methods. However, their underlying change detection and correlation methods, along with the type of network data differ from our approach.

The remaining schemes akin to our correlation methodology are captured by the MetricForensics tool [9]. Our technique span multiple levels of the network graphs, in contrast, MetricForensics applies correlation analysis exclusively at a global level.

3   Scan-Statistics

This section summaries the scan-statistics method. For a full treatment of scan-statistics, we refer the reader to [3]. Scan-statistics is a change detection technique that applies statistical analysis to sub-regions of a network graph. Statistical analysis is performed on graph vertices and vertex-induced subgraphs in order to measure local changes across a time-series of graphs. Whenever the network undergoes significant global change, scan-statistics detects and identifies the network vertices (or subgraphs) which exhibited greatest deviation from prior network behaviours.

In scan-statistics, local graph elements are denoted by their vertex induced k-hop subgraph regions. For every k-hop subgraph region, a *vertex-standardized* locality statistic is measured for that region. In order to monitor changes experienced by these subgraph regions, their locality statistics are measured for every graph throughout the time-series of network graphs. The vertex-standardized statistic $\tilde{\Psi}$ is :

$$\tilde{\Psi}_{k,t}(v) = \frac{\Psi_{k,t}(v) - \hat{\mu}_{k,t,\tau}(v)}{\max(\hat{\sigma}_{k,t,\tau}(v),1)} \tag{1}$$

where k is the number of hops (edges) from vertex v to create the induced subgraph, v is the vertex from which the subgraph is induced from, t is the time denoting the time-series graph, τ is the number (*window*) of previous graphs in the time-series to evaluate against current graph at t, Ψ is the local statistic that provides some measurement of behavioural change exhibited by v, and μ and σ are the mean and variance of Ψ.

The vertex-standardized locality statistic equation (1) above is interpreted as follows. For the network graph at time t, and for each k-hop vertex v induced subgraph, equation (1) measures the local subgraph change statistic Ψ in terms of the number of standard deviations from prior variations.

With the aid of equation (1), scan-statistics detects any subgraph regions whose chosen behavioural characteristics Ψ deviated significantly from its recent history. By applying equation (1) iteratively to every vertex induced subgraph, scan-statistics uncovers local regions within the network that exhibit the greatest deviations from their expected behaviours.

With scan-statistics change detection, typically the subsequent change analysis focuses on individual vertices (or subgraphs) that exhibited greatest deviation from their expected prior behaviours only. Our scan-statistical correlation method bridges this gap by examining all regions of change within the network and their relationships with one another using correlation analysis.

4 Scan-Statistical Correlations

In order to examine correlations between local network changes uncovered by scan-statistics, we use Pearson's ρ correlation. We examine and quantify possible relationships in local behavioural changes between every pair of vertex induced k-hop subgraphs in the network. For every pair of vertices v_1 and v_2 induced subgraphs, we extend scan-statistics with correlation computations using Pearson's ρ equation :

$$\rho_{k,t,\tau}(v_1,v_2) = \frac{\sum_{t=t-\tau}^{t-1}(\Psi_{k,t'}(v_1)-\hat{\mu}_{k,t,\tau}(v_1))(\Psi_{k,t'}(v_2)-\hat{\mu}_{k,t,\tau}(v_2))}{\sqrt{\sum_{t=t-\tau}^{t-1}(\Psi_{k,t'}(v_1)-\hat{\mu}_{k,t,\tau}(v_1))^2}\sqrt{\sum_{t=t-\tau}^{t-1}(\Psi_{k,t'}(v_2)-\hat{\mu}_{k,t,\tau}(v_2))^2}} \tag{2}$$

where k, v, t, τ, Ψ, and $\hat{\mu}$ are defined the same as for (1).

The scan-statistical correlation scheme is outlined in Fig. 1. For every network graph in the time-series, correlations between local vertex (or subgraph) changes are computed according to corresponding vertex behaviours from the recent historical window τ of time-series graphs. The raw correlations data are then populated into an $n{\times}n$ matrix of n vertices from the network graph. This matrix provides a simplistic assessment of positive, low, or possibly opposite correlations in change behaviours.

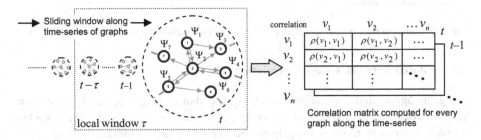

Fig. 1. Correlation is computed for each time-series graph and populated into a matrix

5 Multi-level Correlations Analysis

5.1 Aggregation of Correlation Data

To facilitate analysis of correlations amongst behavioural changes at higher network graph levels, the raw correlation data (i.e. correlation matrix in Fig. 1) is aggregated into other representative results. A number of aggregation schemes were examined. However, compared to basic aggregation methods, spectral, Perron-Frobenius, Eigenvector, and other matrix-based methods did not present any additional benefits and took longer processing times. Hence, for the remainder of this paper, we restrict our discussions to aggregation schemes employing straightforward averaging.

The aggregation of correlation data is described in Fig. 2. In the first step, for each vertex, the vertex's correlation with every other vertex is aggregated together. The outcome is to provide an overall correlation measure for every vertex against the majority of other vertices throughout the network. From the perspective of an individual vertex, this aggregated correlation value indicates if the behavioural change experienced by that vertex is also exhibited by the majority or only a small number of other vertices (discussed further in Section 5.3).

In the second step, using individually aggregated vertex correlation values from Step 1, an overall correlation measure is acquired for the network graph. The network graph correlation indicates if the change experienced by the network is part of a broader graph-wide change, or if the network deviation is due to few local regions.

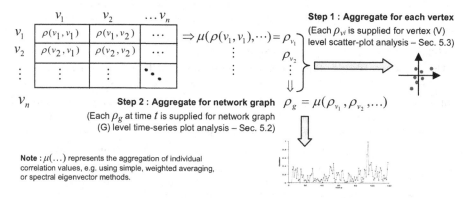

Fig. 2. Correlation data is aggregated to provide results for each individual vertex and the graph

5.2   Global Network Graph Correlation (G)

Using the aggregated correlations values ρ_g, the change in *global* graph correlation levels across the time-series of network graphs can be examined. This enables network analysts to monitor for patterns between the network deviations uncovered from a change detection time-series plot against corresponding graph-wide correlation from the correlation time-series plot. For instance, are significant network deviations due to widespread changes throughout the graph at multiple change-points? In the case of high correlation, this indicates a large majority of network subgraph regions exhibit similar degree of change in network behaviour (as demonstrated in Section 7).

5.3   Vertex Level Correlation (V)

Beneath the global graph level, the aggregated correlation of every vertex to all other vertices is analysed. The aggregated correlation ρ_{vi} is acquired via Step 1 in Fig. 2. For every vertex that undergoes significant change, the aggregated vertex correlation indicates if the change experienced by that vertex is exhibited by the majority or only a few vertices. A high correlation indicates that the change by the vertex was also experienced by other vertices as well. On the other hand, a low correlation signifies the change was likely restricted to that vertex only.

From a change-analysis perspective, besides simply identifying which vertices contributed most to the network change (as per conventional scan-statistics), using vertex level correlations, further insight regarding how these individual deviations relate to the wider network can be deduced. Correlation inspired visualisation techniques may then be employed to observe these changes.

Scatter-Plot Visualisation

To effectively analyse vertex level correlations, a scatter-plot visualisation scheme is employed. The scatter-plots reveal how an individual vertex, groups of vertices, and the overall network vary from one time interval to the next. The two types of scatter-plots are : (i) a scatter-plot of scan-statistic locality deviation value $\tilde{\Psi}(v)$ of every vertex, and (ii) the scatter-plot of aggregated correlation ρ_v of every vertex.

Fig. 3 summarises our scatter-plot concept. To examine how certain vertices of interest vary over time, scatter-plots are created for network graphs that undergo significant network change. For each of these network graph change-points, the deviation (or correlation) results of every vertex from the previous and current graphs (i.e. graphs before and at the change-point) are plotted on the scatter-plot.

On the scatter-plot, every vertex is plotted as a xy-coordinate point. The y-axis represents the vertex deviation statistic or correlation value held by the vertex in the previous graphs, and the x-axis value corresponds to the vertex deviation or correlation of the current graph under examination.

By examining where individual or clusters of vertices appear on the scatter-plots, the vertices that experienced most significant changes are easily identified, and the types of changes can be inferred immediately. Dynamically changing scatter-plots, whereby a scatter-plot is displayed for consecutive time-series graphs also reveal how specific vertices of interest or clustered changes transpire over time.

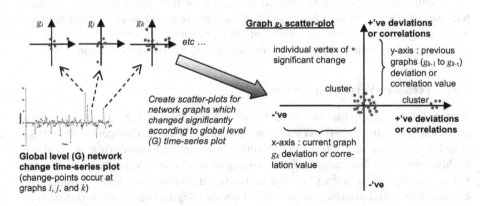

Fig. 3. Concept of vertex (V) level scatter-plots created for significantly deviated graphs

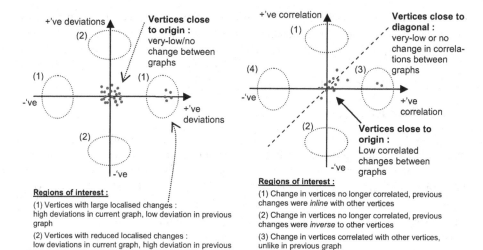

Regions of interest :

(1) Vertices with large localised changes :
high deviations in current graph, low deviation in previous graph

(2) Vertices with reduced localised changes :
low deviations in current graph, high deviation in previous graph (return to *normality* behaviour)

Regions of interest :

(1) Change in vertices no longer correlated, previous changes were *inline* with other vertices

(2) Change in vertices no longer correlated, previous changes were *inverse* to other vertices

(3) Change in vertices correlated with other vertices, unlike in previous graph

(4) Change in vertices inversely correlated with other vertices, unlike in previous graph

Fig. 4. Vertex (V) level deviation scatter-plot   **Fig. 5.** Vertex (V) level correlation scatter-plot

For instance, the above concept for the scan-statistic deviation scatter-plot is shown in Fig. 4. This scatter-plot reveals the change in edge-connectivity (k=0 hop) of vertices; in particular, the extent of edge-connectivity changes and clustering of vertices with similar connectivity variations.

Various *regions of interest* are identified on this scatter-plot and described in Fig. 4. We observe which regions vertices fall into and how these vertices shift across the scatter-plots throughout the time-series of graphs. This allows the connectivity deviations of every vertex (and clusters) relative to the wider network to be examined.

For the correlations scatter-plot (Fig. 5), various similar regions of interests are also identified. This scatter-plot reveal if specific vertices acted alone in exhibiting localised changes, or if their behavioural deviations were part of a collective network-wide change. For example, do single, multiple, clustered vertices exhibit similar or independent deviations in edge-connectivity from prior network behaviours?

5.4   Vertex-to-Vertex Correlation (V×V)

At the lowest level, the raw correlation data matrix in Fig. 1 allows for the examination of individual vertex-to-vertex correlations in change behaviours. A possible use-case of such vertex-to-vertex correlations monitoring is to detect highly similar or duplication of behaviours from multiple vertices. For example, the discovery of a vertex in the network attempting to falsely mimic the characteristics and assume the identity of another legitimate network vertex. Over a sufficient period of time, if the correlations between two vertices are suspiciously maintained as highly correlated, then this may indicate the presence of illegal vertex imposters.

6   A Multi-level Network Change Analysis Scheme

In this section, we bring together the different levels of correlations data and analysis above to outline a scheme for examining network changes uncovered by scan-statistics. The approach is depicted in Fig. 6 as a flow diagram. It involves examining various forms of network correlation data, to gather evidence for establishing possible scenarios and the context in which network changes were triggered.

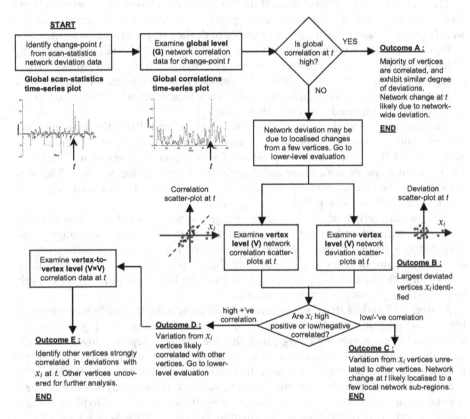

Fig. 6. Multi-level network change analysis process using scan-statistics correlations data

7   Experiments

The scan-statistical correlations techniques have been applied to a variety of network datasets, both internally within and external to our organisation. For demonstration purposes in this paper, we make use of the Enron email dataset [3]. The dataset contains emails from 150 Enron employees including those of senior management between 1999 and 2001, covering events leading up to the collapse of the company. A network graph is extracted from email transactions during each week resulting in a time-series of 120 graphs. In each graph, an edge is established between two vertices if at least one email was sent between them during that weekly period.

Global (G) Level Network Deviations and Correlations

We adopt the multi-level correlations change analysis outlined in Fig. 6. For scan-statistics and correlations evaluations, the $k=0$ hop edge connectivity deviations of every vertex is computed – i.e. the change in number of new emails between individuals and their overall emailing connectivity is our main focus. From preliminary test runs, the window τ of graphs to establish statistical edge-connectivity mean and compute correlations was set at a size of 5.

The global level (G) scan-statistical deviation and correlation time-series plots are shown in Fig. 7 and 8. The x-axis corresponds to network graph change-points at weekly intervals, and the y-axis is the number of deviations or correlation level.

Fig. 7 reveals a number of positive and negative change-spikes when emailing edge-connectivity rose excessively or dropped sharply from prior weeks. These change-spikes indicate when significant increases or decreases in emails were sent/received amongst individuals from one week to another when compared to the recent history of expected emailing behaviours.

The interesting period occurred between weeks 64 and 101. We focus on three change-points, weeks 85, 88, and 94, when new emailing activity escalated significantly. Weeks 85 and 88 corresponds to the periods before and after the resignation of the Enron CEO; who oversaw the price-fixing and illegitimate practices of the company. The week leading up to the investigations by the Securities and Exchange Commission (SEC) into Enron's operations is also highlighted during week 94.

Besides uncovering when significant change events occurred, the scan-statistics global time-series plot does not reveal much. For instance, were these change-points triggered by a single individual vertex, a few or clusters of vertices, or collectively by a majority of the network graph nodes? In Fig. 8, the global (G) correlation time-series plot is the first step in examining how emailing behaviour deviates collectively and individually across all Enron employees.

At weeks 85 and 88, the corresponding global correlation in emailing deviations is low. This suggests the large emailing deviations indicated by Fig. 7 are not widespread. This is not surprising given that the planned stepping down of a CEO concerns highest level executives. As expected, the emailing behaviour of the majority of employees does not change from previous weeks. At week 94, the global correlation is higher, indicating the emailing network change may involve a larger population of employees. To assess this possibility and identify individual vertices that triggered the network change, the emailing behaviour at the vertex level (V) are examined next.

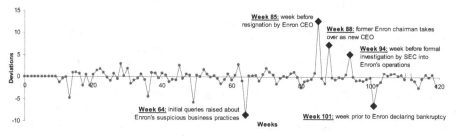

Fig. 7. Global (G) deviation time-series plot : Enron dataset

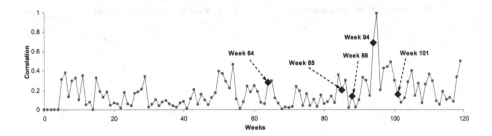

Fig. 8. Global (G) correlation time-series plot : Enron dataset

Vertex (V) Level Network Deviations and Correlations

Fig. 9, 10 and 11 show the scan-statistics deviation and correlation scatter-plots. The deviation units are normalised such that deviations on the scatter-plot are relative to the maximum deviation exhibited from the vertex that deviated the most during the specified week.

For week 85, Fig. 9(a) shows that vertex 118 (and 60) exhibit the largest individual deviation. Their location at the extreme positive x-axis and near-zero y-axis region indicates their emailing activity increased up to 16 times from the prior weeks of low emailing. Relative to these two vertices, the deviation in emailing activity of other vertices remained low, all being clustered around the origin.

Tracing back our vertex labelling, it is no surprise that vertex 118 is the Enron CEO (and vertex 60 is a president of Enron Online Business). Prior to stepping down, it is usual for the CEO to send various emails to large groups of individuals to close off remaining official duties or resolve other matters (e.g. even a company-wide email announcing his resignation). The CEO may also receive many new emails from other employees offering farewell messages. In an organisation such as Enron, even a small proportion of such emailing activity for one individual would cause their emailing edge connectivity to spike up.

However, with vertex 60, suspicious reasoning behind the concurrent spike in emailing with vertex 118 may exist. The Enron online business was a major part of Enron's suspicious practices, hence it would be interesting to establish what anomalous relationship exists between the CEO and the online business president.

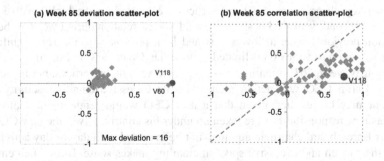

Fig. 9. Vertex (V) level scatter-plots : Enron dataset – Week 85

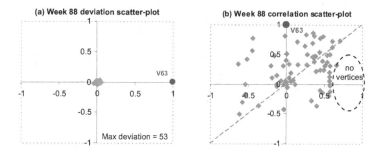

Fig. 10. Vertex (V) level scatter-plots : Enron dataset – Week 88

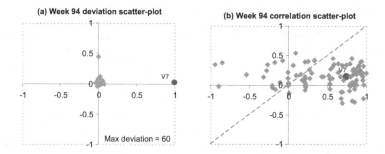

Fig. 11. Vertex (V) level scatter-plots : Enron dataset – Week 94

For week 88, Fig. 10(a) shows the extreme emailing deviation is entirely due to vertex 63, who happens to be the former Enron chairman that took over the new CEO role during that week. For week 94, Fig. 11(a) shows that the network change was dominated by vertex 7, the Enron chief operating officer (COO). These scan-statistics scatter-plots identify vertices that deviated vertices most, as per Outcome B in Fig. 6.

From our deviation scatter-plots, it is clear emailing deviation is dominated by a single (or two) vertex. Deviations of other vertices are much smaller, concentrated at the scatter-plot origin. But it remains beneficial to examine if deviations from the rest of the network are correlated (or disparate) with the dominant single vertex deviation.

From an overall network perspective, the majority of graph vertices on the week 88 correlation scatter-plot (Fig. 10(b)) do not reveal any discernable pattern. However, we make two key observations. First, no vertices are located on the high positive x-axis region; and second, vertex 63 is shown to hold low correlation during week 88 but high correlation previously (i.e. at low x-axis and high positive y-axis). This signifies the extreme deviation of vertex 63 is limited to itself (i.e. Outcome C in Fig. 6).

Previously, vertex 63's emailing was consistent with other vertices, but in week 88, the new Enron CEO was acting alone with its excessive emailing activity. Such behaviour may be justified given that a new CEO would send/receive many more emails as new responsibilities are taken up under his control. Given the new CEO was a former Enron board chairman and may not be involved with day-to-day activities of Enron, the sudden and excessive spike in emailing makes sense. But if such emailing behaviour was detected for other vertices, then this could be deem anomalous.

The correlation scatter-plot in Fig. 11(c) shows the largest deviated vertex 7 (Enron COO) was previously uncorrelated (low y-axis previous graphs correlation), but its extreme deviation is correlated with other vertices during week 94 (high x-axis current graph correlation). In addition, a significant portion of vertices are also located on the low y-axis and higher positive x-axis region. This suggests wider network change occurred at week 94, and vertex 7 was not acting alone.

Whilst other vertices may not have deviated as excessively as vertex 7, they still exhibited the same positive degree of new emailing connectivity as the Enron COO. These vertices may represent employees working closely together to respond to the pending SEC investigations; of which, the Enron COO was likely the coordinator for the company. Intuitively, this accounts for the large spike in new emailing deviation from vertex 7, and associated deviation from other vertices. For week 85, similar correlation analysis as week 94 can be deduced.

8   Conclusions

This paper presented a correlations based network change analysis technique. The correlations between network graph deviations amongst vertices are examined in order to gain greater insight into different scenarios triggering the network changes. We extend scan-statistical change detection with correlations inspired network analytics operating at multiple levels of the network graph. Whilst our technique is beneficial for any networks in general, the Enron dataset was used to demonstrate valuable outcomes using correlations analysis. In the future, our research shall focus on applying higher order statistics to acquire other in-depth network change correlation results.

References

1. Shoubridge, P., Kraetzl, M., Ray, D.: Detection of Abnormal Change in a Time-Series of Graphs. Journal of Interconnection Networks 3(1-2), 85–101 (2002)
2. Bunke, H., Dickinson, P., Kraetzl, M., Wallis, W.: A Graph-Theoretic Approach to Enterprise Network Dynamics, Birkhauser (2007)
3. Priebe, C., Conroy, J., Marchette, D., Park, Y.: Scan Statistics on Enron Graphs. Computational and Mathematical Organization Theory 11(3), 229–247 (2005)
4. Akoglu, L., Faloutsos, C.: Event Detection in Time-series of Mobile Communication Graphs. In: 27th Army Science Conference, pp. 1–8 (2010)
5. Akoglu, L., Dalvi, B.: Structure, Tie Persistence and Event Detection in Large Phone and SMS Networks. In: Mining & Learning with Graphs, pp. 10–17. ACM (2010)
6. Ide, T., Kashima, H.: Eigenspace-based Anomaly Detection in Computer Systems. In: Knowledge Discovery and Data Mining Conference, pp. 440–449. ACM (2005)
7. Ahmed, E., Clark, A.: Characterising Anomalous Events Using Change-Point Correlation on Unsolicited Network Traffic. In: Secure IT Systems, pp. 104–119. Springer (2009)
8. Fukuda, K., Hirotsu, T., Akashi, O., Sugawara, T.: Correlation among Piecewise Unwanted Traffic Time-series. In: IEEE Global Telecommunications Conference, pp. 1–5 (2008)
9. Henderson, K., Eliassi-Rad, T., Faloutsos, C., Akoglu, L., Li, L., Maruhashi, K., Prakash, B., Tong, H.: Metric Forensics: a Multi-level Approach for Mining Volatile Graphs. In: Knowledge Discovery and Data Mining Conference, pp. 163–172. ACM (2010)

Predicting High Impact Academic Papers Using Citation Network Features

Daniel McNamara[1], Paul Wong[2], Peter Christen[1], and Kee Siong Ng[1,3]

[1] Research School of Computer Science
[2] Office of Research Excellence
The Australian National University, Canberra, Australia
[3] EMC Greenplum
dpmcna@gmail.com, {paul.wong,peter.christen}@anu.edu.au,
keesiong.ng@emc.com

Abstract. Predicting future high impact academic papers is of benefit to a range of stakeholders, including governments, universities, aca-
demics, and investors. Being able to predict 'the next big thing' allows
the allocation of resources to fields where these rapid developments are
occurring. This paper develops a new method for predicting a paper's
future impact using features of the paper's neighbourhood in the citation network, including measures of interdisciplinarity. Predictors of high
impact papers include high early citation counts of the paper, high citation counts by the paper, citations of and by highly cited papers, and
interdisciplinary citations of the paper and of papers that cite it. The
Scopus database, consisting of over 24 million publication records from
1996-2010 across a wide range of disciplines, is used to motivate and
evaluate the methods presented.

1 Introduction

This paper seeks to produce a method which, given a database of academic
publications and citations between them, can predict future high impact papers.
The topic of this paper is a part of an effort to provide ongoing analytical support
to decision and policy development for the Commonwealth of Australia [1,2,3].
One aspect of this effort is to develop an 'early warning system' to predict,
anticipate and respond to emerging research trends.

It is amply clear that R&D operates in an increasingly competitive environment, where the traditional US and Europe dominance is under direct challenge
by a number of Asian countries. Australia, with a small population base and
slightly more than 2% GDP spend on R&D [2], will need to compete and stretch
its investment dollar in more creative and efficient ways. Decision and policy
makers thus need to marshal all available resources and intellectual capital to
develop sound strategies to remain competitive on a global scale. The utilisation
of data mining techniques to make predictions about citations of scholarly publications, taken as a proxy for the onset of research breakthroughs, when used
in combination with other relevant leading indicators, can potentially provide

J. Li et al. (Eds.): PAKDD 2013 Workshops, LNAI 7867, pp. 14–25, 2013.

competitive intelligence for strategy development. While Australia may not be able to invest in R&D to the same extent as other economic powerhouses to take advantage of being 'the first mover', with the development of insightful predictive analytics over a range of data sources, it can become an 'early adopter' and develop national research capabilities in an agile and timely manner. The motivation behind this paper is to develop useful predictive models to empower decision and policy making.

This paper is organised in the following way. Section 2 reviews related work, and the Scopus database is presented in Sect. 3. Section 4 covers the methods used in this paper, including a suitable measure of paper impact, predictive features from the paper's citation network neighbourhood, and prediction algorithms. The results of applying these methods to the Scopus database are shown in Sect. 5. Section 6 presents the conclusion and future work.

2   Related Work

There is a rich literature on the topics of defining and predicting the impact of academic papers. Citation counts are the traditional and most straightforward way of measuring the impact of an individual paper. Citation counts have been used to distinguish between 'classic' papers which continue to be cited long after publication, and 'ephemeral' papers which rapidly cease to be cited [4]. We seek to formalise the notion of a classic or high impact paper.

Raw citation counts vary significantly between disciplines, making it a challenge to find an impact measure which is fair to papers from all fields. One approach has been to divide a paper's citations by its disciplinary average [5,6]. A critique found that dividing by disciplinary average still generates different distributions across disciplines [7]. Other studies have instead worked with the disciplinary percentile rank, for example proposing that the top 1% of papers in each discipline should be considered classics [8,9]. As detailed in Sect. 4.1, this paper builds on the percentile rank approach, but explicitly considers the possibility of multiple disciplinary classifications for a single paper, and favours papers with enduring influence using exponential discounting favouring more recent citations.

There are a range of features that can be used as predictors of a paper's future impact. These include citations of a paper soon after it is published [10,11]; measures of network centrality such as average shortest path length, clustering coefficient and betweenness centrality [12]; the paper's authors' previous work [13,14]; and keywords from the text of the paper [15]. The framework of information diffusion emphasises that ideas, like epidemics, spread through networks [16,17]. We therefore expect that a paper's position in the network will be a determinant of the impact of its ideas. The theory of 'preferential attachment' suggests that in evolving networks, new nodes favour connections to existing highly connected nodes [18]. It has been proposed that when nodes span boundaries or 'structural holes' between previously disparate parts of intellectual networks, they induce structural variation and hence become influential [19,20,21].

This paper draws upon and examines these arguments by evaluating whether the number and interdisciplinarity of citations by and of a paper are predictive of its future impact.

Previous research has investigated the effect on future citation counts of paper interdisciplinarity, measured by the proportion of citations made by a paper outside its own discipline [22,23]. This study builds on this approach but additionally distinguishes between closely and distantly related disciplines, allows multiple disciplines per paper, and considers the interdisciplinarity of citations of papers citing and cited by the original paper.

The experiments presented in previous studies using network features to predict academic impact often use datasets from individual fields [12,20] or institutions [24]. This paper is unusual in presenting results over a dataset as large and broad as the Scopus database. Additionally, it incorporates the dynamic nature of the citation network by considering citations disaggregated by year.

3   The Scopus Database

Scopus is a proprietary database of metadata records of academic papers. The database is owned by the publisher Elsevier and is one of a small number of major multidisciplinary bibliometric databases along with Thomson's Web of Science and Google Scholar. The version of Scopus used in this paper contains metadata records for 24,097,496 papers published during the years 1995-2012. The years 1996-2010 are complete, with more recent records yet to be comprehensively added. The records include title, authors including their countries and institutional affiliations, journal, document type, abstract, keywords, subject areas, and citations of and by the paper.

Figure 1 shows the disiplinary coverage of the Scopus database, which focuses on medicine and science. The All Science Journal Classification (ASJC) system is used, with papers hierarchically grouped into 334 disciplines at the 4-digit level and 27 disciplines at the 2-digit level [25]. A given paper may have zero, one, or multiple disciplinary classifications.

4   Methods

We consider the task of predicting the future impact of papers over a horizon of τ years from the present. We assume that citations by the paper of papers published up to κ years before its publication are available. The parameter δ is the number of years of citations of the paper available at the time of prediction.

The database of academic papers considered can be represented as a set N, and an individual paper is represented by $n \in N$. $N_t \subset N$ refers to the set of all papers published in year t. Citations are represented by a_{mn}, which is equal to 1 if paper m cites paper n, and 0 otherwise. The paper impact vector of length $|N|$ is represented as $\mathbf{y}$, where $y_n = y(n)$ is the impact of paper n.

We assume that each paper is classified as belonging to one or more disciplines $k \in K_0$, where K_0 is the set of disciplines. Further, we assume that the elements

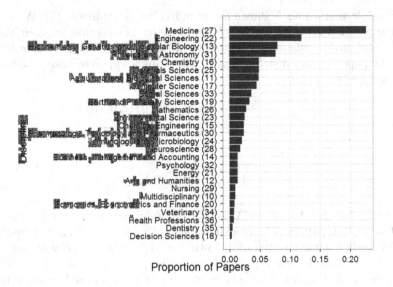

Fig. 1. Scopus coverage by discipline. The 2-digit ASJC codes of each discipline are shown in brackets.

of K_0 may be hierarchically grouped at levels of discipline similarity in the range $i \in [0, \omega]$, where K_i is the set of groups at level i in the hierarchy. At level 0, each code is assigned its own group; at level ω, all codes are in the same group; and at intermediate levels, codes are assigned to groups containing some but not all other codes. In the case of Scopus, $\omega = 2$, K_0 contains a group for each 4-digit ASJC code, K_1 contains the 2-digit ASJC code discipline groups, and K_2 contains all disciplines in one group. Disciplinary classifications are represented by c_{nk}, the proportion of classifications of paper n as discipline k.

4.1 Measuring Paper Impact

Our goal is to predict the impact of a given paper. To do this we must first determine how to measure impact, a topic discussed in Sect. 2. The number of citations of a paper is a good starting point.

We would like to take into account citations over several years, favouring recent citations. This is to find papers that have a lasting influence, rather than those that are popular for only a brief time. We do this using exponential decay in (1). The parameter $r \in [0, 1]$ controls the rate of decay, and can also be called the discount factor.

$$y'(n) = \sum_{t=\delta+1}^{\tau+\delta} r^{\tau+\delta-t} \sum_{m \in N_t} a_{mn} \tag{1}$$

Some disciplines cite more frequently than others. We accommodate this by finding the percentile rank of n across all papers in its discipline(s), including papers from multiple years. This is shown for an individual discipline in (2). We use the indicator function $I(a, b) = 1$ if $a > b, 0$ otherwise. These ranks are combined to a single rank in (3), where y is the paper impact metric. Using percentile rank makes the paper impact distributions of all disciplines approximately uniform in the range $y(n) \in [0, 1]$.

$$y''(n, k) = \frac{\sum\limits_{m \in N} I(y'(n), y'(m)) I(c_{mk}, 0)}{\sum\limits_{m \in N} I(c_{mk}, 0)} \qquad (2)$$

$$y(n) = \sum_{k \in K} c_{nk} y''(n, k) \qquad (3)$$

We propose fixing a threshold λ, such that for a set of papers N, the high impact or classic papers N^* are defined according to (4). A similar approach has previously been suggested [9], identifying high impact or classic papers as the top 1% most highly cited papers in each discipline. Using this 1% threshold corresponds to setting $\lambda = 0.99$. The paper impact $y(n)$, referred to as the target variable in the context of prediction, has the additional advantages that it takes into account papers with multiple classifications, and weights later citations more heavily to measure the ongoing effect of a paper. Note that this definition of classics is relative to the set of papers being considered, so that every set of papers will always have a fixed proportion of classics.

$$N^* = \{n \in N | \frac{1}{|N|} \sum_{m \in N} I(y(n), y(m)) \geq \lambda\} \qquad (4)$$

4.2   Predictive Features

There are many potential predictors of future impact. In this paper only properties of the paper's neighbourhood in the citation network are considered. As described in Sect. 2, this is motivated by the framework of information diffusion which states that a node's position in a network impacts its ability to have intellectual influence. The features f used are specified in Table 1.

The paper's disciplinary classifications and the annual citations of and by the paper are the base citation network neighbourhood features considered. In the case $\delta = 0$, we only have information about papers cited by the paper, whereas if $\delta > 0$ we also have information about papers that cite the paper.

Previous work has proposed that interdisciplinary work is likely to be more influential [20,21,26], since it fills in 'structural holes' in the network. This paper seeks to quantitatively evaluate this hypothesis, extending previous work which measures the interdisciplinarity of a paper using the proportion of its citations that are of papers in other disciplines [22,23]. In this study, individual papers may have multiple disciplinary classifications, and the classifications may be hierarchically grouped at levels in the range $i \in [0, \omega]$. The interdisciplinarity type i means that at least one pair of classifications of the cited and citing

Table 1. Summary of features used for predicting the impact of individual papers. 'b' stands for citations *by* a paper, 'o' stands for citations *of* a paper, and moving outwards from the original paper these citation types are added to the feature set name. K_ν is the set of discipline groups at the hierarchy level ν, ω is the number of levels in the hierarchical grouping of disciplines, κ is the years of citations by the paper available, and δ is the year of prediction relative to the paper's publication.

Feature Set	Feature Set Size	Feature Set Description
c	$\|K_\nu\| - 1$	c_k is the proportion of paper's disciplinary classifications in discipline group k
b	κ	b_t is the number of citations by paper in year t
B	$(\omega + 1)\kappa$	b_{it} is the proportion of cited papers of interdisciplinarity type i published in year t
o	δ	o_t is the number of citations of paper in year t
O	$(\omega + 1)\delta$	o_{it} is the proportion of citing papers of interdisciplinarity type i published in year t
bo	1	Average number of citations of cited papers
bo	$\omega + 1$	bo_i is the average proportion of citations of cited papers of interdisciplinarity type i
oo	1	Average number of citations of citing papers
oo	$\omega + 1$	oo_i is the average proportion of citations of citing papers of interdisciplinarity type i

papers are in the same group at hierarchy level $i \in [0, \omega]$, but not at any lower hierarchy level. In the context of Scopus, interdisciplinarity type 0 indicates that the two papers share a 4-digit ASJC code, type 1 indicates that they share a 2-digit ASJC code but no 4-digit ASJC code, and type 2 indicates that they share no 2-digit ASJC code. The proportions of citations of and by the paper of each interdisciplinary type for each year are used as predictive features.

Going one level further out in the neighbourhood of the paper, the number and interdisciplinarity of citations of those papers cited by and citing the paper are considered. These 'higher order' features are of interest since they measure the effect of citing and being cited by 'authorities'.

4.3 Prediction Algorithms

Several algorithms are used for making predictions of the target variable based on the features outlined in Sect. 4.2. These are linear regression, decision trees and random forests [27]. These were chosen since they are known to be effective prediction algorithms with readily available implementations [28,29,30].

5 Experiments and Discussion

The Scopus Database detailed in Sect. 3 was used to evaluate the methods presented in Sect. 4. A training set with predictors and response variables completely available before the year of prediction is required to train the prediction algorithm. In our experiments, the training set consists of Scopus database papers published in 2000 and the test set consists of papers published in 2005.

Furthermore, the papers considered are restricted to those with at least one ASJC disciplinary classification, and to citations of and by those papers where the other paper also had at least one ASJC disciplinary classification. This is the case in more than 98% of the dataset and eliminates the complexity of dealing with missing data. The final training set consists of 1,184,842 papers and the test set of 1,704,624 papers.

We use the following parameter settings: the prediction horizon $\tau = 3$, a common timeframe for decision-makers; citations of papers up to $\kappa = 4$ before the paper's publication are included to fit into the data available; experiments where $\delta = 0$ and $\delta = 2$ are tried to assess the impact of varying the year of prediction relative to the paper's publication; $\omega = 2$ so that citation interdisciplinarity can be measured using 2-digit and 4-digit ASJC codes; $\nu = 1$ so that the 2-digit ASJC codes of papers are made available to the prediction algorithm; and the discount rate $r = 0.9$ to reward papers with enduring influence.

5.1 Feature Ranking Using Spearman Coefficient

Spearman's rank correlation coefficient ρ, a standard measure of the dependence of two variables using a monotone function, was taken for each of the features described in Sect. 4.2 and the target variable $\mathbf{y}$. The top features ranked by their ρ value with the target variable $\mathbf{y}$ are shown in Table 2. Figure 2 shows a dendogram of the top features, which are hierarchically clustered using the distance metric defined in (5). The unsupervised feature clusters correspond closely to the groupings defined in Table 1.

$$dist(f_1, f_2) = 1 - |\rho(f_1, f_2)| \tag{5}$$

The variables not known at the time of the paper's publication are shown as NA in the ρ_0 column. The feature sets $\mathbf{B}$, $\mathbf{O}$, $\mathbf{bo}$ and $\mathbf{oo}$ are the proportions of citations of a particular interdisciplinarity type (see Table 1 for details). For each of these feature sets, the papers for which there are no such citations are excluded from the Spearman coefficient calculations, since these proportions are not meaningful for these papers. In the prediction algorithms these features are given a value of 0 in these cases, to avoid the problem of missing data.

Table 2 shows that the most predictive variables are o_2 and o_1, the number of citations of the paper 2 years and 1 year after publication respectively, which are also clustered together in Fig. 2. This is intuitive since we would expect citations in early years to have a strong positive correlation with those in later ones.

The next most predictive variables are those in $\mathbf{b}$, the number of citations made by the paper, which also form a cluster in Fig. 2. This suggests that papers which cite more are themselves more highly cited. A high number of citations may suggest that the paper is thoroughly researched, or may be a review paper.

bo, the average number of citations of cited papers, and oo, the average number of citations of citing papers, are both positively correlated with the target

Table 2. Top 10 features, ranked by absolute value of Spearman coefficient ρ for the prediction task where $\delta = 2$. The subscripts 0 and 2 refer to the value of δ used.

Feature	Rank	ρ_2	ρ_0	Description
o_2	1	0.6757	NA	Citations of paper at $t = 2$
o_1	2	0.5887	NA	Citations of paper at $t = 1$
b_{-3}	3	0.4361	0.4463	Citations by paper at $t = -3$
b_{-2}	4	0.4327	0.4489	Citations by paper at $t = -2$
b_{-4}	5	0.4264	0.4325	Citations by paper at $t = -4$
b_{-1}	6	0.3733	0.3919	Citations by paper at $t = -1$
oo	7	0.2735	NA	Average number of citations of citing papers
bo	8	0.2266	0.2594	Average number of citations of cited papers
oo_2	9	0.1346	NA	Proportion of citations of citing papers of most interdisciplinary type
o_{21}	10	0.1341	NA	Proportion of citing papers of most interdisciplinarity type published in year $t = 1$

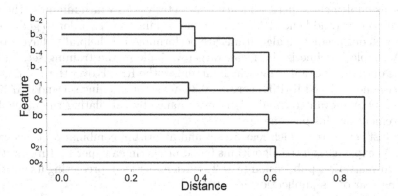

Fig. 2. Dendogram of top 10 features as described in Table 2. The distance between features is given by (5).

variable, and form a cluster in Fig. 2. The first result suggests that citing papers that are 'authorities' is advantageous for future citations. The second suggests that being cited by 'authorities' is also advantageous.

There is also evidence that interdisciplinarity is a predictor of future citations. oo_2, the proportion of citations of citing papers which are most interdisciplinary, is positively correlated with the target variable. So is o_{21}, the proportion of citations of the paper of the most interdisciplinarity type published in year $t = 1$. Other features indicating citations of the most interdisciplinary type fell just outside the top 10 and showed positive correlations. Previous studies have found that interdisciplinarity has a mix of both positive and negative correlations with paper impact depending on the paper's discipline [22,23], and no clear correlation overall [23]. While individual disciplines are not studied here, there are weak positive correlations between features indicating interdisciplinarity and impact overall. A possible reason for this discrepancy is that in this study features of interdisciplinarity are disaggregated by year, and include citations of the paper and citations of cited and citing papers, in addition to citations by the paper as in [22,23].

The correlations with impact calculated from the year of publication follow a similar pattern overall to those with impact calculated from two years after publication. However, citations by a paper matter more to its citations soon after publication than several years after, when other factors become more dominant.

It is possible to test significance of the Spearman coefficients using the null hypothesis that there is no correlation between the target variable and the feature [31]. A test statistic can be generated for a Student's t-distribution with $|N| - 2$ degrees of freedom. The values of this test statistic showed that each of the top 10 features shown in Table 2 were statistically significant.

5.2 Prediction Results

Root mean square error (RMSE) is a standard measure of the accuracy of predictions in a regression context. Linear regression, decision trees and random forests, as implemented here, all learn parameter values which minimise the sum of squares error (and hence RMSE) over the training set. In order to get a sense of how well our prediction algorithms are performing, it is helpful to have a baseline. A simple baseline is the mean target variable of the training set. This is also the optimal constant value which minimises the RMSE over the training set. This baseline achieved RMSE scores of 0.3645 for the training set and 0.3797 for the test set. We evaluate prediction performance by calculating the percentage improvement on this baseline.

The test set score of each feature set and algorithm combination is shown in Fig. 3. As expected, all the algorithms found predicting a paper's future citations from two years after publication ($\delta = 2$) much easier than predicting its citations from the year of its publication ($\delta = 0$).

The best performing algorithm was random forest. For the prediction task where $\delta = 0$, it achieved an 18.38% improvement on the baseline, and for $\delta = 2$, it achieved a 34.44% improvement. It is not surprising that as an ensemble method it performed better than the individual regression methods. It is noticeable that adding more features, particularly in the task predicting from two years after publication, actually made its performance slightly worse. This is likely related to the fact that each split only uses a sample of the features. When more features are added in, it may miss the most important features.

Other metrics offer further insights into the algorithm's performance. Using R^2, which can be interpreted as the proportion of variation in the target variable explained by the prediction, random forest's best test set results were 0.3342 for the $\delta = 0$ task, and 0.5697 for the $\delta = 2$ task. A classification approach, using the definition of classic papers from (4), showed that 8.28% of test set classic papers were successfully predicted for $\delta = 0$, and 38.73% for $\delta = 2$.

In the case of an individual decision tree, its results were not quite as strong as random forest, but were in similar ranges for the two tasks. Linear regression did not perform as well as the other algorithms, though it showed improvement when information about the interdisciplinarity of citations was included.

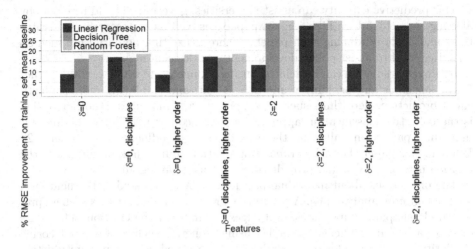

Fig. 3. Performance of prediction algorithms with a range of features, as described in Sect. 4.2

6   Conclusion and Future Work

This paper presented a new method for the prediction of the future impact of individual papers. Predictive features based on a paper's position in the citation network were used, drawing upon and evaluating previous research on information diffusion in networks, which suggests that nodes which are highly connected [18] and span network boundaries [19,20,21] are likely to be more influential. The method was implemented and evaluated using an exceptionally large and broad academic database, Scopus, comprising over 24 million papers from 1996-2010.

The notion of a classic or high impact paper was formalised using a novel metric of paper impact. This is a weighted average of the percentile ranks of citations of a paper across its disciplinary classifications, with an exponential discount rate favouring more recent citations to identify papers with enduring influence. The number of citations of the paper in the early years after publication, the number of citations by the paper, the average number of citations of citing and cited papers, and more interdisciplinary citations of the paper and of citing papers, were found to positively correlate with the paper's future impact.

Three prediction algorithms - linear regression, decision trees and random forest - were proposed to predict the future impact of individual papers. The percentage of RMSE improvement over the training set mean baseline was used to evaluate prediction performance. The results found that random forest was most predictive, achieving an 18% improvement predicting from the year of a paper's publication, and a 34% improvement predicting from two years after it.

This predictive capacity can assist universities, governments and investors by alerting them to future high impact papers, as well as to researchers, institutions and fields producing such papers. There is exciting potential for such an analytical tool to assist policy development and decision making.

Improved prediction can be achieved using a longer time window; adding other features such as author, journal and article text; and employing more sophisticated prediction algorithms such as support vector machines. Another option is the collective classification approach, simultaneously making predictions for individual papers and allowing these predictions to influence each other [32]. While in this paper the task is predicting citation counts, link prediction in the citation network [33] would provide the user with more detail.

The predictions about individual papers may be aggregated at the field level using co-citation analysis [34]. A co-citation graph can be constructed, where predicted classic papers are nodes, and edges occur when the citation behaviours of two papers are sufficiently similar using a metric such as weighted cosine similarity. Emerging fields of research can be predicted using community detection in the co-citation network of predicted high impact papers, for example by extracting the maximal cliques or components of the network. The authors of this paper anticipate a forthcoming publication on this topic, with the goal of creating a powerful tool to aid strategic research investment.

References

1. Australian Government: Australia in the Asian Century White Paper (2012)
2. Department of Industry, Innovation, Science, Research and Tertiary Education: 2012 National Research Investment Plan (2012)
3. Office of the Chief Scientist of Australia: Health of Australian Science (2012)
4. Price, D.: Networks of scientific papers. Science 149(3683), 510–515 (1965)
5. Castellano, C., Radicchi, F.: On the fairness of using relative indicators for comparing citation performance in different disciplines. Archivum Immunologiae et Therapiae Experimentalis 57(2), 85–90 (2009)
6. Radicchi, F., Fortunato, S., Castellano, C.: Universality of citation distributions: Toward an objective measure of scientific impact. Proc. Natl. Acad. Sci. USA 105(45), 17268–17272 (2008)
7. Waltman, L., van Eck, N.J., van Raan, A.F.: Universality of citation distributions revisited. J. Am. Soc. Inf. Sci. Technol. 63(1), 72–77 (2012)
8. Small, H.: Tracking and predicting growth areas in science. Scientometrics 68(3), 595–610 (2006)
9. Upham, S., Small, H.: Emerging research fronts in science and technology: patterns of new knowledge development. Scientometrics 83(1), 15–38 (2010)
10. Adams, J.: Early citation counts correlate with accumulated impact. Scientometrics 63(3), 567–581 (2005)
11. Manjunatha, J.N., Sivaramakrishnan, K.R., Pandey, R.K., Murthy, M.N.: Citation prediction using time series approach KDD cup 2003 (task 1). SIGKDD Explor. Newsl. 5(2), 152–153 (2003)
12. Shibata, N., Kajikawa, Y., Matsushima, K.: Topological analysis of citation networks to discover the future core articles. J. Am. Soc. Inf. Sci. Technol. 58(6), 872–882 (2007)

13. Castillo, C., Donato, D., Gionis, A.: Estimating number of citations using author reputation. In: Ziviani, N., Baeza-Yates, R. (eds.) SPIRE 2007. LNCS, vol. 4726, pp. 107–117. Springer, Heidelberg (2007)

14. Yan, R., Tang, J., Liu, X., Shan, D., Li, X.: Citation count prediction: learning to estimate future citations for literature. In: Proceedings of the 20th ACM International Conference on Information and Knowledge Management, CIKM 2011, pp. 1247–1252 (2011)

15. Yogatama, D., Heilman, M., O'Connor, B., Dyer, C., Routledge, B.R., Smith, N.A.: Predicting a scientific community's response to an article. In: EMNLP 2011, pp. 594–604 (2011)

16. Bettencourt, L., Kaiser, D., Kaur, J., Castillo-Chávez, C., Wojick, D.: Population modeling of the emergence and development of scientific fields. Scientometrics 75(3), 495–518 (2008)

17. Goffman, W., Newill, V.A.: Generalization of epidemic theory: An application to the transmission of ideas. Nature 204(4955), 225–228 (1964)

18. Barabási, A., Albert, R.: Emergence of scaling in random networks. Science 286(5439), 509–512 (1999)

19. Burt, R.S.: Structural holes: the social structure of competition. Harvard University Press, Cambridge (1992)

20. Chen, C.: Predictive effects of structural variation on citation counts. J. Am. Soc. Inf. Sci. Technol. 63(3), 431–449 (2012)

21. Chen, C., Chen, Y., Horowitz, M., Hou, H., Liu, Z., Pellegrino, D.: Towards an explanatory and computational theory of scientific discovery. J. Informetr. 3(3), 191–209 (2009)

22. Adams, J., Jackson, L., Marshall, S.: Bibliometric analysis of interdisciplinary research. Report to Higher Education Funding Council for England (2007)

23. Larivière, V., Gingras, Y.: On the relationship between interdisciplinarity and scientific impact. J. Am. Soc. Inf. Sci. Technol. 61(1), 126–131 (2009)

24. Nankani, E., Simoff, S.: Predictive analytics that takes in account network relations: A case study of research data of a contemporary university. In: Proceedings of the 8th Australasian Data Mining Conference, AusDM 2009, pp. 99–108 (2009)

25. Scopus: Scopus custom technical requirements, Version 2.0 (2009)

26. Guo, H., Weingart, S., Börner, K.: Mixed-indicators model for identifying emerging research areas. Scientometrics 89(1), 421–435 (2011)

27. Breiman, L.: Random forests. Machine Learning 45, 5–32 (2001)

28. Liaw, A., Wiener, M.: Package 'randomForest': Breiman and Cutler's random forests for classification and regression (2012)

29. R Documentation: Fitting linear models (2012)

30. Therneau, T.M., Atkinson, E.: An introduction to recursive partitioning using the RPART routines (2011)

31. R Documentation: Test for association/correlation between paired samples (2012)

32. Sen, P., Namata, G., Bilgic, M., Getoor, L., Galligher, B., Eliassi-Rad, T.: Collective classification in network data. AI Magazine 29(3), 93–106 (2008)

33. Shibata, N., Kajikawa, Y., Sakata, I.: Link prediction in citation networks. J. Am. Soc. Inf. Sci. Technol. 63(1), 78–85 (2012)

34. McNamara, D.: A new method for the prediction of emerging fields of research. Honours thesis, Australian National University (2012)

An OLAP Server for Sensor Networks Using Augmented Statistics Trees

Neil Dunstan

University of New England,
Armidale, Australia
neil@cs.une.edu.au

Abstract. The datacube is a conceptual data structure to support On-Line Analytical Processing (OLAP). It is essentially a series of tables organized according to attributes (called dimensions). Table rows (or cells) contain aggregated information for collections of records that satisfy value constraints for each dimension. The Statistics Tree (ST) uses a tree structure for storing the datacube in memory in order to optimize cell lookup time and handle a variety of types of cell-based queries. An Augmented ST (AST) is proposed with additional list structures within the ST. The additional lists link together the cells that comprise the tables of the datacube. An algorithm that builds table lists requires only a single traversal of the ST. Thus the AST supports both cell-level and table-level queries. Algorithms to build and update datacubes stored as ASTs are shown. A web-based wireless sensor network OLAP server based on the AST is described.

Keywords: Online Analytical Processing, Datacube, Wireless Sensor Network.

1 Introduction

Codd [1] proposed the creation of large datawarehouses for multidimensional data analysis, called Online Analytical Processing (OLAP). An OLAP user can explore the data in summary form by viewing tables by different combinations of dimensions and at different levels of summarization. Descriptive attributes (e.g. Location, Time) are used to select segments of the data for summarizations of numerical attributes (e.g. average daily rainfall). OLAP systems have been used in decision support systems ([2],[3]) and continues to be the subject of research, for example with web applications [4] and visualizations [5].

OLAP is supported by the datacube - a series of tables summarising the raw data. For n attributes (called *dimensions*) there are 2^n tables, being every possible combination of dimensions. The Base table is the most detailed, having entries for every combination of every different dimension value. The Apex is the most summarized table, having a single entry being aggregations over all values of all records. Table entries (rows of the tables) are called *cells*. The number of cells depends on the number of dimensions and their cardinalities. The tables of

J. Li et al. (Eds.): PAKDD 2013 Workshops, LNAI 7867, pp. 26–35, 2013.

the datacube have a "can be derived from" relationship. All tables at higher levels of summarization can be derived from the base table. This relationship is often used when it is prohibitive to pre-compute the whole datacube. Instead, higher level summaries can be generated "on-the-fly" from more detailed pre-computed tables. If the size of the raw data, number of dimensions and cardinalities are small enough, all summarizations can be made "on-the-fly" rather than being pre-computed and stored.

In this paper, the raw data is considered large and continually growing. It is motivated by a real-world application involving a wireless sensor network that provides regular updates of soil and air temperatures, moisture content and other data. The problem requires an OLAP server, that can both provide responses to client queries, as well as amend the datacube contents according to received updates. The size of the raw data prohibits the "on-the-fly" approach. It is assumed the server is able to store the whole datacube in memory, which supports both fast response to queries and fast updating. A ROLAP server uses a relational database approach, typically using a star schema with a fact table and dimension tables. A MOLAP server uses a multidimensional data structured approach [6]. The Statistics Tree (ST) of [7] uses a tree structure. The ST is optimized for handling ad-hoc queries of a cell-based nature - rather than the traditional table-based OLAP operations such as manifesting a whole table. The query handling algorithm CubiST was further developed (and called CubiST++) to use families of STs [8] for dealing with hierarchies of data dimensions. It has been shown that CubiST and the ST has faster performance than ROLAP or MOLAP servers in responding to ad-hoc cell-based datacube queries. It is important to note that CubiST returns aggregation results over all cells in the query, whereas table-based queries return a (perhaps partial) table of cells.

2   The Statistics Tree

The Statistics Tree is a tree structure where each descriptive attribute or dimension is a level of the tree. The leaf nodes hold the aggregations that represent the cells of the datacube. A small example with just three dimensions (A, B and C) will be used to illustrate. A and B are the only descriptive attributes, so the total number of tables in the datacube is $2^2 = 4$. They are AB (the Base table) B, A and the Apex. Dimension A had cardinality 2 and discrete values a_1 and a_2. Dimension B had cardinality 3 and discrete values b_1, b_2 and b_3. Hence the total number of cells in the datacube is $(2 + 1) \times (3 + 1) = 12$. Dimension C is numeric. The cells of the data cube contain aggregated values from dimension C, e.g. count and sum. The cell m_{ij} refers to the aggregated values of all raw data records having a_i as its A dimension value and b_j as its B dimension value. When i or j is $*$ this indicates that values for that dimension have been aggregated. That is, m_{*j} is the aggregation of cells m_{1j} and m_{2j}, or the aggregation of all records where the value for dimension B is j. The datacube as an ST is illustrated in Figure 1.

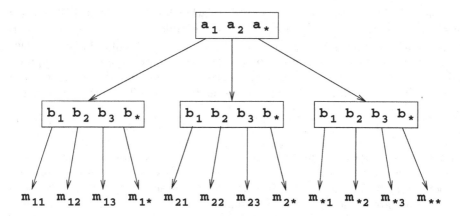

Fig. 1. An example of a datacube as a Statistics Tree

The figures in the papers of Fu and Hammer ([7], [8]) show that the leaf nodes form a linked list, but this feature is not explicitly used in their algorithms. The relevant C data structures are:

```
/* aggregation record */
typedef struct Aggs {
    float sum;
} Aggs;

/* leaf node of the Statistics Tree */
typedef struct Agg_node {
    int count;
    Aggs **ag;              /* array of links to aggregations */
    struct Agg_node *p; /* leaf-node link */
} Anode;

/* non-leaf node of the Statistics Tree */
typedef struct ST_node {
    struct ST_node **p; /* array of links to the next dimension */
    Anode **ap;         /* or last dimension leaf node links */
} STnode;

STnode *ST; /* The Statistics Tree */
```

Meta data required to build the tree includes the number of descriptive dimensions (`Dim`) and their cardinalities, and the number of dimensions used for aggregations (`Ags`). Since no algorithm to build the tree exists in the literature, C code is provided here from a current implementation consistent with the example of Figure 1.

```
void treegen( STnode *T, int level ) {
  int i, j, next;
  Aggs *a = NULL;
  Anode *t = NULL;
  STnode *v = NULL;

  if( level == Dim-1 ) {
    if( ((*T).ap = calloc( sizeof(Anode *),
                    dimension_cards[Dim-1]+1 )) ==  NULL ) {
      printf( "Out of memory\n" );
      exit(1);
    }
    for( i=0; i<dimension_cards[Dim-1]+1; i++ ) {
      t = (*T).ap[i] = (Anode *) malloc( sizeof(Anode) );
      if( t ==  NULL ) {
        printf( "Out of memory\n" );
        exit(1);
      }
      (*(*T).ap[i]).count = 0;
      (*(*T).ap[i]).p = NULL;
      if( ((*(*T).ap[i]).ag = calloc( sizeof(Aggs *),
                                aggregations )) ==  NULL ) {
        printf( "Out of memory\n" );
        exit(1);
      }
      for( j=0; j<Ags; j++ ) {
        a = (*(*T).ap[i]).ag[j] = (Aggs *) malloc( sizeof(Aggs) );
        if( a ==  NULL ) {
          printf( "Out of memory\n" );
          exit(1);
        }
      }
      for( j=0; j<Ags; j++ ) {
        (*(*(*T).ap[i]).ag[j]).min = (*(*(*T).ap[i]).ag[j]).max
                        = (*(*(*T).ap[i]).ag[j]).sum = 0.0;
      }
    }
    return;
  }
  next = level+1;
  if( ((*T).p = calloc( sizeof(STnode *),
                dimension_cards[level]+1 )) ==  NULL ) {
    printf( "Out of memory\n" );
    exit(1);
  }
```

```
  for( i=0; i<dimension_cards[level]+1; i++ ) {
    v = (*T).p[i] = (STnode *) malloc( sizeof(STnode) );
    if( v ==  NULL ) {
      printf( "Out of memory\n" );
      exit(1);
    }
    treegen( (*T).p[i], next );
  }
}
  /* make the tree */
  ST = (STnode *) malloc( sizeof(STnode) );
  treegen( ST, 0 );
```

A recursive algorithm to update the ST for each raw data record is provided in [7]. Here an alternative, iterative algorithm is described that is based on the following observation. The tables of the datacube can be codified, that is, table names can correspond to indices in a datacube table array, where a *merged* dimension has the binary digit 0 and included dimensions have the binary digit 1. The table codes for the example datacube are shown in Table 1, where ∗∗ is the Apex.

Table 1. Table codes and indices

$TableName$	$Index$	$bit0$	$bit1$
∗∗	0	0	0
∗B	1	0	1
A∗	2	1	0
AB	3	1	1

Each record requires updating in each of the tables of the datacube in exactly one cell. For each table, a path through the ST is constructed to the relevant cell. The path is followed, and the cell updated.

```
/* rec has dimension ranks, aggreg has numbers */
void addrec( STnode *T, int rec[Dim], aggreg[Ags] ) {
  int i, j, d, l, index, val[Dim], path[Dim];
  STnode *temp;

  for( i=0; i<cuboids; i++ ) {
    for( index=i,d=Dim-1; d>=0; d-- ) {
      val[d] = index % 2;
      index = index / 2;
    }
    for( d=0; d<Dim; d++ ) {
      if( val[d] &=&  0 )
```

```
            path[d] = dimension_cards[d]+1;
        else
            path[d] = rec[d]+1;
    }
    temp = (*T).p[path[0]-1];
    for( l=1; l<Dim-1; l++ )
        temp = (*temp).p[path[l]-1];
    (*(*temp).ap[path[Dim-1]-1]).count++;
    for( j=0; j<aggregations; j++ ) {
        (*(*(*temp).ap[path[Dim-1]-1]).ag[j]).sum += aggreg[j];
    }
  }
}
```

3 Augmented Statistics Trees

The ST has an inherent ordering. Leaf nodes occur in the order they would in
tables. However, a single left-to-right linked list of leaf nodes (a normal ST) has
table cells intermixed. An inorder traversal of the ST visits leaf nodes in the
order they should appear in tables. The table that a leaf node belongs to can be
derived from its path and is inherent in its name. For example, m_{12} belongs to
table 3 (AB). (m_{*2}) belongs to table 1 ($*B$). The algorithm to augment the ST
with table links uses the corresponding index of the table in an array.

```
Anode *table[cuboids];
```

The ST is traversed inorder, the path to each leaf node is saved in a string.
At each leaf node addtotable(string, nodeptr) adds the node to the table
list indicated by the string.

```
void traverse( STnode *T, int level, char *string ) {
    int i, next;
    char stem[MAXSTR], str[MAXSTR];

    if( level == Dim-1 ) {
        for( i=0; i<dimension_cards[Dim-1]+1; i++ ) {
            if( i < dimension_cards[Dim-1] )
                sprintf( str, "%s %d", string, i+1 );
            else
                sprintf( str, "%s -1", string );
            addtotable( str, (*T).ap[i] );
        }
        return;
    }
    next = level+1;
    sprintf( stem, "%s", string );
```

```
for( i=0; i<dimension_cards[level]+1; i++ ) {
  str[0] = '\0';
  if( i < dimension_cards[level] )
    sprintf( str, "%s %d", stem, i+1 );
  else
    sprintf( str, "%s -1", stem );
  traverse( (*T).p[i], next, str );
}
}
  /* make the table links */
  sprintf( string, "" );
  traverse( ST, 0, string );
```

Figure 2 illustrates the ST of Figure 1 augmented with table links.

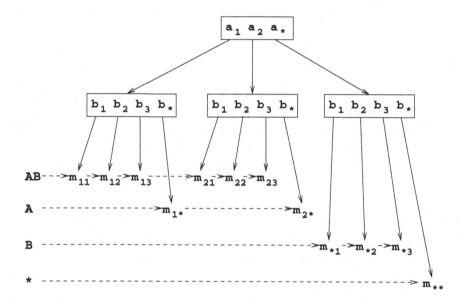

Fig. 2. An example of a datacube as an Augmented Statistics Tree

AST's have explicit support for table-based queries. The CubiST algorithm can still be used for cell-based queries on ASTs. However some range type queries may be more efficiently handled using the table lists. For instance, a range involving only a single dimension is more efficiently handled by following the ST pathway to the starting cell in the range, then following its table list.

4   A Web-Based OLAP Server Application

Wireless sensor networks are becoming increasingly common, particularly in agriculture where sensors are deployed to record and transmit climatic and other measures to a base station. This work is motivated by the development of an OLAP server for web-based clients that provides selected summarized information on continually updated (every 5 minutes) recordings from 100 sensors deployed around a farm. The dimensions of the data include:

- the number of the sensor;
- the time of the sampling;
- the location of the sensor;
- the elevation at the location of the sensor;
- the enclosure at the location of the sensor;
- the current land use in the enclosure;

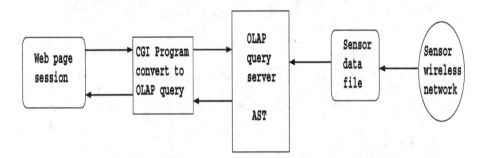

Fig. 3. Dynamic OLAP for a Wireless Sensor Network

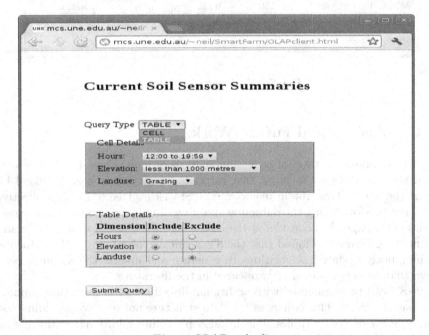

Fig. 4. OLAP web client

- the air temperature;
- the soil temperature;
- the soil moisture level;
- the soil conductivity;
- and more.

Figure 3 shows the system design for a web-based OLAP server of the wireless sensor data.

Figures 4 and 5 show a typical table query and response from the prototype implementation.

Hours	Elevation	Count	Ave. Air Temp.	Ave. Soil Temp.	Ave. Soil VWC	Ave. Soil EC
12:00 to 19:59	< 1000m	20	26.3C	22.5C	9.6%	0.01dS/m
12:00 to 19:59	1000-1099m	68	26.0C	20.3C	9.3%	0.01dS/m
12:00 to 19:59	> 1100m	12	25.6C	20.0C	9.3%	0.02dS/m
20:00 to 03:59	< 1000m	20	16.5C	10.5C	9.7%	0.01dS/m
20:00 to 03:59	1000-1099m	68	15.0C	10.1C	9.7%	0.01dS/m
20:00 to 03:59	> 1100m	12	25.6C	20.0C	9.6%	0.01dS/m
04:00 to 11:59	< 1000m	20	19.1C	11.5C	9.6%	0.01dS/m
04:00 to 11:59	1000-1099m	68	19.0C	11.4C	9.4%	0.01dS/m
04:00 to 11:59	> 1100m	12	17.9C	11.1C	9.3%	0.02dS/m

Fig. 5. OLAP server response

5   Conclusions and Future Work

OLAP is a popular method of providing analysis of multidimensional data sets. When the raw data set is large, fast response to queries is best provided by storing the whole datacube in memory. The Statistics Tree (ST) is an effective data structure for storing the datacube and providing fast response to cell-based queries. This paper has considered the case where the raw data set is large and continually growing and found that the ST is suitable also because the datacube can be quickly updated. Algorithms to generate and update the ST have been shown that have not previously appeared in the literature.

The ST can be augmented with additional linked list structures that support table-based queries. This enhances the data structure not only by providing fast manifestation of whole tables, but by also providing additional pathways by which some range cell-based queries can be processed. An algorithm based on a single inorder traversal of the ST has been shown that generates linked lists for all tables of the datacube to form the Augmented Statistics Tree (AST) data structure.

Hierarchies within dimensions add to the number of tables in the datacube. The ST approach uses additional STs with higher levels of summarization to form Families of STs (FST). Future work will investigate how ASTs can be effective in dealing with dimensional hierarchies. The AST will also be enhanced by further development of linked list structures such as those to support pivoting (reordered tables) without the need for sorting, and links to support customized frequent queries.

Acknowledgments. The wireless sensor network application comes from SmartFarm, a collaborative project of the Commonwealth Science and Industry Research Organization and the University of New England, Australia, supported by the Australian Centre for Broadband Innovation. http://www.sensornets.csiro.au/deployments/684

References

1. Codd, E.F., Codd, S.B., Salley, C.T.: Providing OLAP (Online Analytical Processing) to User-Analysts: An IT Mandate,
   http://www.minet.uni-jena.de/dbis/lehre/ss2005/sem_dwh/lit/Cod93.pdf
2. Moon, S.W., Kim, J.S., Kwon, K.N.: Effectiveness of OLAP-based Cost Data Management in Construction Cost Estimate. Automation in Construction 16(3), 336–344 (2007)
3. Shen, L., Liu, S., Chen, S., Wang, X.: The Application Research of OLAP in Police Intelligence Decision System. Procedia Engineering 29, 397–402 (2012)
4. Hsiao, T., Petchulat, S.: Data Visualization on Web-based OLAP. In: ACM 14th International Workshop on Datawarehousing and OLAP, pp. 75–82. ACM, New York (2011)
5. Ordonez, C., Chen, Z., Garcia-Garcia, J.: Data Visualization on Web-based OLAP. In: ACM 14th International Workshop on Datawarehousing and OLAP, pp. 83–87. ACM, New York (2011)
6. Han, J., Kamber, M., Pei, J.: Data Mining. Morgan Kaufmann, San Francisco (2012)
7. Fu, L., Hammer, J.: CubiST: A New Algorithm for Improving the Performance of Ad-hoc OLAP Queries. In: DOLAP 2000 Proceedings of the 3rd ACM International Workshop on Data Warehousing and OLAP, pp. 72–79. ACM, New York (2000)
8. Hammer, J., Fu, L.: Improving the Performance of OLAP Queries Using Families of Statistics Trees. In: Kambayashi, Y., Winiwarter, W., Arikawa, M. (eds.) DaWaK 2001. LNCS, vol. 2114, pp. 274–283. Springer, Heidelberg (2001)

Indirect Information Linkage for OSINT through Authorship Analysis of Aliases

Robert Layton[1], Charles Perez[2], Babiga Birregah[2], Paul Watters[1], and Marc Lemercier[2]

[1] University of Ballarat, Australia
`r.layton@icsl.com.au,`
`p.watters@ballarat.edu.au`
[2] Université de Technologie de Troyes
{`charles.perez,babiga.birregah,marc.lemercier`}`@utt.fr`

Abstract. In this paper we examine the problem of automatically linking online accounts for open source intelligence gathering. We specifically aim to determine if two social media accounts are shared by the same author, without the use of direct linking evidence. We profile the accounts using authorship analysis and find the best matching guess. We apply this to a series of Twitter accounts identified as malicious by a methodology named SPOT and find several pairs of accounts that belong to the same author, despite no direct evidence linking the two. Overall, our results show that linking aliases is possible with an accuracy of 84%, and using our automated threshold method improves our accuracy to over 90% by removing incorrectly discovered matches.

1 Introduction

In contrast with a more traditional view of intelligence that uses covert and classified sources, open source intelligence (OSINT) analyses publicly available sources to create information. One of the key steps to intelligence gathering is the collection of correlations between sources, in order to combine or fuse together the information from both sources, usable in processes such as Anacapa. We define two classes of the creation of these linkages; direct and indirect. In direct correlation, we look for pieces of information that are shared exactly between two sources, such as the same email address being used for two websites [7, 15]. This type of correlation can be modelled quite easily but can also be easily subverted by knowledgeable attackers.

Indirect linkage aims to find information indicating correlation without direct evidence, such as determining that a suspect was not home at the time a crime was committed. This type of indirect correlation may be defended against using an alibi, but having no such alibi can be seen as a sign of guilt, but not evidence of it. Conceptually, what constitutes an indirect correlation can be difficult to quantify and may lead to a substantial rate of false positives. Computationally, the number of possible events or pieces of information is large for even narrowly restricted circumstances. Comparing all possible pairs with non-trivial

J. Li et al. (Eds.): PAKDD 2013 Workshops, LNAI 7867, pp. 36–46, 2013.

computation can be prohibitive, particularly if an analyst must determine if the correlation is worthy of further investigation. In this research, we investigate authorship analysis to indirectly link aliases.

On the internet, aliases are easy to obtain. Social media accounts, email addresses and forum usernames are just some of the many online aliases available for no cost (and often given with very little proof of identify). Being able to link aliases together using authorship analysis, could provide tangible benefits for analysts gathering intelligence, increasing the number of sources that can be used and further enriching the analysis.

This type of application has recently appeared in the literature. Previous research has proven to be quite successful from a traditional authorship analysis viewpoint. When matching aliases, it is not uncommon to obtain success rates over 90% and a few studies have given results higher than 99%. However the assumptions used in previous studies, while valid for their stated purposes, mean that the results are probably overstated for the purposes of informing OSINT through indirect correlations. In this paper, we investigate this application through this lens, and test empirically a method for matching aliases by author in a way that is robust and automatable, even in different data applications.

In the next section, we review the literature relevant to alias matching using authorship analysis before introducing the context of the application presented. We then propose a method for performing and reporting on indirect correlations through authorship analysis, along with a proof of concept on a corpora of Twitter messages. Finally, we apply the methodology in the real world, to a set of malicious Twitter accounts discovered using the SPOT procedure [16].

As a side note on terminology, we use the term 'author' to refer to an actual person who writes the documents under an alias. We also explicitly use the term 'alias' when referring to the author-chosen pseudonym, such as their account name, and use the term 'sub-alias' when it has been generated by us as researchers, such as by splitting the documents from one alias randomly into two subsets. When two sub-aliases originated from the same alias, they are a 'known match', i.e. we know that those two sub-aliases refer to the same alias. An 'unknown match' is when two sub-aliases (or aliases) are from the same author, but we did not know this in advance. As shown later, our method provides strong evidence that we found some unknown matches in our application experiment.

2   Literature Review

Many works have been proposed to identify malicious actors on social networking platforms, to identify the set of profiles that are responsible of the same malicious activity online. This research problem can contribute to a better defences against these activities on the social networking platform.

The work of [17] proposes to identify connections between 'honey-profiles' from the URLs that they use in their messages. Two profiles that send huge amount of messages pointing to the same URLs will be assumed to belong to the same campaign. As aptly noted in [13], this approach can be limited by the fact that one can create a set of multiple shortened URLs that redirect the user to the same website. An alternative to this approach is to consider, in addition to URLs, the content of messages as described in [4, 3]. [13] proposes a method for detecting malicious profiles that uses keywords to enlarge the audience of their campaign. Looking for the keywords that are ontologically close can help to establish connections between profiles. One of the most used approaches these last decades is the cluster-based algorithms for links detection between profiles. [1] used this approach with a large set of indicators, aiming to link malicious profiles, but it cannot identify more local connections between sets of profiles.

Link farming in social networking sites has been studied by [5, 6], who focus on profiles who use an unusually high number of contacts to raise their influence, benefiting from the popularity of famous profiles. In relation with link detection between malicious profiles, this indicates that the topology of the network can indirectly help to highlight hubs of malicious activity. [2] defines a Socialbot Network (SbN) as a set of social bots that are owned and maintained by a human controller called the botherder. This work presents strategies that can be used to manage an SbN, indicating that to increase the social attractiveness of a socialbot, a solution is to connect in cluster a set of social bots. This approach confirms the possible use of social distance as an indicator of identification of multiple profiles managed by the same person. [8] have proposed a spatio-temporal based solution for the identification of malicious actors. Although this can identify connections between some malicious profiles they assume that malicious actors always communicate with the same spatio-temporal constraints.

Authorship analysis has recently been applied to this problem, first by [14]. Previous work by this group focused on other methods, such as low level features, to link aliases, before discovering the potential for authorship analysis to further inform these linkages. They note that direct attribution is protected by various means of anonymity, while indirect attribution may be possible through authorship analysis. Their research identifies the privacy implications of such methods, both positively and negatively, showing that allowing users to be anonymous can break some models of trust in reputation networks, such as online forums after a user is banned for malicious behaviour.

The method employed by [14] uses five main types of features; bag-of-words, misspellings, punctuation, emoticons and function words, which are common in many authorship analysis studies. They experimented by splitting the documents of each of 100 aliases into two, creating two new sub-aliases for each alias, creating 200 sub-aliases, each with a 'known match'. Their method was able to correctly identify the known match 87% of the time, which is a considerably higher value than most other supervised authorship analysis studies.

In a single document there is a high degree of variance, noise, in the writing which is reduced when combining documents to form 'author profiles' [9]. For unsupervised, we compare only documents to documents, and therefore experience a high amount of noise. For supervised, we often compare a document to an author, reducing the noise. In alias-matching, we compare authors to authors (technically sub-alias to sub-alias), and therefore should expect much lower noise and better quality in the results.

In recent work, [10] identified that splitting aliases based on topic lowers the quality of all authorship methods, however Local n-gram methods, using character n-grams, were more robust than feature based approaches. The ideology behind this paper was mainly concerned with protecting websites against attack, but also as a warning mechanism for those who wish to remain anonymous online, as their authorship style may be used against them.

3   Application Context

In this paper, we propose a method for determining if two aliases belong to the same author, which has several applications.

- Automating Open Source Intelligence, by finding evidence to link profiles that could lead to an increase in available information about a person.
- Website administration, through the identifying of previously banned users.
- Demographic surveying, increasing awareness of the use of social media and removing noise in datasets created by authors having multiple aliases.

Previous research in this field has run experiments that take the assumption that each alias in their database will have a corresponding alias that belongs to the same author - a 'known match', which can be made because the dataset itself it created artificially by the researchers. In this research, we do not take this assumption. We suggest this is a more difficult problem; not only do we need to find the *best candidate match* but also determine if it is a match or not.

4   Proposed Method

One approach to solving the problem posed in the previous section would be to profile all aliases, determine the nearest matching alias for each and then determine if the distance between them is less than some threshold t. If the distance is less than t, we suggest that these two aliases are a match. If the distance is more than t, suggest that the two aliases, despite being 'nearest neighbours', are not a match. The problem with this approach is finding an appropriate value for t, particularly considering most authorship studies require retraining to find parameter values. Examples of this include the n values for character n-grams in authorship, which is often linked loosely to the casualness of the language used [12]. To date, there is little evidence that there are parameters with 'fixed' values for authorship studies. We propose a method to solve this problem based on artificial sub-alias creation to determine a threshold value.

1. Given a set of documents D, each document belonging to an alias in A, create a set of sub-aliases S by splitting the lists of documents in D belonging to each alias $a \in A$ into two subsets.

2. Each sub-alias in S now has a 'known match', i.e. the other sub-alias originating from the same alias $a \in A$.
3. For each (unique) pair of sub-alias $s_i, s_j \in S : i \neq j$, calculate the distance between the sub-alias pairs, and call this d_{s_i,s_j}.

The output of the above method is a sorted list L of distance values. Given a new pair of sub-aliases, we can determine the likelihood that they are an 'unknown match'[1]. The empirical likelihood that a pair of sub-aliases $s_i, s_j \in S$ is an unknown match can be estimated using the following equation:

$$P(s_i \text{ is an unknown match of } s_j) = \frac{|L_k \in L : L_k \geq d(s_i, s_j)|}{|L|} \quad (1)$$

The likelihood of two sub-aliases being an unknown match is the percentage of *known matches* with a distance greater than the distance between the proposed match. We can set this as a hard limit threshold t or can derive it from the data itself. In the section, we identify a method for deriving a threshold value by taking the 'second nearest' likelihood value for correct guesses.

We begin our analysis of this method by first using a proof of concept on a dataset with artificially created aliases. We then apply this in a real world scenario, specifically the output of the SPOT algorithm After obtaining the alias pairs that this procedure considers a match, we then analyse them manually to determine the quality of the approach.

5   Proof of Concept Experiment

As a proof of concept, we create some artificial known and unknown matches in a dataset. We use the Twitter dataset described in [11] for this experiment, selecting 100 aliases at random with at least 200 documents each. For the authorship analysis method, we used the RLP method with n=5 and L=500, due to the high performance of this method on this dataset in the past [10]. First, we performed the following preprocessing steps on the data:

1. Remove all URLs from tweets.
2. Remove all 'at-tags', leaving only the   character
3. Remove any retweet
4. Remove any documents shorter than 50 characters
5. Remove any profiles that had fewer than 50 tweets remaining.

We then applied a ten-fold cross-validation evaluation methodology. The sub-aliases was split into ten 'folds', and ten iterations of tests were undertaken in which each fold was used as the testing fold and not used in the training. This gives a training set of 180 sub-aliases and a testing set of 20 sub-aliases. For each fold, the method proposed in section 4 was applied to the training set, generating

---

[1] They belong to the same alias/author, but we did not know this beforehand in the training set.

the list L of sorted known match distances. The sub-aliases in the testing set were then compared against all matches. Importantly, there was no assurance that the known match of one of the testing sub-aliases was in the training set, as both sub-aliases of the pair may be in the training set.

5.1 Results

For the results for the proof of concept, we first measured the overall accuracy of the method, i.e. the number of 'next-nearest sub-aliases' that were the actual match. The accuracy for this method was 0.8400, which is quite good for 200 authors using this dataset.

Examining the likelihood values of these matches, we found the following median likelihoods under different categories:

- Correct predictions: 0.9960
- 'Second-nearest sub-alias' when the prediction is correct: 0.6889
- Incorrect predictions: 0.7164
- Correct match when the prediction was originally incorrect: 0.5716

The results indicate that when a prediction is correct, the likelihood is much higher than for incorrect predictions and that when the method is wrong, we are less confident in this match. Further, when the correct prediction is given, the second match, i.e. the closest incorrect match, is much less likely to be a match. These 'second matches' have similar values to the closest match for incorrect predictions, with a comparison median likelihood of 0.6889 to 0.7164, indicating that the problem with these incorrect predictions is that the actual match looks incorrect (and not that a wrong match appears to be correct). We can use a threshold value equivalent to the median 'second match' likelihood value for determining if we are to 'believe' a match or not.

In comparison to a 'standard' value of 0.9, this threshold obtains quite good results, with 90% of the above threshold matches correctly identified and 71% of the below threshold matches identified. As the threshold increases, we obtain a higher precision but lower recall.

We therefore suggest using the median second match likelihood for correct predictions to determine the threshold value, which we will test further in the next section.

Threshold: 0.6889 (median second match likelihood)
162/179 above threshold and correct (0.9050)
17/179 above threshold and incorrect (0.0950)
6/21 below threshold and correct (0.2857)
15/21 below threshold and incorrect (0.7143)
Threshold: 0.9
154/162 above threshold and correct (0.9506)
8/162 above threshold and incorrect (0.0494)
14/38 below threshold and correct (0.3684)
24/38 below threshold and incorrect (0.6316)

6   Application

The application of this work is based on a tool for detecting malicious profiles on social networking sites named SPOT 1.0 [16], which collects data from the Twitter stream API in real time. For each profile, a set of characteristics is synthesised such as the frequency of messages, the number of reference, keywords, and the URLs posted. The tool detects suspicious profiles based on profiles with characteristics deviating from the norm. The suspicious profiles are then further analysed, with each URL from a suspicious profiles evaluated and profiles containing malicious URLs are identified as malicious profiles. SPOT then profiles the malicious users in three dimensions; visibility as an indicator of the potential audience of an attack carried out by a profile, aggressiveness which represents the frequency with which the attack was carried out and danger is the real danger brought by the profile on the social networking site.

In this section we apply the presented method to a real world dataset and a real world application. The goal is to identify the profiles classified by the SPOT platform which are originating from the same author. The input to this application is a set of malicious Twitter profiles, which have been pre-processed using the procedure described above. Overall we have analysed 29,706 documents across 210 classes, giving a mean number of documents per class of 141.5.

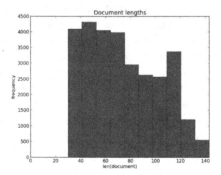

Fig. 1. Histogram of document lengths in characters, after preprocessing

The experimental methodology for this application differs slightly from the proof of concept, to account for the fact that we do not, in advance, know if there are any matches in our dataset. To compensate for this problem, we generate a dataset using the malicious profiles using a similar procedure to the proof of concept. We take the aliases with more than 200 tweets and split them into two sub-aliases. Then we calculate the accuracy and likelihood values for this subset of the data to derive at threshold value. We then rerun the analysis on the original dataset with this threshold and without any sub-aliases. Any matches above this threshold are considered an 'unknown match' and are manually analysed by an expert in authorship to determine the quality of the results.

7   Results

7.1   Malicious Profile Sub-aliases

In the first phase of the application, we repeated the experiment above on the final dataset. The dataset used in this phase was the tweets from each of the Twitter accounts marked as malicious by the SPOT program. After preprocessing, this dataset composed of 132 Twitter accounts and a total of 19,718 tweets.

We created two subaliases for each account and then applied the method proposed earlier. Overall, the accuracy of this method was 0.8712, with a median likelihood value of 0.9980 for correct matches. The second threshold was 0.9889, which was above the median threshold of incorrect matches, 0.9896. This was above the median likelihood for the correct match when an incorrect match was predicted, which was 0.9801. These results further given evidence to our hypothesis that incorrect matches are not because other authors match the query author, but instead the known match is highly different. When using the 'second match likelihood' from before as our threshold value (0.9889), we obtained the following results:

209/226 above threshold and correct (0.9248)
17/226 above threshold and incorrect (0.0752)
21/38 below threshold and correct (0.5526)
17/38 below threshold and incorrect (0.4474)

7.2   Full Dataset with Expert Analysis

On applying the method to the full dataset, we used a threshold value of 0.9889 obtained from the previous experiment. After the calculations had completed, we obtained 40 possible matches which were above the threshold, from 132 possible matches. Of these matches, there was a median likelihood value of 0.9976, mean of 0.9966 and standard deviation of 0.003) (see figure 2).

An expert in authorship then examined each of the matches individually, giving a mark of 'Yes, definite match', 'Maybe, a potential match' and 'No, not a match'. Overall, 11 of the matches were marked as 'Yes', 9 were marked as 'Maybe' and the other 20 marked as 'No'. Overall, this method was able to find 11 matches from over 132 pairs of accounts, which would not have been feasible if an expert was required to manually assess all of the data.

The result of the procedure is visualised as a graph in the figure 7.2, where the set of nodes is the set of sub-alias. An edge between two nodes represents that a matching occurred. The edges are coloured in grey and black. Grey edges represent connections between sub-aliases that belongs to the same alias, while black edges identify the connections that are newly highlighted by the authorship attribution method. Running a strongly connected component algorithm leads to identify three main clusters of malicious profiles.

We then performed a manual deeper analysis on the three strongest components identified above in figure 8. This will help to validate new insights given by our approach. The first cluster composed of nodes {327,255, 372} is composed of profiles that tweet in English using large amount of Bible quotations.

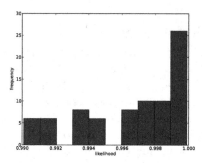

Fig. 2. Likelihood distribution for application experiment

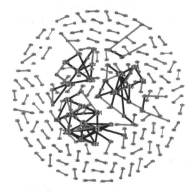

Fig. 3. Graph of highlighted connections between malicious profiles

Such a behaviour illustrates the originality of malicious profiles to bypass Twitter limitations. The Twitter platform forbids the repetition of the same tweets from a single profiles. Thus, this set of profiles rely on semi-automatic importation of Bible quotation to overcome this limitation and manage automatically their profiles. We have noticed that they also include hashtags in their tweets in order to increase their audience. The second cluster composed of nodes {233,5203}, and were profiles in Spanish containing journalistic information. All of their tweets are composed by a simple prototype of sentence: passive subject + verb + agent. Once again this strategy reveals some category of profiles which pretends to be normal, but which finally remain on other sources of information to generate high level of trust for users. The third cluster composed of nodes {208,334,124,152} contains profiles that use very crude English language, containing many retweets and possess a particularity to multiply occurrence of some letters or couple of letter (e.g. o,.,!,=,RT). This observation can reveal an underlying mechanism of tweet generation that ensure the non duplicate of messages by adding a pseudo random repetition of characters. This section highlighted that beyond the capability of the approach to identify direct authors of tweets, it is also capable to identify groups of malicious profiles that may be automated

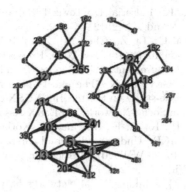

Fig. 4. Strongly connected components

based on the same underlying strategy defined by the creator. This observation gives interesting perspectives to our work, when applied at a larger scale. First, how many distinct strategies can we observe for malicious Twitter users, second is there a unique malicious person beyond these profiles, third can we easily cross platforms to identify multi-platform based malicious users.

8   Conclusions

In this paper we examined the use of authorship analysis to discover when malicious profiles were authored by the same person. In our proof of concept, the method obtained a base accuracy of 0.8400, and given a threshold value using the 'second match' for correct guesses, the method obtained 0.9050 accuracy. We were also able to show that incorrect guesses do not look like correct guesses (on average) by using this threshold value.

In our application to malicious profiles, our method found 11 definite matches between 132 possible malicious Twitter accounts. There were also 9 potential matches, that the expert had inadequate evidence for one way or another. This discovery would not have been possible without an automated method, and shows a significant amount of potential for use in automated open source intelligence, usable to link profiles together indirectly. We plan to build on these results, creating more robust methods for authorship through the use of ensembles.

References

[1] Ahmed, F., Abulaish, M.: An MCL-Based Approach for Spam Profile Detection in Online Social Networks. In: IEEE 11th International Conference on Trust, Security and Privacy in Computing and Communications, pp. 1–7 (June 2012)

[2] Boshmaf, Y., Muslukhov, I., Beznosov, K., Ripeanu, M.: The socialbot network: when bots socialize for fame and money. In: ACSAC 2011: Proceedings of the 27th Annual Computer Security Applications Conference. ACM Request Permissions (December 2011)

[3] Gao, H., Chen, Y., Lee, K., Palsetia, D.: Towards online spam filtering in social networks. ... on Network and ... (2012)

[4] Gao, H., Hu, J., Wilson, C., Li, Z., Chen, Y., Zhao, B.Y.: Detecting and characterizing social spam campaigns. In: IMC 2010: Proceedings of the 10th Annual Conference on Internet measurement. ACM Request Permissions (November 2010)

[5] Ghosh, S., Korlam, G., Ganguly, N.: The effects of restrictions on number of connections in OSNs: a case-study on twitter. In: WOSN 2010: Proceedings of the 3rd Conference on Online Social Networks. USENIX Association (June 2010)

[6] Ghosh, S., Viswanath, B., Kooti, F., Sharma, N., Korlam, G., Benevenuto, F., Ganguly, N., Gummadi, K.P.: Understanding and combating link farming in the twitter social network. In: WWW 2012: Proceedings of the 21st International Conference on World Wide Web (2012)

[7] Golbeck, J., Rothstein, M.: Linking Social Networks on the Web with FOAF: A Semantic Web Case Study.. In: Proceedings of the Twenty-Third Conference on Artificial Intelligence, AAAI 2008 (2008)

[8] Halim, Z., Gul, M., ul Hassan, N., Baig, R., Rehman, S., Naz, F.: Malicious users' circle detection in social network based on spatio-temporal co-occurrence. In: 2011 International Conference on Computer Networks and Information Technology (ICCNIT), pp. 35–39 (2011)

[9] Layton, R., Watters, P., Dazeley, R.: Automated unsupervised authorship analysis using evidence accumulation clustering. Natural Language Engineering 1(1), 1–26 (2011)

[10] Layton, R., Watters, P., Dazeley, R.: The effect of topic on alias matching for online communications (2012) (submitted)

[11] Layton, R., Watters, P., Dazeley, R.: Authorship Attribution for Twitter in 140 Characters or Less. In: 2010 Second Cybercrime and Trustworthy Computing Workshop, pp. 1–8. IEEE (July 2010),
http://www.computer.org/portal/web/csdl/doi/10.1109/CTC.2010.17,
http://ieeexplore.ieee.org/xpls/abs_all.jsp?arnumber=5615152,
http://ieeexplore.ieee.org/lpdocs/epic03/wrapper.htm?arnumber=5615152

[12] Layton, R., Watters, P., Dazeley, R.: Recentred Local Profiles for Authorship Attribution. Journal of Natural Language Engineering (2011); available on CJO 2011

[13] Lee, K., Caverlee, J., Kamath, K.Y., Cheng, Z.: Detecting collective attention spam. In: WebQuality 2012: Proceedings of the 2nd Joint WICOW/AIRWeb Workshop on Web Quality. ACM Request Permissions (April 2012)

[14] Novak, J., Raghavan, P., Tomkins, A.: Anti-aliasing on the web. In: Proceedings of the 13th Conference on World Wide Web - WWW 2004, p. 30 (2004),
http://portal.acm.org/citation.cfm?doid=988672.988678

[15] Perez, C., Birregah, B., Lemercier, M.: The multi-layer imbrication for data leakage prevention from mobile devices. In: 2012 IEEE 11th International Conference on Trust, Security and Privacy in Computing and Communications (TrustCom), pp. 813–819. IEEE (2012)

[16] Perez, C., Lemercier, M., Birregah, B., Corpel, A.: Spot 1.0: Scoring suspicious profiles on twitter. In: 2011 International Conference on Advances in Social Networks Analysis and Mining (ASONAM), pp. 377–381. IEEE (2011)

[17] Stringhini, G., Kruegel, C., Vigna, G.: Detecting spammers on social networks. In: ACSAC 2010: Proceedings of the 26th Annual Computer Security Applications Conference, pp. 1–9. ACM Request Permissions (July 2012)

Dynamic Similarity-Aware Inverted Indexing for Real-Time Entity Resolution*

Banda Ramadan[1], Peter Christen[1], Huizhi Liang[1], Ross W. Gayler[2], and David Hawking[1,3]

[1] Research School of Computer Science, The Australian National University,
Canberra ACT 0200, Australia
{banda.ramadan,peter.christen,huizhi.liang,david.hawking}@anu.edu.au
[2] Veda, Melbourne VIC 3000, Australia
ross.gayler@veda.com.au
[3] Funnelback Pty. Ltd., Canberra ACT 2601, Australia
david.hawking@acm.org

Abstract. Entity resolution is the process of identifying groups of records in a single or multiple data sources that represent the same real-world entity. It is an important tool in data de-duplication, in linking records across databases, and in matching query records against a database of existing entities. Most existing entity resolution techniques complete the resolution process offline and on static databases. However, real-world databases are often dynamic, and increasingly organizations need to resolve entities in real-time. Thus, there is a need for new techniques that facilitate working with dynamic databases in real-time. In this paper, we propose a dynamic similarity-aware inverted indexing technique (DySimII) that meets these requirements. We also propose a frequency-filtered indexing technique where only the most frequent attribute values are indexed. We experimentally evaluate our techniques on a large real-world voter database. The results show that when the index size grows no appreciable increase is found in the average record insertion time (around 0.1 msec) and in the average query time (less than 0.1 sec). We also find that applying the frequency-filtered approach reduces the index size with only a slight drop in recall.

Keywords: Dynamic indexing, real-time query, record linkage, data matching, duplicate detection, frequency-filtered indexing.

1 Introduction

Massive amounts of data are being collected by most business and government organizations. Given that many of these organizations rely on information in their day-to-day operations, the quality of the collected data has a direct impact on the quality of the produced outcomes [7,13]. Various data validation and

---

* This research was funded by the Australian Research Council (ARC), Veda, and Funnelback Pty. Ltd., under Linkage Project LP100200079.

J. Li et al. (Eds.): PAKDD 2013 Workshops, LNAI 7867, pp. 47–58, 2013.

cleaning practices are employed to improve the collected data. One important practice in data cleaning and data integration is the identification of all records that refer to the same real-world entity [13]. This process is called *entity resolution* [7], and can be applied to a single or to multiple data sources (within a single data source the process is called *de-duplication*). A real-world entity could be a person (e.g. customer, patient or student), a product, a business, or any other object that exists in the real world.

Examples of duplicates may be a patient who is represented several times in a hospital database, a product that is inserted many times in an inventory list, or a voter who is registered more than once in an election roll. These duplicates, if not removed or merged, can lead to serious consequences for organizations or individuals. A patient's information could for example be dispersed between their duplicated records, leaving medical staff unaware of the patient's overall condition and affecting diagnosis and treatment. In another example, duplicate records in an election roll could allow voting irregularities.

In many cases, organizations need to perform the entity resolution process in real-time in order to be able to complete their operations. For example, social services need to identify individuals on the spot even if their social security number is not available. Police officers also need to identify individuals within seconds when they do an identity check on a suspect, using their personal details. Real-time matching can be achieved using indexes that reside in main memory rather than using disk-based indexes, and by reducing the size of those indexes.

The databases used by most organizations and businesses are not static but are modified constantly by adding, deleting, or updating records. This makes the entity resolution process more challenging, since most entity resolution techniques currently available are only suitable for static databases. This is because most of these techniques are based on batch algorithms that resolve all records rather than resolving those relating to a single query record. There is an urgent need to develop new techniques that support real-time entity resolution for dynamic large databases.

In this paper we develop and investigate a dynamic similarity-aware inverted indexing technique [5] for real-time entity resolution on dynamic databases. Our contribution is two-fold. The first is to dynamically update the inverted index after every query record rather than leaving the index out-of-date between periodic batch updates. The second is to investigate reducing the size of the inverted index using frequency-based filtering where only the attribute values that occur most frequently in a database are inserted into the index.

2   Related Work

The entity resolution process encompasses several steps [7]: *Data Preprocessing*, which cleans and standardizes the data to be used; *Indexing*, which creates candidate records that potentially correspond to matches; *Record Pair Comparison*, which compares the candidate records using one or more similarity matching functions [10]; *Classification*, where candidate record pairs are classified into matches and non-matches; and finally, *Evaluation*, where the entity resolution process is evaluated using a variety of measures [4].

This paper is concerned with the indexing step, which is a vital step in entity resolution as it reduces the number of records that need to be compared in detail to resolve the matching of a given query record. Different indexing techniques are summarized in [6]. Standard blocking [11] segregates records into blocks according to a certain criteria, and subsequently compares only records that are in the same block. Usually this criteria, called blocking key, is based on one or more attributes [7]. This approach has the disadvantage of assigning records into the wrong block in case of errors in attribute values (i.e. dirty data). To avoid this from occurring, iterative blocking [17] can be applied where multiple blocking keys are used and each record is inserted into more than one block.

The sorted neighbourhood method (SNM) [12] sorts all records in the database using a key that is based on attribute values. Then a fixed size widow is used to slide over the sorted records comparing only records within the window. The main drawback of this method is that using a fixed size window potentially leads to missed true matches if the window size is too small, and unnecessary pair comparisons if the window size is too large. To avoid this an adaptive SNM [9,19] can be used where the window size can grow or shrink adaptively.

Another approach is q-gram based indexing. The idea behind this technique is to convert the values of the blocking key into a list of q-grams (a q-gram is a sequence of q continuous characters generated from a string). Based on these generated lists of q-grams, each attribute is inserted into more than one block to reduce the effect of errors that might occur in attribute values. Although this approach achieves better quality blocking than traditional blocking and the SNM [2], it is computationally expensive and therefore is not suitable for large databases or real-time entity resolution.

Canopy clustering [15] on the other hand is a technique that aims at speeding up the process of blocking records for large databases. This technique uses a computationally cheap clustering approach to create high dimensional overlapping clusters called *canopies*, from which block of candidate record pairs can then be generated. Another idea of indexing is to use a sorted suffix array [1] of all the subsequences of tokens that appear in a string. These tokens are used as blocking keys allowing records to be inserted into several blocks.

Existing entity resolution techniques focus on improving the accuracy and the efficiency of the entity resolution process. However, most of these techniques are aimed at offline processing of static databases. Not much research has concentrated on real-time entity resolution (where a stream of query records arrive that need to be resolved against the records in the database in real-time) or on entity resolution for dynamic databases. The first query-time entity resolution approach was based on a collective classification approach [3]. The idea behind this approach is to only use a subset of records in a database for resolving queries, by extracting records related to a query and then resolving this query using only these records. Although this approach can improve matching quality, experiments showed an average time of 31.28 sec was needed on a database with

831,991 records. Thus, this approach is not suitable for real-time entity resolution, nor it is scalable to large databases since it is computationally expensive.

The similarity-aware inverted indexing technique [5] described in Sect. 3 proposes a real-time entity resolution approach that is very fast. Although it has an average query time of 0.1 sec for a query record on a database that contains nearly 7 million records, the approach only works on static databases. Another real-time entity resolution approach that works on static databases is proposed by Dey et al. [8]. It is based on using a matching tree to limit the amount of communication required for matching records between disparate databases held at different locations, where a matching decision can be made without the need of comparing all attribute values between records. This approach is shown to reduce the communication overhead, without affecting the matching quality.

Ioannou et al. [14] on the other hand propose an approach that provides entity resolution in real-time, and works on dynamic databases. Their method is based on using links between the entities in a database combined with a probabilistic database for resolving entities. The approach uses existing entity resolution techniques to find possible matches of a query, and instead of using these possible matches to make an offline resolution decision, it stores the possible matches alongside with a probability weight in a dynamic index data structure. This stored information is then used at query time to perform entity resolution in real-time. The approach is reported to have an average time of 70 msec for a query record on a database of 51,222 records. This query time is almost constant and does not increase when the database get larger.

Another dynamic entity resolution approach is proposed by Whang and Garcia-Molina [18] that allows matching rules to evolve over time when new records become available. This approach aims at using materialized entity resolution results (which are a set of records that are classified as matches) to save redundant work, and does not require running the entity resolution process from scratch. The authors report that this rule evolution approach can be faster than the naive approach by up to several orders of magnitude [18].

3   Dynamic Similarity-Aware Inverted Indexing

The similarity-aware inverted index proposed in [5] aims at providing real-time entity resolution for a stream of query records. The main idea behind this approach is to pre-calculate similarities between attribute values that are in the same block. These pre-calculated similarities are stored in main memory to be used later in the query resolution process. Avoiding similarity calculations at query time significantly reduces the time needed for matching a query record. This approach was shown to be two orders of magnitude faster than traditional approaches [5], which makes it suitable for real-time entity resolution.

To use this approach, three indexes are needed as shown in Fig. 1. The first index, called the Block Index (**BI**), is an inverted index that stores unique attribute values and their associated blocking key values (generated using traditional encoding techniques such as Soundex, Phonex, or Double-Metaphone [7]). Keys

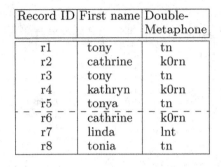 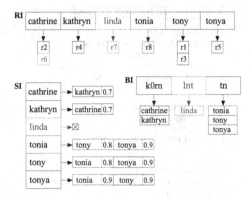

Fig. 1. The Dynamic Similarity-aware Inverted Index created from the example records in the table on the left. The example records contain first name values and their Double Metaphone encodings used as blocking key values. **RI** is the record identifier index, **BI** is the block index and **SI** is the similarity index.

of this index are the blocking key values, while each key points to a list of all attribute values that have this blocking key value. The second index, called the Similarity Index (**SI**), stores the pre-calculated similarities between attribute values that are in the same block (similarities are calculated using comparison functions such as Winkler or Jaccard [7]). Keys for the **SI** are unique attribute values, while each key points to a list of pre-calculated similarities between this value and all other values that are in the same block (similarity values range between 0 and 1, where 1 means exact match). Finally, the Record Index (**RI**) stores all unique attribute values and their associated record identifiers. Keys of this index are the unique attribute values, while each key points to a list of all record identifiers that have the same attribute value.

To overcome the limitation of the original similarity-aware inverted indexing technique that works only with static databases, we modify the original technique to be used with dynamic databases. The main difference between the two techniques is that in the original technique indexes are static, and once they are created no more records and attribute values are added to them. On the other hand, the proposed dynamic indexing technique (DySimII) is more flexible and values are added whenever a new query is being processed. The following section describes the proposed techniques in detail.

3.1 Indexing Dynamic Databases

Building the Indexes. We start with three empty indexes. First, unique attribute values for records are added to the three indexes as described in [5]. Adding attribute values to the inverted indexes is based on two cases: the first case occurs when an attribute value is new and it does not exist in the inverted indexes (r7 and r8 in Fig. 1). The second case occurs when an attribute value has been indexed previously and it exists in the inverted indexes (r6 in Fig. 1).

Algorithm 1: *DySimII - Overall*

Input:
- Database: **D**
- Number of attributes of **D** used: n
- Encoding functions: $\mathbf{E}_a, a = 1 \ldots n$
- Similarity functions: $\mathbf{S}_a, a = 1 \ldots n$
- Stream of query records: **Q**

Output:
- Record index: **RI**
- Similarity index: **SI**
- Block index: **BI**
- Ranked list of matches: **M**

1: Initialise **RI** = {}
2: Initialise **SI** = {}
3: Initialise **BI** = {}
4: **for r** ∈ **D**:
5:     **for** $a = 1 \ldots n$:
6:         $Insert(\mathbf{r}.a, \mathbf{r}.id, \mathbf{E}_a, \mathbf{S}_a)$
7: **for q** ∈ **Q**:
8:     $Query(\mathbf{q}, \mathbf{E}_a, \mathbf{S}_a)$

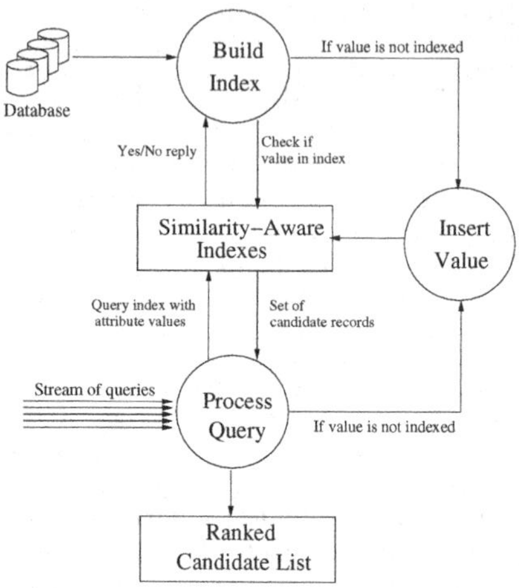

Fig. 2. Algorithm 1 illustrates the overall process of the DySimII technique. The right side illustrates the framework of the DySimII technique, as described in Sect. 3.1.

1. In the first case, an attribute value is first inserted into the **RI** with its associated record identifier. Then its encoded value is calculated to decide into which block it should be added. If the block of that encoded value exists then the attribute value will be inserted into that block in the **BI**. Otherwise, a new block for the encoded value is created and this attribute value is inserted. If this value is added into an existing block, the similarities between this new attribute value and all other values within this block are calculated. These similarities are then stored in **SI**.
2. In the second case, where a value has been indexed previously, the only action needed is to add the identifier of this query record that holds this attribute value into the corresponding record list in the **RI**.

The process of loading and indexing attribute values will continue until we reach the last record in the database. As a result we will have three inverted indexes (**BI**, **SI**, and **RI**). In the original similarity-aware indexing technique, building the indexes will stop at this point. If new values arrive, these values cannot be added to the indexes. However, this issue is handled in DySimII allowing more values to be added to the indexes. If a new record arrives, its attribute values are loaded, encoded values are calculated, and the steps described above will take place adding any new value to the previously built indexes. The overall DySimII framework is illustrated in Fig 2.

The process of inserting a new attribute value **r**.*a* (Algorithm 2) requires the identifier of the record of this attribute, **r**.*id*, the encoding function, the similarity comparison function, and the inverted indexes **RI**, **SI**, and **BI** as input. The process starts with inserting **r**.*id* into the **RI** (line 1). If this attribute value does not exist in the **SI** (line 2), the following steps are conducted. First, the encoding

Algorithm 2: *DySimII - Insert*	Algorithm 3: *DySimII - Query*
Input:	Input:
- Attribute value: $\mathbf{r}.a$	- Query record: $\mathbf{q}$
- Record identifier: $\mathbf{r}.id$	- Number of attributes of $\mathbf{D}$ used: n
- Encoding functions: $\mathbf{E}_a, a = 1 \ldots n$	- Encoding functions: $\mathbf{E}_a, a = 1 \ldots n$
- Similarity functions: $\mathbf{S}_a, a = 1 \ldots n$	- Similarity functions: $\mathbf{S}_a, a = 1 \ldots n$
- Indexes: $\mathbf{RI}, \mathbf{SI}, \mathbf{BI}$	- Indexes: $\mathbf{RI}, \mathbf{SI}, \mathbf{BI}$
Output:	Output:
- Updated indexes: $\mathbf{RI}, \mathbf{SI}, \mathbf{BI}$	- Ranked list of matches: $\mathbf{M}$
1: Append $\mathbf{r}.id$ to $\mathbf{RI}[\mathbf{r}.a]$	1: Initialise $\mathbf{M} = ()$
2: if $\mathbf{r}.a \notin \mathbf{SI}$:	2: for $a = 1 \ldots n$:
3: $c = \mathbf{E}_a(\mathbf{r}.a)$	3: if $\mathbf{q}.a \notin \mathbf{RI}$:
4: $b = \mathbf{BI}[c]$	4: $Insert(\mathbf{q}.a, \mathbf{q}.id, \mathbf{E}_a, \mathbf{S}_a)$
5: Append $\mathbf{r}.a$ to b	5: else:
6: $\mathbf{BI}[c] = b$	6: Append $\mathbf{q}.id$ to $\mathbf{RI}[\mathbf{q}.a]$
7: Initialise inverted index list $\mathbf{si} = ()$	7: $\mathbf{ri} = \mathbf{RI}[\mathbf{q}.a]$
8: for $v \in b$:	8: for $\mathbf{r}.id \in \mathbf{ri}$:
9: $s = \mathbf{S}_a(\mathbf{r}.a, v)$	9: $\mathbf{M}[\mathbf{r}.id] = \mathbf{M}[\mathbf{r}.id] + 1.0$
10: Append (v, s) to $\mathbf{si}$	10: $\mathbf{si} = \mathbf{SI}[\mathbf{r}.a]$
11: $\mathbf{oi} = \mathbf{SI}[v]$	11: for $(\mathbf{r}.a, s) \in \mathbf{si}$:
12: Append $(\mathbf{r}.a, s)$ to $\mathbf{oi}$	12: $\mathbf{ri} = \mathbf{RI}[\mathbf{r}.a]$
13: $\mathbf{SI}[v] = \mathbf{oi}$	13: for $\mathbf{r}.id \in \mathbf{ri}$:
14: $\mathbf{SI}[\mathbf{r}.a] = \mathbf{si}$	14: $\mathbf{M}[\mathbf{r}.id] = \mathbf{M}[\mathbf{r}.id] + s$
	15: Sort $\mathbf{M}$ according to similarities

Fig. 3. Algorithm 2 illustrates the process of inserting an attribute value into the index structures, and Algorithm 3 the process of querying an attribute value

value c is calculated and all other values in its block are retrieved from the **BI**. The new value is then added into the inverted index list b of this block, and the updated list is stored back into **BI** (lines 3-6). Next the similarities between the new attribute value $\mathbf{r}.a$ and all attribute values v that already exist in this block are calculated (line 8), and inserted into both the new value's similarity list $\mathbf{si}$ (line 10) and the other value's list $\mathbf{oi}$ (line 12). Finally, the similarity list $\mathbf{si}$ of the new value $\mathbf{r}.a$ is added to **SI** in line 14.

Querying in Real-Time. Since similarities between attribute values that are located in the same block are pre-calculated and stored in the **SI**, the process of resolving queries is faster than with traditional entity resolution techniques [5]. However, in the original similarity-aware inverted indexing approach, after resolving and matching a certain query record it is not added into the inverted index data structures. As a result, when a previously resolved attribute value arrives in another query record we would again have to do the similarity calculations to resolve that query. To avoid such repeated unnecessary computations, the DySimII approach adds any new attribute value from a query record into the indexes. Therefore, if the same attribute value occurs in several query records the encoding and similarity computations need to be performed only the first time. Algorithm 3 illustrates how the query is handled in the DySimII.

First an accumulator **M**, which is a data structure that contains record identifiers and their similarities with the query record, is initialized (line 1). Then for every attribute value in the query, the algorithm checks if this value is in the **RI** (lines 2 and 3). If it is not in the **RI**, then it will be inserted into the three

Table (a).

First Name (118,565)		Second Name (189,890)	
james	41,022	smith	28,243
michael	37,536	williams	23,247
john	34,141	johnson	22,100
robert	33,241	jones	19,807
william	31,918	brown	16,256
david	30,126	davis	15,002
mary	22,993	moore	10,968
christopher	20,590	miller	10,435
jenifer	19,468	wilson	10,254
charles	17,438	harris	9,380

Table (b).	Frequency = 1	Frequency <= 10
First Name	67.72%	93.63
Last Name	47.14%	90.76%

Fig. 4. Table (a) represents a list of the top 10 most frequent first/last names in the North Carolina (NC) voter database. Table (b) illustrates the percentage of uncommon first/last names. The right plot illustrates the distribution of attribute values.

indexes as described in Algorithm 1 (line 4). In lines 5 to 7, the identifiers $r.id$ of all other records that have the same attribute value are retrieved and their similarities (exactly 1, as they have the same attribute value) are added into the accumulator $\mathbf{M}$. A new element for record identifier $r.id$ will be added to the accumulator if it does not exist. Next, all other attribute values in the same block and their similarities with the query attribute value are retrieved from the $\mathbf{SI}$ (line 8). For each of these values, their record identifiers are retrieved from the $\mathbf{RI}$ and their similarities are added into the accumulator in line 12. Finally, in line 13, the accumulator is sorted such that the records with largest similarities are located at the beginning, and this sorted list is returned.

3.2   Frequency-Filtered Indexing

The original similarity-aware inverted indexing technique is based on building the inverted indexes for all unique attribute values in a database. However, some attribute values may be uncommon and have low frequencies. Indexing such rare values might not be of use. For instance, the first name *John* in the voter database that we use for our experiments (see Sect. 4) is a common name and it has a frequency of 34,141 in this database, while a first name like *Juvena* is uncommon and only occurs once in the same database. This suggests that the probability of receiving a query with the first name value *John* is much higher than the probability of receiving a query with the value *Juvena*. Figure 4 illustrates the frequency distributions of the four attributes that are in this database (i.e. first name, last name, city, and zip-code). It can be seen that only a small number of attribute values have a high frequency, while most have low frequencies.

Many databases that contains values such as personal details are found to have a frequency distribution that follow Zipf's law [20], which states that in a list of words ranked according to their frequencies, the word at rank r has a relative frequency that corresponds to $1/r$. Distributions in which the relative frequency approximates $1/r^\alpha$ are considered Zipfian, even if $\alpha \neq 1$. This means that the number of uncommon values in many databases is large, and since these values are taking space in the inverted index while they are not queried very often, we suggest indexing only the most frequent attribute values.

We therefore investigate the effect of indexing only a certain percentage $x\%$ of the most frequent attribute values where $0 < x\% < 100$. This requires a list of frequent values, which can be generated for example from an online telephone book. Before we add any value into the index structures, we check if this value is in the $x\%$ of most frequent values. If this is the case, the value is added to the index structures, otherwise it will not. This process is expected to reduce the size of the index structures since we are only indexing the most frequent values.

4   Experimental Evaluation

In our experimental evaluation, we use a large real-world voter registration database from North Carolina (NC) in the US [16]. We downloaded this database every two months since October 2011 to build a compound temporal database. This database contains the names, addresses, and ages of more 2.5 million voters, as well as their unique voter registration numbers. Each record has a time-stamp attached which corresponds to the date a voter originally registered, or when any of their details have changed. This database therefore contains realistic temporal information about a large number of people. We identified 39,967 individuals with two records, 553 with three, and 9 with four records in this database.

The attributes used in our experiments are: first name, last name, city, and zip-code. An exploration of the database has shown that many of the changes in the first name attribute are corrections of nicknames and small typographical mistakes, while changes in last name and address attributes are mostly genuine changes that occur when people get married or move address. Our analysis also shows that this database approximately follows a Zipfian frequency distribution for the first name and last name attributes, and that most attribute values have low frequencies, as can be seen in Fig. 4.

We implemented our approach using Python (version 2.7.3), and ran experiments on a server with 128 GBytes of main memory and two 6-core Intel Xeon CPUs running at 2.4 GHz. For the encoding (blocking) functions $\mathbf{E}_a$, the Double Metaphone [7] technique was used for the first name, last name, and city attributes, while the last 4 digits were used for the zip-code. For the string comparison functions $\mathbf{S}_a$, the Winkler function was used [7] for the first three attributes, while for the zip-code the similarity was calculated by counting the number of matching digits divided by the length of the zip-code.

In our first set of experiments, we evaluate whether the proposed approach facilitates real-time querying and updating of dynamic databases. We use the first 10% of the database to build the inverted index data structures, and we treat the remaining records as queries. When these query records are processed,

(a)   (b)

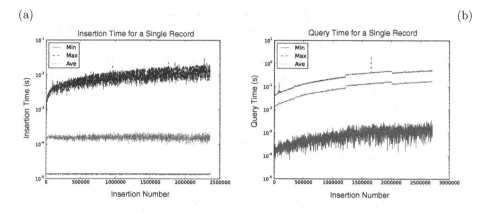

Fig. 5. Plot (a) illustrates the time needed for a single record insertion into the index. Plot (b) illustrates the average time required for querying the growing index.

Measure	x% of the most frequent attribute values indexed									
	10	20	30	40	50	60	70	70	90	100
Coverage	0.73	0.85	0.92	0.95	0.98	0.98	0.99	0.99	0.99	1.00
Recall (%)	64	81	92	95	98	99	100	100	100	100
Memory (MB)	1,026	1,086	1,151	1,222	1,299	1,395	1,489	1,595	1,710	1,828

Fig. 6. Recall, query coverage, and memory usage when indexing only x% of the most frequent attribute values using the original similarity-aware indexing technique

they are added to the already existing index data structures. The record insertion time, the average query time and the memory usage are measured for the growing size of the index structures.

In our second set of experiments, we evaluate the frequency-filtered indexing and investigate its effect on the original static similarity-aware inverted indexing technique [5]. The investigation includes the effect on recall (i.e. found number of true matches over total number of true matches), memory requirements, and query coverage (i.e. the ratio between the number of times an attribute value of a query is available in the index and the number of times that it is not available). In this set of experiments we index the most frequent $x\%$ of attribute values where x ranges from 10% to 100%. A value of $x = 10\%$ means that only the most frequent 10% of the attribute values from the NC database are added to the index structures. A list of all distinct values and their frequencies in the NC database has been generated earlier to be used in the decision of adding an attribute value to the index structures or not. We finally apply the frequency-filtered indexing approach to the dynamic similarity-aware indexing technique to see if it has the same effect as on the original static approach.

5   Results and Discussions

The results from running the first set of experiments are illustrated in Fig. 5. In plot (a), it is shown that the average time needed for a single record insertion into the index structures is almost constant. This implies that even if the index structures grow dynamically when new values are added to it, it does not affect the time required for inserting a single record. The plot shows that the maximum insertion time for a single record is around 10 msec, the average insertion time is around 0.1 msec, and the minimum insertion time is around 0.01 msec. In plot (b), it can be seen that the query time is not affected by the growing size of the index structures. The plot shows that the maximum query time for a single record is less than 0.5 sec, the average query time is less than 0.1 sec, and the minimum query time is around 1 msec.

The memory required for building the index structures for the whole database was 3,641 MB. This memory required was only a tiny fraction of the amount available on the experimental machine, indicating that our implementation would be viable even for much larger databases. If the size of the problem increased substantially relative to the physical memory, a possible approach is to prune low-frequency attributes from the index structures.

A summary of the results for the second set of experiments is illustrated in Fig. 6. As seen in this table, the query coverage is very high for all values of $x\%$. For example when we index only 30% of the most frequent attribute values from the NC voter database, 92% of the arriving queries are actually found in the index. Recall drops only slightly when we do not index all attribute values. For example, when we index 50% of the most frequent attribute values, the recall drops only by 2%. The acceptability of this drop in recall depends on who is using the proposed approach. For example, a 2% drop in recall might be acceptable for a general business company, but not for a national security organization. The experiments also show that memory requirements drop by around 43% when we index only 10% of the most frequent attribute values in the database. When applying the frequency-filtered approach on the DySimII technique, similar effect occurs where the recall remains almost the same for all different values of $x\%$, and the required memory decreases by half when we index only 10% of the most frequent attribute values in the voter database.

6   Conclusions

In this paper, a dynamic similarity-aware inverted indexing technique for real-time entity resolution on dynamic databases was presented, and a frequency-filtered indexing was investigated where only the most frequent attribute values are indexed. The two approaches were evaluated using a large real-world database. The experiments showed that the growing size of the dynamic index structures proposed in our approach does not affect the time required to insert new records into the index structures, and it does not affect the time required to resolve query records. It was also shown that the frequency-filtered approach reduces the size of the index structures with only a slight drop in recall. Our future work aims at conducting a theoretical analysis of scalability to much larger databases and investigating the use of this approach in a parallel environment.

References

1. Aizawa, A., Oyama, K.: A Fast Linkage Detection Scheme for Multi-Source Information Integration. In: WIRI, Tokyo, pp. 30–39 (2005)
2. Baxter, R., Christen, P., Churches, T.: A Comparison of fast blocking methods for record linkage. In: ACM SIGKDD Workshop on Data Cleaning, Record Linkage and Object Consolidation, Washington DC (2003)
3. Bhattacharya, I., Getoor, L.: Collective Entity Resolution. Journal of Artificial Intelligence Research 30, 621–657 (2007)
4. Christen, P., Goiser, K.: Quality and Complexity Measures for Data Linkage and Deduplication. In: Guillet, F., Hamilton, H.J. (eds.) Studies in Computational Intelligence (SCI), vol. 43, pp. 127–151. Springer, Heidelberg (2007)
5. Christen, P., Gayler, R., Hawking, D.: Similarity-Aware Indexing for Real-Time Entity Resolution. In: ACM CIKM, Hong Kong, pp. 1565–1568 (2009)
6. Christen, P.: A Survey of Indexing Techniques for Scalable Record Linkage and Deduplication. IEEE Transactions on Knowledge and Data Engineering (2012)
7. Christen, P.: Data Matching: Concepts and Techniques for Record Linkage, Entity Resolution and Duplicate Detection. Springer, Canberra (2012)
8. Dey, D., Mookerjee, V., Liu, D.: Efficient Techniques for Online Record linkage. IEEE Transactions on Knowledge and Data Engineering 23(3), 373–387 (2010)
9. Draisbach, U., Naumann, F., Szott, S., Wonneberg, O.: Adaptive Windows for Duplicate Detection. In: International Conference on Data Engineering. IEEE (2012)
10. Elmagarmid, A.K., Ipeirotis, P.G., Verykios, V.S.: Duplicate Record Detection: A Survey. Knowledge and Data Engineering 19(1), 1–16 (2007)
11. Fellegi, I.P., Sunter, A.B.: A Theory for Record Linkage. Journal of the American Statistical Association 64, 1183–1210 (1969)
12. Hernandez, M.A., Stolfo, S.J.: The Merge/Purge Problem for Large Databases. In: ACM SIGMOD, San Jose, pp. 127–138 (1995)
13. Herzog, T.N., Scheuren, F.J., Winkler, W.E.: Data Quality and Record Linkage Techniques. Springer, New York (2007)
14. Ioannou, E., Nejdl, W., Niederee, C., Velegrakis, Y.: On-the-fly entity-aware query processing in the presence of linkage. Proceeding of the VLDB Endowment 3 (2010)
15. McCallum, A., Nigam, K., Ungar, L.H.: Efficient Clustering of High-Dimensional Data Sets with Application to Reference Matching. In: ACM SIGKDD, Boston, pp. 169–178 (2000)
16. North Carolina State Board of Elections, NC voter registration database, ftp://www.app.sboe.state.nc.us/
17. Whang, S.E., Menestrina, D., Koutrika, G., Theobald, M., Garcia-Molina, H.: Entity Resolution with Iterative Blocking. In: Proceedings of the 35th SIGMOD International Conference on Management of Data (2009)
18. Whang, S.E., Garcia-Molina, H.: Entity Resolution with Evolving Rules. Proceeding of the VLDB Endowment 3(1-2), 1326–1337 (2010)
19. Yan, S., Lee, D., Kan, M.Y., Giles, L.C.: Adaptive Sorted Neighborhood Methods for Efficient Record Linkage. In: ACM/IEEE-CS Joint Conference on Digital Libraries, pp. 185–119 (2007)
20. Zipf, G.K.: Human Behavior and the Principle of Least Effort. Addison-Wesley (1949)

Identifying Dominant Economic Sectors and Stock Markets: A Social Network Mining Approach

Ram Babu Roy[1] and Uttam Kumar Sarkar[2,*]

[1] Indian Institute of Technology Kharagpur, Kharagpur, India, 721 302
rbroy@iitkgp.ac.in
[2] Indian Institute of Management Calcutta, Kolkata, India, 700 104
uttam@iimcal.ac.in

Abstract. We propose a method to identify dominant economic sectors and stock markets using a social network approach to mining stock market data. Closing price data from January 1998 through January 2011 of 2698 stocks selected from 17 major stock market indices have been used in the analysis. A Minimum Spanning Tree (MST) has been constructed using the cross-correlations between weekly returns of the stocks. The MST has been chosen to obtain a simplified but connected network having linkages among similarly behaving stocks and it constitutes a social network of stocks for our study. The macroscopic interdependence networks among economic sectors as well as among stock markets have been derived from the microscopic linkages among stocks in the MST. The analysis of these derived macroscopic networks demonstrates that the European and the North American stock markets and Financial, Industrials, Materials, and Consumer Discretionary economic sectors dominate in the global stock markets.

Keywords: Social Network Mining, Minimum Spanning Tree, Centrality, Correlation Coefficient, Global Stock Market, Economic Sectors.

1 Introduction

Stock prices are usually governed by economic fundamentals of the firms and several other factors such as geographical proximity of investors, opinion of market analysts, important news and extreme events (Hatemi-J and Roca 2005; Aydemir and Demirhan 2009; Wang, Wang et al. 2010). The dynamic interdependence and interaction involving a large number of heterogeneous agents make financial market an intriguing example of a complex adaptive system (Mauboussin 2002; Markose 2005). Interdependence between developed and developing countries reduces the benefits of international diversification of portfolio (Dicle, Beyhan et al. 2010). The structure of interdependence among stock markets of various countries emerges due to increasing degree of integration of major stock markets in the world (Bessler and Yang 2003). There is a need to understand the factors driving financial market integration (Büttner and Hayo 2011). Economists and policy makers have started recognizing the

---

J. Li et al. (Eds.): PAKDD 2013 Workshops, LNAI 7867, pp. 59–70, 2013.

limitations of equilibrium-based conventional tools for modeling out-of-equilibrium behavior of financial and economic systems (Buchanan 2009; Farmer and Foley 2009). A network based model of stock markets has gained attention to facilitate insights into the internal structure of interdependence among various stock markets in the world (Eryiğit and Eryiğit 2009). The network model provides a visual representation of the interrelations, in which the nodes represent stocks or stock indices and the edges represent interrelationships among them.

Recently, several studies on the topological properties of stock market networks of various countries have been reported in the literature (Boginski, Butenko et al. 2006; Huang, Zhuang et al. 2009; Caraiani 2012). Stock market networks have been shown to display properties of both the scale-free and 'small world' networks (Tse, Liu et al. 2010). The scale free property of a network facilitates the fastest growth and diffusion of innovations throughout the network (Lin and Li 2010) and hence makes the stock market network vulnerable to shocks. Many real-world networks from quite different domains have exhibited scale-free property. Since, the structure and the evolution of networks are inseparable (Barabási 2009), researchers are investigating why this particular network configuration is prevalent for so many diverse types of networks. Some of the stocks may occupy relatively advantageous positions in a stock market network by virtue of their emergent interdependence among other stocks. These dominant stocks may have connections with stocks in distant geographical locations. They are crucial in integrating the stock markets from across the globe as a connected network. Such inter-market interconnections increase the risk of contagion spreading from one region of a network to the entire network. Therefore, it becomes important to understand the underlying interdependence among economic sectors as well as among stock markets for investment decisions and portfolio management.

The rest of the paper is organized as follows. We have presented some related studies in Section 2. Section 3 describes the data sets used and Section 4 describes the methodology to derive stock market network and identification of dominant economic sectors and stock markets from such a network. Section 5 gives the empirical results and associated discussions and finally, we present some concluding remarks in Section 6.

2   Some Related Studies

Social network analysis and mining techniques have been used to understand the social structure and its influence on the behavior of individual agents in the network (Christakis and Fowler 2008; Rosen, Barnett et al. 2010). The opinion and behavior within a group are observed to be more homogeneous than that of between the groups (Burt 2004). People who are connected across several groups (e.g. international investors in a stock market) may behave differently than those with only local connections. The roles of individuals can be inferred from the pattern of relations that emerge due to the types of role played by the individual in the social network (Wasserman and Faust 1994). Freeman has defined three types of centrality measures, namely degree, betweenness and closeness centrality to understand the potential importance of individual nodes in a network (Freeman 1979). These measures are derived from the relative position of an individual node compared to other nodes in the network. Eigenvector centrality measures the overall influence or dominance of a node in the network based on the entire pattern of connections in the network (Bonacich 1987).

Recent interests in social network research emphasize its potential applications in diverse domains (Bakker, Hare et al. 2010; Scott 2011; Jin, Lin et al. 2012). Social processes are context dependent leading to strong overlap between the relational and physical space. There is an opportunity of research on underdeveloped area of formal integration of social network and spatial network (Adams, Faust et al. 2012). The literature on network based models of stock markets has mainly focused on the behavior of the regional stock markets that is unable to capture the interdependence structure of global stock markets. The importance of a stock is normally represented by financial parameter such as market capitalization. The comovement of stock returns in the emergent social network of stocks is often not taken into account while judging their importance. Therefore, we have incorporated the concepts of social network analysis and mining for analyzing stock market data to understand their interdependence structure and their evolutionary behavior. Our aim is to look for the answers to some of the following questions regarding the way stocks from different parts of the world cluster together. Do the stocks from same economic sector from across the globe tend to cluster together? Do the stocks from same geographical region (irrespective of the economic sectors they belong to) tend to cluster together? How are the economic sectors and stock markets of various countries inter-related? How to identify the dominant economic sectors and stock markets in the global stock market?

Counterintuitive and even intriguing results appear from such study. The stock market networks from different regions show their own characteristic evolutionary patterns (Roy and Sarkar 2010). The social network of stocks and stock indices in the global stock markets were studied for identifying dominant stocks (Roy and Sarkar 2011a) and stock indices (Roy and Sarkar 2011) respectively. Methods developed to detect changes in the stock market network structure (Roy and Sarkar 2012) show that the network of stock market indices shows relatively more decentralized structure in the period following the bankruptcy filing by Lehman Brothers. The insights gained by these works lead to an opportunity to extend them for identifying dominant economic sectors and stock markets. In this paper, we have taken a bottom up approach to investigate the macroscopic behaviors of emergent interdependence among stock markets and economic sectors by analyzing the microscopic comovement of stock returns. One of the twin objectives of this paper is to present a method to derive an emergent interdependence network of economic sectors and stock markets as inferred from the microscopic interdependence network of stocks. The other one is to use this network to identify the dominant economic sectors and stock markets.

3   Data Description

The closing price of 2698 stocks selected from 17 stock indices of the major economies of the world for a period of 13 years from January 1998 through January 2011, obtained from Bloomberg, have been used. The value of missing data for any calendar

Table 1. Number of stocks belonging to various stock indices and economic sectors

Stock Index	Number of Stocks		Stock Index	Number of Stocks	GICS Economic Sector	Number of Stocks
AS52	136		NMX	192	Consumer Discretionary	486
CNX500	303		NZSE50FG	26	Consumer Staples	229
FSSTI	19		SBF250	140	Energy	128
HDAX	38		SET	285	Financials	408
HSI	25		SHCOMP	382	Health Care	146
IBOV	27		SPTSX	147	Industrials	512
KRX100	65		SPX	384	Information Technology	234
MEXBOL	24		TWSE	313	Materials	425
NKY	192				Telecommunication Services	36
					Utilities	94
Total	**829**		**Total**	**1869**	**Grand Total**	**2698**

day is assumed to be the same as the nearest available data for any previous day. The number of stocks belonging to different stock indices and different economic sectors per Global Industry Classification Standard (GICS) is given in Table 1.

4   Methodology

The weekly return $R_i(t)$ of stock i over the period from $(t-7)$ to t is given by

$$R_i(t) = \ln\left(\frac{P_i(t)}{P_i(t-7)}\right) \tag{1}$$

Where $P_i(t)$ is the closing price of the stock i at time t and t represents time in calendar days. The correlation coefficient of the returns of stocks i and j is given by the standard formula (Boginski, Butenko et al. 2006).

$$C_{ij} = \frac{\langle R_i R_j \rangle - \langle R_i \rangle \langle R_j \rangle}{\sqrt{\left(\langle R_i^2 \rangle - \langle R_i \rangle^2\right)\left(\langle R_j^2 \rangle - \langle R_j \rangle^2\right)}} \tag{2}$$

Where $\langle R_i \rangle$ represents the average return of the stock i over a specified time period T consisting of say, N days i.e. $\langle R_i \rangle = \dfrac{1}{N}\sum\limits_{t=1}^{N} R_i(t)$. C_{ij} is dependent on the specified time period T. The geodesic distance d_{ij} between stocks i and j required for constructing the MST is computed from the correlation C_{ij} between the returns of stocks i and j using Equation 3 (Garas and Argyrakis 2007).

$$d_{ij} = \sqrt{2(1 - C_{ij})}, \qquad 0 \le d_{ij} \le 2, \tag{3}$$

Recent work using S&P 100 stocks highlights the role of MST in analyzing industry level clustering in stock market network (Lyócsa, Výrost et al. 2012). We explain briefly the process of MST creation from raw data using a small hypothetical example. Let us assume that we have four stocks S1, S2, S3, and S4. We calculate their weekly returns over a specified time period T and the correlations between the returns. These correlations C_{ij} represent the strength of interdependence among them as shown in Figure 1(a) using dotted lines. Further, we compute the geodesic distance d_{ij} between these stocks to measure the similarity between their behavior. Finally, we use Prim's algorithm (Weiss 1997) to construct the MST (links constructing the MST have been depicted using solid lines) as shown in Figure 1(b). The real and huge stock market data sets, from Bloomberg, have been used to carry out the experiments and to draw conclusions. We have constructed an MST of all the 2698 stocks using the entire thirteen year data. This provides us a simplified connected network of stocks for further analysis, in which the stocks having similar behavior are connected together.

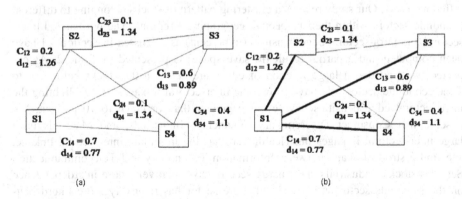

Fig. 1. Illustration of MST creation using cross-correlation between stock returns

4.1   Identification of Dominant Economic Sectors and Stock Markets

The constructed MST connects similarly behaving stocks and serves as an emergent social network of stocks in our study on link analysis. Since the numbers of stocks in different indices and economic sectors are not the same, we derived the networks of economic sectors and stock markets using normalized edge densities in the MST. The normalized intra-sectoral edge density (in percent) is computed as the ratio of the number of edges between the stocks of the particular sector and the maximum number of possible edges between the stocks of that particular sector in the MST. Similarly, the inter-sectoral edge density is the ratio of the number of edges between the stocks of the two different sectors and the maximum number of possible edges between the stocks of those two sectors in the MST. The maximum value for intra-sectoral edges in the MST is n-1 where n is the number of stocks of that particular sector. The maximum value for inter-sectoral edges is min (n_1, n_2) where n_1 and n_2 are the number of stocks belonging to the two sectors. A network of economic sectors using these edge densities as weights has been constructed. Further, the eigenvector centralities of the nodes, representing economic sectors, have been computed to rank the economic sectors in order to identify dominant economic sectors. Similar procedure has been followed to identify dominant stock markets after computing the inter-index and intra-index edge densities.

5   Empirical Findings and Discussions

The work discussed in (Roy and Sarkar 2011a) has been extended to investigate the networks of stock markets and economic sectors derived from the MST of stocks shown in Figure 2. The stocks belonging to different geographical regions have been depicted using different shapes such as triangle for Asian, circle for North American, ellipse of South American, boxes for European, and diamond for Australian stock markets. The stocks belonging to different economic sectors have been shown using different colors. Our study reveals a clustering pattern of stocks belonging to different economic sectors within their respective geographical regions. The normalized inter-sectoral and intra-sectoral edge densities (in percent) as discussed in Section 4.1 have been computed and a partial result (to save space) is presented in Table 2. As expected, we find that a large fraction of edges are between the stocks belonging to same economic sector. We have shown the intersectoral linkages by highlighting the inter-sectoral edge densities having value greater than or equal to 10 percent. We observe that Consumer Discretionary, Financials, Industrials, and Materials have large inter-sectoral linkages but Health Care has the minimum intersectoral linkage. We find a strong linkage between Information Technology and Telecommunication Services stocks. Industrials and Energy sectors have relatively more interdependence on the Materials sector and the Health Care sector has relatively more interdependence with Financials. The network of economic sectors is shown in Figure 3(a). The Figure clearly shows the dominance of Financial, Materials, and Consumer Discretionary sectors in linking the stocks from various other sectors in the network.

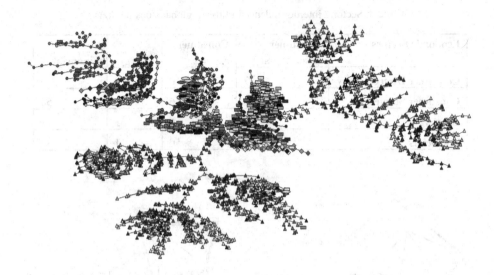

Fig. 2. MST showing dominance of geographical proximity over economic sector

Further, we have investigated whether the stocks providing cross country linkages are from the same or different economic sectors. A partial result of the normalized edge densities (in percent) based on the number of edges linking stocks belonging to various economic sectors as well as providing cross-country linkages are shown in Table 3. The linkages based on the normalized edge density greater than or equal to 10 percent (highlighted using shades in Table 3) between the economic sectors linking the international stock markets only are shown in Figure 3(b). The ranks of economic sectors based on eigenvector centrality computed from the weighted inter-sectoral linkages in the entire MST network as well as inter-index linkages only are presented in Table 4. We find that Financial, Industrials, Materials, and Consumer Discretionary sectors dominate in linking the stocks from various other sectors while Industrial, Financial, Materials and Utilities sectors play major role in linking the cross-country stock markets.

Table 2. Inter-sectoral and intra-sectoral normalized edge density in the MST

Economic Sectors	Consumer Discretionary	Consumer Staples	Energy	Financials
Consumer Discretionary	46	17	4	23
Consumer Staples	17	38	4	20
Energy	4	4	69	9
Financials	23	20	9	83

Table 3. Sectoral interdependence in linking global stock markets

Economic Sectors	Consumer Discretionary	Consumer Staples	Energy	Financials
Consumer Discretionary	37	10	0	18
Consumer Staples	10	16	6	50
Energy	0	6	53	11
Financials	18	50	11	37

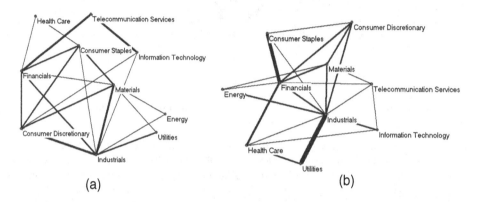

(a)   (b)

Fig. 3. Network of economic sectors (a) entire data set, (b) inter-index linkage

Table 4. Ranks of economic sectors based on inter-sectoral linkages

Rank	Based on the entire MST network		Based on the inter-index linkages	
	Economic Sector	Eigenvector Centrality	Economic Sector	Eigenvector Centrality
1	Financials	0.4785	Industrials	0.4738
2	Industrials	0.4042	Financials	0.4575
3	Materials	0.3795	Materials	0.3105
4	Consumer Discretionary	0.3449	Utilities	0.2921
5	Information Technology	0.2962	Health Care	0.2886
6	Consumer Staples	0.2702	Consumer Staples	0.2747
7	Telecom Services	0.2694	Consumer Discretionary	0.2685
8	Utilities	0.2002	Information Technology	0.2306
9	Energy	0.1957	Telecom Services	0.225
10	Health Care	0.1817	Energy	0.2232

Similarly, a partial result (to save space) of the inter-index and intra-index normalized edge densities (in percent) are presented in Table 5 to highlight the regional interdependence among stock indices. We observe that the intra-index normalized edge densities are very high compared to the inter-index normalized edge densities. We have shown the inter-index linkages by highlighting the densities having value greater than or equal to 1 percent. This demonstrates the fact that stocks have more resemblance to their geographic neighbours as compared to their distant neighbours. The interdependence structure (binary i.e. linking indices with inter-index edge density greater than or equal to 1 percent) of global stock market indices based on the similarity in evolutionary behavior of their component stocks is shown in Figure 4(a).

Table 5. Inter-index and intra-index edge density in the MST

Index	AS52	CNX500	FSSTI	HDAX	HSI	IBOV
AS52	79	1	0	8	8	0
CNX500	1	100	0	0	4	4
FSSTI	0	0	89	0	16	0
HDAX	8	0	0	62	0	0
HSI	8	4	16	0	100	0
IBOV	0	4	0	0	0	96

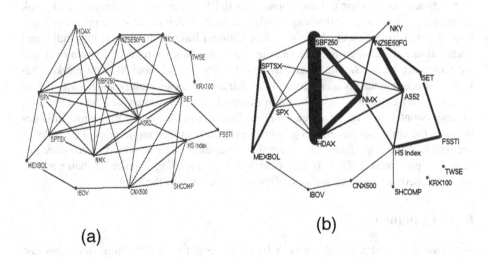

(a)   (b)

Fig. 4. Network of stock market indices (a) binary, (b) weighted

Table 6. Ranks of stock indices based on their global linkages

Rank	Index	Country	Eigenvector Centrality	Rank	Index	Country	Eigenvector Centrality
1	SBF250	France	0.6381	10	MEXBOL	Mexico	0.0423
2	HDAX	Germany	0.5938	11	CNX500	India	0.0353
3	NMX	UK	0.393	12	NKY	Japan	0.0289
4	SPX	USA	0.1523	13	FSSTI	Singapore	0.0208
5	AS52	Australia	0.1517	14	SHCOMP	China	0.0048
6	NZSE50FG	New Zealand	0.1248	15	IBOV	Brazil	0.0043
7	SPTSX	Canada	0.1112	16	TWSE	Taiwan	0.0004
8	HSI	Hong Kong	0.071	17	KRX100	South Korea	0
9	SET	Thailand	0.0465				

Since different indices in our study belong to different countries, the network of indices approximately reveals the interrelationship among stock markets of corresponding countries. Among the three major Asian economies China, Japan and India, we notice that India and Japan are well connected to the regional markets but are weakly connected to the developed stock markets from the western economy. This might give them an advantageous position due to relative immunity from western economy in case of any financial crisis originating in that region. Japan shows stronger links to developed economies than that with the regional developing economies (e.g. Chinese and Indian). This emphasizes the importance of economic trade link dominating the regional influence as reflected in the behavior of stock prices of Japanese stocks. Chinese stocks have very few regional links with Hong Kong, India, and Thailand and no linkage to western countries indicating its relative immunity to the western stock markets. The triad between the US, Canada and Mexico markets reveals a stronger interlinkages between the markets of these countries. The network of indices with weighted edge is shown in Figure 4(b) that captures the relative strength of inter-country ties in the stock market. The network captures the dense linkages between the countries having geographical proximity and economic ties. The ranks of the indices based on eigenvector centrality computed from weighted inter-index linkages are presented in Table 6. European indices are leading in terms of their ranks in the social network of stock indices followed by the SPX of the USA.

6   Conclusions

We have proposed a social network based method to identify dominant economic sectors and dominant stock markets in the emergent social network structure of stocks. Our findings indicate that the Financial, Industrials, Materials, and Consumer Discretionary sectors emerge as dominating economic sectors in influencing the behavior of global stock market. The French, German, and UK stock markets from Europe followed by the US stock market emerge as dominating stock markets in the social network of the global stock markets. The observed tendency of stocks from same economic sectors and having geographical proximity to cluster together into various sub-groups has potential use in classification of stocks for portfolio management. An interesting extension to this work could be capturing causal relationship among economic sectors and stock markets using some suitable method and subsequently applying the Google page rank algorithm as discussed in (Perra and Fortunato 2008) to determine their dominance in the global stock market network. The research can be extended to study the interdependence of economic sectors after filtering out the global and country-level market effects on the correlations. Further, it would be intriguing to explore the evolution of the dominance using more complicated network structure, instead of MST, to capture the relations among the markets and sectors.

Acknowledgments. The authors thank the anonymous reviewers whose comments and suggestions helped in significantly improving the readability of the paper.

References

1. Adams, J., Faust, K., et al.: Capturing context: Integrating spatial and social network analyses. Social Networks 34(1), 1–5 (2012)
2. Aydemir, O., Demirhan, E.: The Relationship between Stock Prices and Exchange Rates: Evidence from Turkey. International Research Journal of Finance and Economics, 207–215 (2009) ISSN 1450-2887(23)
3. Bakker, L., Hare, W., et al.: A social network model of investment behavior in the stock market. Physica A 389, 1223–1229 (2010)
4. Barabási, A.L.: Scale-Free Networks: A Decade and Beyond. Science 325(5939), 412–413 (2009), doi:10.1126/science.1173299
5. Bessler, D.A., Yang, J.: The structure of interdependence in international stock markets. Journal of International Money and Finance 22, 261–287 (2003)
6. Boginski, V., Butenko, S., et al.: Mining market data: A network approach. Computers & Operations Research 33, 3171–3184 (2006)
7. Bonacich, P.: Power and Centrality: A Family of Measures. The American Journal of Sociology 92(5), 1170–1182 (1987)
8. Buchanan, M.: Meltdown Modelling. Nature 460(6), 680–682 (2009)
9. Burt, R.S.: Structural Holes and Good Ideas. American Journal of Sociology 110(2), 349–399 (2004)
10. Büttner, D., Hayo, B.: Determinants of European stock market integration. Economic Systems 35(4), 574–585 (2011)
11. Caraiani, P.: Characterizing emerging European stock markets through complex networks: From local properties to self-similar characteristics. Physica A: Statistical Mechanics and its Applications 391(13), 3629–3637 (2012)
12. Christakis, N., Fowler, J.: The collective dynamics of smoking in a large social network. New England Journal of Medicine 358(21), 2249–2258 (2008)
13. Dicle, M.F., Beyhan, A., et al.: Market Efficiency and International Diversification: Evidence from India. International Review of Economics and Finance 19, 313–339 (2010)
14. Eryiğit, M., Eryiğit, R.: Network structure of cross-correlations among the world market indices. Physica A: Statistical Mechanics and its Applications 388(17), 3551–3562 (2009)
15. Farmer, J.D., Foley, D.: The economy needs agent-based modelling. Nature 460(6), 685–686 (2009)

16. Freeman, L.C.: Centrality in social networks: Conceptual clarification. Social Networks 1(3), 215–239 (1979)
17. Garas, A., Argyrakis, P.: Correlation study of the Athens Stock Exchange. Physics A 380, 399–410 (2007)
18. Hatemi-J, A., Roca, E.: Exchange rates and stock prices interaction during good and bad times: evidence from the ASEAN4 countries. Applied Financial Economics 15(8), 539–546 (2005)
19. Huang, W.-Q., Zhuang, X.-T., et al.: A network analysis of the Chinese stock market. Physica A 388, 2956–2964 (2009)
20. Jin, Y., Lin, C.-Y., et al.: Mining dynamic social networks from public news articles for company value prediction. Social Network Analysis and Mining (2012), doi:10.1007/s13278-011-0045-5
21. Lin, M., Li, N.: Scale-free network provides an optimal pattern for knowledge transfer. Physica A: Statistical Mechanics and its Applications 389(3), 473–480 (2010)
22. Lyócsa, Š., Výrost, T., et al.: Stock market networks: The dynamic conditional correlation approach. Physica A 391(16), 4147–4158 (2012)
23. Markose, S.M.: Computability and Evolutionary Complexity: Markets as Complex Adaptive Systems (CAS). The Economic Journal 115, F159–F192 (2005)
24. Mauboussin, M.J.: Revisiting Market Efficiency: The Stock Market as a Complex Adaptive System. Journal of Applied Corporate Finance 14(4), 8–16 (2002)
25. Perra, N., Fortunato, S.: Spectral centrality measures in complex networks. Physical Review E 78, 036107; arXiv:0805.3322v2 [physics.soc-ph] (2008)
26. Rosen, D., Barnett, G.A., et al.: Social networks and online environments: when science and practice co-evolve. Social Network Analysis and Mining 1(1), 27–42 (2010)
27. Roy, R.B., Sarkar, U.K.: Capturing Early Warning Signal for Financial Crisis from the Dynamics of Stock Market Networks: Evidence from North American and Asian Stock Markets. In: Society for Computational Economics 16th International Conference on Computing in Economics and Finance, London, UK (2010)
28. Roy, R.B., Sarkar, U.K.: Identifying influential stock indices from global stock markets: A social network analysis approach. In: The 2nd International Conference on Ambient Systems, Networks and Technologies (ANT), Ontario, Canada. Procedia Computer Science, vol. 5, pp. 442–449 (2011)
29. Roy, R.B., Sarkar, U.K.: A social network approach to examine the role of influential stocks in shaping interdependence structure in global stock markets. In: International Conference on Advances in Social Network Analysis and Mining (ASONAM), Kaohsiung, Taiwan, pp. 567–569 (2011a), doi:10.1109/ASONAM.2011.87
30. Roy, R.B., Sarkar, U.K.: A social network approach to change detection in the interdependence structure of global stock markets. Social Network Analysis and Mining (2012), doi:10.1007/s13278-012-0063-y
31. Scott, J.: Social network analysis: developments, advances, and prospects. Social Network Analysis and Mining 1(1), 21–26 (2011), doi:10.1007/s13278-010-0012-6
32. Tse, C.K., Liu, J., et al.: A network perspective of the stock market. Journal of Empirical Finance (2010), doi:10.1016/j.jempfin.2010.04.008
33. Wang, M.L., Wang, C.P., et al.: Relationships among Oil Price, Gold Price, Exchange Rate and International Stock Markets. International Research Journal of Finance and Economics, 83–92 (2010) ISSN 1450-2887(47)
34. Wasserman, S., Faust, K.: Social Network Analysis: Methods and Applications, pp. 461–502. Cambridge University Press (1994)
35. Weiss, M.A.: Data Structures and Algorithm Analysis in C, 2nd edn., pp. 330–332 (1997)

Ensemble Learning Model for Petroleum Reservoir Characterization: A Case of Feed-Forward Back-Propagation Neural Networks

Fatai Anifowose[1], Jane Labadin[1], and Abdulazeez Abdulraheem[2]

[1] Faculty of Computer Science and Information Technology, Universiti Malaysia Sarawak
fanifowose@gmail.com, ljane@fit.unimas.edu.my
[2] Department Petroleum Engineering, King Fahd University of Petroleum and Minerals
aazeez@kfupm.edu.sa

Abstract. Conventional machine learning methods are incapable of handling several hypotheses. This is the main strength of the ensemble learning paradigm. The petroleum industry is in great need of this new learning methodology due to the persistent quest for better prediction accuracies of reservoir properties for improved exploration and production activities. This paper proposes an ensemble model of Artificial Neural Networks (ANN) that incorporates various expert opinions on the optimal number of hidden neurons in the prediction of petroleum reservoir properties. The performance of the ensemble model was evaluated using standard decision rules and compared with those of ANN-Ensemble with the conventional Bootstrap Aggregation method and Random Forest. The results showed that the proposed method outperformed the others with the highest correlation coefficient and the least errors. The study also confirmed that ensemble models perform better than the average performance of individual base learners. This study demonstrated the great potential for the application of ensemble learning paradigm in petroleum reservoir characterization.

Keywords: Ensemble, artificial neural networks, hidden neurons, reservoir characterization, porosity, permeability.

1 Introduction

The degree of application of Computational Intelligence (CI) in petroleum engineering over the years is an indication of the relative increase in the level of awareness and interest in the concept [1]. Gradually, researchers in the petroleum industry have moved from the use of empirical correlations and linear regression models to the use of CI [2]. Interestingly, the application of CI in the industry has majorly been limited to Artificial Neural Networks (ANN) [3]. However, ANN has a number of deficiencies [4]. Recently, the interest of CI researchers in hybrids and ensembles of these techniques has increased. Reports have showed that the performance of hybrid CI models is better than that of each of its components [5 - 7] while ensemble models have not been applied in oil and gas reservoir characterization.

J. Li et al. (Eds.): PAKDD 2013 Workshops, LNAI 7867, pp. 71–82, 2013.

The ensemble learning paradigm is an imitation of the human social learning behavior of seeking several opinions before making a decision. With the successful application and superior performance of ensemble models over individual learners in areas outside the petroleum industry [8 - 10], petroleum engineers need to embrace this technology and maximize its utility in the modeling and prediction of petroleum reservoir properties. Ensemble models are especially suitable for the petroleum industry where data are usually scarce and the few available ones are noisy.

Reservoir characterization is an essential process in the petroleum industry in which various properties of petroleum reservoirs are determined. This, in turn, helps in more successful reservoir exploration, production and management. As the quest for increased performance of predictive models in reservoir characterization continues to increase, the ensemble methodology offers a great potential for better and more robust predictive models. Among the various reservoir properties that are of interest to petroleum engineers, this paper focuses on the prediction of porosity and permeability using a novel ANN ensemble model based on diverse expert opinions on the optimal number of hidden neurons. Porosity and permeability were chosen because they are the key indicators of the potential volume and quality of a reservoir. Almost nothing can be done without accurate values of these properties. The choice of ANN as the basis for our proposed ensemble algorithm is due to its popular use by petroleum professionals.

This paper attempts to achieve the following objectives:

- To establish a premise for ensemble learning application in petroleum engineering.
- To implement an ANN ensemble model with different number of hidden neurons.
- To demonstrate the superiority of the ensemble model over existing techniques.
- To further demonstrate the superiority of our proposed ensemble algorithm over those of ANN using the conventional Bootstrap Aggregation (bagging) method and the Random Forest technique.

To achieve these objectives, an overview of the ensemble learning methodology is given in Section 2, a detailed research methodology explaining the experimental set up and implementation strategies is presented in section 3, results are presented and discussed in section 4 while conclusions are drawn in section 5.

2   Literature Review

2.1   Overview of Ensemble Learning Methodology

Ensemble learning is the methodology by which diverse multiple expert hypotheses are strategically incorporated and smartly combined to solve a problem. The idea of combining the opinions of different "experts" to obtain an overall "ensemble" decision is justified by its association with human behavior where the judgment of a committee is believed to be superior to those of individuals, provided the individuals have reasonable competence [11]. The ensemble method was initially introduced for classification and clustering purposes. This is the reason for having a large number of its applications in protein synthesis [8], genes expression [11], bio-informatics [12] and other classification and clustering tasks. It was later extended and applied to time series prediction problems [13]. The ensemble learning paradigm is basically used to improve the performance of a model by utilizing the best instance of expert knowledge while reducing the possibility of an unfortunate emergence of a poor decision.

For regression tasks, the conventional ensemble method is the bagging [14]. This method trains a set of weak learners and combines their outputs using any of the algebraic combination rules. The traditional combination rule is the Mean which is equivalent to the Mode rule in classification problems. The first implementation of the bagging method is found in Random Forest, an ensemble model made up of several instances of Decision Tree models [15]. This technique begins with building a single Decision Tree (DT) model and then creating more instances of this Tree by taking random samples (with replacement) of a portion of the dataset to train each Tree and the remaining portion for testing. This goes on for each Tree until the minimum node count is reached in order to avoid overfitting that comes with larger number of Trees. Thus, the collection of these Tree models makes the Forest. The results of all Trees are combined and the averages of all the performance criteria become the performance indices of the ensemble Forest.

2.2   Review of Applications of Ensemble Learning

Petroleum reservoir characterization has benefited immensely from the application of CI and hybrid CI techniques, most commonly ANN [1, 2, 16]. However, the ensemble learning method is still very new and not yet adequately explored in petroleum engineering. The only work found in the petroleum industry-related literature was [17] that proposed an ensemble model of ANN in the prediction of open-hole triple-combos. This is no more a challenge as the triple combos can now be easily measured with simple coring tools. In view of this, this paper is the first attempt in the application of a novel ensemble method in the prediction of petroleum reservoir properties. The successful application of this new learning methodology in non-petroleum fields is our major motivation for this attempt to apply it in the petroleum industry.

Most of the successful applications of the ensemble learning method are found in classification and clustering tasks. A significantly superior performance of an SVM ensemble model over an individual SVM model in the prediction of financial distress was reported by [10]. Ensembles of SVM to classify IRIS data and to detect the occurrence of road accidents were proposed by [18] and [19] respectively. They both reported that the ensemble models outperformed their respective individual SVM models. In bio-informatics, [20] and later [21] presented an ensemble of SVM and ANN classifiers respectively for the classification of microarray gene data. They also reported that their respective ensemble techniques performed better than using the individual SVM and ANN techniques. [8] proposed an ensemble of SVM classifiers for the prediction of bacterial virulent proteins. They showed that the ensemble model outperformed the individual SVM used with the usual feature extraction method.

Similar positive conclusions were made in [12] and [22] about SVM ensemble models for Glycosylation site prediction and cancer recognition respectively. Though the available literature indicates that the ensemble learning paradigm has been successful in various fields, it has not been harnessed in the prediction of petroleum reservoir properties.

2.3   Overview of Artificial Neural Networks

ANN is a CI technique that is modeled after the biological nervous system. It is made up of several layers of neurons interconnected by links using weights. The ANN architecture is mathematically expressed as:

$$y_i = f\left(\sum_k w_{ik} x_k + \mu_i\right) \tag{1}$$

where x_k are inputs to the input neuron k, w_{ik} are weights attached to the inputs of the neuron k, μ_i is a threshold, offset or bias, $f(\bullet)$ is a transfer function and y_i is the output of a sample of k neurons. The transfer function $f(\bullet)$ can be any of: linear, non-linear, piece-wise linear, sigmoidal, tangent hyperbolic and polynomial functions.

The multi-layer feed-forward back-propagation Neural Network is the most popular and widely used ANN paradigm especially in petroleum engineering research. It comprises one input layer, one output layer and one or more intermediate hidden layers. During the training process, signals, composed of the input data multiplied by the weights and added to a possible bias, pass through the network in the forward direction. Starting from the input layer, they move to the hidden layer (or layers) and then to the output layer where the results are evaluated. This is the "forward" pass. The "back-propagation" pass occurs when, based on the unsatisfactory evaluation of the training performance at the output layer, the signals are sent back to the input layer where the weights are re-adjusted for another forward propagation through the subsequent layers. This cycle continues until either the error goal is achieved or the pre-defined number of training epochs is reached, whichever occurs first.

In the hidden and output layers, each neuron sums up the weighted values (signals) from the previous layer and passes the result through a transfer function, which is also called activation function, to give a scalar output value (the impulse signal) [4]. More technical details of the ANN technique can be found in [4, 23]. A number of applications of ANN can also be found in [1 - 3, 5, 6].

2.4   Justification for the Proposed Ensemble Method

Despite the wide application of ANN in petroleum engineering, it suffers from a number of deficiencies [4] which include:

- Lack of general framework to design the appropriate network for a specific task.
- The number of hidden layers and neurons are determined mostly by trial and error.
- A large number of parameters are usually required to fit a good network structure.

- ANN needs large samples of data to attain a good training performance.
- It easily gets caught up in local optima. Hence, the occurrence of several "optimal" numbers of hidden neurons.

Various studies to address these problems through the development of other algorithms such as the Cascade Correlation and Radial Basis Function neural networks did not improve the overall performance of the ANN technique [24]. The deficiencies of ANN, stated above, are the justifications for seeking a better model in terms of performance for the prediction of porosity and permeability of petroleum reservoirs while still being close to the technique of most interest to petroleum engineers. Since these two properties are key indicators of reservoir quality and are also used for the estimation of other properties, a marginal improvement in their prediction accuracy will lead to the improvement in the accuracy of those other reservoir properties whose values depend on these two that are used in this study.

Another interesting justification for the proposal of this ensemble of ANN technique stems out of the diverse reports of different optimal number of hidden neurons for different applications. The determination of this parameter is very important to ensure that a problem is solved with the right amount of "energy" from the model. Using too little neurons for a complex problem leads to underfitting while using too much neurons for a simple problem leads to overfitting. The challenge has been to strike a balance between the two phenomena [25]. For example, [26] used 10 neurons in a single-layer ANN model while [27] used 8 neurons in a similar ANN model for a time series prediction problem and both were presented to be optimal. An example related to Extreme Learning Machine, an advanced version of ANN, is found in [26] and [28] where 21 and 77 hidden neurons were respectively claimed to be optimal. An ensemble model is most applicable to automatically incorporate all these diverse expert opinions without using trial-and-error methods.

3   Research Methodology

3.1   Description of Data

A total of six core and well log datasets for porosity and permeability were used for the design, implementation, testing and validation of this study. The three datasets for porosity were obtained from a drilling site in the Northern Marion Platform of North America and the three datasets for permeability were obtained from a giant carbonate reservoir in the Middle East. The porosity datasets have five predictor variables viz. Top Interval, Grain Density, Grain Volume, Length and Diameter while the permeability datasets have eight predictor variables viz. Gamma Ray, Porosity, Density, Water Saturation, Deep Resistivity, Microspherically Focused, Neutron and Caliper Logs.

In petroleum reservoir characterization, there are two possible ways to apply machine learning concepts for improved results: using the data of the cored section of a well for training a model to predict the properties of uncored sections, and using the data of the cored sections of a field for training to predict the properties of the uncored sections of other fields. The first is more realistic. In order to have a snapshot idea of a prospective well, some sections of it are usually cored by taking samples from randomly selection depths. Taking core samples from the entire sections of a well is expensive. The complete data of the cored sections would then be used to predict the properties of the uncored section. However, the second requires that the training dataset be representative of the entire field, which is often difficult to achieve. It is also counter-intuitive to train a model with a data from a field to predict the properties of another field with different geological, geophysical and petrophysical composition.

Following the standard machine learning paradigm, the data for each well was divided into training and test subsets using a stratified sampling technique where 70% of the entire data were randomly selected for training, and the remaining 30% for testing. Thus the 70% represents the cored sections of the reservoir while the 30% represents the uncored sections. The choice of this stratification method is based on its popularity for fairness and ensuring high confidence of results [7, 16].

3.2   Model Evaluation Criteria and Ensemble Combination Rules

For effective evaluation and comparison of the performances of the proposed ANN ensemble with respect to those of its base learners, we applied the standard and commonly used criteria viz. correlation coefficient (R-square), root mean-squared error (RMSE), mean absolute error (MAE), and Execution Time (ET). R-square measures the statistical correlation or the degree of closeness between the predicted and actual output values. RMSE is one of the most commonly used error measures of success for numeric prediction. It computes the average of the squared differences between each predicted value and its corresponding actual value. MAE takes the average of all the individual absolute errors between the actual and predicted target values. The mathematical bases for these criteria can be found in literature [3, 4, 7 - 9, 10, 13, 16]. The ET is a measure of the time taken to execute the algorithms from beginning to the end. It is simply the difference of the finish time and the start time.

While using the above measures to evaluate the performance of the individual ANN models, the ensemble models were evolved using the algebraic rules: Max() and Mean() rules for R-square, and Min() and Mean() for the error measures. With these rules, the output of the base learner with the highest R-square, which mostly corresponds to that with the least error, is chosen to be the output of the ensemble model. Hence the performance of the ensemble models were the combined result of all the base learners in terms of the highest R-square and the lowest RMSE/MAE measures. The "combination" rules, except the Mean(), are essentially "selection" rules. The Mode() rule is similar to the Majority Vote rule in classification tasks. All of them are generally called "combination" rules.

A distinction and relationship among our proposed algorithm, bagging method and the Random Forest technique is as follows: our proposed algorithm is a novel ensemble approach that applies to any neuron-based computational intelligence technique as it utilizes the diversity in the result of using different number of neurons to evolve a robust ensemble technique. The bagging method is an ensemble algorithm that is based on the assumption that the mean of a diverse set of outputs is most reasonable to represent an ensemble model. The Random Forest is an implementation of the bagging method in

Decision Trees. The bagging method can be applied on any CI technique. In this study, we applied the bagging method on ANN for effective comparison with our novel algorithm and the conventional implementation in random Forest.

3.3   Design of Expert Opinions and Implementation of the Ensemble Models

Taking into consideration all the divergent "expert opinions" discussed in Section 2.4 and since the optimal number of hidden neurons is best determined from the nature of the problem, we first performed a sample run of a simple 2-layer ANN model with all the parameters set to values that have been reported to work well in previous studies [3, 5, 6] while varying the number hidden neurons between 1 and 50. The choice of this architecture and this range for determining the optimal number of hidden neurons is based on the suggestion of [23] that most problems can be solved with a 2-layer architecture and with no more than 50 neurons in each hidden layer. With each selected number of hidden neurons, a new random division of the dataset into training and testing sets was made. This was done to further increase the diversity of the results. The implemented ANN model consisted of two hidden layers, *sigmoid* activation function at the hidden layers, *purelin* activation function at output layer, *Levenberg-Marquardt* (*trainlm*) training algorithm, and random initialization for weights.

It would be noted that the aim of this procedure is not to find the optimal number of hidden neurons. Rather, we are using it as a premise to show that the choice of the number of hidden neurons is problem/data dependent, hence calling for an ensemble solution. We established in this sample run that even choosing the best number of hidden neurons for an instance of a problem does not work well for another instance of the same problem. The result for another problem would be worse. This is a major requirement for an ensemble solution. Results for one porosity and one permeability dataset are shown in Figure 1 and 2. It was observed that several points in each plot could qualify for the optimal number of neurons using the criterion of the highest points with the closest distance between the training and testing lines. This procedure achieved two objectives: (1) it established the diversity in the opinions on the optimal number of neurons, which is the basic requirement for an ensemble model [29]; (2) it used the above as the basis for the implementation of our proposed ensemble model.

The traditional way of handling this problem is to make several runs of ANN with different number of neurons, later compare them and choose the one that gave the best performance. This approach has two problems: (1) it is time wasting; (2) there is no guarantee that the best result obtained is a global optima [4]. Another option is to use evolutionary approaches such as Genetic Algorithm to obtain the optimized number of neurons. There are three problems with this as well: (1) it is time wasting as these algorithms use exhaustive search techniques; (2) it is memory-intensive; (3) sometimes, it does not give optimal results [30, 31]. The best solution lies in the ensemble learning method that creates several instances of ANN with different locally optimal number of neurons, combines the results of all instances and ensures that the best instance is used to solve the problem. Using the established diversity as the basis of our proposed ensemble algorithm, we implemented the model using the following procedure:

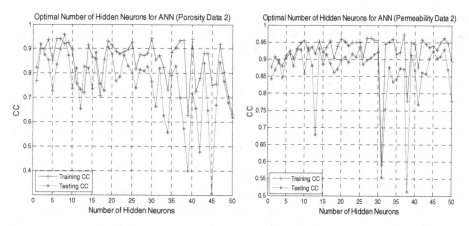

Fig. 1. Diversity Indicated by Different Number of Neurons (Porosity Data)

Fig. 2. Diversity Indicated by Different Number of Neurons (Permeability Data)

```
Start with the other stated parameters
Do for k = 1 to 6 //there are 6 datasets
   Do for n = 1 to 10 //there are 10 instances of ANN
      Randomly divide data into training and testing
      Do for m = 1 to 50 //try different number of neurons
         Use the training data to train the base learner, Sₙ
         Use the testing data to predict the target
         Update result of each run, m
      Continue
      Select the best of the m values
   Continue
   Keep the result of the above as Hypothesis, Hₙ
Continue
Compute the best performance of all hypotheses, H_final (x) =
argₙᵐᵃˣ μⱼ(x)
```

By using the decision rules as follows:

a. Mean rule: $\mu_j(x) = \frac{1}{n} \sum \sum_1^n H_n(x)$

b. Maximum rule: $\mu_j(x) = {}_{i=1,\ldots n}^{max} H_n(x)$

c. Minimum rule: $\mu_j(x) = {}_{i=1,\ldots n}^{min} H_n(x)$

Next, we implemented another ANN ensemble model using the conventional bagging method [14]. Finally, for effective comparison of our proposed algorithm with an existing ensemble-based technique, we also applied the Random Forest [15]. The Random Forest model contained 500 tree instances.

4   Results and Discussion

After the 10 instances of the ANN model making up the proposed ensemble-based technique were applied on the 6 datasets, the results of the comparison of our proposed model with the ANN conventional ensemble and the Random Forest technique are shown in Figure 3 - 5 and Table 1.

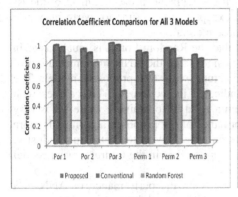

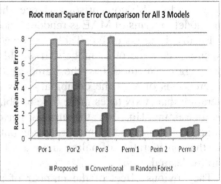

Fig. 3. Correlation Coefficient Comparison of all Ensemble Models on all Datasets

Fig. 4. Root Mean Square Error Comparison of all Ensemble Models on all Datasets

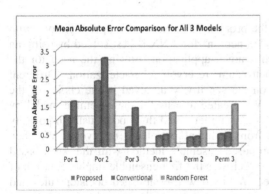

Fig. 5. Mean Absolute Error Comparison of all Ensemble Models on all Datasets

Table 1. Execution Time Comparison on all datasets

	Execution Time (s)	
Dataset	Proposed/ Conventional	Random Forest
Por 1	118.60	0.59
Por 2	113.04	0.43
Por 3	34.26	0.29
Perm 1	165.13	0.62
Perm 2	198.19	0.78
Perm 3	200.66	0.68

Figure 3 clearly showed that our proposed ensemble model outperformed the ANN-based conventional bagging method and Random Forest technique with the highest R-square. Random Forest showed the least performance. The R-square comparison also showed that the ANN-based bagging method performed better than Random Forest. This, in turn, indicates the better performance of the ANN model over the Decision Tree model which makes up the Random Forest technique.

In terms of RMSE, Figure 4 also showed clearly the superiority of our proposed algorithm having the least error. Random Forest also showed the least performance. The ANN-based bagging method performed better than Random Forest. With the mean absolute error (Figure 5), our proposed algorithm emerged as the best performing in four out of the six cases of the datasets used. In the other two cases, our model performed better than the ANN-based bagging method but less than the Random Forest technique. However, with the inconsistency shown in the MAE comparison result, we gave more weight to the agreement in the judgment of the R-square and RMSE comparisons. Hence, the exception to the superior performance of our model in terms of MAE is rendered inconsequential.

Finally, in terms of ET, Table 1 showed that the Random Forest is much faster in execution than the other models. It would be noted that the ANN implementation of the bagging method has the same architecture with the proposed model. The difference is only in the combination as indicated in section 3.3. This agrees with literature that ANN takes more time to obtain a good fit for training while DT is very fast in training. However, the superior performance of our proposed algorithm is more attractive and desired than a faster computation especially in the petroleum industry. For the consideration of online and real-time applications in the future, a faster model will be desired.

The obvious effect of the number of neurons on the performance of ANN is a confirmation of the diversity of this parameter and the need for an ensemble solution for optimal performance. This is also a proof that our proposed ensemble model met the major requirement of the ensemble learning paradigm.

5   Conclusion

In this paper, we have showed that the problem of diversity in expert opinions with respect to the optimal number of hidden neurons for ANN is best solved by using an ensemble model. We have presented a novel application showing the need for the ensemble learning paradigm in petroleum reservoir characterization. Different opinions of experts were presented on the sensitivity involved in the choice of the number of hidden neurons of ANN. We created a basis for the ensemble model by determining the diverse optimal values and implemented the models using 6 porosity and permeability datasets obtained from different petroleum reservoirs. We then compared the performance of our proposed ensemble method with the ANN-based bagging method and Random Forest, which was the first ensemble implementation of the bagging method in Decision Tree. We used well-established decision rules and standard evaluation criteria to evaluate the performance of the ensemble models.

The conclusions reached on the results of this study are presented as follows:

- Our proposed ensemble model outperformed the other models.
- The ANN-based bagging method performed better than the Random Forest model.
- The results are in perfect agreement with literature on the superiority of ensemble models over their individual base learners.
- Our study shows a great potential for more successful applications of the ensemble method in petroleum engineering.

- The petroleum industry will gain immensely from this novel application since a marginal improvement in the prediction of reservoir properties will lead to a huge increase in the efficiency of exploration and production of energy.

With the success of this study, more ensemble models of ANN using different activation functions and learning algorithms are proposed in our future studies.

Acknowledgements. The authors would like to thank the Universiti Malaysia Sarawak and King Fahd University of Petroleum and Minerals for providing the resources used in the conduct of this study.

References

1. Anifowose, F., Abdulraheem, A.: Artificial Intelligence Application in Reservoir Characterization and Modeling: Whitening the Black Box. In: SPE 2011 Young Professional Technical Symposium, Dhahran, Saudi Arabia (2011)
2. Ali, J.K.: Neural Networks: A New Tool for the Petroleum Industry? In: SPE European Petroleum Computer Conference, Aberdeen, pp. 217–231 (1994)
3. Jong-Se, L.: Reservoir Properties Determination using Fuzzy Logic and Neural Networks from Well Data in Offshore Korea. J. of Petroleum Sci. & Eng. 49, 182–192 (2005)
4. Petrus, J.B., Thuijsman, F., Weijters, A.J.: Artificial Neural Networks: An Introduction to ANN Theory and Practice. Springer, Heidelberg (1995)
5. Abe, S.: Fuzzy LP-SVMs for Multiclass Problems. In: European Symposium on Artificial Neural Networks, Belgium, pp. 429–434 (2004)
6. Mohsen, S., Morteza, A., Ali, Y.V.: Design of Neural Networks using Genetic Algorithm for the Permeability Estimation of the Reservoir. J. of Petroleum Sci. & Eng. 59, 97–105 (2007)
7. Anifowose, F., Labadin, J., Abdulraheem, A.: A Hybrid of Functional Networks and Support Vector Machine Models for the Prediction of Petroleum Reservoir Properties. In: 11th International Conference on Hybrid Intelligent Systems, Melaka, Malaysia, pp. 85–90. IEEExplore, New York (2011)
8. Nanni, L., Lumini, A.: An Ensemble of Support Vector Machines for Predicting Virulent Proteins. Expert Systems with Applications 36, 7458–7462 (2009)
9. Zaier, I., Shu, C., Ouarda, T.B.M.J., Seidou, O., Chebana, F.: Estimation of Ice Thickness on Lakes using Artificial Neural Network Ensembles. J. of Hydrology 383, 330–340 (2010)
10. Sun, J., Li, H.: Financial Distress Prediction Using Support Vector Machines: Ensemble vs. Individual. Applied Soft Computing 12(8), 2254–2265 (2012)
11. Re, M., Valentini, G.: Simple Ensemble Methods are Competitive with State-of-the-Art Data Integration Methods for Gene Function Prediction. J. of Machine Learn. Res. 8, 98–111 (2010)
12. Caragea, C., Sinapov, J., Silvescu, A., Dobbs, D., Honavar, V.: Glycosylation Site Prediction using Ensembles of Support Vector Machine Classifiers. BMC Bioinformatics 8(2), 438 (2007)
13. Landassuri-Moreno, V., Bullinaria, J.A.: Neural Network Ensembles For Time Series Forecasting. In: Genetic and Evolutionary Computation Conference (GECCO), Montréal Québec, Canada (2009)
14. Breiman, L.: Bagging Predictors. Machine Learning 24(2), 123–140 (1996)

15. Breiman, L.: Random Forests. Machine Learning 45(1), 5–32 (2001)
16. Anifowose, F., Abdulraheem, A.: Fuzzy Logic-Driven and SVM-Driven Hybrid Computational Intelligence Models Applied to Oil and Gas Reservoir Characterization. J. Nat. Gas Sci. & Eng. 3, 505–517 (2011)
17. Chen, D., Quirein, J., Hamid, H., Smith, H., Grable, J.: Neural Network Ensemble Selection using Multiobjective Genetic Algorithm in Processing Pulsed Neutron Data. In: SPWLA 45th Annual Logging Symposium, June 6-9 (2004)
18. Kim, H., Pang, S., Je, H., Kim, D., Bang, S.Y.: Constructing Support Vector Machine Ensemble. Pattern Recognition 36, 2757–2767 (2003)
19. Chen, S., Wang, W., Zuylen, H.: Construct Support Vector Machine Ensemble to Detect Traffic Incident. Expert Systems with Applications 36, 10976–10986 (2009)
20. Peng, Y.: A Novel Ensemble Machine Learning for Robust Microarray Data Classification. Computers in Biology and Medicine 36, 553–573 (2006)
21. Chen, Y., Zhao, Y.: A Novel Ensemble of Classifiers for Microarray Data Classification. Applied Soft Computing 8, 1664–1669 (2008)
22. Valentini, G., Muselli, M., Ruffino, F.: Cancer Recognition with Bagged Ensembles of Support Vector Machines. Neurocomputing 56, 461–466 (2004)
23. Demuth, H., Beale, M., Hagan, M.: Neural Network Toolbox™ 6 User's Guide. The MathWorks Inc., New York (2009)
24. Bruen, M., Yang, J.: Functional Networks in Real-Time Flood Forecasting: A Novel Application. Advances in Water Resources 28, 899–909 (2005)
25. Aalst, W.M.P., Rubin, V., Verbeek, H.M.W., Dongen, B.F., Kindler, E., Günther, C.W.: Process Mining: A Two-Step Approach to Balance Between Underfitting and Overfitting. Software System Modeling 9, 87–111 (2010)
26. Fei, H., De-Shuang, H.: Improved Extreme Learning Machine for Function Approximation by Encoding a Priori Information. Neurocomputing 69, 2369–2373 (2006)
27. Fei, H., Qing-Hua, L., De-Shuang, H.: Modified Constrained Learning Algorithms Incorporating Additional Functional Constraints into Neural Networks. Information Science 178(3), 907–919 (2008)
28. Singh, R., Balasundaram, S.: Application of Extreme Learning Machine Method for Time Series Analysis. Int. J. Intell. Sys. & Tech. 2(4), 256–262 (2007)
29. Polikar, R.: Ensemble Based Systems in Decision Making. IEEE Circuits & Sys. Mag. 3, 21–45 (2006)
30. Hassan, R., Cohanim, B., Weck, O.: A Comparison of Particle Swarm Optimization and the Genetic Algorithm. J. American Institute of Aeronautics and Astronautics, 1–13 (2004)
31. Maertens, K., Baerdemaeker, J.D., Babuska, R.: Genetic Polynomial Regression as Input Selection Algorithm for Non-Linear Identification. J. Soft Comp. 10, 785–795 (2006)

Visual Data Mining Methods
for Kernel Smoothed Estimates
of Cox Processes

David Rohde[1], Ruth Huang[2], Jonathan Corcoran[2], and Gentry White[2]

[1] Instituto de Matemática, Universidade Federal do Rio de Janeiro,
Rio de Janeiro, Brazil
[2] School of Geography, Planning and Environmental Management,
University of Queensland, Brisbane Australia

Abstract. Real world planning of complex logistical organisations such
as the fire service is a complex task requiring synthesis of many different
computational techniques, from artificial intelligence and statistical or
machine learning to geographical information systems and visualization.
A particularly promising approach is to apply established data mining
techniques in order to produce a model and make forecasts. The nature of
the forecast can then be rendered using visualization techniques in order
to assess operational decisions, simultaneously benefiting from generic
and powerful data mining techniques, and using visualization to understand these results in the context of the actual problem of interest which
may be very specific. Previous approaches to visualization in similar contexts use iso surfaces to visualize densities, these methods ignore recent
improvements in interactive 3D visualization such as volume rendering
and cut-planes, these methods also ignore what is often a key problem
of interest comparing two different stochastic processes, finally previous
methods have not paid sufficient attention to differences between estimation of densities and point processes (or Cox processes). This paper
seeks to address all of these shortcomings and make recommendations for
the trade-offs between visualization techniques for operational decision
making. Finally we also demonstrate the ability to include interactive
3D plots within a paper by rendering an iso surface using 3D portable
document format (PDF).

1 Introduction

Real world planning of logisticly complex organisations such as the fire service is
a complex task that requires a synthesis of skills including intelligent data analysis techniques, geographical information systems and visualization. A promising
way to harness the growing literature on sophisticated, but general data mining
techniques with highly specific operational concerns is to use visual data mining
techniques in order to communicate the important trends the data mining algorithms have identified [13] these methods have proved powerful for the analysis
of spatial [9] and spatial-temporal data [2].

J. Li et al. (Eds.): PAKDD 2013 Workshops, LNAI 7867, pp. 83–94, 2013.

An important class of problems for managing operational concerns is the Cox process or point process which is a model of events. Event modelling is of importance for many applications, the one pertinent to this study is modelling the occurrence in space and time of malicious hoax call fire events. An important contribution in combining data mining with visualization in this area was [4] which proposed a kernel smoothing method for estimating spatial diurnal (i.e. hour of day) aspects of a dataset and visualizing the model using 3D rendering of iso surfaces. While this work proposed a new kernel and demonstrated the utility of 3D visualization it had some shortcomings in that it left a number of important aspects of the model implicit including the distinction between Cox process estimation and density estimation and properties of smoothing in space time. In addition to this technology in 3D rendering has improved significantly in recent times. It is the goal of this paper to investigate the properties of kernel smoothing algorithms for Cox processes, and the relative merits of different visualization approaches, using the python [7] bindings for the Mayavi [11] visualization library and also demonstrating the capabilities of 3D PDF in latest PDF readers[1]. We also expand on previous work by considering visual methods for comparing estimated stochastic processes.

In Section 2 we discuss kernel smoothing techniques for spatial-diurnal estimation of Cox processes. The method described is essentially that developed in [4], but we do make make explicit some aspects of the model including noting some of the important differences between estimating a Cox process and a density and illustrating lines of equal distance in space-time. In Section 3 implementation details are given for the statistical kernel smoothing and visualization methods using Mayavi and 3D portable document format (pdf). In Section 4 the spatial-diurnal Cox process is estimated for a dataset of hoax call fire events occurring in Australia. Visualization is carried out using three methods for rendering a scalar field, iso surfaces, volume rendering and cut planes. The ability of these algorithms to compare differences between stochastic processes is also evaluated. In Section 5 a discussion of the main findings are presented. Section 6 concludes.

2   Non-parametric estimation of Spatial-Diurnal Cox Processes

2.1   Kernel Smoothing for Density Estimation and Estimating Cox Processes

Kernel smoothing is a popular method originating and most popular when applied to density estimation [12] but which has also been demonstrated for the estimation of Cox processes [6].

When applied to density estimation a kernel smoothing algorithm applied to N data points is

---

[1] e.g. Adobe Acrobat reader 8 or later.

$$P(X_{N+1}|X_1, ..., X_N) \approx \frac{1}{N} \sum_{n=1}^{N} \mathcal{K}(X_{N+1}, X_n, \sigma^2)$$

The kernel function $\mathcal{K}()$ measures the distance between X_{N+1} and all previous points i.e. is high for low values and decays to zero. Smoothing is achieved such that points close to observed points are more probable. In general the kernel can be viewed as computing distances between pairs of points or alternatively as placing a probability distribution on top of every previously observed point.

A Cox process or a Point process [5] has some important similarities and differences with a standard density. A Cox process is a stochastic process, the practical significance is that under a stochastic process you must specify the space of interest, in our application this is metropolitan Australia in a given region of time (and different regions will be of interest when estimating and forecasting the Cox process). Once the region of interest is specified an integral must be computed under the region of interest under an intensity function, once this integral is computed Poisson distributions on quantities of interest can be specified. The fact that two integrals need to be computed to determine probabilities one under the intensity function and one under the density produced means that this model is referred to as 'doubly stochastic'.

A Cox process models the count of incidents q within a region of time and space R as a Poisson distribution with the expectation of the Poisson model specified as an integral under the intensity function $\lambda(s)$ where s specifies a point in 2D space and diurnal time.

$$q \sim \text{Poisson} \left(\int_R \lambda(r) dr \right)$$

If two or more disjoint regions are specified then the Poisson distributions for the respective regions must be independent.

Like a density the intensity function of a Cox process is non-negative, although it need not integrate to one. An important contribution of [6] is that standard density estimation algorithms can be applied in order to estimate Cox process intensity functions. Although the density approach has been shown to be effective there are a number of alternatives such as Bayesian mixture models [10], Bayesian Gaussian Cox Processes [1] which employ other models and sophisticated computational techniques such as Markov chain Monte Carlo.

2.2   Kernel Smoothing in Euclidean Space

First we consider kernel smoothing using standard Euclidean space and ignoring the diurnal component. Distance in space follows from simple geometry where the distance between $\mathbf{x}_1 = (x_1, y_1)$ and $\mathbf{x}_2 = (x_2, y_2)$ is given by:

$$d(\mathbf{x}_1, \mathbf{x}_2) = \sqrt{(x_1 - x_2)^2 + (y_1 - y_2)^2}.$$

A line of constant distance is given by a circle. A kernel smoothing algorithm is obtained by specifying a bandwidth σ and computing

$$f(x_1, y_1; x_2, y_2)$$
$$= e^{-\frac{1}{2\sigma}^2 d(x_1, y_1; x_2, y_2)^2}$$
$$= \mathcal{N}(x_1 - x_2; 0, \sigma^2) \mathcal{N}(y_1 - y_2; 0, \sigma^2)$$

where $\mathcal{N}()$ is the normal distribution, this results in the standard kernel smoothing algorithm using spherical Gaussian kernels.

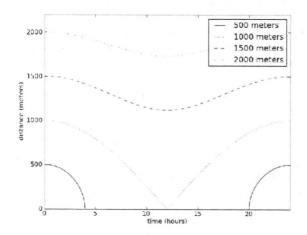

Fig. 1. Plots of equal distance using the proposed space time distance function. Note that 500 meters away is equivalent to 4 hours away. The maximum possible distance in time (12 hours) is 1000m.

2.3   Kernel Smoothing in Euclidean Diurnal Space

We now imagine that an additional diurnal variable is available and as such we have $x_1 = (x_1, y_1, t_1)$ and $x_2 = (x_2, y_2, t_2)$. Where time is a time given in hours, it is a real value although we will only model the periodic hourly component. In order to extend the model to include periodic time we define a periodic function which maps a diurnal hour of day variable to be between zero and one:

$$\Delta(t_1, t_2) = 1/2 - \frac{1}{2} \cos(2\pi/24(t_1 - t_2)).$$

This function returns 1 if $t_1 - t_2$ is an even multiple of 12 hours (the maximum possible) and zero if $t_1 - t_2$ is an even multiple of 24 hours. This represents a distance in time in order to be able to smooth in time space in order to achieve this we introduce the constant c which gives an equivalent distance in meters equivalent to a distance in time of 12 hours. We will see shortly that if we adopt

the following distance kernel that we will obtain the kernel smoothing algorithm
applying the Von-Mises kernel in the time dimension

$$d(x_1, y_1, t_1; x_2, y_2, t_2) = \sqrt{(x_1 - x_2)^2 + (y_1 - y_2)^2 + c^2 \Delta(t_1, t_2)}.$$

We can explain the presence of squares for the Euclidean distance, but the
absence of squares for the periodic component by the fact that we need a nonnegative distance and the proposed periodic distance function is already nonnegative.

Intuition about this function can be gained by plotting lines of constant distance in space-time i.e. taking one spatial dimension and one dimension in time.
This is demonstrated in Figure 1 with $c = 1000m$. From this plot we can see
that a zero distance in space and a distance of 4 hours in time is equivalent
to a distance of 500 meters in space and 0 hours in time. Similarly as a direct
consequence of setting $c = 1000m$ a distance of 0 meters in space and 12 hours in
time is equivalent to a distance of 1000m in space and 0 hours in time. It is also
illustrative to consider distances larger than 1000m for which it is impossible to
achieve such a large distance without some contribution in space as the largest
distance time can contribute is 1000m. Another point to note about this kernel
is that it is periodic and therefore points that are near 0 hours are correctly
smoothed to points near 23.9 hours. In real smoothing situations assuming data
is plentiful a bandwidth σ may be set to a relatively small value, this means that
the tail behavior i.e. the behavior at large distances might correspond to many
multiples of σ and therefore have negligible effect on the smoothing. Therefore
the behavior at large distances while interesting is of relatively little importance
and the most important contribution of this distance function is its periodic
nature.

Kernel smoothing can be developed by analogous to Euclidean space considering the exponential of the negative square of the distance function.

$$f(x_1, y_1, t_1; x_2, y_2, t_2)$$
$$\propto e^{-\frac{1}{2\sigma^2} d(x_1, y_1, t_1; x_2, y_2, t_2)^2}$$
$$\propto N(x_1 - x_2; 0, \sigma^2) N(y_1 - y_2; 0, \sigma^2) \mathcal{V}(2\pi(t_1 - t_2)/24; 0, c^2/(2\sigma^2))$$

where $\mathcal{V}()$ is the Von Mises distribution (see [8] for details) which has a period
of 2π and is defined

$$\mathcal{V}(\theta; \vartheta, \gamma) \propto e^{\gamma \cos(\theta - \vartheta)}.$$

The normalization constant is available in analytical form if you employ a special
function (the Bessel function) although this is not important for our purposes.

This kernel was applied to a Cox process in [4] with 3D iso surfaces, but
the discussion neglected to identify the role of the c parameter, the distinction
between density estimation and Cox processes and did not consider more modern
visualization techniques nor differences between different intensity functions.

3   Implementation

Both the statistical model and the visualization were implemented in a Python environment [7] using [11] for visualization. Kernel density estimation was achieved by adding the Von Mises kernel to existing scientific python (scipy) libraries to produce a three dimensional kernel surface. We set a distance of 12 hours to be equivalent to a distance of 100km, the bandwidth was set to 10km. An intensity function was estimated for the data combined and for weekends and weekdays separately.

Mayavi approximates a 3D scalar field by the use of a three dimensional array with samples taken at intervals, this structure was created by evaluating the kernel estimate over the grid. Modifications of existing Mayavi examples means it is relatively easy to render the density with iso surfaces, volume rendering and cut planes. Both the densities and their differences were rendered. A coastline of Australia was added in order to improve the visualization.

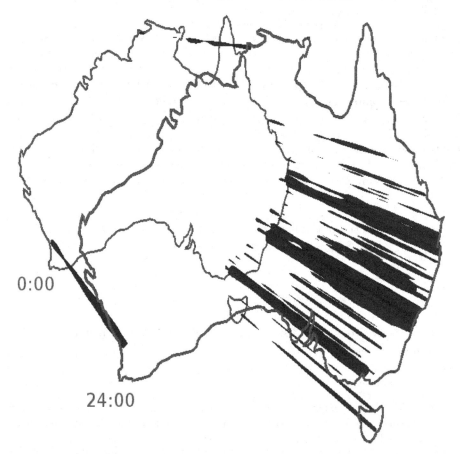

Fig. 2. Iso surface for all fire events, the contour represents the highest 90% . Please click in order to rotate (requires Acrobat Reader 8 or greater).

The rendering of the iso surfaces for all the data was also converted to 3D PDF format. This involved saving the data in wavefront (obj) format from Mayavi and then converting to universal 3D (u3d) format finally for importing into latex with the movie15 package. Judging from comments by other researchers the software for producing these files is improving, although it remains non-trivial. The result is shown in Fig 2 and requires a recent PDF viewer.

4   Visualization of Estimates

An iso surface estimate of the intensity function identifying the highest 90% of the intensity function is demonstrated in an interactive figure in Figure 2. There are some obvious advantages in presenting the visualization to the reader in such a way with potential draw backs being that Mayavi remains a better visualization environment and there remain technological issues in both the creation and viewing of such figures. File size requirements being one such limitation which restricts the inclusion of any more 3D figures in this document.

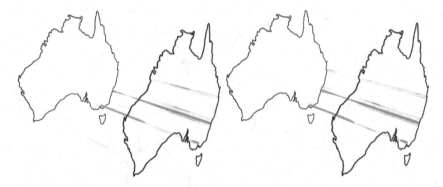

Fig. 3. Iso surface showing the contours covering 67% and 50% of the intensity function for weekends (top) and weekdays (bottom)

The fire incidence datasets were implemented to visualize the incident regions in time and space with 67% and 50 % of probability contour. The kernel smoothing technique is applied to estimate the weekend and weekday fire incidence datasets from malicious hoax calls and accompanied by the 3D visualizing iso surface (Figure 3) using the Mayavi library. This method allows visualizing and identifying the intensity of the fire risk at certain locations and times. For example in Figure 3 (top) in Brisbane, there are more fire incidents happening approximately during 12:00 to 18:00 of the day which shows the higher intensity on the weekday than the weekend (see Figure 4 for location of cities). It is also confirmed by Figure 5 that between 12:00 to 18:00 time period in Brisbane, it shows yellow colour which refers to the higher fire incidents during the weekday than the weekend. By using two different colours to refer to the higher

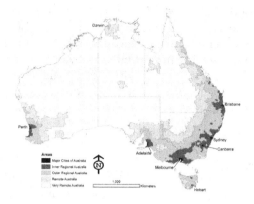

Fig. 4. Map of Australia

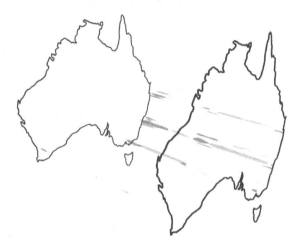

Fig. 5. The difference between weekends and weekdays i.e. Fig 3 (top) and (bottom). The pink colour area is represented for the probability density of the fire incidence during the weekend occurred more than during the weekday, yellow represents the incidence during the weekday occurred more than the weekend.

fire incidents during the weekend or weekday, it can be easily visualized and given the information including the time of the day, the location and intensities of the incident. It also can represent the comparison of these two datasets (weekends and weekdays) by subtracting the kernel (Figure 5) as well as the volume rendering (Figure 6). The volume rending is generated by using the kernel smoothing identifies the difference of spatial-time between two datasets with the same colour.

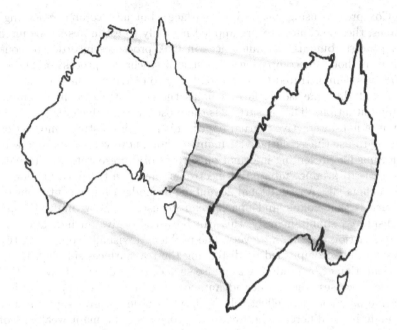

Fig. 6. Volume rendering showing the difference between (a) and (b) with the kernel smoothing using the Normal-Normal-von Mises kernel. Rendering used the Mayavi library.

5   Discussion

Kernel smoothing is a simple, but very powerful data mining technique for non-parametric analysis of large datasets. Kernel smoothing refers to two similar techniques, the first and most common is density estimation, the second is estimation of a Cox process, which is a significantly more complex 'doubly stochastic' model. Methodologically these can be considered identical, but the treatment of time in particular in a Cox process is more subtle. In a density estimation scenario a kernel smoothed surface can be seen as a summary of history that can be used to forecast the future. A spatial temporal Cox process is a stochastic process indexed by both space and more importantly time, as the stochastic process is indexed by time, it is not in general meaningful to use a smoothed history to forecast future events. A way around this problem is to use only the hour of day or diurnal component of time as in [4], this simplifies the problem such that under reasonable assumptions a smoothed history in space and periodic time can be used for making forecasts using the insight in [6] that kernel density estimation techniques can also be applied to Cox processes. The visualization of the intensity surfaces using iso surfaces was also demonstrated in [4].

In this work we have made use of the space circular-time kernel in [4] and made explicit some of the issues of applying kernel smoothing to Cox processes estimation rather than to density estimation. We also considered visualization of the Cox process using not only iso surfaces, but also volume rendering and cut planes, these techniques were applied not only to estimates of the intensity of Cox process, but also to differences in Cox processes in order to consider graphical methods for comparing estimates of stochastic processes. The use of 3D PDF was demonstrated to be a useful way to distribute these results.

We found that the iso surface remains the tool of choice in a number of important situations. The iso surface is the most interpretable of the graphics to display in a non-interactive journal paper, this provides a strong motivation for continuing to use the iso surface for many authors, however there are now many other forums for presenting information such as oral presentations alternatively it is possible to produce interactive electronic papers in the portable document format such as [3] . An additional advantage of modern implementations of the iso surface is that colour and opacity can be used to allow multiple surfaces to be displayed simultaneously, this can be used to give an indication of the intensity function at different levels. The problem of visually comparing two iso surfaces can be accomplished by displaying the two surfaces side by side at the same orientation or by rendering as an iso surface the difference between the two stochastic processes. Yet another advantage of the iso surface is apparent for this application as colour can effectively be used in order to give sign information when rendering a difference between cox processes. The main weakness of iso surfaces is that information is only available at a fixed number and perhaps a single threshold of the intensity surface, this means that some details of the intensity surface are necessarily absent from the display. Volume rendering and cut planes suffer less from this particular problem.

Volume rendering also showed promise for a range of scientific visualization. It is arguably more difficult to interpret a static display of a intensity surface, but some information is still apparent from displaying a static volume rendering image, particularly if colour is available. While there are no arbitrary thresholding in volume rendering, the colour scheme itself is arbitrary and the image can be difficult to interpret in a precise way. The appeal of volume rendering seems to be in an interactive display to get an overall intuition about the nature of the intensity function of the Cox process. Volume rendering offers the advantages over iso surfaces of being more intuitive and requiring no arbitrary thresholds, but should primarily be used in interactive settings and in preliminary parts of the study where precision on the intensity function is not critical. Volume rendering can also be used for comparison of stochastic processes again by side by side display or by considering differences between intensity functions. While colour could in principle be used to represent a signed difference between intensities, our experience was that this was not very intuitive and we recommend that volume rendering only be used for unsigned differences.

Cut planes are primarily an interactive way to visually explore a Cox process, static realizations of a cut plane are neither interpretable or very attractive. The advantage of a cut plane is that like volume rendering and unlike the iso surface there are no arbitrary thresholds although again like volume rendering an arbitrary colour mapping is required, but this mapping is made much more explicitly as a color bar is available and transparency does not confuse the colour at any given location. The cut plane is the most difficult to use in an interactive environment and some orientations of the cut plane do not seem very interpretable in this application i.e. if the plane sweeps through time-space the meaning of the plane is not necessarily very clear.

6   Conclusion

Visualization of intensity of spatial-diurnal Cox processes estimated with kernel smoothing is a technique which combines powerful data mining approaches with sophisticated 3D visualization in order to assist real world decision makers. Previous work demonstrated the effectiveness of this technique with application to rendering spatial-diurnal Cox processes. Here we considered the same kernel, articulated some of its underlying assumptions in terms of identifying lines of constant distance in space-time and discussed some of the subtle differences between density estimation a Cox process estimation.

Despite requiring one or more arbitrary thresholds be chosen iso surfaces are likely to be 3D visualization tool of choice for visualizing Cox processes, however alternatives such as volume rendering and cut planes are likely to see an expanded role in scientific visualization particularly in interactive environments. In terms of rendering differences between the intensity functions of Cox processes, the iso surface again shows advantages in representing signed differences, but volume rendering in particular shows promise in visualizing absolute differences. It was argued that operational decisions could be evaluated using these visualization techniques.

Improvements in graphical software will make more widespread application of 3D visualization techniques possible. Our experience with Mayavi has been very positive, and its flexible licensing terms and easy integration into scientific python are both big advantages, as is the possibility to change between different methods for rendering a scalar field.

An obvious route to consider for future work is in applying visualization techniques to other statistical methods for Cox process. A potential advantage of some other modeling techniques is to allow a more sophisticated treatment of time within the model, we are currently investigating these models.

Acknowledgements. This paper is based on research conducted on a project funded by the Australian Research Council Linkage program grant LP120100172. David Rohde acknowledges partial support from Coordenação de Aperfeiçoamento de Pessoal de Nível Superior (CAPES, Brasil).

References

[1] Adams, R.P., Murray, I., MacKay, D.J.C.: Tractable nonparametric Bayesian inference in poisson processes with Gaussian process intensities. In: Proceedings of the 26th International Conference on Machine Learning (ICML 2009), Montreal, Quebec (2009)

[2] Andrienko, G., Andrienko, N., Gatalsky, P.: Visual mining of spatial time series data. In: Boulicaut, J.-F., Esposito, F., Giannotti, F., Pedreschi, D. (eds.) PKDD 2004. LNCS (LNAI), vol. 3202, pp. 524–527. Springer, Heidelberg (2004)

[3] Barnes, D.G., Fluke, C.J.: Incorporating interactive three-dimensional graphics in astronomy research papers. New Astronomy 13(8), 599–605 (2008)

[4] Brunsdon, C., Corcoran, J., Higgs, G.: Visualising space and time in crime patterns: A comparison of methods. Computers, Environment and Urban Systems 31(1), 52–75 (2007)

[5] Cox, D.R.: Some Statistical Methods Connected with Series of Events. Journal of the Royal Statistical Society, Series B 17(2), 129–164 (1955)

[6] Diggle, P.J.: A kernel method for smoothing point process data. Applied Statistics 34, 138–147 (1985)

[7] Dubois, P.F.: Guest editors introduction: Python: Batteries included. Computing in Science and Engineering 9(3), 7–9 (2007)

[8] Fisher, N.I.: Statistical Analysis of Circular Data. Cambridge University Press (1996)

[9] Keim, D.A., Panse, C., Sips, M., North, S.C.: Visual data mining in large geospatial point sets. IEEE Comput. Graph. Appl. 24(5), 36–44 (2004)

[10] Kottas, A., Sansó, B.: Bayesian mixture modeling for spatial poisson process intensities, with applications to extreme value analysis. Journal of Statistical Planning and Inference 137, 3151–3163 (2009)

[11] Ramachandran, P., Varoquaux, G.: Mayavi: 3d visualisation of scientific data. Computing in Science & Engineering 13(2), 40–51 (2011)

[12] Scott, D.W.: Multivariate density estimation: theory, practice, and visualization. Wiley series in probability and mathematical statistics: Applied probability and statistics. Wiley (1992)

[13] Zhao, K., Liu, B., Tirpak, T.M., Xiao, W.: A visual data mining framework for convenient identification of useful knowledge. In: Proceedings of the Fifth IEEE International Conference on Data Mining, ICDM 2005, pp. 530–537. IEEE Computer Society, Washington, DC (2005)

Real-Time Television ROI Tracking
Using Mirrored Experimental Designs

Brendan Kitts, Dyng Au, and Brian Burdick

PrecisionDemand, 821 Second Avenue, Suite 700, Seattle, WA 98104, USA
{bkitts,dau,bburdick}@precisiondemand.com

Abstract. Real-time conversion tracking is the holy grail of TV advertisers. We show how to use thousands of tiny areas available via commercial cable and satellite systems to create low cost tracking cells. These areas are created as "mirrors" of a national campaign, and run in parallel with it. With properly controlled areas, it is possible to calculate national effects due to TV using statistical methods. We show performance of the method on a large-scale TV advertising campaign where it was used successfully to maintain a real-time CPA target of $60 for 179 days.

Keywords: Television, ROI, Conversion Tracking.

1 Introduction

Tracking ROI from Television is an unsolved problem for advertising. There are no physical mechanisms that allow for tracking a viewer from the view event to a purchase in a store, dealership, or over the web. This has led many marketers to be unable to allocate rational budgets towards TV advertising. This paper describes a method for using TV cable and satellite systems to track conversions due to TV. This is the first time that we have seen real-time TV ROI reported that is not using a panel-based approach, and is unique in that it can be implemented cost-effectively and using today's TV infrastructure.

2 Prior Work

There have been many attempts to track the revenue being generated from TV advertising.

2.1 IPTV

Many commentators have written that efforts such as IPTV will eventually enable TV conversions to be tracked via conversion tracking pixels similar to those in place today throughout the web. IPTVs obtain their TV content from the internet and use HTTP protocol for requesting content. In addition to TVs, Mobile phones such as the iPhone may be able to control the TV, and possibly click on on-screen ad content. However there are many technical challenges before this becomes a reality. Today

J. Li et al. (Eds.): PAKDD 2013 Workshops, LNAI 7867, pp. 95–108, 2013.

only 8% of US TV households have IP enabled TV. Attempts to introduce IPTVs such as Google TV and Apple TV have met with only lukewarm interest, as evidenced by Logitec first announcing the GoogleTV-compatible, Revue Set Top Box, and then halting manufacturing only two years later. Even if web-like conversion tracking becomes possible using TV, it still won't capture all of the activity such as delayed conversions, and purchasing at retail stores. In fact [18] have noted that TV disproportionately reaches low brand users, and so immediate ad response conversions may not be a good measure of TV effects.

2.2   RFI Systems

Some companies have experimented with methods for enabling existing TVs to be able to support a direct "purchase" or "Request For Information" (RFI) actions from "the lounge" using present-day Set Top Box systems and hand-held TV remote controls. The QUBE system, piloted in the 1970s, was an early example. In 2010 Backchannel Media developed an on-screen "bug" that appeared at the bottom of the screen and asked the consumer if they would want more information or a coupon. The consumer could click on their remote control to accept. Dish and DirecTV have also experimented with interactive capabilities. Although promising, adoption of remote control RFI systems is constrained by lack of hardware support and standards. Canoe Ventures – a joint venture with 6 MSOs - was tasked with developing these standards, but in 2012 laid off 120 of 150 employees including its CEO, and closed its New York office. These systems also have the same disadvantages of IPTV, in being unable to track delayed conversions.

2.3   TV Broadcast Time Alignment

Some authors have proposed a "Broadcast Time Alignment" strategy in which TV broadcasts are aligned with website activity within a few seconds of the TV airing [7], [8], [13]. For example, [13] show close time alignment between movie Super Bowl ads and searches for the same movie name. Unfortunately for regular TV ads, few people visit websites right after an ad airs, and due to web traffic noise, this method can have difficulty attributing small TV broadcasts [8]. In addition the method is unable to provide insight into delayed conversions.

2.4   Panels

One of the most common fallbacks, when faced with difficult-to-measure effects, is to use volunteer, paid panels to find out what people do after they see the ads. There are several companies that use panels to try to track TV exposures to sales. These include the Nielsen, IRI and TRA panels. One advantage of this method is real-time tracking is possible. However, in all cases, the small size of the panel (e.g. Nielsen 25,000 people) presents formidable challenges for extrapolation and difficulty finding enough transactions to reliably measure sales. Another problem with the panel approach is the cost of maintaining the panels[1].

---

[1] The authors are working on another approach to television tracking that is panel-like but which uses Set Top Boxes. Further details can be found in [9].

2.5   Mix Models

If data from previous campaigns has been collected, then it may be possible to regress the historical marketing channel activity (e.g. impressions bought on TV ads, Radio ads, web ads, print, etc) against future sales [8]. Unfortunately, such an approach offers no help if the relationships change in the future – it certainly is not real-time tracking! In addition, historical factors are rarely orthogonal - for example, retailers often execute coordinated advertising across multiple channels correlated in time on purpose in order to exploit seasonal events. This can lead to a historical factors matrix that aliases interactions and even main effects. Even if there are observations in which all main effects vary orthogonally, there may be too few cases for estimation.

2.6   Market Tests

Market Tests overcome the problems of aliasing by creating orthogonal experimental designs to study the phenomena under question. They also overcome the problem of historical data by using conventional scientific testing methods to run TV in some geographic areas and not others, and then compare the sales between the two [5], [11], [16], [17].

An added benefit of Market Tests is that they are easy for independent parties to validate. Mix models are ultimately black boxes which are determining how many conversions to attribute to TV versus other channels – a contentious decision since it impacts other channels, teams and marketing budgets. This can make it difficult for an organization to get behind this kind of attribution. Market Tests, on the other hand, allow the lift from TV to be directly observable by just comparing the number of conversions in treatments to controls, and so this is an easier measurement device to deploy (since one team with a marketing budget can do it) and get acceptance around (as the results are directly observable). The answer to the question of "how do you know TV is working" is to point to the area that has had TV applied, and its sales data in comparison to its controls.

The problem with Market Tests is their inability to be used during a national campaign, since there are no longer any controls that aren't receiving the TV signal. Therefore, after getting a nice "research binder" showing the value of TV, once the advertiser starts up their national campaign, they are once again running "by the seat of their pants".

2.7   Mirrored Tracking

The method we describe will update the market testing concept to make it work with national campaigns and using current TV infrastructure. This is the first that we know of to provide for real-time tracking across all advertiser sales channels without a panel. The method is considerably more scalable than other methods (e.g. limited sample of households available in panels) and is able to utilize larger populations, and is implementable by advertisers using their own data without any panel costs.

3   Mirrored Tracking Overview

Our problem is as follows: There is a national television ad campaign underway which is injecting $I_N(N)$ impressions into all national areas, and we want to measure its sales effects $Q(N)$. Our strategy for this problem will be to use local ad insertion systems to add impressions $I_L(d)$ to some of the local areas d. We need to add the impressions carefully to ensure that the impression nationally has exactly the same viewership as an equivalent impression locally. This process is what we refer to as "mirroring" and involves careful matching of treatment areas to national, and of local impressions to national. Using each day's observed injected impressions and additional quantity, we can then calculate what impressions are causing in terms of quantity in general.

4   TV Hardware

One of the key aspects of our approach is the use of existing TV capabilities in order to create mirrored tracking cells. A TV video stream is generally compressed using MPEG-2 format with possibly some other embedded instructions. National advertisements can be inserted into national video stream by electronically or manually trafficking the ads and rotation logic to the Network (e.g. ABC, CBS, Fox, NBC, CW) or cable station (e.g. CNN)   directly.

Local ad insertion is more complex. This requires local content to be spliced into a national video stream. Local insertion has been used for many years to create screen overlay "bugs" such as semi-transparent icons at the bottom of the screen that identify the station on news reports. It also allows local stations to splice in their station information to comply with FCC rules which require hourly station identification. Local insertion has also been used to inject ads; in the past this was primarily for local businesses such as local car dealers. We will co-opt the infrastructure to create a mirrored design for a major national campaign.

For Cable stations, the Cable MSO itself inserts the ad into the video stream, and has 2 minutes per hour of possible ads to insert, so approximately 13% of ad inventory. The MSO has multiple levels of signal control. This includes the Cable Interconnect – which cover Direct Marketing Association (DMA) areas, Zone – a collection of about 10,000 households.

For Broadcast stations, local ad insertion is handled by the local station (e.g. KOMO). 4 minutes per hour of time are provided for local station IDs, as well as local ads, so about 26% of ad inventory is available to be purchased locally.

There are approximately 2,000 cable zone areas that can be purchased, and over 2,500 local broadcast stations, providing considerable ability to create representative treatment mirrors.

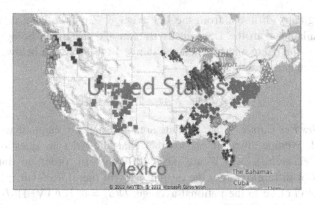

Fig. 1. Geographic distribution of Cable Zones from Comcast

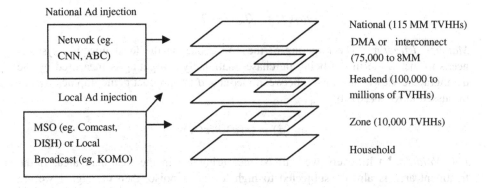

Fig. 2. Local and National ad Insertion for Cable Systems

5   Treatment Area Selection

There are 2,000 cable and broadcast areas d available. Which should we select for local ad injection? The key objective for selecting good treatment areas is to find areas that match national well enough so that they allow for accurate extrapolation to national. Ideally the local areas and national are homogenous populations, and so ads displayed locally have the same effect as is occurring nationally. In order to maximize the chances of homogeneity in the local areas to national, the area needs to meet several criteria:

5.1   Treatment Fitness Criteria

Low Census Disparity from US Average: The mean absolute difference between the ith US population census demographic $x_i(N)$, and the demographic reading $x_i(d)$ of a particular region d needs to be as low as possible. A lower value indicates that the area is not greatly different from the US average. Zip-code-level demographics are publicly available from the US Census Bureau and these can be aggregated to the same level as the cable and broadcast systems. In the formula below w_i is a weight applied to each demographic.

$$m_1(d) = \sum_i w_i \cdot |x_i(d) - x_i(N)|$$

Average Sales Per Capita: If a candidate area has sales per capita that are higher than the national average, then it is possible that the area in question might have advertising elasticities which are also different. In order to introduce fewer assumptions or differences into the design, we will therefore favor areas which have sales per capita close to the national average. $Q(d) = q(d) / \text{TVHH}(d) =$ conversions per capita in area d. $q(d)$ is the quantity of conversions generated in area d. $\text{TVHH}(d)$ are the number of TV Households in area d. $\text{TVHH}(N) = 112,000,000$ are the number of TV Households nationally.

$$m_2(d) = |Q(d) - Q(N)|$$

Matched Targeting: The targeting of the TV media via the local injection systems needs to match the media being purchased nationally. Targeting is measured by the demographic viewership match between media and the product demographics $r(d)$ as discussed in Kitts (2013b).

$$m_3(d) = |r(d) - r(N)|$$

Low Volatility: Ultimately we will be measuring lift in the treatment area. If the treatment area is already subjected to high levels of noise, then the signal we are trying to measure may not be detectable against the area's organic background noise. We measure this as the variance of sales per capita per day in the area.

$$m_4(d) = \frac{1}{T}\sum_t (Q(d,t) - E[Q(d,t)])^2$$

High Geographic Dispersion from other Experimental Areas: It is important to avoid areas which are too close together. Multiple test cells all in the same general geographic area increases the threat that some unique factor in this particular region is influencing sales and elasticities. By spreading out the test cells over a wider area, this threat can be reduced. In addition, increasing the dispersion of tracking cells also even helps avoid spillover of TV broadcasts into neighboring areas, avoiding contamination of other treatment cells. Let the set of possible geographic areas be G, and already selected areas $S \subseteq G$. We use the Great Circle method [23] to find the closest already-selected treatment area in Earth Surface distance kilometers, and report this as dispersion from previously selected areas. In the definition below, latitude and longitude are both converted from Cartesian to radians; $d_{lat} = \frac{d_{lat}}{180/\pi}$, and $K = 6378$ is the Earth radius in kilometers.

$$m_0(d_j) = \min\big(ESD(d_j, e): \forall e \in d_{1..j-1}\big);$$

$$ESD(d, e) = \text{acos}[\sin(d_{lat})\sin(e_{lat}) + \cos(d_{lat})\cos(e_{lat})\cos(e_{lon}-d_{lon})] \cdot K$$

Low Cost: Cheaper areas allow for more media to be run for the same price. Prices of areas are available from companies which monitor the clearing price of all ad buys on TV. Smaller geographic areas tend to be less in demand and have lower prices, and so are favored for testing over areas such as New York.

$$m_6(d) = TVHH(d) \cdot CPM(d)/1000$$

Average Cable and Satellite Penetration: Some areas of the country have lower numbers of cable TVs. We try to avoid selecting areas with unusually low cable adoption rates.

$$m_7(d) = |pen(d) - pen(N)| < PEN$$

Minimum Number of Insertible Networks: Insertible networks are stations that can have ads inserted to them. If the number of insertible networks becomes too low, then local inventory may not be able to match national.

$$m_8(d) = \text{sgn}(insert(d) \geq INS)$$

5.2   Treatment Selection Algorithm

Using the factors above, a weighted fitness score is calculated. Other researchers have discussed either "caliper" matching in which only subjects that meet particular significance testing criteria are selected, and "nearest neighbor matching" where subjects that have the closest match to ideal are selected [2], [15], [20]. We favor the nearest neighbor method, and we effectively pick the best N areas for mirrored cells.

In order to select areas we use an interactive procedure similar to Leader Clustering [3] in which the first area with best fitness is selected, and then subsequent areas are selected until all treatment cells are selected. Iterative recalculation is needed because the GeoDispersion metric is dependent upon areas already selected. In the formula below, R converts the raw number into a percentile, m_k is a criteria and M_k the weight of that criteria.

$$d_j: \min\left(\sum_k M_k \cdot R\big(m_k(d_j)\big): d_j \notin d_{1..j-1}\right)$$

6   Control Area Selection

We will be measuring treatment change in quantity per capita versus control change in quantity per capita over the same period of time. In order for this comparison to show differences due to TV (and not other factors), it is critical to ensure that the control area purchase behavior, demographics, and responsiveness to advertising are all as close as possible to the treatment areas [19]. The only difference between the areas should be the application of additional media. Various authors have referred to this as minimizing "threats to validity" or "matching" controls to treatments [2], [15], [20]. We use the following criteria to attempt to ensure homogeneity across multiple dimensions between the control and treatment areas.

6.1   Control Fitness Criteria

Demographic Similarity: Controls should have similar demographics to their treatment group. The D_Jth area to be selected has the following match difference:

$$u_1(D_J, d) = \sum_i \left| \left(\frac{1}{J} \sum_{j=1}^{J} x_i(D_j) \right) - x_i(d) \right|$$

Geographic Proximity: Whereas treatments were ideally geographically dispersed, the controls should be geographically close to their treatment areas. This helps to ensure that treatment and control areas have the same climactic factors (temperature, precipitation), economic characteristics, population attributes, and so on.

$$u_2(D_J, d) = ESD(D_J, d)$$

Matched Movement: The control and treatment areas should both show coordinated movement in sales for an extended period prior to the start of the experiment. When the experimental area has high sales, the control area should have high sales, and vica versa. Systematic variation is a strong test for relatedness since it suggests that the two areas are responding in the same way to changes in environmental conditions, promotions, and other events that can affect sales. In the definition below, the error is proportional to the absolute difference between treatment and the sum of control areas by day. The difference of difference method will also scale the error by national sales, and so we also multiply the difference by national $Q(N, t)^\eta$.

$$u_3(D_J, d) = \sum_t Q(N, t)^\eta \cdot \left[Q(d, t) - \frac{\sum_j q(D_j, t)}{\sum_j TVHH(D_j, t)} \right]^\delta$$

6.2   Control Selection Algorithm

Treatment areas need to utilize local ad injection systems, which restricts feasible treatments to the 2,000 broadcast and cable zone service areas discussed above. However controls – which don't require any media - are under no such obligations. Any controls in the country can be selected. This is useful because it means that controls can be selected at a finer-grain than the treatments. Treatments utilized 2,000 zones, averaging about 55,000 TV households each. Controls can be built from over 30,000 zipcodes, averaging just 3,800 TV Households. Our objective is therefore to assemble a set of controls that match very precisely the demographics of the treatments that we are running in.

The algorithm for selecting controls is iterative, similar to the treatment selection. However, one important difference is that multiple controls are selected for each treatment, and the set of controls are "assembled" to collectively match the treatment. The method starts by selecting the best matching control. Let's say that this control matches well, but has too few African Americans. When selecting the next control area, the error function is the match between the total controls, including the new candidate control, and the treatment. As a result, if one of the candidate controls causes the African American quota to move closer to the treatment, then this control will be favored. As a result, the iterative procedure "self-corrects" and successively selects areas which together have demographics and sales which match the treatment area.

This produces very useful behavior in practice. Figure 5 shows areas chosen after 4 iterations. After 100 iterations, the system has "self-corrected".

The best controls $D(d)$ for each treatment group d are selected based on the score below.

$$D_J: \min \left(\sum_k U_k \cdot R \left(u_k(D_j, d) \right) : D_J \notin d_{1..j} \wedge D_J \notin D_{1..J-1} \right)$$

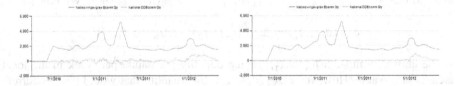

Fig. 3. (left) Estimated conversions due to TV for 4 best matching zip control areas (based on closeness to control). (right) 9 zip control areas.

We have found real situations in practice where better matched controls help to improve measurement fidelity. During one ROI Tracking campaign, we noticed that areas not running TV seemed to increase upwards, whereas treatments remained steady. After analyzing the bump we determined that African Americans as a group were lifting much higher than others. It turned out that Whitney Houston died on February 11, 2012, and the Grammy Music Awards were also held on February 12, 2012 and were largely dedicated to Whitney Houston. The bump seemed to be due to large numbers of older, African American, females increasing spontaneously, unrelated to TV. Without well matched controls, we would be reporting negative lift from a large TV campaign when actually the campaign was performing very well.

7   Real-Time Mirrored Estimation

We have now selected treatment areas d_i and multiple control areas $D_j(d_i)$ for each treatment. We will now run additional advertising I_L in the local area d_i. Our objective is to create a detectible increase in the sales per capita in area d, compared to the control areas. Based on the size of the increase, we can then measure how TV advertising is driving sales, and then estimate the unknown (but simultaneously executing) national effects.

Let $\Delta Q_N(d, t_1, t_2)$ be the quantity per capita per week that is being generated in area d between time t_1 and t_2 due to I_N impressions of national TV. This is what we want to estimate. Let E be the quantity per capita per week that is occurring in a local area d without TV; possibly due to other marketing programs and also due to noise. The total quantity that we observe in area d is therefore $Q_{N+}(d, t_1, t_2) = E + \Delta Q_N$. The quantity per capita per week produced by I_N is an unknown function that we will refer to as f. Our objective is to report on ΔQ_N – the quantity due to TV - each week due to running media.

$$\Delta Q_{N+}(d, t_1, t_2) = \Delta Q_N(d, t_1, t_2) + E = f(I_N) + E$$

In order to make the quantity measurable, we will inject an additional amount of local impressions per capita per week I_L into a local area d using the local ad insertion systems which produce local revenue per capita per week of $\Delta Q_L(d, t_1, t_2)$. Let $\Delta Q_{L+}(d, t_1, t_2)$ be the total revenue now observed in the local area inclusive of local and national ads. $Q_{L+}(d, t_1, t_2) = \Delta Q_L(d, t_1, t_2) + \Delta Q_N(d, t_1, t_2) + E$ We now have:

$$\Delta Q_L(d, t_1, t_2) = \Delta Q_{L+}(d, t_1, t_2) - \Delta Q_{N+}(d, t_1, t_2)$$

In the above formula, $\Delta Q_{L+}(d, t_1, t_2)$, the quantity per capita per week in the local area, is observable. However $\Delta Q_{N+}(d, t_1, t_2)$, the quantity that would have occurred, is not directly observable since we over-concentrated in d. However, if we now find matched areas $D(d)$ that are homogenous with d, then we can use their performance (which is only based on national ad insertion) for ΔQ_{N+} since it is observable. We now have:

$$\Delta Q_L(d, t_1, t_2) = \Delta Q_{L+}(d, t_1, t_2) - \Delta Q_{N+}(D(d), t_1, t_2)$$

$$\Delta Q_L(d, t_1, t_2) = \Delta Q_{L+}(d, t_2) - \Delta Q_{L+}(d, t_2) - \Delta Q_{N+}(D(d), t_2) - \Delta Q_{N+}(D(d), t_1)$$

Where Q_{L+} and Q_{N+} are both observable and we injected $\Delta I_L(d)$ impression concentration. We therefore have an observation between impressions and quantity a point "higher" than the national impressions. We want to try to infer the same relationship, but at a point "lower". In order to infer ΔQ_N , which is running with $\Delta I_N(N)$, we need to know something about the shape of the TV impression to quantity function f. One property that we can determine *a priori* is that $f(0) = 0$. If 0 impressions are injected into an area, then the revenue due to those 0 ad injections will also be zero. We can also assert that $f(I_N) \leq Q_{N+}(d, t_1, t_2)$ since it is not possible to produce more quantity than what were observed.

What shape should we assume for f? There is a large body of advertising research which shows diminishing returns at higher levels of advertising [4], [6], [22], [24]. Ordinarily, a linear assumption for an advertising response function would lead to unrealistically optimistic estimates. However, in this case, we are actually "extrapolating downwards" and the diminishing returns observation works to our advantage. Assuming diminishing returns as advertising impressions increase, a linear fit to the observed data at the higher concentration level, actually becomes a lower bound on the lift produced by the national ad impressions (which are at lower concentrations). Therefore, the simple linear model results in conservative – and in fact lower bound - estimates of TV effects! This is a convenient result that allows us to be more confident than usual about our TV effects.

In accordance with the observations above, a linear function should be intercept-less and so we have a function form of $f(I) = cI$, we can calculate an estimate for the function as follows:

$$\Delta Q_N(t_1, t_2) = c \cdot I_N \text{ where } c = \frac{\Delta Q_L(d_j, t_1, t_2)}{I_L}$$

$$\text{if } \Delta Q_N \leq 0 \text{ then } \Delta Q_N = 0 \text{ ; if } \Delta Q_N \geq \Delta Q_{N+} \text{ then } \Delta Q_N = \Delta Q_{N+}$$

8   Experiment

We used the technique to achieve a television-drive-to-web Cost Per Acquisition (CPA) goal from September 10, 2012 to March 1, 2013: a period of 172 days.

The client's CPA objective was to spend $45 per signup on their website. This kind of goal is typical for online advertising with cookie based conversion tracking systems, but for TV, it is virtually unheard of to be able to actively target and achieve a CPA.

Our tracking markets consisted of three areas in sequence (a) Lacrosse,WI-MN, (b) Tulsa, OK and Charleston, SC, (c) Harrisburg, PA and Milwaukee, WI. We used Lacrosse from 9/10/2012 to 10/31/2012, Tulsa and Charleston from 11/12/2012 to 1/6/2013, and Harrisburg and Milwaukee from 1/7/2013 to 3/1/2013. All areas were near the 50th percentile for sales per capita and better than 30th percentile for census disparity to US. Each area was matched to 300 zip controls.

The reason for using three areas was because we found that over time the lift in the areas began to decline. In order to ensure our lift readings remained accurate for national, we rotated the tracking areas every couple of months.

Local ads were targeted to match the tratios of the national campaign, by selecting relevant programming to run the ads during. The disparity between tratio of local and national was negligible – both were about tratio = 0.265.

National media was maintained at approximately 345 impressions per thousand households and approximately $8,500 per day, although we increased this significantly over Christmas. Local markets were executed at approximately 400 impressions per thousand households and matched tratio.

Our initial market Lacrosse performed relatively poorly. It quickly lost lift after two weeks, and we brought Tulsa and Charleston online starting in November.

Overall, inclusive of LaCrosse, we produced 29,811 signups from $1.797 million dollars in media spending at a CPA of $60.29. The 29,911 signups boosted sales by nearly 11%. We also recorded a CPA of $45 after November.

In addition, because of our use of treatment-control tracking markets, after leaving the tracking markets we were able to monitor delayed conversions in the form of elevated lift after switching off TV. By summing incremental conversions versus controls, we were able to report that conversions added 3.3 times the number of initially injected conversion by the end of year, dropping their ultimate CPA to $18.27.

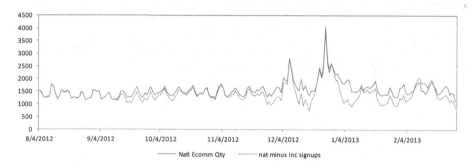

Fig. 4. Web conversions versus web conversions without TV. The method provides a way to report daily on the conversions being generated due to TV.

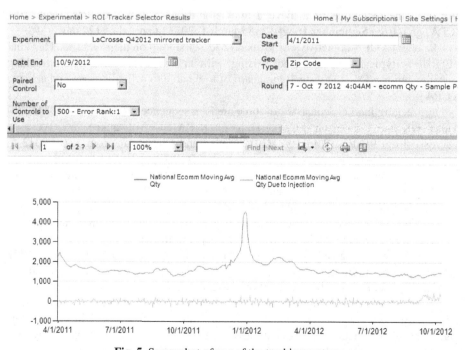

Fig. 5. Screenshot of one of the tracking systems

9   Conclusion

We have described a method for tracking Television ROI in real-time. The method does not rely upon panels, and can be implemented by an advertiser using existing television infrastructure and without their own sales data. The technique also measures delayed conversions, which is a key aspect of television campaigns. So far we have implemented six of these mirrored tracking deployments with major, multi-million dollar national TV campaigns, and the results in all cases are good. We believe that this is an important technique for tracking ROI in what is otherwise an untrackable medium.

References

1. Angrist, J., Pischke, J.: Mostly Harmless Econometrics. Princeton University Press (2010)
2. D'Agostino, R.: Tutorial In Biostatistics: Propensity Score Methods for Bias Reduction in the Comparison of a Treatment to a Non-Randomized Control Group. Statistics in Medicine 17, 2265–2281 (1998)
3. Duda, R., Hart, P., Stork, D.: Pattern Classification, 2nd edn. Wiley (2000)
4. Hanssens, D., Parsons, L., Schultz, R.: Market Response Models: Econometric and Time Series Analysis. Kluwer Academic Press, Boston (2001)
5. Hu, Y., Lodish, L., Krieger, M.: An Analysis of Real World TV Advertising Tests: a 15 year update. Journal of Advertising Research 47(3), 341–353 (2007)
6. Johansson, J.K.: Advertising and the S-Curve: A New Approach. Journal of Marketing Research 16(3), 346–354 (1979)
7. Joo, M., Wilbur, K., Zhu, Y.: Television Advertising and Online Search, SSRN Working paper (2012), http://ssrn.com/abstract=1720713
8. Kitts, B., Wei, L., Au, D., Powter, A., Burdick, B.: Attribution of Conversion Events to Multi-Channel Media. In: Proceedings of the Tenth IEEE International Conference on Data Mining, December 14-17 (2010)
9. Kitts, B., Au, D., Burdick, B.: Television Conversion Tracking using Anonymized Set Top Box Data (unpublished, 2013)
10. Kokernak, M.: What's Television's Next Business Model? Media Post Daily News, March 17 (2010)
11. Lambert, D., Pregibon, D.: Online effects of Offline Ads. In: Proceedings of the Second International Workshop on Dataa Mining and Audience Intelligence for Advertising. ACM Press, New York (2008)
12. Leaders. In: Praise of Television: The great survivor. The Economist (April 2010)
13. Lewis, R., Reiley, D.: Down-to-the-Minute Effects of Super Bowl Advertising on Online Search Behavior. Working Paper (2010),
    http://davidreiley.com/papers/DownToTheMinute.pdf
14. Lewis, R., Rao, J.: On the Near Impossibility of Measuring Advertising Effectiveness, Yahoo! Research working paper (2011),
    http://justinmrao.com/lewis_rao_nearimpossibility.pdf
15. Little, R., Rubin, D.: Causal Effects in Clinical and Epidemiological Studies Via Potential Outcomes: Concepts and Analytical Approaches. Annual Review of Public Health 21, 121–145 (2000)

16. Lodish, L., Abraham, M., Kalmenson, S., Livelsberger, J., Lubetkin, B., Richardson, B., Stevens, M.: How T.V. Advertising Works: A Meta-Analysis of 389 Real World Split Cable T.V. Advertising Experiments. Journal of Marketing Research 32(2), 125–139 (1995a)
17. Lodish, L., Abraham, M., Kalmenson, S., Livelsberger, J., Lubetkin, B., Richardson, B., Stevens, M.: A Summary of Fifty-five In-Market Experimetns on the Long-term Effect of TV Advertising. Marketing Science 14(3), 133–140 (1995b)
18. Nelson-Field, K., Riebe, E., Sharp, B.: What's Not To Like?; Can a Facebook Fan Base give a Brand the Advertising Reach it needs? Journal of Advertising Research (2012)
19. Rosenbaum, P., Rubin, D.: Constructing a Control Group Using Multivariate Matched Sampling Methods That Incorporate the Propensity Score. The American Statistician 39(1) (1985)
20. Rubin, D.: Estimating Causal Effects of Treatments in Randomized and Nonrandomized Studies. Journal of Educational Psychology 66(5), 688–701 (1974)
21. Simon, H.: Price Management. North-Holland Publishing Company, Amsterdam (1989)
22. Simon, J.L., Arndt, J.: The Shape of the Advertising Response Function. Journal of Advertising Research 20(4), 767 (2002)
23. Sinnott, R.: Virtues of the Haversine. Sky and Telescope 68(2), 159 (1984)
24. Vakratsas, D., Feinberg, F., Bass, F., Kalyanaram, G.: Advertising Response Functions Revisited. Marketing Science 23(1), 109–119 (2004)

On the Evaluation of the Homogeneous Ensembles with CV-Passports

Vladimir Nikulin[1], Aneesha Bakharia[2], and Tian-Hsiang Huang[3]

[1] Department of Mathematical Methods in Economy,
Vyatka State University, Kirov, Russia
vnikulin.uq@gmail.com
[2] Faculty of Science and Engineering
Queensland University of Technology, Australia
aneesha.bakharia@gmail.com
[3] Cloud Computing Research Center, National Sun Yat-Sen University, Taiwan
huangtx@gmail.com

Abstract. Ensembles are often capable of greater prediction accuracy than any of their individual members. As a consequence of the diversity between individual base-learners, an ensemble will not suffer from overfitting. In this regard, development of a systematic and automatic approach for the evaluation of ensemble solutions is particularly important. Based on the mechanism of homogeneous ensembling (known, also, as bagging), we can construct a passport of the solution as a unified validation trajectory against all available training data. Assuming that passports mimic closely the corresponding test solutions, we can use them for the consideration of many tasks including optimizations of blends and ensembles, calculation of the biases and any other tests as required. The reported results were obtained online during the International PAKDD data mining competition in 2010, where we were awarded a certificate for the fourth best result. We, also, report results from the second most popular contest on the Kaggle platform named "Credit", where we demonstrate one of the best results.

Keywords: ensemble and base learner, cross-validation, decision trees, boosting, classification, data mining competitions, financial credit risk assessment.

1 Introduction

Ensemble (including voting and averaged) classifiers are learning algorithms that construct a set of many elementary classifiers (called base-learners) [1]. In most cases, base-learners are combined to classify test data points by sample average, and it is now well-known that ensembles are often much more accurate than the base-learners that make them up [2], [3]. Tree ensemble called "random forests" was introduced in [4] and represents an example of a successful classifier. Another example, the bagging support vector machine (SVM) [5] is very important because direct application of the SVM to the whole data set may not be possible.

J. Li et al. (Eds.): PAKDD 2013 Workshops, LNAI 7867, pp. 109–120, 2013.

In the case of SVM, we are interested to deal with limited sample size, which is equal to the dimension of the corresponding kernel matrix. The well known bagging technique [6] is relevant here. According to this technique, each base-learner used in the ensemble is trained with data that are randomly selected from the training sample (without replacement).

Our approach was motivated by [6], and represents a compromise between two major considerations. On the one hand, we would like to deal with balanced data. On the other hand, we are interested in exploiting all available information. We consider a large number m of balanced subsets of available data, where any single subset includes two parts 1) nearly all "positive" instances (minority) and 2) randomly selected "negative" instances. The method of balanced random sets (RS) is general and maybe used in conjunction with different base-learners.

In the experimental section we report test-results against real-world financial data of the PAKDD2010 Data Mining Competition[1].

This paper is organised as follows: Section 2 describes the PAKDD2010 data-mining Contest. Section 3 discusses method of Mean-Variance Filtering (MVF) for feature selection. Section 4 explains the experimental procedure with homogeneous ensembling, where the definition of the CV-passports for evaluation of the homogeneous ensembles (as a main proposed novelty) is given in Section 4.2. Section 5 describes one exceptionally popular contest on the Kaggle platform, which, also, is relevant to financial modelling and credit-rating assessment. Finally, Section 6 concludes the paper.

2   PAKDD2010 Challenge and Data

The Challenge datasets were collected during period from 2006 to 2009, and came from a private label credit card operation of a Brazilian credit company.

Three datasets were made available to the participants: 1) modelling (50,000 samples), 2) leaderboard (20,000 samples) and 3) prediction (20,000 samples), where labels were given only for the modelling set, which has 13,041 or 26.08% of "bad" clients. The client was labelled as bad (target variable=1) if he/she made 60 days delay in any payment of the bills contracted along the first year after the credit has been granted.

The important aspect to emphasize is that modelling set includes approved customers only, leaderboard and prediction sets were extracted from over one and two years later and contain randomly selected applicants, who have had their applications rejected by the credit scoring system. However, for the purpose of monitoring the decision support system's performance and collecting data for future model re-calibration, these clients have received the credit they had applied for.

2.1   Data Pre-processing

The original datasets contain 52 features, where feature "ID.Client" was not counted. Those features, which have only one value in the absolute majority of

---

[1] http://sede.neurotech.com.br/PAKDD2010/

Table 1. List of 40 original features, where values index=1 and 2 indicate categorical and numerical variables; k - number of corresponding values or secondary variables (see Section 2.1); rates "SUM" and "MEAN" (multiplied by 100) were computed according to the secondary coefficients, see for details Section 3.

Feature	Index	k	SUM	MEAN
AGE	2	58	3.5446	6.1113
PROFESSIONAL.ZIP	1	80	1.8374	2.2968
RESIDENCIAL.ZIP	1	80	1.8366	2.2957
RESIDENCIAL.PHONE.AREA.CODE	1	60	1.6651	2.7752
RESIDENCIAL.CITY	1	39	1.3988	3.5867
PROFESSIONAL.PHONE.AREA.CODE	1	37	1.0885	2.9419
RESIDENCIAL.STATE	1	26	0.739	2.8422
PROFESSIONAL.CITY	1	27	0.6837	2.5322
CITY.OF.BIRTH	1	19	0.5947	3.1298
STATE.OF.BIRTH	1	27	0.5454	2.0198
PROFESSIONAL.STATE	1	24	0.3751	1.5629
PAYMENT.DAY	1	5	0.3065	6.1309
RESIDENCIAL.BOROUGH	1	9	0.288	3.2002
PROFESSION.CODE	1	12	0.2868	2.3903
QUANT.DEPENDANTS	2	7	0.2324	3.3195
PROFESSIONAL.BOROUGH	1	7	0.2117	3.0236
RESIDENCE.TYPE	1	6	0.2063	3.4386
MONTHS.IN.RESIDENCE	2	11	0.1861	1.6916
MARITAL.STATUS	1	7	0.1548	2.211
PERSONAL.MONTHLY.INCOME	2	10	0.1473	1.4734
EDUCATION.LEVEL	1	5	0.1397	2.7945
MATE.PROFESSION.CODE	1	6	0.1302	2.1697
OCCUPATION.TYPE	1	6	0.123	2.0507
APPLICATION.SUBMISSION.TYPE	1	2	0.0998	4.9891
FLAG.RESIDENCIAL.PHONE	1	1	0.0777	7.7735
PERSONAL.ASSETS.VALUE	2	4	0.0697	1.7417
FLAG.MASTERCARD	1	1	0.0677	6.7678
PRODUCT	1	2	0.0655	3.2764
SEX	1	2	0.0488	2.4411
NACIONALITY	1	2	0.0412	2.0617
QUANT.BANKING.ACCOUNTS	1	2	0.0321	1.6028
QUANT.SPECIAL.BANKING.ACCOUNTS	1	2	0.032	1.5982
MONTHS.IN.THE.JOB	1	1	0.0247	2.473
POSTAL.ADDRESS.TYPE	1	1	0.0234	2.3422
FLAG.PROFESSIONAL.PHONE	1	1	0.0229	2.295
COMPANY	1	1	0.0208	2.0815
OTHER.INCOMES	2	2	0.0192	0.9583
QUANT.CARS	1	1	0.0088	0.8811
FLAG.EMAIL	1	1	0.0026	0.2591
FLAG.VISA	1	1	0.0016	0.1584

all cases (more than 99.5%), were automatically excluded. As an outcome, the number of features was reduced to 40 (see Table 1). Among them 6 are numerical (*Index = 2*), while others are categorical. An effective way to link information contained in numerical and categorical variables is to transfer the numerical variables to a binary format. We used the most basic method of subintervals. The splitting points were defined manually based on the visual consideration of the corresponding averages of labels.

As a next step, we considered all possible values for the remaining categorical variables, and found those values which occurred frequently enough (the range from 100 to 200 was used as a threshold) to be considered as independent

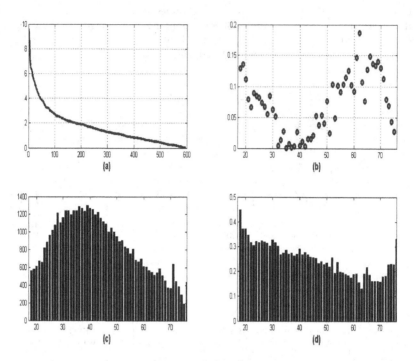

Fig. 1. (a) secondary rates sorted in a decreasing order; (b) secondary coefficients for the feature "Age" (see Section 3); (c) numbers of customers per age-group; (d) empirical probabilities per age-group

binary (secondary) variables. Otherwise, values were removed from any further consideration.

As an outcome of the pre-processing, we got a set with 595 binary (secondary) features. This popular format is well known as a sparse format. Column "k" in Table 1 represents the numbers of secondary binary features per corresponding primary feature.

As a consequence of the above pre-processing transformation/treatment, we produced two completely numerical matrices (for training and for testing) with 40 features each and without any missing values.

3   Mean-Variance Filtering with Linear Regression

Regularised linear regression (RLR) represents the most simple example of a classification model. The main target of such a model is to produce a decision function, which is able to rank observations from the unlabelled test dataset.

By definition, regression coefficients may be regarded as natural measurements of influence of the corresponding features. In our case we have m vectors of regression coefficients (which correspond to m balanced random sets), and we can use them to investigate the stability of the influence of corresponding features. The proper feature selection may reduce overfitting significantly [7]. We remove features with unstable coefficients, and recompute the classifiers. Note that stability of the coefficients may be measured using different methods. For example, we can apply the t-statistic given by the ratio of the mean to the standard deviation [8]. We computed MVF-rates for the 595 secondary binary features as described in Section 2.1. Figure 1(a) represents the corresponding rates sorted in a decreasing order. According to our evaluation, feature "Age" is the most influential, and Figure 1(b) shows average coefficients for the related 58 dummy (binary, secondary) variables.

Rates for the primary features (see column "SUM" in Table 1) were computed as sums of the relevant secondary coefficients. In addition, we presented averages of the secondary coefficients (see column "MEAN" in Table 1).

Figure 1(c) presents the numbers of customers within particular age-groups. According to the following Figure 1(d), the bad-rates (or empirical probabilities) among young and older people are higher, and it is expected that the corresponding bad-rates increase in the prediction set generally. This observation is very interesting as a graphical explanation why non-linear classifiers (decision trees, for example) are more efficient compared to the simple linear regression.

4   Homogeneous Ensembling with Balances Random Sets

In many cases, ensembles have significantly better prediction accuracy compared to their individual members [3]. As a consequence of the diversity between individual base-learners, an ensemble will not suffer from overfitting. On the other hand, in many cases we are dealing with imbalanced data and a classifier which was built using all the data has tendency to ignore minority classes. As a solution to the problem, we propose to consider a large number of relatively small and balanced subsets where representatives from both patterns are to be selected randomly [9].

4.1   On the Boosting Principles Applied to the Selection of the Balanced Subsets

In our previous publications [9], [10], we used a sequence of balanced subsets, which were selected from the training set independently (one subset was completely independent from the next, and so on). However, it appears to be logical to apply here the principles of boosting [11] based on the latest solution (known, also, as the solution corresponding to a base-learner).

Principle of Complexity in Application to the Labelled Data. Let us describe the proposed boosting model in more details. Suppose that $y_t \in \{0, 1\}$ is the target variable and $s_t^{(\alpha)} \in [0, \ldots, 1]$ is the training solution corresponding to the sample t, α is a sequential index of the balanced random subset. Then, we shall select sample t as a prospective to be included in the following balanced subset $\alpha + 1$ subject to the following conditions

$$\xi \leq \xi_1 \ if \ y_t = 1; \tag{1a}$$

$$\xi \leq \xi_2, \ otherwise, \tag{1b}$$

where

$$\xi_i = c_{i1} + (c_{i2} + c_{i3} \cdot \phi) \cdot w(y_t, s_t^{(\alpha)}), i = 1, \ldots, 2, \tag{2}$$

$$w(y, s) = |y - s|^{\beta}, \tag{3}$$

where ξ and $\phi \in [0, \ldots, 1]$ are standard uniform random variables, $\beta > 0$ and $c_{ij} > 0, i = 1, \ldots, 2, j = 1, \ldots, 3$, are regulation parameters. For example, we can select $\beta = 0.35$, and the recommended values (based on our extensive experiments) for coefficients c are given in Table 2.

Table 2. PAKDD2010 Challenge: recommended values for the matrix of coefficients $c_{ij} > 0, i = 1, \ldots, 2, j = 1, \ldots, 3$, in (2)

minority (label=1):	0.55	0.2	0.15
majority (label=0):	0.16	0.08	0.06

Remark 1. We can see that values in the first row of Table 2, which correspond to the minority class (1a) are much bigger compared to the second row, which corresponds to the majority class (1b). As a direct consequence, selection according to (1a) and (1b) will create relatively balanced subset. However, we considered selection in accordance with (1a) and (1b) as just a preliminary. After that, we conducted final adjustment to ensure that the relation between positives and negatives is exactly as required.

Remark 2. The function (3) in (2) represents a very important boosting multiplier to ensure that "difficult" samples will be given higher probability to be selected.

Principle of Simplicity in Application to the Unlabelled Data. We can extend selection (1a) and (1b) to the unlabelled test set. However, there is a fundamental difference between treatment of labelled and unlabelled data. In the case of labelled data, we shall be selecting more complex samples, but in the case of unlabelled data, we shall be selecting simpler samples with stronger indication regarding their classification in accordance with available training solution. We used this semi-supervised approach in application to the Credit Challenge on the Kaggle platform (see Section 5), where the data had stronger imbalance and the quality of classification according to the AUC was significantly higher compared to the PAKDD2010 Challenge.

4.2   Main Novelty of Our Method: Calculation of the CV-Passports as a Validation Trajectories Against all Training Data

In accordance with the principles of homogeneous ensembling, it appears to be natural to consider calculation of the decision function as an average of the large number of the single learners (or base classifiers), where any single learner is based on the randomly selected subsamples of observations and features. Note that feature selection maybe conducted according to the MVF criterion as described in Section 3.

Let us describe the proposed method in more details. Suppose that we are using about 75% of the available data for training. Then, remaining 25% of the data maybe used for the validation control. In line with the principles of cross-validation, we shall test stability of the validation results by considering a sequence of the random splittings.

The main novelty of our method: we are proposing to accumulate the validation results against all training samples in line with construction of the homogeneous ensemble. We shall call averaged validation trajectory as a CV-passport of the corresponding homogeneous ensemble.

The validation results corresponding to the CV-passports with different base-learners (Models) are given in Table 3

Table 3. Some selected experimental results, where second and third columns represent results in terms of the AUCs corresponding to the CV-passport and to the validation set

Model	CV-passport	Leaderboard	ENS1	ENS2
GBM	0.6626	0.6259	10	10
RF	0.6474	0.6166	7	2
GLM	0.6397	0.6106	4	0
RLR+RS	0.6413	0.6107	2	0
ADA	0.6313	0.6224	1	5

Further, we calculated an ensemble solution as a linear combination of five solutions (see Table 3), where four solutions were adjusted to the scale of the leading solution GBM, using an ensemble constructor [12] (the linear weight coefficients without normalisation are given in the column $ENS1$). The observed corresponding result on the Leaderboard was 0.6283. Based on the separate submissions of the particular solutions to the Leaderboard, we created a second ensemble with the linear coefficients, which are given in the column $ENS2$. The observed result on the Leaderboard was 0.6357.

The final solution to the Prediction set was created using hundreds of balanced and imbalanced random sets, where GBM and ADA were used as a primary base learners.

Table 4. Descriptions for the Credit database, where the target variable is given in the first row, the following 10 sections, separated by the horizontal lines present features

Target: person experienced 90 days past due delinquency or worse.
Var1: total balance on credit cards and personal lines of credit divided by the sum of credit limits.
Var2: age of borrower in years.
Var3: number of times borrower has been 30-59 days past due but no worse in the last 2 years.
Var4: monthly debt payments, alimony,living costs divided by monthy gross income.
Var5: monthly income
Var6: number of Open loans and Lines of credit (e.g. credit cards).
Var7: number of times borrower has been 90 days or more past due.
Var8: number of mortgage and real estate loans including home equity lines of credit.
Var9: number of times borrower has been 60-89 days past due but no worse in the last 2 years.
Var10: number of dependents in family excluding themselves (spouse, children etc.)

5   Credit Challenge on the Kaggle Platform

Banks play a crucial role in market economies. They decide who can get finance and on what terms, and can make or break investment decisions[2]. Credit scoring algorithms, which make a prediction on the probability of default, are the methods banks use to determine whether or not a loan should be granted. The Credit Challenge on the Kaggle Platform required participants to improve on the state of the art in credit scoring, by predicting the probability that somebody will experience financial distress in the next two years.

The duration of the Credit competition was 87 days and it was ran from the 19th September 2011 to 15th December 2011. The related database includes two parts 1) training with 150000 samples, where 10026 or 6.68% are positive (that means problematic), and all the other samples are negative (that means normal); 2) testing with 101503 samples (unlabelled).

The subject of the Credit contest is a well related to the PAKDD2010 competition (see Table 4), and we used similar methods during both contests (in the sense of general structure). The "Credit" data are strongly imbalanced compared to the PAKDD2010 data and the second row of Table 5 reflects this very important property.

Table 4 represents binary target variable in the first row, and ten explanatory variables, which maybe classified into three types: 1) percent (N1 and N4); 2) integer (NN2-3 and NN6-10); 3) real (N5).

We are interested to investigate how objective is evaluation of the homogeneous ensemble by the corresponding CV-passports. Accordingly, we conducted

---

[2] http://www.kaggle.com

Table 5. Credit contest: recommended values for the matrix of coefficients $c_{ij} > 0, i = 1, \ldots, 2, j = 1, \ldots, 3$, in (2)

minority (label=1):	0.65	0.2	0.15
majority (label=0):	0.045	0.02	0.01

Table 6. Evaluations with CV-passports (Part1) and testing (Part2 and Part3) in the terms of AUC, where column "Outcome" indicates relation of the CV-passport with test results. Column "LeaderBoard" presents results, which were obtained against the Contest final test set using an opportunity of the post-challenge submissions.

CV-passport (Part1)	Outcome	Part2	Part3	LeaderBoard
0.86444	1	0.865093	0.861744	0.86227
0.862213	1	0.861325	0.867946	0.861799
0.861863	1	0.867841	0.86037	0.862734
0.860872	0	0.86616	0.864002	0.863231
0.866882	2	0.864535	0.858622	0.862771
0.863608	1	0.862083	0.867613	0.86371
0.862468	0	0.864618	0.864311	0.862201
0.865894	2	0.862112	0.864984	0.862818
0.862137	0	0.864673	0.863647	0.860718
0.863792	0	0.864619	0.864232	0.862716

the following experiment. We split randomly available training data into 3 equal size parts with 50000 samples each, where first part was used for training and for evaluation with CV-passport (used 300 random sets, as described in Section 4). Two other parts were used for testing. Results of this experiment, corresponding to the 10 independent splittings are presented in Table 6.

Remark 3. We can see a quite close correspondence between first column "CV-passport" v_1 and columns 3 and 4 (v_2 and v_3), which represent test results. The evaluation by the CV-passport is rather a conservative: in 4 cases we observed that

$$\min(v_2, v_3) < v_1 < \max(v_2, v_3)$$

(Outcome=1), and in 4 other cases

$$v_1 < \min(v_2, v_3),$$

(Outcome=0), and in only 2 remaining cases we have Outcome=2.

Remark 4. The results presented in Table 6 were obtained using GBM as a base learner are very competitive taking into account the fact that winning result in the Credit contest was 0.869558. This observation is a very interesting taking into account the fact that in order to produce results of Table 6 we used only one third of the available training data. Further improvement maybe achieved using semi-supervised approach as described in Section 4.1, or we can create secondary (more informative) features as functions of the given (or original) features (see Section 5.1).

Remark 5. The average of the ten solutions presented in Table 6 produced on the LeaderBoard a significant improvement: 0.867536 (post-challenge submissions) - rank 81 out of 926.

5.1   Secondary Features in the Credit Contest

The features Var3, Var7 and Var9 (see Table 4) represent some problems with debt repayments in the past, and we had noticed that those features are very informative. Accordingly, we can generate some secondary features as sums or products of original features:

$$Var3 + Var7, Var3 + Var9, Var7 + Var9, Var3 + Var7 + Var9,$$

$$Var3 \cdot Var7, Var3 \cdot Var9, Var7 \cdot Var9, Var3 \cdot Var7 \cdot Var9.$$

In addition, we can generate synthetic secondary features using method as presented in [13], where we described our successful online experience, obtained during another very popular data-mining competition of the Kaggle platform named Carvana. Coincidently, both competitions Credit and Carvana were active at about the same time (December 2011 - January 2012).

Remark 6. Our best result in Public LeaderBoard (validation phase based on 30% of the test data) was 0.863904, which corresponds to the rank N1 out of 926. Our final result (in Private LeaderBoard, remaining 70% of the test data: best out of the five selected) was 0.868942, which corresponds to the rank N9. It is interesting to note that Private result was better compared to the Public result. This fact is a very unusual and indicates that, probably, more complex samples were selected specially for the preliminary (Public) testing. However, the competitors were not notified about it by the Organisers.

6   Concluding Remarks

Selection bias [14] or overfitting represents a very important and challenging problem. As it was noticed in [15], if the improvement of a quantitative criterion such as the error rate is the main contribution of a paper, the superiority of a new algorithms should always be demonstrated on independent validation data. In this sense, the importance of data mining contests is unquestionable. The rapid popularity growth of the data mining challenges [16] demonstrates with confidence that it is the best known way to evaluate different models and systems. Based on our own experience, cross-validation (CV) can easily overfit as a consequence of the intensive experiments. Further developments such as nested CV [17] are computationally too expensive [15], plus very sensitive to the particular design, and should not be used until it is absolutely necessary, because nested CV may generate secondary serious problems as a result of 1) the dealing with an intense computations, and 2) very complex software (and, consequently, high level of probability to make some mistakes) used for the implementation of the nested CV. Moreover, we do believe that in most of the cases scientific results produced with the nested CV are not reproducible (in the sense of an absolutely fresh data, which were not used prior).

Homogeneous ensemble, where any single learner is based on the randomly selected fractions of the available samples and features represents a very efficient barrier against traps by a local maximum. Accordingly the solutions obtained using method of the homogeneous ensembles are more stable and reliable. However, in general terms, to ensure a high quality of the ensemble, we have to consider a large number of the single learners, and, accordingly, the related computation process maybe very expensive. The proposed in this paper definition of the CV-passports naturally fits the mechanism of the construction of the ensemble and doesn't require any extra computation time. Based on the fundamental principles of our approach CV-passport will naturally accompany any homogeneous ensemble.

Essentially, the CV-passports are computed against not some particular parts (as in the cases of ordinary cross-validation), but against the whole training set, and reflect very closely the particular design of the corresponding ensemble. Note that the CV-passports maybe used not only as a self-targets, but, also, as a base-ground for the variety of important secondary tasks such as construction of heterogeneous ensembles and definition of the cutting points to transfer decision functions into decision rules.

Generally, we are satisfied with our results, which were obtained online during the PAKDD and Credit data mining contests. Note, that using a conceptually similar method to that described in this paper, we were able to achieve best results (in absolute sense) in another Kaggle-based contest named "Boehringer" [18].

Acknowledgment. Tian-Hsiang Huang was supported in part by the Ministry of Economic Affairs (MOEA) of Taiwan, under Grant number MOEA 101-EC-17-A-03-S1-214.

References

[1] Djukova, E.V., Zhuravlev, Y.I., Sotnezov, R.M.: Construction of an ensemble of logical correctors on the basis of elementary classifiers. Pattern Recognition and Image Analysis 21(4), 599–605 (2011)
[2] Biau, G., Devroye, L., Lugosi, G.: Consistency of random forests and other averaging classifiers. Journal of Machine Learning Research 9, 2015–2033 (2007)
[3] Wang, W.: Some fundamental issues in ensemble methods. In: World Congress on Computational Intelligence, pp. 2244–2251. IEEE, Hong Kong (2008)
[4] Breiman, L.: Random forests. Machine Learning 45(1), 5–32 (2001)
[5] Zhang, B.-L., Pham, T.D., Zhang, Y.: Bagging support vector machine for classification of SELDI-toF mass spectra of ovarian cancer serum samples. In: Orgun, M.A., Thornton, J. (eds.) AI 2007. LNCS (LNAI), vol. 4830, pp. 820–826. Springer, Heidelberg (2007)

[6] Breiman, L.: Bagging predictors. Machine Learning 24, 123–140 (1996)

[7] Guyon, I., Weston, J., Barnhill, S., Vapnik, V.: Gene selection for cancer classification using support vector machines. Machine Learning 46, 389–422 (2002)

[8] Nikulin, V.: Learning with mean-variance filtering, SVM and gradient-based optimization. In: International Joint Conference on Neural Networks, Vancouver, BC, Canada, July 16-21, pp. 4195–4202. IEEE (2006)

[9] Nikulin, V.: Classification of imbalanced data with random sets and mean-variance filtering. International Journal of Data Warehousing and Mining 4(2), 63–78 (2008)

[10] Nikulin, V., McLachlan, G.J., Ng, S.K.: Ensemble approach for the classification of imbalanced data. In: Nicholson, A., Li, X. (eds.) AI 2009. LNCS, vol. 5866, pp. 291–300. Springer, Heidelberg (2009)

[11] Freund, Y., Schapire, R.: A decision-theoretic generalization of on-line learning and an application to boosting. Journal of Computer and System Sciences 55, 119–139 (1997)

[12] Nikulin, V., McLachlan, J.: Classification of imbalanced marketing data with balanced random sets. JMLR: Workshop and Conference Proceedings 7, 89–100 (2009)

[13] Nikulin, V.: On the homogeneous ensembling with balanced random sets and boosting. In: Yao, J., Yang, Y., Słowiński, R., Greco, S., Li, H., Mitra, S., Polkowski, L. (eds.) RSCTC 2012. LNCS, vol. 7413, pp. 180–189. Springer, Heidelberg (2012)

[14] Heckerman, J.: Sample selection bias as a specification error. Econometrica 47(1), 153–161 (1979)

[15] Jelizarow, M., Guillemot, V., Tenenhaus, A., Strimmer, K., Boulesteix, A.L.: Over-optimism in bioinformatics: an illustration. Bioinformatics 26(16), 1990–1998 (2010)

[16] Carpenter, J.: the best analyst win. Science 331, 698–699 (2011)

[17] Cudeck, R., Browne, M.: Cross-validation of covariance structures. Multivariate Behavioral Research 18(2), 147–167 (1983)

[18] Efimov, D., Nikulin, V.: Prediction of a biological response of molecules from their chemical properties. Advanced Science (published in Russian by Vyatka State University) 2(2), 107–123 (2013)

Parallel Sentiment Polarity Classification Method with Substring Feature Reduction

Yaowen Zhang, Xiaojun Xiang, Cunyan Yin, and Lin Shang

State Key Laboratory of Novel Software Technology, Nanjing University,
Nanjing 210046, China

Abstract. Sentiment analysis is an important issue in machine learning, which aims to identify the emotion expressed in corpus. However, sentiment analysis is a difficult task, especially in large-scale data, where feature reduction is needed. In this paper, we propose a parallel feature reduction algorithm for sentiment polarity classification based on a substring method. Specifically, the proposed algorithm is based on parallel computing under the Hadoop platform. The proposed algorithm is examined on a large data set and a K-nearest neighbor algorithm and a Rocchio algorithm are used for classification. Experimental results show that the proposed algorithm outperforms other commonly used methods in terms of the classification performance and the computational cost.

Keywords: Sentiment polarity, Feature extraction, Parallelization.

1 Introduction

Text information can be divided into facts and opinions [8]. A fact is objective expression about some existing things while an opinion is subjective feelings about things [8]. With the development of E-commerce, more and more users to express their opinions about a product or products, news and blog content, etc al. Sentiment Analysis or Opinion Mining is used to identify sentimental tendency so as to understand consumers' spending habits and analyze the public opinion towards hot issues, etc. Therefore, sentiment analysis is an important issue in E-commerce and it is needed to develop an effective sentiment analysis approach.

Obviously, sentiment polarity is dependent on topics or domains. Much work has been done in detecting topics [2][5][6]. However, such work only focused on discovering and analyzing topics of document, and did not conduct sentiment analysis in the text. In such cases, the mining results were not fully used. Some of the existing works, have solved the problem of sentiment classification in many different ways (i.e. from word/phrase level, to sentence and document level) [17][4][13][28][15]. Meanwhile, sentiment classification methond used well in one domain might not work well in another domain [6].

In sentiment classification, feature extraction is an important part of text processing. Ngram, Substring, Substring-group, key-Substring-group and sentiment dictionary are common used feature extraction methods [18]. It has been shown

J. Li et al. (Eds.): PAKDD 2013 Workshops, LNAI 7867, pp. 121–132, 2013.

that sentiment dictionary, bigram and substring feature extraction methonds have good perfomances in sentiment classification [9][19]. As sentiment word identifies the dominant in sentiment classification [25], It is natural to use the existing dictionary as sentiment classification features. Ngram is very popular in text classification [26][27]. For example, "I like maths" can be represented by unigram form: I/like/maths. In bigram form, it can be represented as: I like/like maths. Unigrams are widely used for representing documents in classical text classification tasks, but a unigram appears to be inadequate in description in the case of sentiment analysis [3].

The motivation of this research is to mix features for representing expressions of sentiment. We aim to make full use of richer features to describe complex and subtle expressions of emotion by using a substring reduction feature extraction algorithm. For example,the meaning of a unigram "good" will change the polarity held by the expression "not good" captured by bigram. It will also change the polarity by the expression "not so good" captured by trigram. In order to achieve this, we will propose a new feature reduction algorithm based on a substring method. The proposed algorithm employs the Hadoop platform to complete parallelization algorithms including Rocchio algorithm and K-nearest neighbor (kNN) algorithm, which provides a more stable idea to feature.

2   Preliminary of Sentiment Classification and Feature Extraction

2.1   Sentiment Classification

Sentiment classification is an extensive research topic in sentiment analysis. Sentiment classification is to distinguish the polarity of the subjective evaluation of the text, which can be generally divided into positive and negative (in some cases, there is neutral in this category) [8]. What sentiment classification cares is the view expressed in the text, rather than its subject. sentiment classification is a challenging task.

Document-level sentiment classification can be broadly divided into three categories, which are non-supervised learning, semi-supervised learning and supervised learning. The unsupervised methods identified semantic orientation of each word or phrase, then counted the number of each document semantic orientation of words or phrases. Hu et al [9] classified customers' view using a complete dictionary. Turney [10] used Pointwise Mutual Information to determine the phrases of semantic orientation. Based on Turney's method, Zhang et al [11] has made some improvements, and proposed an Internet-based method for the excavation of the Chinese product reviews. Semi-supervised learning method was combined with the labeled sample and non-labeled sample to learn. Xiaojun et al [12] use English Sentiment classification to solve the problem of Chinese sentiment classification.

It is difficult to find the appropriate emotion dictionary for unsupervised learning and all semi-supervised learning methods require strong assumption. Therefore, unsupervised learning and semi-supervised learning methods achieve low accuracy. Bo Pang et al [15] first reviewed sentiment analysis in document-level with machine learning methods using Nave Bayes, Max Entropy, Support Vector Machine classification algorithm in 2002. Turney [15] used the average value of tendency comment word's occurrences to represent the tendency of the entire review. In 2005, Pang et al [19] further expanded their work by using machine learning methods to 3 star or 4 star movie review . Pang et al [19] use the Nave Bayes and SVM classification methonds with unigrams to classify movie review with the acurracy of 81% and 82.9%. Li et al [20]compared the performance of four machine learning methods in sentiment classification of Chinese comment using N-gram as feature extraction method. A lot of sentiment classification research focused on feature selection methods in recent years [21][22][23][24].

2.2 Feature Extraction

Feature extraction is an important part of text processing, which influence the overall performance of sentiment classification. Ngram, Substring, Substring-group, key-Substring-group and sentiment dictionary are common used feature extraction methods [18]. In this section, we focus on sentiment dictionary, bigram and substring feature extraction methods that have good perfomances in sentiment classification.

Sentiment Word Feature. The methods to process Chinese sentiment polarity have three steps. Firstly, the segmentation tool is used to convert the text into a feature vector. Secondly, the training data is loaded to the algorithm. Thirdly, the test data is put to the trained classifier and get results.

Ngram Feature. Unigram, bigram and trigram are commonly used among Ngram models. Bigram feature extraction, which is shown to be better than other Ngram model in performance [24], is used here.

3 Our Proposed Sentiment Classification Method

In this paper, we propose a new method for sentiment classification. The method has three main procedures: feature extraction algorithm, vector weighted algorithm and sentiment classification procedure, which can be seen in Fig. 1 [24]. We have introduced feature extraction algorithm in section 2, we will continue the following details of the framework.

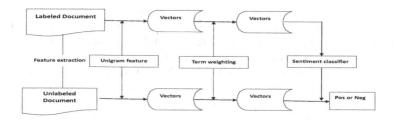

Fig. 1. The sentiment classification framework based on supervised learning method

3.1 Vector Weighted Procedure

The formulation of a problem has a great influence on the accuracy of a learning system [30]. Documents are usually composed of a string by words, so the document must be converted into the form of an appropriate formula for learning algorithms and classification tasks. These algorithms are based on mathematical model that can be measured. Each feature is corresponding to each dimension.

Feature weighted algorithms can be broadly divided into two categories. One is based on its presence, and the other is based on its frequency. In our proposed sentiment algorithm, we use two typical feature weighting algorithms, Bool algorithm and TF-IDF algorithm.

Bool Algorithm. Although algorithms based on frequency is popular, algorithms based on presence achieved better performance [32]. Therefore, we use the algorithm based on presence in this study.

TF-IDF Algorithm. Term Frequency Inverse Document Frequency (TF-IDF) [31], is a common weighting technique for information retrieval and text mining. In a given document, TF (term-frequency) refers to the number of occurrences of a given word in the file of the normalized (the same words, regardless of the importance or not, may have a higher number of words in the long file than the short file).

Bool algorithm is simple, clear and efficient, but it doesn't have weighting mechanism .you can not specify A is more important than B [1]. While TF-IDF has weighting mechanism, it considers the local word frequency (TF) and global word frequency (IDF). TF-IDF is an effective and efficient algorithm to deal with large-scale document applications [1].

3.2 Classification Algorithm

There are many classification algorithms, such as Nave Bayes, decision tree, KNN, neural networks and support vector machine [16]. Among them, the support vector machine is widely used because it can achieve good classification performance. However, its training process is more complicated and computationally more expensive, especially in a distributed environment, and its parallelization method, which involves the iteration of the algorithm, is hard to achieve. So in our method, we choose two more efficient algorithms: Rocchio algorithm and KNN.

Rocchio Algorithm. Rocchio relevance feedback algorithm[32] put forward by Rocchio in 1971 is one of the widely used algorithm in information retrieval. It is initially used optimize relevance feedback query but it can also be used for text classification. The algorithm's advantage lies in its efficiency and it is suitable for use in distributed environment.

k-Nearest Neighbors. k-Nearest Neighbor classification algorithm[33] is one of the easiest machine learning algorithms. KNN methods mainly rely on the limited surrounding neighboring samples, but do not depend on the method of discriminant class field to determine the category. For class field intersecting or overlapping set of samples, KNN method is more appropriate than other methods. Distance can be measured by euclidean distance, cosine similarity et al. Cosine similarity is more suitable for text processing, so we use the cosine similarity as distance metric.

4   Substring Feature Reduction Method

Although substring feature is rarely used in text classification, it has many potential advantages [29]. Firstly, sub-word and super-word can be extracted, and it makes sense to non-theme text classification. Secondly, it avoids tedious segmentation task. Thirdly, different types of documents can be dealt with in a unified approach. Algorithm pseudo code is shown in Algorithm 1. S[j] refers to the jth element of S string. S refers to the phrase split by punctuation. It can be observed from the pseudo code that substring features are actually a collection of all n-gram featues.

Algorithm 1. pseudo of substring feature extraction algorithm

---

Require:
    Input S[1,...,l];
    Output F[1,...,p],p=$\frac{l(l+1)}{2}$;
Ensure:
1: for n = 1 to l do
2:    for i = 1 to l-n+1 do
3:       F.insert(S[i,...,i+n-1]);
4:    end for
5: end for

Note that substring feature dimension is very high, and there are a lot of redundant or meaningless features. We will propose a substring feature reduction algorithm: RemoveRedundance algorithm.

First, in order to filter out meaningless features, we remove the high-frequency words and low-frequency words. We define two parameters, H and L. Features with frequency lower than L are removed, and features with frequency higher than H are also removed. Low frequency features are those infrequent substring and often do not have practical significance. High frequency features are those stop words, and often can not represent a document.

In addition to these meaningless features, there is also a large number of redundant features. For example, "give" and "up" always come in pairs in a corpus. "give" and "up" are redundant features, because we only need a "give up" feature that can represent these three features.

After such a feature reduction procedure, the computational complexity is reduced from $O(n^2)$ to O(n). Algorithm's pseudo-code is shown in Algorithm 2.

Algorithm 2. Substring feature algorithm for attributes reduction

Require:
    FeatureData,L,H;
    ReductFeatureData;
Ensure:
    1: For all features F[1,...,p],compute their frequency TF[1,...,p]
    2: For all features F[1,...,p],if TF(i) < L ,remove F[i]
    3:    else if TF(i) > H,remove F(i)
    4: For remaining features F[1,...,q], if F(i) ⊆ F(j) && TF(i) == TF(j)
    5: remove F(j)

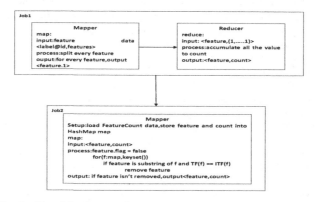

Fig. 2. Algorithm's pseudo-code of MapReduce implementation

With the development of web, the data generated by users is becoming larger and larger. According to some survey results, people send more than 200 million tweets per day. It's hard to find useful information in the large data. At the same time, it is also difficult to process the data in one single computer. In this paper, we use the cloud computing platform Hadoop to parallel our algorithms to process the large-scale data. This algorithm MapReduce implementation process is shown in Fig. 2.

5 Experiments

We have conducted experiments to show the performance of our proposed method on sentiment analysis and compare each algorithm's time complexity and accuracy. We firstly experiment a few corpus using various freeature extraction method combined with two classical classification algorithms (KNN,Rocchio) in the platform Hadoop 0.20.2 [7]. The results are collected in table form to show the performance of our proposed.

5.1 Data Sets

The data set used in this paper is arranged by Excavation and Security of Web Search Laboratory of Beijing Institute of Technology [14]. The data set involves three areas of hotels, notebooks and books. There are four corpus:

Table 1. The number of features of four corpus in three kinds of feature extraction algorithms

Corpus \ Feature Extraction Algorithm	Sentiment Lexicon	Bigram Feature	Substring Feature	
			Before Feature Reduction	After Feature Reduction
ChnSentiCorp-Htl-ba-2000	933	46114	853360	23118
ChnSentiCorp-Htl-del-4000	1256	82701	2037015	42780
ChnSentiCorp-Book-del-4000	1887	94138	2601610	39763
ChnSentiCorp-NB-del-4000	754	41726	825397	15522

1. ChnSentiCorp-Htl-ba-2000,hotel field,positive and negative class 1000 documents with no removed duplicates corpus.
2. ChnSentiCorp-Htl-del-4000,hotel field,positive and negative class 2000 documents with removed duplicates corpus.
3. ChnSentiCorp-Book-del-4000,book field,positive and negative class 2000 documents.
4. ChnSentiCorp-NB-del-4000,notebook field,positive and negative class 2000 documents.

Users can choose to upload their own data,and the data must meet the following requirements:data is a series of Chinese text documents and each document is a comment. The naming of the document must be "neg or pos.documentid.txt".

5.2 Our Feature Reduction Experiment Results

After three features extraction algorithm,which substring features have been reduced and the number of features in the four corpus are shown in Table 1.

From Table 1, it can be seen that the number of features extracted based on sentiment words are much smaller than other feature extraction algorithms.

Substring feature dimension is high, and if we do not do feature reduction, there will be difficulties in the subsequent processing. Meanwhile, useless features and redundant features will reduce the classification accuracy and increase the computational cost. Training data are also based on the reduction features.

5.3   Algorithm Accuracy Analysis

We compare the proposed algorithm with several different methods in feature extraction, feature vector weighting and classification and analyse the classification accuracies.

In KNN, we take k = 5. In substring feature reduction algorithm, we set L = 3 and H is set as half of the total number of documents. Table 2-5 show the classification accuracies of the used algorithms.

Table 2. ChnSentiCorp-Htl-ba-2000: classification accuracy

Feature Extration Method	Feature Vector Weighting Method	Classification Method	Accuracy
Bigram	Bool	Knn	80.0%
Bigram	Bool	Rocchio	88.0%
Bigram	TF-IDF	Knn	83.0%
Bigram	TF-IDF	Rocchio	91.5%
Sentiment Lexicon	Bool	Knn	78.0%
Sentiment Lexicon	Bool	Rocchio	82.0%
Sentiment Lexicon	TF-IDF	Knn	74.5%
Sentiment Lexicon	TF-IDF	Rocchio	87.5%
Substring	Bool	Knn	82.5%
Substring	Bool	Rocchio	86.0%
Substring	TF-IDF	Knn	84.5%
Substring	TF-IDF	Rocchio	91.5%

From Tables 3, 4 and 5, it can be seen that the extraction of features in sentiment words fails to achieve high precision despite that it is the most primitive and intuitive algorithm. This is because the comment itself is very short, and it is not common sentiment word. Meanwhile, it is hard to find out all the sentiment words when there are new sentiment words appear.

From Tables 1-5, we can see that Bigram and Substring feature extraction method is superior to the sentiment word feature extraction method. Sometimes Bigram performs not well (in ChnSentiCorp-Book-del-4000, combined with Knn, its accuracy is only %46), which means it is not very stable and it varies with classification methods. Meanwhilek, substring feature reduction method performs good with every method in our paper. In feature vector weighting algorithm, TF-IDF is superior to Bool algorithm, and in classification algorithm, Rocchio is better than kNN algorithm. Methonds using TF-IDF or Rocchio will obtain a relatively high classification accuracy regardless of the feature extraction methods.

Table 3. ChnSentiCorp-Htl-del-4000:classification accuracy

Feature Extration Method	Feature Vector Weighting Method	Classification Method	Accuracy
Bigram	Bool	Knn	77.2%
Bigram	Bool	Rocchio	84.3%
Bigram	TF-IDF	Knn	80.0%
Bigram	TF-IDF	Rocchio	86.4%
Sentiment Lexicon	Bool	Knn	75.6%
Sentiment Lexicon	Bool	Rocchio	78.7%
Sentiment Lexicon	TF-IDF	Knn	73.2%
Sentiment Lexicon	TF-IDF	Rocchio	84.5%
Substring	Bool	Knn	81.1%
Substring	Bool	Rocchio	87.1%
Substring	TF-IDF	Knn	82.6%
Substring	TF-IDF	Rocchio	85.3%

Table 4. ChnSentiCorp-Book-del-4000:classification accuracy

Feature Extration Method	Feature Vector Weighting Method	Classification Method	Accuracy
Bigram	Bool	Knn	46.0%
Bigram	Bool	Rocchio	89.5%
Bigram	TF-IDF	Knn	68.0%
Bigram	TF-IDF	Rocchio	91.0%
Sentiment Lexicon	Bool	Knn	70.8%
Sentiment Lexicon	Bool	Rocchio	71.3%
Sentiment Lexicon	TF-IDF	Knn	64.7%
Sentiment Lexicon	TF-IDF	Rocchio	65.0%
Substring	Bool	Knn	86.1%
Substring	Bool	Rocchio	87.1%
Substring	TF-IDF	Knn	74.9%
Substring	TF-IDF	Rocchio	90.0%

Table 5. ChnSentiCorp-NB-del-4000:classification accuracy

Feature Extration Method	Feature Vector Weighting Method	Classification Method	Accuracy
Bigram	Bool	Knn	84.0%
Bigram	Bool	Rocchio	82.9%
Bigram	TF-IDF	Knn	78.4%
Bigram	TF-IDF	Rocchio	87.7%
Sentiment Lexicon	Bool	Knn	78.9%
Sentiment Lexicon	Bool	Rocchio	78.4%
Sentiment Lexicon	TF-IDF	Knn	74.1%
Sentiment Lexicon	TF-IDF	Rocchio	81.6%
Substring	Bool	Knn	79.5%
Substring	Bool	Rocchio	68.8%
Substring	TF-IDF	Knn	82.9%
Substring	TF-IDF	Rocchio	85.3%

Table 6. Time cost on feature extraction algorithm.unit:second

Feature Extraction Algorithm Corpus	Sentiment Lexicon	Bigram Feature	Substring Feature	
			Extraction Time(s)	Reduction Time(s)
ChnSentiCorp-Htl-ba-2000	25	18	27	813
ChnSentiCorp-Htl-del-4000	66	34	39	2736
ChnSentiCorp-Book-del-4000	33	36	24	2682

Table 7. Time cost on feature vector weighting algorithm.unit:second

Feature Extraction Algorithm Corpus	Bool	Tfidf
ChnSentiCorp-Htl-ba-2000	77	107
ChnSentiCorp-Htl-del-4000	92	131
ChnSentiCorp-Book-del-4000	90	107
ChnSentiCorp-NB-del-4000	80	104

Table 8. Time cost on classification algorithm. unit: second

Classification Algorithm Corpus	Knn	Rocchio
ChnSentiCorp-Htl-ba-2000	43	80
ChnSentiCorp-Htl-del-4000	59	90
ChnSentiCorp-Book-del-4000	59	83
ChnSentiCorp-NB-del-4000	60	83

5.4   Time Cost Analysis

We calculated the time cost of algorithms, then we analyze the pros and cons of each algorithm in time cost perspective. The computational cost of each method is shown in Table 6.

It can be seen in Table 6, the Bigram feature extraction used the shortest time while substring feature extraction method used the longest computational time. Because substring feature takes all Ngram into consideration. Suppose k is the total number of words in the corpus. All Ngram words will have k^N words. The data processed by substring method is very large. That's why substring method costs so much time.

The Table 7 shows that Bool algorithm used shorter time than TF-IDF. It is recommended to choose the TF-IDF when taking into account both the time and the classification accuracy.

Table 8 shows that KNN used shorter time than Rocchio.

As can be seen from the tables, the performance of the proposed algorithm is good in the data set and can be extended to a massive data mining. If the data is very large, we can choose an efficient algorithm to accomplish the task. If the data is small, the computational cost of different algorithms is not significant. Therefore, it is better to choose an algorithm with a high classification accuracy.

6 Conclusions

This paper aimed to proposed a feature extraction method in sentiment classification problems. We propose a a parallelization feature extraction method on Hadoop platform and compare the proposed method with widely used methods in terms of the classification accuracy and time cost. Experimental results show that the proposed parallelization classification algorithms are suitable for massive data mining. By the description of the process and performance of the algorithm, we conduct experiments to verify the effectiveness of these algorithms.

Acknowledgments. We would like to acknowledge the support from the National Science Foundation of China (No. 61170180), and the Key Program of Natural Science Foundation of Jiangsu Province, China (Grant No. BK2011005).

References

1. Baeza-Yates, R., Ribeiro-Neto, B.: Modern information retrieval. ACM press, New York (1999)
2. Blei, D.M., Ng, A.Y., Jordan, M.I.: Latent dirichlet allocation. J. Mach. Learn. Res. 3, 993–1022 (2003)
3. Dzogang, F., Lesot, M.J., Rfqi, M., Meunier, B.B.: Early Fusion of Low Level Features for Emotion Mining. Biomedical Informatics Insights 5 (2012)
4. Choi, Y., Cardie, C., Riloff, E., Patwardhan, S.: Identifying sources of opinions with conditional random fields and extraction patterns. In: Proceedings of Human Language Technology Conference and Conference on Empirical Methods in Natural Language Processing, Vancouver, British Columbia, Canada, pp. 355–362. Association for Computational Linguistics (October 2005)
5. Titov, I., McDonald, R.: Modeling online reviews 383 with multi-grain topic models. In: WWW 2008: Proceeding of the 17th International Conference on World Wide Web, pp. 111–120. ACM, New York (2008)
6. Lin, C., He, Y.: Joint Sentiment/Topic Model for Sentiment Analysis. In: Proceedings of the 18th ACM Conference on Information and Knowledge Management, pp. 375–384
7. Boss, G., Malladi, P., Quan, D., et al.: Cloud computing. IBM white paper, 1369 (2007)
8. Liu, B.: Web Data Mining: Exploring Hyperlinks,Contents, and Usage Data (Data-Centric Systems and Applications). Springer (2007)
9. Liu, H.M.B.: Mining and summarizing customer reviews. In: Proceedings of the tenth ACM SIGKDD International Conference on Knowledge Discovery and Data Mining, pp. 168–177 (2004)
10. Littman, T.P.M.: Unsupervised Learning of Semantic Orientation from a Hundred-Billion-Word Corpus, in Technical Report ERB-1094, National Research Council Canada (2002)
11. Zhang, Z.Q., Li, Y.J., Ye, Q., Law, R.: Sentiment Classification for Chinese Product Reviews Using an Unsupervised Internet-based Method. In: Proceeding of International Conference on Management Science & Engineering, pp. 3–9 (2008)

12. Wan, X.: Co-Training for Cross-Lingual Sentiment Classification. In: Wan, X. (ed.) Proceedings of the 47th Annual Meeting of the ACL and the 4th IJCNLP of the AFNLP, pp. 235–243 (2009)
13. Kim, S.-M., Hovy, E.: Determining the sentiment of opinions. In: COLING 2004: Proceedings of the 20th International Conference on Computational Linguistics, Morristown, NJ, USA, p. 1367. Association for Computational Linguistics (2004)
14. http://www.datatang.com/member/6880/t02-p1
15. Pang, B., Lee, L., Vaithyanathan, S.: Thumbs up? Sentiment Classification Using Machine Learning Techniques. In: Proceedings of the EMNLP 2002, pp. 79–86 (2002)
16. Michelle, T.M.:Machine Learning. McGraw-Hill Companies, Inc. (1997)
17. Blitzer, J., Dredze, M., Pereira, F.: Biographies, bollywood, boom-boxes and blenders: Domain adaptation for sentiment classification. In: Proceedings of the 45th Annual Meeting of the Association of Computational Linguistics, Prague, Czech Republic, pp. 440–447. Association for Computational Linguistics (June 2007)
18. Pang, B., Lee, L.: Opinion Mining and Sentiment Analysis. Foundations and TrendsR in Information Retrieval 2(12), 1135c (2008), doi:10.1561/1500000001
19. Pang, B., Lee, L.: Seeing stars: Exploiting class relationships for sentiment categorization with respect to rating scales. In: Proceedings of the ACL, pp. 115–124 (2005)
20. Li, J., Sun, M.: Experimental Study on Sentiment Classification of Chinese Review using Machine Learning Techniques. In: Proceedings of IEEE NLP-KE (2007)
21. Pang, B., Lee, L.: A Sentimental Education:Sentiment Analysis Using Subjectivity Summarization Based on Minimum Cuts. In: Proceeding of ACL, pp. 271–278 (2004)
22. Pang, B., Lee, L.: Seeing stars: Exploiting class relationships for sentiment categorization with respect to rating scales. In: Proceedings of the ACL, pp. 115–124 (2005)
23. Phyu Shein, K.P., Nyunt, T.T.S.: Sentiment classification based on Ontology and SVM Classifier. In: Proceedings of ICCSN, pp. 169–172 (2010)
24. Zhai, Z.W., Xu, H., Kang, B., Jia, P.: Exploiting effective features for Chinese sentiment classification. Expert. Syst. Appl. 38(8), 9139–9146 (2011)
25. Liu, B.: Handbook of natural language processing. Sentiment Analysis and Subjectivity, 627–667 (2010)
26. Raaijmakers, S., Kraaij, W.: A shallow approach to subjectivity classification. In: Proceedings of ICWSM, pp. 216–217 (2008)
27. Tan, S., Zhang, J.: An empirical study of sentiment analysis for chinese documents. Expert Systems with Applications 34(4), 2622–2629 (2008)
28. Pang, B., Lee, L.: A sentimental education: sentiment analysis using subjectivity summarization based on minimum cuts. In: ACL 2004: Proceedings of the 42nd Annual Meeting on Association for Computational Linguistics, Morristown, NJ, USA, p. 271. Association for Computational Linguistics (2004)
29. Zhang, D., Lee, W.: Extracting key-Substring-group features for text classification, pp. 474–483. ACM, New York (2006)
30. Joachims, T.: A probabilistic analysis of the Rocchio algorithm with TF-IDF for text categorization. In: Proceedings of ICML, pp. 143–151 (1997)
31. Salton, G., Buckley, C.: Term Weighting Approaches in Automatic Text Retrieval. Information Processing and Management 24(5), 513–523 (1988)
32. Rocchio: Relevance Feedback in Information Retrieval. In: Salton (ed.) The SMART Retrieval System: Experiments. In Automatic Document Processing, ch. 14, pages 313–323. Prentice-Hall (1971)
33. Cover, T.M., Hart, P.E.: Nearest neighbor pattern classification. IEEE Transactions on Information Theory 13(1), 21–27 (1967)

Identifying Authoritative and Reliable Contents in Community Question Answering with Domain Knowledge

Lifan Guo and Xiaohua Hu

College of Information Science and Technology, Drexel University
3141 Chestnut Street, Philadelphia, PA19104, USA
{lg367,xh29}@drexel.edu

Abstract. Community Question Answering (CQA) has emerged as a popular forum for users to ask and answer questions. Over the last few years, CQA portals such as Yahoo answers and Baidu Zhidao have exploded in popularity, and now provide a viable alternative to general purpose Web search. A number of answers submitted to address questions on CQA sites compose a valuable knowledge repository, which could be a gold mine for information retrieval as well as text mining. Two important questions in CQA research are focused on the quality of contents and the reputation of the answerers. Previous approaches for retrieving relevant and high quality content have been proposed, but not much work has been done on providing an integrated framework to solve these two problems. Besides, no research work has used both text and link information in their methods via leveraging existing ratings of answers and questions. In this paper, we present a novel approach to analyze questions and answers based on the topic modeling framework with Dirichlet forest priors (LDA-DF)[8]. We utilize information obtained from LDA-DF to construct a joint topical and link model to identify authorities and reliable answers on a CQA site.We evaluate our methods in a dataset obtained from Yahoo! Answers. With the new representation of topical structures on CQA datasets, using a limited amount of web resource, we show significant improvements over the state-of-art methods LDA-DF, LDA, and HLDA on performance of authority identification and answer ranking.

Keywords: Answer Ranking, Authority Ranking, Community Question Answering.

1   Introduction

Community Question Answering (CQA) sites have emerged in the past few years as Web 2.0 becomes more and more popular such as Yahoo! Answers, Baidu Zhidao and Live QnA. The reasons behind this boom are: 1. Traditional QA System is not able to satisfy user's information demand in various domains 2. Online users are preferred to be involved. 3. Answers for a certain question need to be generated in real time response by anyone in the community and trust is based on intimacy [9,13,25]. The

J. Li et al. (Eds.): PAKDD 2013 Workshops, LNAI 7867, pp. 133–142, 2013.
© Springer-Verlag Berlin Heidelberg 2013

volume of questions answered on CQA site so far exceeds the number of questions answered by library reference services [8]. In CQA, users exchange and share their knowledge explicitly by asking questions or answering questions in all predefined categories. After enough number of answers is collected during this process, the best answer would be chosen by the asker and all answers would be rated by thumbs up or thumbs down. Then this question would be closed. The resulting question and answer archives are numerous knowledge repositories.[7] With such valuable knowledge repositories, information seeking based on these repositories has proven to be more effective and successful compared to general web search.

Considering the quality issues of questions and answers as well as the reputations of users, two major tasks had attracted a lot of researches. They are: how to identify reliable answers in CQA [1,2,3,14,17,20,26,27] and how to identify authorities in CQA [6,7,9,10,16,17,21,23,24,34]. However, a major problem of those approaches is that they ignore the importance of topical information in questions answering community For example, to identify reliable answers, a question asking "Chinese Buffet" in "Philadelphia" would only be well responded by the answer that response to "Chinese Buffet" and "Philadelphia" accurately and succinctly, such as "Ruby Buffet in Columbus Blvd". Any other answers lacking such information would be an inaccurate answer, such as "IHOP" or "restaurant in DC". Therefore, applying such topical analysis of questions and answers would help to identify good answers. On the other hand, to identify authorities, an expert in History may not give good suggestions in Gardening. Obviously, it would be better to give authority score based on different topics. Besides, existing approaches ignore utilization of existing questions and answers repository. Such invaluable domain knowledge extracted from existing Q/A pairs should be further utilized for topic analysis, which in turn help to identify reliable answers and identify authorities. In fact, such relationships between terms achieve two links Must-Link (ML) and Cannot-Link (CL) in a novel topic modeling framework LDA with Dirichlet Forest priors [8]. This paper aims to address identifying authoritative and reliable contents in CQA. First we rely on existing Q/A pairs to extract ML and CL relationships between n-grams in Q/A. Next we integrate the learned knowledge into LDA-DF as domain knowledge to discover latent topics in contents of questions, associated answers, and latent topic interests of users. Then we use this information as new features in existing methods to help to achieve better performance in answers ranking and authority ranking. The experimental results demonstrate that learned information improves the performance of answer ranking and authority ranking.

The remainder of this paper is organized as follows: Section 2 reviews related work. Section 3 introduces the proposed method of constructing ML and CL relationships. In Section 4, we present and discuss experimental results. Finally, we conclude the paper in section 5.

2   Related Work

In recent years, Question Answering research has shifted its focus from generic question answering task [1, 33] to Community Question Answering since the explosion of Web 2.0. According to Shal et al. [29], Community Question Answering consists of three components: a system for users to submit questions and answers, a mechanism to evaluate questions and answers, a social network. CQA has already attracted a great deal of attention for different research tasks. In general, two primary tasks are mapped out [6] research on the content of CQA sites, including analyses of the content of questions and answers [16][18][20], in which authors are trying to evaluate quality of questions and answers, and research on prediction of authorities in Question Answering Community, in which authors are analyzing the reputation systems in these sites.

On the other hand, topic models, such as Latent Dirichlet Allocation (LDA) [9], have achieved success in discovering latent topics from text documents. Recently, a lot of research is focused on developing better topic model algorithms with more information. Particularly, some topic models are employed in CQA domain in the purpose of utilizing underlying topics of text to address those challenges. One direction of topic modeling in CQA is to give a general generative model for the whole activities incurred in CQA. For example, Liu et al. [38] developed a general generative topic model for questions and answers in CQA by adding link information between users. Another study of topic modeling in CQA is to utilize existing topic models to generate additional features of questions, answers and users. Experiments demonstrate that those features would help boost performance in addressing challenges in CQA. For example, Asli el.at [1] used LDA model and hierarchical LDA to uncovering underlying topic information of questions and answers, then calculate the similarity between questions and answers. Hong el.at [18] used pLSA as topic model and added the features learned into PageRank algorithm to rank authorities of answerers. Their methods, however, did not use existing rated questions and answers as domain knowledge. To the best of our knowledge, there is no research work to use such information. In topic models domain, Andrzejesski el.at [8] had incorporated domain knowledge using a novel Dirichlet Forest prior in a Latent Dirichlet Allocation framework. Experiments demonstrated that their model is able to follow and generalize beyond user specific domain knowledge. Their method, however, has not been used for CQA domain tasks and also lacks a mechanism to automatically extract domain information.

In our approach, we will extract domain information automatically from existing Q/A pairs and then incorporate that knowledge into LDA-DF to uncover topical information. And then use topical information to address reliable answers and authority.

3   Methodology of Incorporating Knowledge into Answer and Authority Ranking

Incorporating domain knowledge into CQA is our major contribution. Therefore, how to retrieve domain knowledge from existing q/a pairs is important. We first define two different kinds of Q/A pairs: best answer and inappropriate answer. Best answer is the answer rated by users as the best in the community; inappropriate answer is the most unfavorable answer being selected by users through ratings. Then we define methods to construct ML and CL relations of terms from these kinds of q/a pairs. Based on these two different kinds of knowledge, we use LDA-DF to generate topical feature vectors for questions and answers. Feature vectors are used to measure the degree of similarity [1] between each q/a pair for the purpose of reliable contents identification. Finally, the topical information would be used for authority ranking by using topical HITS algorithm [18]. A proper extracting method is crucial for incorporating knowledge into LDA-DF. In our research, we borrow the idea of two different kinds of relations defined in [8] for incorporating knowledge. Our contribution is that we extend their work by applying it into CQA domain and constructing domain knowledge automatically. The details of the process are described below.

3.1   Automatically Construct Must Link Relations of Terms in Existing Best Q/A Pairs

Leveraging Wikipedia and Search Engine to Extract Important N-Grams
The goal of this step is to extract all terms from questions and the corresponding best answers for further analysis. We only use the best answers for questions since we believe the best answer could respond every topic emerged in the question, thus provides domain knowledge we need.

For example, a question with subject: Looking for best Chinese Buffet in Philly and with content:Q:"I have been to several in the area that I've enjoyed at first. However, for one reason or another, eventually have been turned off-waiters coughing around tables, low class clientele getting loud and disruptive, dirty restrooms, things of that nature I want to visit one tonight, so maybe someone can recommend a place I haven't been to yet. I 'd like recent review, not ones from things I find on websites."

Best answer: "The Ruby Buffet on Columnbs Blvd is a great Chinese buffet. The food always seems fresh and they have a nice variety. They have custom lo mein."

All possible n-grams are extracted from Q/A pairs. And those n-grams are searched in Wikipedia article titles. We use search engine and Wikipedia instead of POS tools since some meaningful and important terms in QA, like "Ruby might be ignored by POS tools.

Leveraging Search Engine to Set ML Constrains
A popular and effective way to calculate the semantic distance between terms is the Normalized Google Distance [26]. Specifically, the normalized Google distance between two search terms x and y is:

$$NGD(x,y) = \frac{Max(\log f(x), \log f(y), \log f(x,y))}{\log M \times \min(\log f(x), \log f(y))} \tag{1}$$

Where M is the total number of web pages searched by Google and we set M as 500000000000.00 in the experiment. f(x) is the number of return pages searched by Google. Larger NGD value indicates a stronger semantic relation.

3.2   Automatically Construct ML Relations of Terms in Existing Q/A Pairs.

Four rules are applied here to construct ML relations. Rule 1: ML constrains are transitive. {A,B} and {B,C} infer {A,B,C} Rule 2: If n-grams in question and answers have overlapping terms, then we set ML for them. As for the example above, we have ML constraint of {"rubby buffet", "buffet", "Chinese"}. After we eliminate those n-grams in Rule 1, we get the semantic distance between n-grams in the Q/A pair. And we selected the largest pairs compared to the others. Rule 3: We calculate mean square error of each row, if that value is too low, it indicates that that term is too general. As for the example above, "great", "waiters" are eliminated. Rule 4: for the remaining tokens, the pair of tokens with the highest value is picked up and set ML constrain for them. After applying these four rules, two ML relations are automatically constructed.   {"rubby buffet", "buffet", "Chinese buffet", "Chinese","lo mein"}, {"philly","Columbus blvd"}.

3.3   Automatically Construct Cannot Link Relations of Terms in Existing Inappropriate Q/A Pairs

After ratings, each answer has "thumbs up" and "thumbs down" to reflect its acceptance by the users. Inappropriate answer is defined as the answer has the most negative value in term of "thumbs down" number subtract "thumbs up number".For example:Q: "Do you think that "man" is to blame for global warming, or is nature taking its course?"Inappropriate Answer:" No, God is preparing to fry us!!"In this example, this answer received 5 thumbs down rating on that. We present a method to automatically extract CL relations from this example as below:

3.4   Leveraging Wikipedia and Search Engine to Extract Important N-Grams.

We want to extract important tokens from questions and answers to generate CL relations. We only consider noun phrases to simplify the problem Therefore, we use part-of-speech tool to process both questions and answers to choose tokens based on three criteria: (1), tokens in answers containing terms that not appeared in the question, (2), tokens should be tagged as NN in the tool, (3) Tokens are either in Wikipeadia titles or able to have search results in the search engine.For the example above, we have:
Q: global, warming, natural, global warming

3.5   Leveraging Search Engine to Set CL Constrains

We constructed a matrix of these tokens for Q/A pairs and we can choose God and global warming since they have 0.9 similarity.Similarly, we calculated the mean square error of each row, if the value is too low, it indicates the semantic relations of these two terms are too weak. Therefore, we would set CL constrain on them.Besides, for some Q/A pairs, if there is no search result from the search engine, we would set CL constrain on them.Finally if CL constrains conflicts with ML constrains. CL constrains has priority to be considered. In this example, "global warming" and "God" are set as CL constrains. After we have this ML and CL, we applied those domain knowledge directly to DF-LDA model.[8]. After applying LDA-DF with incorporating domain knowledge, we have global topic distribution of each n-gram in the dataset and topic distribution of each q/a pair. We use these features for ranking answers, we borrowed the idea from [1] to calculate the similarity between every pair of Q/A based on two measures via topical information generated by LDA-DF. we apply the model to in [1] to rank answers to questions based on the extracted topical information from LDA-DF.

3.6   Topical Link Analysis for User Reputation

For ranking For ranking authorities, each user has discrete topical distribution, which is calculated as the sum of topical distribution of all questions and answers that users gave in the community Therefore, for user ui $\sum_{d \in D(ui)} P(z|d)$ Where, d denotes a question or an answer. D(ui) represents all the questions and answers user i produces. In the Topical HITS model [18], each node represents the user in CQA. A user answering another user's question creates an in-link to itself, vice versa. Each node has hub value H(ui), authority value A(ui) over topics and topical distribution value P(z|ui).The interaction between nodes can be represented based on the following mutual reinforcement relations. The advantage of this approach is that we can consider topical authority of each user.In details, the random walk model in Topical HITS is a multi-surfer scheme represented in [18]. Where, u denotes the nodes v links to; α is the probability of staying in the same topic; A(u) and H(v) represents the vector of authority and hub value on each topic, respectively; I(u) and O(v) are   the number of in-links that u has and the number of out-links that v has, respectively.

4   Experiments

In this section, we conduct the experimental study using data from Yahoo! Answers. We mainly use LDA-DF to extract topical features from questions, answers and users and add those features to rank answers and authorities. Therefore, we compare other topic models, like LDA and HLDA with LDA-DF in feature extraction step. Then use those features to rank answers. As for ranking authorities, we not only compare different features extracted from LDA, LDA-DF and HLDA, but also compare Z-score [16], HITS algorithm and Topical HITS algorithm with different topical features. We use 10 cross-validation methods.

4.1   Yahoo! Answers Data

In our test data set, there are 216,563 questions, 1,981,992 answers, 171,676 users and 100 categories extract from Yahoo! Answer Data. Two different categories: Biology and History are used in the experiment considering they contain more domain knowledge.

4.2   Evaluation Metrics

For ranking answers, we use:

Average Precision $@K$ in CQA: To leverage the ratings of answers, we assume that good answers will have more positive number of thumbs up. Therefore, for a given question, it is to measure the mean fraction of thumbs up number received in relevant answers ranked in the top K results compare to entire thumbs up number received in all the answers; the higher the precision the better the performance is:

$$\text{precision}@k = \frac{\sum(\textit{thumbs up number of K relevant answers})}{\sum(\textit{thumbs up number of all answers})} \tag{2}$$

Mean Reciprocal Rank: The MRR of an individual query is the reciprocal of the rank at which the best answer is returned, or 0 if none of the top K results contain the best answer. For ranking authorities, we use percentage of best answers in top K authorities with different method to evaluate the performance. The idea behind this is that top K authorities should be able to give better answers in the community.

4.3   Answer Ranking Results

Table 4 shows the results of applying LDA-DF into ranking answers in the community via automatically learning ML and CL constrains, compared to applying LDA and HLDA method. The bold values in table are improved results compared to the baseline. From Table 4, we can see that applying LDA-DF always gets the best results across two different datasets. In most cases, they can significantly improve the performance of ranking answers. This indicates that integrating knowledge into ranking answers could help us to find better answers.

4.4   Authority Ranking Results

Table 5 shows the result of using topical information in Topical HITS algorithm to rank authorities. We compare z-score, HITS algorithm and Topical HITS algorithm, where in Topic HITS algorithm we use topical information generated from LDA, HLDA and LDA-DF respectivelyTable 6 displays the best answer percentage for top k authorities evaluated of the baselines and Topical HITS algorithm with LDA-DF. Overall, the best Topical HITS algorithm variant consistently outperforms other baselines across all different evaluation metrics. Particularly, when we select top 2 authorities in the ranking list, the best answer percentage improves dramatically in Topical HITS algorithm with LDA and HLDA. The average percent of best answers for top 5 users with high authority values is often significantly higher than the average for all users in the category. However, the adoption of which topical model as features in HITS algorithm is better is still subject to different category.

Table 1. Answer Ranking Results

	MMR	Precision@1	Precision@5
Biology_LDA	42.7	20.1	64.4
Biology_HLDA	55.8	33.1	71
Biology_DF_LDA	**70.1**	**48.3**	82
History_LDA	48.3	53.1	84.0
History_HLDA	59.3	61.2	84.0
History_DF_LDA	**68.4**	**80.3**	84.0

Table 2. Authority Ranking Results

	Top_1	Top_2	Top_5	Average best answers for all users (History)	Average best answers for all users (Biology)
Z_S@H	11%	20%	24%	15%	N/A
H_A@H	8%	11%	40%	15%	N/A
T_H_LDA@H	12%	**30%**	45%	15%	N/A
T_H_HLDA@H	10%	21%	**50%**	15%	N/A
T_H_DF_LDA@H	**13%**	8%	42%	15%	N/A
Z_S@B	15%	17%	30%	N/A	23%
H_A@B	13%	15%	45%	N/A	23%
T_H_LDA@B	14%	32%	**50%**	N/A	23%
T_H_HLDA@B	12%	**60%**	43%	N/A	23%
T_H_DF_LDA@B	8%	16%	30%	N/A	23%

5   Conclusion and Future Work

In this paper, we present a general framework for leveraging existing question answer pair and their ratings in the community to improve answers ranking and authority ranking performance. Based on two different constrains, Must-Link constrains and Cannot-Link constrains, we are able to create topical features for questions, answers and users. They are used as extra information in existing models to evaluate the performance.For answers ranking, the proposed framework is tested with LDA-DF, LDA, and HLDA to evaluate the similarity of question answer pairs. For authority ranking, the proposed framework is tested with Z-score, HITs algorithm and Topical HITs Algorithm on two datasets: biology category and history category. Based on the empirical results, we can draw the following conclusions: (1) Ratings of questions and answers could be invaluable repository to generate domain knowledge automatically. (2)Incorporating domain knowledge generated in the community could help to boost performance of answers ranking dramatically. (3) Incorporating topical information in the users could help to boost performance of authority ranking.We believe that our findings can be extended to other applications in the Community Question Answers, such as similar question search and new category exploration. Besides, the constructed ML and CL rules could be further used in the evaluation of new question and answers. For future work, we will further use more existing questions and answers data with ratings in the construction of ML and CL constrains, we will explore how to utilize that information for other applications in other domains.

References

1. Celikyilmaz, A., Hakkani-Tur, D., Tur, G.: LDA based similarity modeling for question answering. In: Proceedings of the NAACL HLT 2010 Workshop on Semantic Search (2010)
2. Hickl, A.: Answering questions with authority. In: Proceeding of the 17th ACM Conference on Information and Knowledge Management, pp. 1261–1270 (2008)
3. Pal, A., Counts, S.: Identifying topical authorities in microblogs. In: Proceedings of the Fourth ACM International Conference on Web Search and Data Mining, pp. 45–54
4. McCallum, A., Corrada-Emmanuel, A., Wang, X.: Topic and role discovery in social networks. Journal of Artificial Intelligence Research, 786–791 (2005)
5. Rasmussen, C.E.: The infinite Gaussian mixture model. Advances in Neural Information Processing Systems 12, 554–560 (2000)
6. Shah, C., Pomerantz, J.: Evaluating and predicting answer quality in community QA. In: Proceeding of the 33rd International ACM SIGIR Conference on Research and Development in Information Retrieval, pp. 411–418
7. Andrzejewski, D., Zhu, X., Craven, M.: Incorporating domain knowledge into topic modeling via Dirichlet Forest priors. In: Proceedings of the 26th Annual International Conference on Machine Learning, Montreal, Quebec, Canada, June 14-18, pp. 25–32 (2009)
8. Horowitz, D., Kamvar, S.D.: The anatomy of a large-scale social search engine. In: Proceedings of the 19th International Conference on World Wide Web, pp. 431–440
9. Blei, D.M., Ng, A.Y., Jordan, M.I.: Latent dirichlet allocation. The Journal of Machine Learning Research 3, 993–1022 (2003)
10. Agichtein, E., Liu, Y., Bian, J.: Modeling information-seeker satisfaction in community question answering. ACM Transactions on Knowledge Discovery from Data (TKDD) 3, 10 (2009)
11. Agichtein, E., Castillo, C., Donato, D., Gionis, A., Mishne, G.: Finding high-quality content in social media. In: Proceedings of the International Conference on Web Search and Web Data Mining 2008, pp. 183–194 (2008)
12. Zhang, J., Ackerman, M.S., Adamic, L.: Expertise networks in online communities: structure and algorithms. In: Proceedings of the 16th International Conference on World Wide Web 2007, pp. 221–230 (2007)
13. Kleinberg, J.M.: Authoritative sources in a hyperlinked environment. Journal of the ACM (JACM) 46, 604–632 (1999)
14. Hong, L., Yang, Z.: Incorporating participant reputation in community-driven question answering systems. In: Symposium on Social Intelligence and Networking (2009)
15. Bian, J., Liu, Y., Zhou, D., Agichtein, E., Zha, H.: Learning to recognize reliable users and content in social media with coupled mutual reinforcement. In: Proceedings of the 16th International Conference on World Wide Web 2009, pp. 51–60 (2009)
16. Ko, J., Nyberg, E., Si, L.: A probabilistic graphical model for joint answer ranking in question answering. In: Proceedings of the 30th Annual International ACM SIGIR Conference on Research and Development in Information Retrieval 2007, pp. 343–350 (2007)

17. Sun, K., Cao, Y., Song, X., Song, Y.I., Wang, X., Lin, C.Y.: Learning to recommend questions based on user ratings. In: Proceeding of the 18th ACM Conference on Information and Knowledge Management 2009, pp. 751–758 (2009)
18. Adamic, L.A., Zhang, J., Bakshy, E., Ackerman, M.S.: Knowledge sharing and yahoo answers: everyone knows something. In: Proceeding of the 17th International Conference on World Wide Web 2008, pp. 665–674 (2008)
19. Page, L.: S. Brin The PageRank citation ranking: bring order to the Web. Technical report, Stanford Digital Library Technologies Project (1998)
20. Nie, L., Davison, B.D., Qi, X.: f. In: Proceedings of the 29th Annual International ACM SIGIR Conference on Research and Development in Information Retrieval 2006, pp. 91–98 (2006)
21. Bilotti, M.W., Ogilvie, P., Callan, J., Nyberg, E.: Structured retrieval for question answering. In: Proceedings of the 30th Annual International ACM SIGIR Conference on Research and Development in Information Retrieval 2007, pp. 351–358 (2007)
22. Suryanto, M.A., Lim, E.P., Sun, A., Chiang, R.H.L.: Quality-aware collaborative question answering: methods and evaluation. In: Proceedings of the 32th Annual International ACM SIGIR Conference on Research and Development in Information Retrieval 2009, pp. 142–151 (2009)
23. Bouguessa, M., Dumoulin, B., Wang, S.: Identifying authoritative actors in question-answering forums: the case of yahoo! answers. In: Proceeding of the 14th ACM SIGKDD International Conference on Knowledge Discovery and Data Mining 2008, pp. 866–874 (2008)
24. Jurczyk, P., Agichtein, E.: Discovering authorities in question answer communities by using link analysis. In: Proceedings of the Sixteenth ACM Conference on Conference on Information and Knowledge Management 2007, pp. 919–922 (2007)
25. Han, K.S., Song, Y.I., Rim, H.C.: Probabilistic model for definitional question answering. In: Proceedings of the 29th Annual International ACM SIGIR Conference on Research and Development in Information Retrieval 2006, pp. 212–219 (2006)
26. Cilibrasi, R., Vitanyi, P.: Automatic Meaning Discovery Using Google (2004), http://xxx.lanl.gov/abs/cs.CL/0412098
27. Griffiths, T.L., Steyvers, M.: Finding scientific topics. Proceedings of the National Academy of Sciences of the United States of America 101, 5228 (2004)
28. Kao, W.C., Liu, D.R., Wang, S.W.: Expert finding in question-answering websites: a novel hybrid approach. In: Proceedings of the 2010 ACM Symposium on Applied Computing, pp. 867–871 (2010)
29. Noguchi, Y.: Web searches go low-tech: You ask, a person answers. Washington Post, page A 1 (2006)
30. Liu, Y., Niculescu-Mizil, A., Gryc, W.: Topic-link LDA: joint models of topic and author community. In: Proceedings of the 26th Annual International Conference on Machine Learning, Montreal, Quebec, Canada, June 14-18, pp. 665–672 (2009)
31. Gyongyi, Z., Koutrika, G., Pedersen, J., Garcia-Molina, H.: Questioning Yahoo! Answers. In: Proceedings of the 28th Annual International ACM SIGIR Conference on Research and Development in Information Retrieval (2007)

On the Application of Multi-class Classification in Physical Therapy Recommendation

Jing Zhang[1], Douglas Gross[2], and Osmar R. Zaïane[1]

[1] Department of Computing Science
[2] Department of Physical Therapy,
University of Alberta, Edmonton, Alberta, Canada
{jzhang14,dgross,zaiane}@ualberta.ca

Abstract. Recommending optimal rehabilitation intervention for injured workers that would lead to successful return-to-work (RTW) is a challenge for clinicians. Currently, the clinicians are unable to identify with complete confidence which intervention is best for a patient and the referral is often made in trial and error fashion. Only 58% recommendations are successful in our dataset. We aim to develop an interpretable decision support system using machine learning to assist the clinicians. We use various re-sampling techniques to tackle the multi-class imbalance and class overlap problem in real world application data. The final model has shown promising potential in classification compared to human baseline and has been integrated into a web-based decision-support tool that requires additional validation in a clinical sample.

Keywords: multi-class imbalance, re-sampling, clinical decision-support, rule-based learning.

1 Introduction

Decision support systems (DSS) in clinical prognosis have received increased attention from researchers. In this paper, we develop a system to help clinicians categorize injured workers and recommend appropriate rehabilitation programs based on the unique characteristics of individual worker.

Our system is a web application consisting of a user interface and a knowledge base. Unlike many DSS using knowledge bases developed manually by domain experts, we use rule-based machine learning algorithms to learn a set of rules from data. The rules can be further modified and tuned by the experts. By doing so, the experts can inject their own knowledge into the discovered rule set.

The major challenge of generating the knowledge base is the presence of multi-class imbalance and class overlap in our real clinical dataset. Directly using off-the-shelf classifiers is not a solution since these classifiers would be biased with class imbalance. Typically, since most classifiers assume a balanced training set, data distribution is altered before training by over-sampling a minority class and under-sampling a majority class. However, it is not realistic to simply balancing the dataset with complex class overlap. We compare and analyze various data

J. Li et al. (Eds.): PAKDD 2013 Workshops, LNAI 7867, pp. 143–154, 2013.

re-sampling and cleaning methods to tackle these problems. We find that the combination of SMOTE [4] with Tomek Link [1] and RIPPER [6] can produce meaningful recommendation rules as evaluated by our domain expert. Moreover, the combination of class decomposition and data processing method can help the classification on the minority class examples.

The rest of the paper is organized as follows: We provide the background of the project in Section 2, and describe the system design methods, model and implementation in Section 3. In Section 4, we discuss the evaluation of our model and conclude in Section 5 with a summary and future study.

2   Background

Work-related musculoskeletal conditions are some of the most burdensome health conditions in terms of personal, societal and economic costs[8,7,3]. Low back pain is a leading cause of work disability and was recently identified as the sixth most disabling health condition worldwide in terms of overall disease burden[5].

In general, each injured worker receives a return-to-work (RTW) assessment and a following rehabilitation treatment. This is a classification process which involves assigning patients to appropriate rehabilitation programs that lead to successful return-to-work (RTW) based on their clinical and work-related characteristics (obtained from the assessment). There are five types of rehabilitation programs in total labeled as prog0, prog3, prog4, prog5 and prog6.

Each rehabilitation program has two possible outcomes:

- The program leads to successful return-to-work at a pre-determined time.
- An unsuccessful result at that pre-determined time followed by subsequent rehabilitation programs.

Although it is possible that multiple rehabilitation programs can lead to return-to-work for a patient, we cannot determine them since we cannot possibly let a patient go through multiple programs at once to observe the outcomes. Therefore, an important assumption is that for each patient there exists only one appropriate program. If patients are correctly categorized into the true appropriate program, they return to work. Otherwise, there will be no successful RTW. Under the assumption above, we could determine a patient's return-to-work status in advance based on the classification result. The main idea here is to build a classification model that categorizes an injured worker into the appropriate rehabilitation program leading to RTW.

3   System Design and Implementation

3.1   System Requirements

The system we are developing has the following requirements:

- The classification model should be interpretable. The users should be able to see the evidence supporting the recommendations made by the system. Rule-based algorithms are more desirable.
- The system should provide multiple predictions with support evidence (e.g., supporting rules or guidelines) so the users can choose the most appropriate one under different considerations.
- The system should include a limited number of variables.

3.2 Data Analysis

The dataset is from an outcome evaluation database managed by the Workers' Compensation Board Alberta. This includes data on workers in the province of Alberta who filed compensation claims for musculoskeletal injuries and who were referred to rehabilitation facilities for Return-to-Work assessment. WCB-Alberta's administrative database was augmented by clinical data from rehabilitation providers who are contracted to file reports at time of claimants' admission and discharge from rehabilitation programs.

The dataset of mainly the year of 2010 contains 14484 cases of injured workers, of which 8611 were unique cases and included in further analysis. To train a classification model that predicts successful interventions, we extract only the successful cases. The successful outcome is when the injured worker receives no compensation at 30 days after the assessment admission. In total, 4859 cases are extracted. The new dataset is highly-skewed as shown in Table 1. The rest of the data consisting of unsuccessful cases is used to train a negative model. The dataset includes 200 features. We consulted the experts from the Department of Physical Therapy to check each variable and eliminate those that are absolutely irrelevant from the perspective of clinical practice. 59 features are selected for further investigation.

Table 1. Class Distribution of the Final Dataset

Class	prog0	prog3	prog4	prog5	prog6
num of records	1828	84	2286	96	582

3.3 Method

The class distribution in the dataset is severely imbalanced as shown in Table 1. With class imbalance, the classifier becomes biased towards the majority classes over-shadowing the minority classes. Possible solutions for this problem are cost-sensitive learning, attaching costs to misclassifications, and re-sampling techniques, adjusting the data distribution. Since we cannot obtain the costs of misclassifications, we focus on the re-sampling techniques.

We use a variety of known re-sampling techniques including 1) over-sampling: SMOTE [4] and 2) data cleaning (under-sampling) methods: Tomek Link [1],

Edited Nearest Neighbor (ENN) [11] and Neighbor Cleaning Rule (NCR) [9]. These are used to mitigate the imbalance and to weed out noise in the data.

However, these methods are only validated in the literature on binary datasets (2 classes). Their effectiveness is unknown for multi-class imbalance problems. We apply the re-sampling techniques directly on the dataset as well as combining class decomposition with the re-sampling techniques The details of each method are described below:

SMOTE: SMOTE stands for Synthetic Minority Over-sampling Technique. It manipulates the feature values of data examples that are nearest neighbors to each other in order to form new synthetic minority class examples. It generalizes the data space and thus can avoid overfitting to some extent.

Tomek Links: If two data examples from different classes are the 1 nearest neighbors to each other, they form a Tomek Link. Either both of them are borderline points, or one of them is noise invading the data space of the other class. Generally, we can remove both points in a Tomek Link.

Neighborhood Cleaning Rule(NRC): Unlike ENN, NCR finds each data example whose class label differs from the class of at least two of its three nearest neighbors. If this example belongs to the majority class, remove it. Otherwise, remove its nearest neighbors which belong to the majority class.

SMOTE + Tomek Link: The main reason for this combination is that the synthetic data from a minority class might invade the majority class too deeply and with the cleaning of Tomek Links, we could avoid potential overfitting.

3.4   Algorithms

Naive Bayes, C4.5 and RIPPER classifiers were all investigated; however, the best results were obtained with RIPPER. We briefly present these methods.

Naive Bayes: The Naive Bayes algorithm applies the Bayes theorem to compute the likelihood that an unseen object belongs to a certain class C_i $(i = 1, 2, ..., k)$ given the attribute values in the object. Then the algorithm assigns the object to the class with the maximum likelihood. The algorithm relies on a naive assumption that given the class label, all attributes are mutually independent. Although the assumption seems over-simplified, it has shown its competitiveness in many practical situations.

Equation 1 shows that given a test case t with values of f_1 to f_n, we can use Bayes rule to calculate the probability of class C_i $(i = 1, 2, ..., k)$.

$$p(C_i|f_1, f_2, f_3, ..., f_n) = \frac{p(C_i)p(f_1, f_2, f_3, ..., f_n|C_i)}{p(f_1, f_2, f_3, ..., f_n)} \tag{1}$$

Based on the assumption of conditional independence, Equation 1 can be represented by Equation 2 as followed.

$$p(C_i|f_1, f_2, f_3, ..., f_n) = \frac{p(C_i) \prod_{j=1}^{n} p(f_j|C_i)}{p(f_1, f_2, f_3, ..., f_n)} \tag{2}$$

Then according to the maximum a posteriori (MAP) decision rule, one can classify a test instance t using Equation 3 as followed.

$$classification(t) = arg\,max\,p(C_i) \prod_{j=1}^{n} p(f_j|C_i) \tag{3}$$

C4.5: C4.5 [10] is a well-known decision tree induction algorithm. Each node in the tree represents a selected feature and the tree branches out based on the values in the node. The leaf node represents a class. A new instance is classified by testing against the feature at each node and following the branch of the tree based on the observed value in the instance. This process repeats until the instance reaches the leaf node and is assigned to the class of the leaf.

Associative Classification: Associative classification is based on the association rule mining. It only discovers associations between a set of features and a class label. We use the Associative Rule Classification-By Category (ARC-BC) [12] algorithm. ARC-BC mines rules in each class separately and is shown to be less affected by class imbalance. The rules that pass through a local threshold are grouped together to build a final classifier. The classifier may assign multiple class labels to a new instance, the final decision is made by measuring and comparing the quality of each prediction.

Repeated Incremental Pruning to Produce Error Reduction (RIPPER): RIPPER [6] is an inductive rule-based learner that generates Disjunctive Normal Form (DNF) rules to identify classes while minimising the error defined by the number of misclassified training example by the rule. Each classification rule has a conjunction of attribute values as antecedent and a class as consequent.

$$r : (Rule\ Antecedent) \rightarrow y \tag{4}$$

In a multi-class situation, the rules generated from the RIPPER algorithm are ranked in ascending order based on the number of examples in the class. An unknown instance is tested against the rules in that order. The first rule that covers the test instance fires and the testing phase ends.

The default RIPPER algorithm makes only one prediction. It fires the first rule that covers the test instance. To make multiple predictions, we make the following modifications and refer to the modified algorithm as ARIPPER (Alternate RIPPER) in the rest of the paper: for each test instance, we gather all the rules covering it and group the rules together that predict the same program and rank these predictions based on their quality. Such quality can be computed by measuring the quality of the underlying supporting rules. We consider four types of measurements:

- **Highest Average Rule Confidence (HAvgRCF):** calculate the average rule confidence of all rules supporting each recommendation. The one with the highest average rule confidence is the final prediction.
- **Single Rule with Highest Confidence (SRHCF):** the rule with the highest confidence makes the final prediction.

- **Highest Average Weighted Chi-Square (HAvgCS):** HAvgCS is a measurement adopted from CMAR, i.e., Classification based on Multiple Association Rules [2]. It calculates the weighted rule Chi-Square value of all rules supporting each recommendation.
- **Single Rule with Highest Weighted Chi-Square (SRHCS):** SRHCS looks at the Chi-Square of each single rule and uses the one with the highest Chi-Square value as the quality of a recommendation.

3.5   Evaluation Measurements

To evaluate the performance of the physicians (human baseline), we use the successful rate as our measurement. It is the only measurement we can use for the human baseline. The successful rate of the physicians is defined as the number of successful recommendations (patient returns to work by receiving this recommendation) made by a physician over the number of all cases in the dataset. This is similar to the overall classification accuracy measurement. With class imbalance, this is not a good measurement. However, since we do not know the true class label of unsuccessful cases, it is neither possible to obtain the confusion matrix to use other measurements like Precision and F-measure, nor to know the measurements of each class. Therefore, we can only use overall classification accuracy in comparison with the human baseline, however, we do include other measurements for completeness.

- **Sensitivity:** sensitivity describes the proportion of actual positive examples that are correctly identified.
- **Specificity:** specificity measures the proportion of actual negative examples that are correctly identified.
- **Geometric Mean (G-mean):** There is a trade-off between sensitivity and specificity. G-mean is a more harmonic measurement defined as

$$\sqrt{sensitivity * specifity}. \tag{5}$$

3.6   Experiment Design

We conducted a variety of experiments and only those giving meaningful results are presented here. We explain one experiment in detail. The rest of them are described briefly since most experiments use the same strategy with the only difference being the underlying method for sampling.

SMOTE + Tomek Link + DataSet1 (direct approach): To mitigate the class imbalance, we use a progressive sampling approach to change the class distribution:

1. Choose one minority class and fix the rest.
2. Increase the size of the selected class by a certain percentage P.

3. Train an ARIPPER classifier on the sampled dataset. If the true positive rate of the selected class increases significantly, undo the sampling and repeat step 2 with a larger percentage P and step 3. However, if the size of the sampled class is greater than that of the largest class in the dataset or the increase is less than 2%, stop the sampling process.
4. Choose P as the final sampling percentage.

The final sampling percentage obtained for each minority class is 900%, 900% and 300% respectively. Figure 1 shows the class distribution before and after the sampling. We can visualize the sampled dataset using Principal Component Analysis (PCA) with the first two components as shown in Figure 2-a. We can see that on the left side class 3 has a minor overlap with class 6 while class 5 has invaded class 6. On the right side, class 0 and 4 are mixed together.

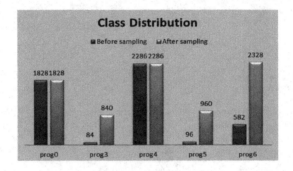

Fig. 1. Class Distribution Before and After Sampling-Final Dataset

To make it easier for any algorithm to build a good classification model, a data cleaning stage is desirable to clean up the borders between each class. We apply the Tomek Link Cleaning method to weed out noise. Data points from different classes that form a Tomek Link are considered as borderline or noisy points, and generally can be removed. The details of the cleaning process are stated as follows:

1. Extract each pair of classes.
2. Identify the Tomek links between these two classes.
3. Remove noise or borderline points. If such cleaning improves the overall performance of the model, merge the cleaned up classes back to the whole dataset. Otherwise, undo the cleaning.
4. Repeat step 1 to 3 until all possible pairs of classes is processed.

Figure 2-b visualizes the dataset after Tomek Link cleaning. We can see that data points from Class 0 are completely mixed with Class 4. It is possible that the current selected features cannot separate these two classes effectively. Since feature selection is data dependent, we further sampled on prog0 as a possible solution for the class overlap. It is possible that we can select new and effective features to separate Class 0 and 4. Sampling on Class 0 may cause further overlapping between Class 0 and 4. But those points will be removed later as noise while the useful examples will be reinforced. We choose to sample 60% on class 0 and apply the same procedures above. 19 features are selected and the visualization using PCA is shown in Figure 2-c.

Clearly, we can see that part of Class 0 is now separable from Class 4. We then apply the Tomek Link cleaning on the new dataset. Figure 2-d visualizes the dataset after the cleaning. Those points from class 0 mixing with class 4 are removed while those separable remain in the data space. We then build a model using both ARIPPER and associative classification learner on this dataset. The evaluation is detailed in the next section.

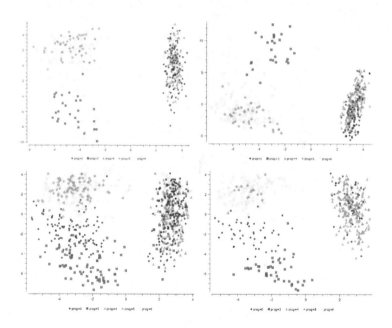

Fig. 2. Dataset Visualization a)left top: after SMOTE, b)right top: after Tomek Link cleaning, c)left bottom: after resampling, d)right bottom: after cleaning in second round

Class Decomposition + SMOTE + NCR (OVA: One-vs-All): In this approach we first decompose the dataset into 5 binary datasets. Each binary dataset contains the data from one positive class and all other classes are considered as one negative class. We use SMOTE to sample on the minority class in each binary dataset. The size of the minority class should be close to but smaller than that of the majority class. Then we use Neighborhood Cleaning Rule (NCR) as a data cleaning method to clean the data space. After the cleaning, five binary classifiers are created using different learning algorithms. To make a prediction for an unknown instance, each classifier generates a probability of that instance belonging to the positive class. We use the imbalance rate to combine the probability prediction of all 5 classifiers: we take the product of prediction probability and the imbalance rate of its corresponding class as a final weight. The test instance belongs to the class with the highest weight.

4   Evaluation and Discussion

4.1   Experiment Evaluation

As mentioned in the System Requirement Section, our system should make multiple recommendations for the users to choose from. Since this is a Decision **Support** System, our goal is to help the physicians but not to replace them. The physicians can view the rules supporting the recommendations and make their own decisions from the recommendation pool.

However, from a computer science perspective, this is not sufficient. For a multi-class classification problem, the model has to finalize its prediction. Therefore, for each dataset obtained by using different data preprocessing strategies, we train a model from it using different algorithms and then evaluate their performance on the test set.

SMOTE + Tomek Link + DataSet1 (Direct Approach): We first train a model using the ARIPPER algorithm. The rules obtained from this model were evaluated by experts from the Department of Physical Therapy and considered as meaningful rule sets. Our prototype system is implemented based on these rules. Table 2 shows the prediction evaluation on the test set using these four measurements: The potential means that if any of the predictions matches with the true label, we count it as a correct prediction. Note that in rules generated from the RIPPER algorithm, there is a default rule with empty rule body and neither confidence nor Chi Square is applicable. So for each test instance, we assign to it both the selected prediction and the default prediction. If either of them matches with the true label, we count it as a correct prediction.

Table 2. Evaluation On the Test Set (ARIPPER)

Criterion	HAvgRCF	SRHCF	HAvgCS	SRHCS	Potential
Accuracy	0.73	0.72	0.48	0.48	0.78

We then train three other classifiers using the Naive Bayes algorithm, C4.5 algorithm and ARC-BC respectively. Table 3 to 5 show the evaluation of each algorithm on the test set. The overall accuracy is 0.385, 0.478, and 0.470 respectively.

Class Decomposition + SMOTE + NCR (OVA): for the decomposition approach, we are using two base learners for each binary classifier Naive Bayes and RIPPER (original RIPPER). Table 6 and 7 show the confusion matrix of the evaluation on the test set using base learner Naive Bayes and RIPPER.

Table 3. Evaluation On the Test Set (Naive Bayes)

	Sensitivity	Specificity	G-Mean
Prog0	0.071	0.961	0.261
Prog3	0.000	1.000	0.000
Prog4	0.969	0.069	0.260
Prog5	0.000	1.000	0.000
Prog6	0.000	1.000	0.000
Overall	0.482	0.870	0.647

Table 4. Evaluation On the Test Set (C4.5)

	Sensitivity	Specificity	G- Mean
Prog0	0.05	0.98	0.22
Prog3	0	1	0
Prog4	0.98	0.04	0.199
Prog5	0	1	0
Prog6	0	1	0
Overall	0.478	0.869	0.645

4.2   Discussion

In this section, we discuss the evaluation in the former section. Note that the evaluation here has its own limitations as we mentioned in the earlier section.

For the direct approach with ARIPPER algorithm, we can see that by choosing the prediction with rule confidence measurement, the prediction accuracy reaches around 72%. Unfortunately, since each instance has two predictions, we cannot analyze other measurement using the confusion matrix. The accuracy on test set using Naive Bayes, C4.5 and ARC-BC algorithms is lower than the human baseline. However, ARC-BC does slightly better than the other two on predicting minority class examples. For the class decomposition approach, the overall accuracy is also lower than the human baseline. However, one thing worth noticing is that by using Naive Bayes as the base learner, the model makes good predictions of the minority classes. But it is difficult to ensure good classification results on both the majority and minority classes at the same time. This is a common tradeoff with the presence of class imbalance.

The nature of the rehabilitation program is also somewhat responsible for the misclassification between the majority classes. As we are informed by the experts, prog0 and prog4 are similar to each other. A large portion of people receiving prog4 actually does not need prog4. But in order to make sure that people do return to work, they are assigned with prog4 in the end. Additionally, prog6 is a hybrid program of prog4 and prog5, which makes it even more complicated in classification. The data visualization in earlier section also confirms this issue as we can see the overlap between these classes. Currently our prototype system implements the ARIPPER model trained from the first experiment since the rules are considered

Table 5. Evaluation On the Test Set (ARC-BC)

	Sensitivity	Specificity	G- Mean
Prog0	0.132	0.958	0.355
Prog3	0.588	0.458	0.519
Prog4	0.856	0.274	0.484
Prog5	0.105	0.969	0.319
Prog6	0.069	0.952	0.256
Overall	0.471	0.747	0.593

Table 6. Evaluation On the Test Set (Naive Bayes)

	Sensitivity	Specificity	G- Mean
Prog0	0.08	0.931	0.276
Prog3	1	0.732	0.856
Prog4	0.284	0.849	0.491
Prog5	0.556	0.666	0.608
Prog6	0.06	0.902	0.249
Overall	0.201	0.8	0.401

Table 7. Evaluation On the Test Set (RIPPER)

	Sensitivity	Specificity	G- Mean
Prog0	0.846	0.308	0.511
Prog3	0.444	0.987	0.662
Prog4	0.314	0.857	0.519
Prog5	0	0.994	0
Prog6	0	1	0
Overall	0.473	0.868	0.641

to be very meaningful from clinical perspective. This rule set shows a high potential on the test evaluation. As a decision *support* system, this should be sufficient since the clinician is the one who makes the final decision. To further evaluate the system, we need to do additional validations in real clinical settings.

5   Summary

In this work we build a decision support system with a knowledge base generated by machine learning algorithms. To tackle the multi-class imbalance and class overlap due to the nature of this clinical dataset, we apply several data re-sampling techniques to make it easier for the learning stage. Our results show that the direct approach SMOTE + Tomek Link + ARIPPER generates a meaningful rule-based model whose prediction ability is comparable to the clinicians. Moreover, combining class decomposition with data re-sampling is a better way to effectively classify minority class examples than applying the data re-sampling directly.

Since our system provides human readable rules and presents these rules as evidence of any recommendation, a feedback loop is conceivable allowing an expert user to change these rules by directly injecting domain knowledge in the model initially automatically derived from the data.

As for future study, we plan to find a solution to determine the right prediction between the default prediction and the other one as discussed in experiment 1. Building a binary classifier between these two predictions would be a good start. Another extension to our work is to integrate the negative model into the evaluation of the positive model such as canceling conflicting predictions under certain circumstances. To evaluate the system from a clinical perspective, additional validation in random clinical trials is required.

References

1. Two modifications of cnn. IEEE Transactions on Systems, Man and Cybernetics SMC-6(11), 769–772 (November 1976)
2. CMAR: accurate and efficient classification based on multiple class-association rules (2001)
3. Martin, B.I., Deyo, R.A., Mirza, S.K., Turner, J.A., Comstock, B.A., Hollingworth, W., Sullivan, S.: Expenditures and health status among adults with back and neck problems. JAMA 299, 656–664 (2008)
4. Chawla, N.V., Bowyer, K.W., Hall, L.O., Kegelmeyer, W.P.: Smote: synthetic minority over-sampling technique. J. Artif. Int. Res. 16(1), 321–357 (2002)
5. Murray, C.J., Vos, T., Lozano, R., Naghavi, M., Flaxman, A., Michaud, C., et al.: Disability-adjusted life years (dalys) for 291 diseases and injuries in 21 regions, 1990-2010: a systematic analysis for the global burden of disease study 2010. Lancet 380(9859), 2197–2223 (2012)
6. Cohen, W.W.: Fast effective rule induction. In: Proceedings of the Twelfth International Conference on Machine Learning, pp. 115–123 (1995)
7. Hadler, N.M.: Occupational musculoskeletal disorders, 3rd edn. Lippincott Williams & Wilkins, Philadelphia (2005)
8. Lane, R., Desjardins, S.: Canada. population and public health branch. Strategic policy directorate. Policy research division. Economic burden of illness in Canada [Ottawa], Health Canada (2002)
9. Laurikkala, J.: Improving Identification of Difficult Small Classes by Balancing Class Distribution. In: Quaglini, S., Barahona, P., Andreassen, S. (eds.) AIME 2001. LNCS (LNAI), vol. 2101, pp. 63–66. Springer, Heidelberg (2001)
10. Ross Quinlan, J.: C4.5: programs for machine learning. Morgan Kaufmann Publishers Inc., San Francisco (1993)
11. Wilson, D.L.: Asymptotic properties of nearest neighbor rules using edited data. IEEE Transactions on Systems, Man and Cybernetics 2(3), 408–421 (1972)
12. Zaïane, O.R., Antonie, M.-L.: Classifying text documents by associating terms with text categories. In: Proceedings of the 13th Australasian Database Conference, ADC 2002, Darlinghurst, Australia, vol. 5, pp. 215–222. Australian Computer Society, Inc. (2002)

EEG-MINE: Mining and Understanding Epilepsy Data

SunHee Kim[1], Christos Faloutsos[1], and Hyung-Jeong Yang[2]

[1] School of Computer Science, Carnegie Mellon University
[2] Department of Computer Science, Chonnam National University
{wkdal749,christos}@cs.cmu.edu,hjyang@jnu.ac.kr

Abstract. Given electroencephalogram time series data from patients with epilepsy, can we find patterns and regularities? The typical approach thus far is to use tensors or dynamical systems. Here, we present EEG-MINE, a non-linear, chaos-based "gray box model", that blends domain knowledge with data observations. When applied to numerous, real EEG sequences, EEG-MINE (a) can successfully reconstruct the signals with high accuracy; (b) can spot surprising patterns within seizure EEG signals; and (c) may provide early warning of epileptic seizures.

Keywords: electroencephalogram, epilepsy seizure, chaos neuron, neural network, oscillatory cortex.

1   Introduction

Epilepsy entails seizures, during which the brain activities are abnormal, and the patient suffers strange sensations, convulsions, muscle spasms, loss of consciousness and even death, often caused by injury during the spasms [17]. The exact mechanism(s) that cause seizures are still under study, but it is known that seizures are correlated to settings such as low oxygen levels (for example chronic obstructive pulmonary disease, severe asthma), meningitis, encephalitis, and brain tumors, etc. Epilepsy diagnosis and management is very important: There are more than 2 million epilepsy patients in United States. In the UK, the number of epilepsy patients is approximately 600,000. Among these patients, 500 have died each year by sudden seizure [1].

Detection and classification of epileptic seizures are important components for the analysis and diagnosis of epilepsy. We propose the EEG-MINE model, based on non-linear dynamics and chaos technique for analysis. Working within a short time frame, our model requires only 5 parameters. Those parameters exhibit regularities that seem to correlate well with the type of brain activity.

Fig. 1 gives more details. It shows two carefully-chosen parameters of our model (C1 and C2), to detect pattern of epilepsy signals. In a nutshell, we fit our EEG-MINE model in each 1-second window W1, W2, etc. extracting the 5 parameters of the model; we draw the scatter plot for the first two (C1 and C2) as shown in Fig. 1(b), (c), and (d). All windows before the onset of seizure (manually marked) are marked with the blue circle symbol, and windows after the onset of seizure indicated by the red star symbol. In the scatter plot of Fig. 1, we can confirm that the markers of the parameter separates into two group.

J. Li et al. (Eds.): PAKDD 2013 Workshops, LNAI 7867, pp. 155–167, 2013.
© Springer-Verlag Berlin Heidelberg 2013

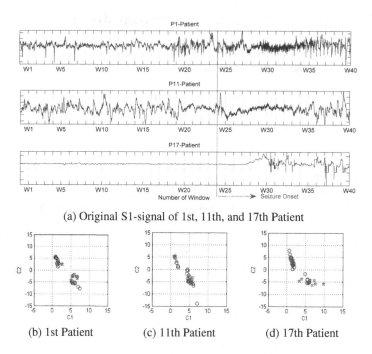

(a) Original S1-signal of 1st, 11th, and 17th Patient

(b) 1st Patient   (c) 11th Patient   (d) 17th Patient

Fig. 1. Mining by EEG-MINE model: (a) shows one of the signals ('S1') of our 1st, 11th, and patient, divided into 40 windows of 256 time-ticks (=1 second) each (dotted vertical lines). Seizure onset is marked manually (red arrow, 25-th window, at 6144). (b) shows the scatter plot of C1, C2 for all 40 windows of the signals ('S1') of our 1st patient. The windows before the onset of seizure marked as blue circles, and seizure windows marked as red stars. (c) is scatter plot of the signals ('S1') of our 1 th patient. (d) shows the scatter plot of C1, C2 for all 40 windows of 17th patient.

Fig. 1(b) is a scatter plot of the 1st patient. In this case, the parameter marker is before the onset of seizure which appears in the positive region, and the windows of seizure signal mostly indicates in the negative region of parameter C2. However, there are a few exceptions though: windows W5, W6 and a few others, are outside the positive region. These deviate from the positive region when the signal has broad amplitude compared with periphery signal. In contrast, in case of the small the amplitude compared with periphery signal, the parameter of the seizure appears in the positive region. The original signal of Fig. 1(c) (11th patient) show amplitude of drastic change in signal before the onset of seizure. In the scatter plot (Fig. 1(c)), parameter markers of normal signal indicates in negative region of parameter C2. In the case of Fig. 1(d), signal before onset and after onset commonly appears in positive and negative region, respectively.

We use the same convention in all such upcoming figures.

Our contributions are the following:

– *Accuracy* of model: Our EEG-MINE model gives a good approximation with respect to; Mean Square Error between the actual and the estimated signals.

- *Surprising pattern discovery*: we show that our model parameters obey some patterns: The C2 parameter can separate typically in the positive and negative region of all windows. Analogous patterns govern the remaining C1, C3, C4 and P parameters, for numerous patients and for numerous signals (= brain locations).
- *Warning Possibility*: Our EEG-MINE model parameters, especially C1 and C2, seem possible of distinguishing between interictal and ictal windows of activity, which may suggest early warning signs.

The outline of the paper is typical: In the next sections, we respectively give: the related work, proposed method, experiments, and conclusions.

2   Related Work

In recent years, several techniques for detection, prediction and classification of epileptic seizures have been proposed and used a variety concepts and theories, such as linear analysis, nonlinear analysis, and chaos [6]. The dynamical analysis techniques have been used for seizure detection from epilepsy EEG. Ghosh-Dastidar et al. [9] developed a novel wavelet-chaos-neural network methodology for classification healthy, ictal, and interictal EEGs. Alvarado et al. [4] proposed a seizure prediction method that based on a measure of brain excitability, and was applied 20 patients with partial epilepsy. Sahu et al. [13] proposed a method that are chaos based parameters as entropy, the largest Lyapunow exponent (LLE), correlation dimension (CD), and capacity dimension (CAD) for EEG signal classification. Li and Ouyang [12] proposed the dynamical similarity measure based on a similarity index to predict epileptic seizures. However, this method is only related to diseases diagnosis by classification. Therefore, it is difficult to pre-warn the epileptic. Also, mentioned above the methods must be divided into training and testing data, consequently a lot of execution time for learning is required. Therefore, these methods need large amounts of data and computationally expensive.

Tensor and multi-way analysis has been applied in various filed like tucker decomposition, parallel factor analysis, and bilinear PCA [16]. Juan et al. [18] applied parallel factor analysis (PARAFAC) and wavelets to distinguish between chronic pain and pain-free individuals. Latchoumane et al. [11] used a multi-way analysis to detect the spatial-frequency characteristics for classification of Alzheimer disease (AD). Alaa et al. [10] detected epileptic seizure from IEEG (intracranial EEG) using a machine-learning approach. Shengkun et al [20] proposed new detection schemes to diagnosis of epilepsy and to detect the onset of epileptic seizures using a dynamic principle component analysis (PCA). However, this method requires a lot of time for training to learn the data, plus when new pattern of seizures arise, the detection rate drop considerably, because it only can detect patterns similar to known seizure such as, one or two.

Our method is based on the nonlinear neuron population model (chaos theory) that can generate estimated signal and detect the pattern of complex epilepsy EEG data. Through this model, we can obtain five parameters, and these can use to pre-warn to epilepsy patient or health care provider. Also, EEG-MINE model can give execution time of $O(T \times n \times r(LM repetition))$ to estimate signal.

3   Proposed Method

In this section, we describe the EEG-MINE model, and our parameter fitting. The our goal is to forewarn the epileptic seizure to patients or medical professionals using few parameters that obtained from each window set. For this, we demonstrated an EEG-MINE system which generate the signal by five optimal parameters.

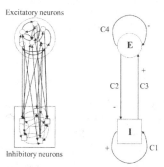

(a) Chaos neuron population (b) Simplified network

Fig. 2. Neural network of oscillatory cortex: Chaos neuron population comprises "E" and "I" neurons set (E: set of excitatory neurons, I: set of inhibitory neurons). E and I neurons interact, with strengths C1, C2, C3, and C4.

3.1   Background

First we describe an elaborate model (Eq 1,2) that involves a large population of neurons, and in the next subsection, we present the EEG-MINE model that we actually use.

Full model (not used here): A successful model for brain activity assumes a population of neurons, some of which are excitatory (E) and the rest are being inhibitory (I) neurons with synaptic connections [15] (Fig. 2(a)). A neural system is composed of two groups of excitatory and inhibitory neurons. Both groups exhibit self-excitation (with coefficients C1 and C4), and cross-excitation (coefficients C2 and C3). The states of neurons are given as follows, respectively: $e_k(t)$, $k = 1, ..., N_e$, $i_l(t)$, $l = 1, ..., N_i$. $e_k(t)$ denotes the energy of $k = 1, ..., N_e$ excitatory neurons and $i_l(t)$ is for the inhibitory one at time t. The dynamic interaction of neuron population can be described by means of the neuron system as shown in Eq.(1) and (2), where $k = 1, ..., N_e$ and $k = 1, ..., N_i$, respectively:

$$\frac{de_k}{dt} = -e_k + S(\frac{1}{N_e}\sum_{l=1}^{N_e}u_{kl}e_l - \frac{1}{N_i}\sum_{l=1}^{N_i}v_{kl}i_l - \theta_k^e + p_k) \tag{1}$$

$$\frac{di_k}{dt} = -i_k + S(\frac{1}{N_e}\sum_{l=1}^{N_e}w_{kl}e_l - \frac{1}{N_i}\sum_{l=1}^{N_i}z_{kl}i_l - \theta_k^i) \tag{2}$$

where t denotes time, S exhibits the sigmoid function as $S(x) = [1 + exp^{(-x)}]^{-1}$.

Algorithm 1. EEG-MINE Model

Input: Observed Epilepsy EEG data sequence: x_{t-1}
Output:
    Estimated sequence: $\hat{x}_t$
    Updated Model parameters: $\theta^{new} := C1, C2, C3, C4, P$

    Initialize $C1, C2, C3, C4, P$ Parameters;
    Initialize Θ^e and Θ^i to semisaturation constants of excitatory and inhibitory;
    $\theta \leftarrow C1, C2, C3, C4, P$

repeat
    1. Objective Function
        Estimate $\hat{E}_k(t)$ using Eq. 3
        Estimate $\hat{I}_k(t)$ using Eq. 4
        Estimate $\hat{x}(t)$ using Eq. 3 - Eq. 4
        //Estimated signal
        Compute sum of squares of error inputs

    2. Parameter Updating //Levenberg-Marquardt
        if the new sum of squared errors has not decreased **then**
            Discard the new weights, increase λ
            and go to 2.1.
        else
            decrease λ and go to 1.
            $\theta^{new} \leftarrow \theta + h$ (h= variation)
        end if
until Converge

This model has the several interactions that are coupled with self-interactions and cross-interactions. It is expressed by u_{kl}, v_{kl}, w_{kl}, and z_{kl}. The external input p_k are switched off, and all activities are simply decayed exponentially to zero. The threshold θ_k^e and θ_k^i should be large enough. The detailed descriptions of this model are shown in [14] [19].

3.2 Method

The above Eq.(1) and (2) can be simplified [14], if we assume only one excitatory and only one inhibitory neuron for each location k ($k = 1, 2, \ldots$), as shown in Fig. 2(b). This simplification leads to Eq.(3) and (4), which we shall refer to the "EEG-MINE Model". Table 1 lists the symbols and definitions.

Given an activity $E_k(t)$ of the excitatory neuron at location k and time t, and the activity $I_k(t)$ of the inhibitory neuron at the same location at time t, we have Eq.(3) and (4):

$$\frac{dE_k(t)}{dt} = -E_k(t) + S_\mu(c_1 E_k(t) - c_2 I_k(t) - \Theta^e + p), \qquad (3)$$

Table 1. Symbols and Definitions

Symbol	Definition
$E_k(t)$	Excitatory at channel k, at time $t(k = 1, ..., n)$
$I_k(t)$	Inhibitory at channel k, at time t
$\hat{E}_k(t), \hat{I}_k(t)$	Our estimates of Excitatory and Inhibitory
Θ^e, Θ^i	Threshold of Excitatory and Inhibitory
$S_k(t)$	Value of k-th $E_k(t) - I_k(t)$ at time t
$\hat{S}_k(t)$	Estimated value of k-th signal

$$\frac{dI_k(t)}{dt} = -I_k(t) + S_\mu(c_3 E_k(t) - c_4 I_k(t) - \Theta^i), \qquad (4)$$

In detail, to generate our estimates using the above two equations, we set the initial values of $E_k(0)$ and $I_k(0)$, to 0. We obtained our estimate $\hat{E}_k(t)$ from Eq.(3), and then we use it in Eq.(4), to estimate $\hat{I}_k(t)$, the new activity of the inhibitory neuron at time t. The output of the model is $\hat{S}(t) = \hat{E}_k(t) - \hat{I}_k(t)$[3], the estimate for the activity signal.

We do the above calculations when the parameter values (C1, C2, etc) are known. If they are not, then we use Levenberg-Marquardt, to minimize the mean squared error (MSE). In the sigmoid function $S_\mu(K)$, μ is the control parameter.

To demonstrate our model, we define the initial parameters at the following plausible values: C1 (self-interaction of Inhibitory) = 3, C2 (cross-interaction from Excitatory to Inhibitory) = 2, C3 (cross-interaction from Inhibitory to Excitatory) = -10, C4 (self-interactions of Excitatory) = 0.2, and P (external inputs) = 1. In addition, the semisaturation constants will be assigned as the values $\Theta^e = 2$, $\Theta^i = 3.5$ from [14].

EEG-MINE model uses the real signal x_{t-1} to generate the estimated signal $\hat{x}_t$. That is, our model generates the new estimate signal to reflect the past values from epilepsy signals. Parameters are updated to minimize the sum of squares of the errors between original signals and the estimated signals. EEG-MINE model can be applied in the various dataset having temporal-dependence similar to the epilepsy EEG data. As we show later, EEG-MINE model has several desirable properties: (a) it gives accurate estimates; (b) it can provide surprising invariants (c) its parameters (especially C2) may can help discriminate between interictal and ictal signal.

3.3 Parameter Fitting

We estimate the parameters using the Levenberg-Marquardt algorithms [8] which is a standard technique to solve nonlinear at least square problems. The Levenberg-Marquardt algorithm is based on the Gauss-Newton method. Weighted adjustment by Gauss-Newton is as follows: $[J^T W J + \lambda diag(J^T W J)]h = J^T W(y - \hat{y})$. J is $m \times n$ Jacobian matrix. It is represented as $[(d\hat{y})/dp]$ by function output $\hat{y}$ to variation in the parameters p. p is a parameter vector which includes C1, C2, C3, C4, and P(external input). The weight matrix W is diagonal with $W_{ii} = 1/w_i^2$. λ is the Levenberg's damping factor. λ would start as a small value such as 0.1. If the function output $\hat{y}$ is nonlinear, the minimization of difference D_{val} for two values with respect to the parameters must be done iteratively. The purpose of iteration is to find a perturbation h to the parameter p that reduces $D_{val} = 1/2 \sum_{i=1}^{m} [y(t_i) - \hat{y}(t_i; p)/w_i]^2$. The Levenberg-Marquardt algorithm is approximated using $J_{i,j} = d\hat{y}_i/dp_j = \hat{y}(t_i; p + \delta p) - \hat{y}(t_i; p)/|\delta p_j|$. The j-th element of δp_j is the only non-zero element and is set to $\epsilon_2(1 + |p_j|)$. During iteration for $D_{val}(p) - D_{val}(p+h) > \epsilon_3 h^T(\lambda h + J^T W(y - \hat{y}))$, parameter vector p is replaced by $p + h$. λ is adaptively decreased (see [8] for more details). The overall process is described in Algorithm 1.

4   Experiments

Experiment Data: Experiment data were recorded at the Epilepsy Center of the University Hospital of Freiburg, Germany [2]. The data contain the 21 patient dataset with medically intractable epilepsy. This EEG data were acquired using an EEG system with 6 signals and 256 Hz sampling rate. Electrodes 1 to 3 are focal electrodes, electrodes 4 to 6 are extra focal electrodes. Each dataset contains signals of epileptic seizures. Dataset were recorded from intracranial grid, strip, and depth-electrodes. Among 21 patients, eleven patients were located epileptic focus in neocortical brain structures. Eight patients were in the hippocampus, and two patients were located in both. We used 21 patients dataset that include epileptic seizure(ictal) signals for the experiments. The patient's data consist of 8 male and 13 female, and age groups of patients is diverse from 12 to 50 years old. Each patient has epileptic seizure between 2 and 5, and interictal signals are recorded during at least 24 hours without seizure activity.

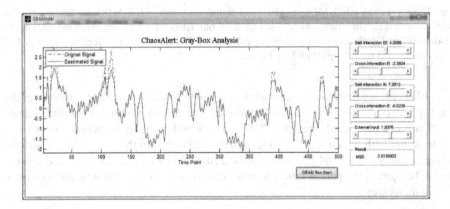

Fig. 3. Estimated Signal by EEG-Mine system - screen-shot: Dashed blue: original; solid red: our estimation (using *only* 5 parameters and Levenberg-Marquardt to fit them). The sliders on the right allow one to further fine-tune the parameters, or check 'what if' scenarios.

Next, we present experiments to answer the following questions:

– *Q1: Accuracy*: How well does our model match real signals, after suitable parameter fitting?

- *Q2: Surprising Pattern Discovery*: What invariants can the model discover?
- *Q3: Warning Possibility*: How can our model be applied to warn of oncoming seizures?

4.1   Q1: Accuracy of EEG-MINE Model

For experiments, we reconfigured the sample data to the combined signals of ictal and interictal. Also we separated the experiment data by a window unit. One window has 256 time points and it means one second. Each signal consists of 40 seconds so that we have 40 windows. The combined dataset includes partial epileptic seizure (ictal) across the entire signals. Therefore, normal and abnormal (seizure) signals are mixed together in a window. All patients include epileptic seizure from the 25, 26, 27, and 28th window, respectively. We applied EEG-MINE model in each window signal and obtained a few parameters and estimated signals. We found the optimal parameters for each window signal to reduce MSE.

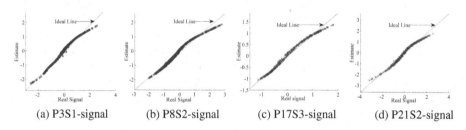

| (a) P3S1-signal | (b) P8S2-signal | (c) P17S3-signal | (d) P21S2-signal |

Fig. 4. Accuracy of EEG-MINE model: total signal on x-axis, EEG-MINE model estimate on y-axis, for several time-ticks notice that most of our EEG-MINE model estimates are on the 45-degree line (ideal). (a) S1-signal of 3rd Patient, (b) S2-signal of 8th Patient, (c) S3-signal of 17th Patient, and (d) S2-signal of 21th-Patient.

For brevity, we omit a table with all the parameter values for all our patients, for the healthy (interictal) and seizure (ictal) portions. The signals are aligned, so that signals of P1 are healthy signals until the 24th window and P1 includes ictal (seizure) signal from the 25th window. P8 includes seizure activity from the 26th window, and the seizure signals of P17 and P21 begin in the 27th window and the 28th window respectively. The rest of the patients include seizure activity from the 25th window. The main observations are:

- The majority of healthy signals lead to parameters C1/C2/C3 that have values in the positive range (C1>5, C2>0, C3>10).
- The majority of seizure signals lead to parameters C1/C2/C3 such as C1<5, C2<0, and C3<10.
- The C4 parameter is near-constant (-5 to -7), for both healthy and seizure cases.
- The MSE of our fitting is small, typically about 0.02

Fig. 3 shows the estimated signal that is generated by five optimal parameters from our model. In EEG-MINE model simulator, a dotted line is original signal, and solid line exhibits estimated signal. In EEG-MINE model simulator, Self-interactions EE means the parameter C1 and Cross-interactions EI is parameter C2 from excitatory to inhibitory. Self-interactions IN indicates parameter C4, Cross-interactions IE signifies parameter C3 from inhibitory to excitatory. Finally, external inputs is parameter P of excitatory neurons. The details of the parameters discussed in Section 4.2. Fig. 4 shows the errors between original signals and the estimated signals by our model. It means the accuracy of EEG-MINE model. Blue cross-maker and red line mean the differences and ideal line, respectively. Fig. 4(a) shows the result of P3S1 by EEG-MINE model. Fig. 4(b) exhibits the results of P8S2. Fig. 4(c) and Fig. 4(d) show accuracy of P17S3 and P21S2, respectively. In plots, the red line is the ideal line which means 0 percent of error rate. As a result, two signals (real and estimated signal) are plotted very similarly, since MSE of each signal is very low. Thus, our model can provide high accuracy rate by generating estimated signals by EEG-MINE model.

4.2   Q2: Surprising Pattern Discovery

EEG-MINE model is required several parameters to simulate EEG signals because it is based on Excitatory-Inhibitory population model[14]. The parameters of EEG-MINE model are very important to seizure analysis. Therefore, we closely observed each parameter as Fig. 5. Fig. 5 shows the parameter plots and original signal(Top of Fig. 5) that combined interictal signal and ictal signal of P3S2. In original signal of Fig. 5, red vertical line means seizure onset. We applied EEG-MINE model in each window of P3, and we obtained optimal parameters. Four parameter plots are displayed from the second row of Fig. 5. The left plot in the second row is parameter C1 vs. C2 where x-axis is C2, and y-axis means C1. They are clearly classified into two groups by parameter C2, and C2 parameter can separate by 0 standards. That is, one group is placed in positive value region (C2 > 0) and the other group is appeared in negative value region (C2 $<$ 0). In case of the C1, all values are parameter located in positive region. In C2 vs. C3 plot, all of parameter C3 were presented in positive value region. When parameter C2 appears in negative value region, parameter C3 has low positive values. On the contrary to this, values of parameter C3 are exhibited in high positive region while values of parameter C2 are located in positive region. All values of parameter C4 are appeared in negative region (around -5 or -7) as C2 vs. C4 plot, and parameter values of external input P are located around 0. As mentioned earlier (in Section 4.1), parameter values of C2 which are healthy (interictal) signals appear in positive value region, and parameters of seizure(ictal) signal mostly appear in the negative region. However, some of parameters of C2 of seizure signal are presented in positive region despite they are seizure signals. This may means that seizure signals contain a small healthy signals (interictal). Also, we can confirm that a few parameters are away from most parameter region of interictal signal. It can be interpreted that healthy signals also include fast frequency as ictal signals or noise.

4.3   Q3: Warning Possibility

Seizure warning signs are important because patients can be protected from the risk of epileptic seizure. Our work may provide early warning signs of seizures to a patient or

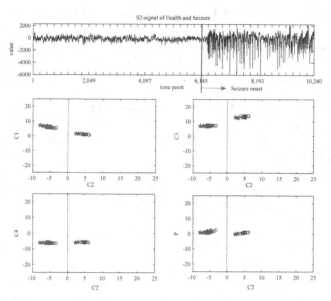

Fig. 5. Bi-modal behavior: original signal of P3S2 (patient#3, signal#2) with seizure onset manually marked by the red arrow at 6145; and scatter-plots of EEG-MINE model parameters vs. C2. Before-/after- onset windows are with blue-circles / red-stars, respectively. Notice the bi-modal behavior, separating at C2=0 (dotted vertical lines).

an expert of epilepsy before it occurs. We cautiously assumed that healthy signals appears in positive region by C2, and seizure signals indicates in negative region through observation of parameters value of several patients so far. For visualization, we show the scatter plot of C1 vs. C2, for each window W_i, of patient P and Signal S as Fig. 6. In plots, we assumed that square of black dotted line is the interictal parameter region, and square of red is ictal parameter region. Fig. 6(a) shows parameter scatter plot of 8th patient. In case of P8 dataset, seizure activity begins on 26th window signal. The blue circles represent the measured parameters in P8 before epileptic seizure (until the 25th window). It includes seven windows deviated from the interictal region, and first exception appeared in the parameter of P8-S3W4 marked in the red line square. In case of the ictal signal, three star symbols of red color appeared inside of interictal region (in the 31, 32 and the 34th window signals). It is the time windows measured during the epileptic seizure. However, except these cases, most windows were located inside or around the red square which is the ictal region. (b) of Fig. 6 is results of P17 dataset. In this case, epileptic seizure begins from the 27th window. In signal S1 of P17, the first exception is appeared in the 6th window, and total six exception are expressed before epileptic seizure onset. During epileptic seizure, one of time windows appeared in interictal region (in the 35th window signal), but the remainder of the windows are marked inside or around of the ictal region. In several experiment dataset, ictal region (red color square) was separated from interictal region. We may use these 'exception' parameter to warn of seizures. Before an epileptic seizure occurs, we may provide warning signs of the seizure by detecting the 'exception' window that appear outside of interictal region.

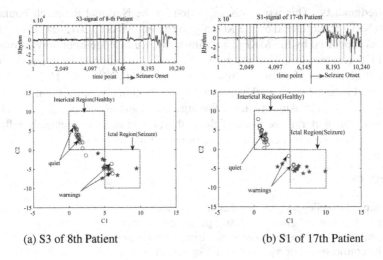

(a) S3 of 8th Patient   (b) S1 of 17th Patient

Fig. 6. Warnings by EEG-MINE model: (a) shows the S3-signal of a 8th Patient, that is divided to 40 windows, each of 256 time-ticks long (1 seconds). Seizure onset marked manually (26th window)(dotted vertical red lines); first warning shows in window W4 before seizure. (b) shows six warning signs before seizure (in red square) that are away from interictal parameter region.

5 Conclusions

We focused on the problem of mining epilepsy EEG data for classification and for detection of epileptic seizure. For this purpose, we use the EEG-MINE model, treating each signal (electrode) as if it focused on one, independent, neuron, and report our contributions:

- *Model Accuracy:* The proposed model is succinct, yet it gives low MSE rates between original and estimated signals, after we fit it with 5 parameters.
- *Surprising Pattern Discovery:* The parameter C2 (from Excitatory to Inhibitory) seems to have separated into the positive and negative region. The parameter C4 is surprisingly stable at -5, for all settings we studied, for all patients, for all signals! Moreover, interictal windows seem to have $0 < C1, C2 > 0$.
- *Warning Possibility:* Our analysis shows that the combination of C1 and C2 parameters of EEG-MINE model may help give early warnings, whenever they deviate from the region ($C2 > 0$).

In the future work, the proposed method will be compared with existing methods as tensor and dynamical systems in order to verify the effectiveness of our proposed method. Furthermore, we will broaden our research to involve different types of data such as similar multiple physiological data in a time series model.

Acknowledgments. This work was supported by the National Research Foundation of Korea(NRF) grant funded by the Korea government(MEST)(2012-047759), This research was supported by the MKE(The Ministry of Knowledge Economy), Korea, under the ITRC(Information Technology Research Center) support program supervised by the NIPA(National IT Industry Promotion Agency)" (NIPA-2012-H0301-12-3005), This material is based upon work supported by the National Science Foundation under Grant No. IIS1017415 Any opinions, findings, and conclusions or recommendations expressed in this material are those of the author(s) and do not necessarily reflect the views of the National Science Foundation, or other funding parties.

References

1. Background to epilepsy and national epilepsy guidance,
   `http://www.epilepsy.org.uk/professionals/`
   `healthcare/primary-care-resource-pack/section-1/`
   `background-epilepsy-national-guidance`
2. Epilepsy data set,
   `http://www.fdmold.uni-freiburg.de/epilepsydata/download/`
3. Computation by Excitatory and Inhibitory Networks,
   `http://www.math.pitt.edu/~bard/classes/compneuro/Chapter7.pdf`
4. Alvarado-Rojas, C., Valderrama, M., Witon, A., Navarro, V., Le, V.Q.M.: Probing cortical excitability using cross-frequency coupling in intracranial eeg recordings: a new method for seizure prediction. In: The 33rd Annual International Conference of the IEEE Engineering in Medicine and Biology Society, pp. 1632–1635 (2011)
5. Chaovalitwongse, W., Iasemidis, L.D., Pardalos, P.M., Carney, P.R., Shiau, D.S., Sackellares, J.C.: Performance of a seizure warning algorithm based on the dynamics of intracranial eeg. Epilepsy. Res. 93, 93–113 (2005)
6. Haibin, C., Pang-ning, T., Christopher, P., Steven, K.: Detection and characterization of anomalies in multivariate time series. In: The 9th SIAM International Conference on Data Mining, pp. 413–424 (2009)
7. Deburchgraeve, W., Cherian, P.J., De, V.M., Swarte, R.M., Blok, J.H., Visser, G.H., Govaert, P., Van, H.S.: Neonatal seizure localization using parafac decomposition. Clin. Neurophysiol. 120, 1787–1796 (2009)
8. Henri, G.: The Levenberg-Marquardt method for nonlinear least squares curve-fitting problems, `http://www.duke.edu/~hpgavin/ce281/lm.pdf`
9. Ghosh-Dastidar, S., Adeli, H.: Chaos in the brain: Novel methodologies for epilepsy diagnosis and seizure detection. Topics on Chaotic Systems, 138–148 (2008)
10. Kharbouch, A., Shoeb, A., Guttag, J., Cash, S.S.: An algorithm for seizure onset detection using intracranial eeg. Epilepsy Behav. 22, S29–S35 (2011)
11. Latchoumane, C.-F.V., Vialatte, E., Cichocki, A., Jeong, J.: Multiway analysis of alzheimers disease: Classification based on space-frequency characteristics of eeg time series. In: WCE. 2, pp. 3–7 (2008)
12. Xiaoli, L., Ouyang, G.: Nonlinear similarity analysis for epileptic seizures prediction. Nonlinear Anal. Theor. 64, 1666–1678 (2006)
13. Sahu, R., Parija, T., Mohapatra, B., Rout, B., Sahu, S., Panda, R., Pal, P., Gandhi, T.: Chaos based nonlinear analysis of epileptic seizure. In: The 3rd International Conference on Emerging Trends in Engineering and Technology, pp. 594–598 (2010)
14. Schuster, H.G., Wagner, P.: A model for neuronal oscillations in the visual cortex 1. Mean-field theory and derivation of the phase equations. Biol. Cybern. 64, 77–82 (1990)

15. Ricard, S., Brian, G.: Signs of Life: How Complexity Pervades Biology. Perseus Books Group, New York (2000)
16. Jimeng, S., Dacheng, T., Christos, F.: Beyond streams and graphs: dynamic tensor analysis. In: ACM SIGKDD, pp. 374–383 (2006)
17. Vegni, E., Leone, D., Canevini, M., Tinuper, P., Moja, E.: Sudden unexpected death in epilepsy (sudep): a pilot study on truth telling among italian epileptologists. Neurological Sciences 32, 331–335 (2011)
18. Wang, J., Li, X., Lu, C., Voss, L.J., Barnard, J.P.M., Sleigh, J.W.: Characteristics of evoked potential multiple eeg recordings in patients with chronic pain by means of parallel factor analysis. Comput. Math. Methods. Med. ID279560 (2012)
19. Hugh, R.W., Jack, D.C.: Excitatory and inhibitory interactions in localized populations of model neurons. Biophysical Journal 12, 1–24 (1972)
20. Shengkun, X., Lawniczak, A.T., Yuedong, S., Lio, P.: Feature extraction via dynamic pca for epilepsy diagnosis and epileptic seizure detection. In: IEEE International Workshop on Machine Learning for Signal Processing, pp. 337–342 (2010)

A Constraint and Rule in an Enhancement of Binary Particle Swarm Optimization to Select Informative Genes for Cancer Classification

Mohd Saberi Mohamad[1,*], Sigeru Omatu[2], Safaai Deris[1], and Michifumi Yoshioka[3]

[1] Artificial Intelligence and Bioinformatics Research Group, Faculty of Computing,
Universiti Teknologi Malaysia, 81310, Skudai, Johor, Malaysia
{saberi,safaai}@utm.my
[2] Department of Electronics, Information and Communication Engineering,
Osaka Institute of Technology, Osaka 535-8585, Japan
omatu@rsh.oit.ac.jp
[3] Department of Computer Science and Intelligent Systems, Graduate School of Engineering,
Osaka Prefecture University, Sakai, Osaka 599-8531, Japan
yoshioka@cs.osakafu-u.ac.jp

Abstract. Gene expression data have been analyzing by many researchers by using a range of computational intelligence methods. From the gene expression data, selecting a small subset of informative genes can do cancer classification. Nevertheless, many of the computational methods face difficulties in selecting small subset since the small number of samples needs to be compared to the huge number of genes (high-dimension), irrelevant genes and noisy genes. Hence, to choose the small subset of informative genes that is significant for the cancer classification, an enhanced binary particle swarm optimization is proposed. Here, the constraint of the elements of particle velocity vectors is introduced and a rule for updating particle's position is proposed. Experiments were performed on five different gene expression data. As a result, in terms of classification accuracy and the number of selected genes, the performance of the introduced method is superior compared to the conventional version of binary particle swarm optimization (BPSO). The other significant finding is lower running times compared to BPSO for this proposed method.

Keywords: Binary particle swarm optimization, gene selection, gene expression data, optimization.

1 Introduction

Advances in microarray technology allow scientists to measure the expression levels of thousands of genes simultaneously in biological organisms and have made it possible to create databases of cancerous tissues. It finally produces gene expression data that contain useful information of genomic, diagnostic, and prognostic for researchers

---

* Corresponding author.

J. Li et al. (Eds.): PAKDD 2013 Workshops, LNAI 7867, pp. 168–178, 2013.

[3]. Thus, there is a need to select informative genes that contribute to a cancerous state [5]. However, the gene selection process poses a major challenge because of the following characteristics of the data: the huge number of genes compared to the small number of samples (high-dimensional data), irrelevant genes, and noisy data. To overcome this challenge, a gene selection method is used to select a subset of informative genes that maximizes classifier's ability to classify samples more accurately [6]. In computational intelligence domains, gene selection is called feature selection.

Recently, several gene selection methods based on particle swarm optimization (PSO) have been proposed to select informative genes from gene expression data [4],[7]-[10]. PSO is a new evolutionary technique proposed by Kennedy and Eberhart [1]. Shen *et al.* have proposed a hybrid of PSO and tabu search approaches for gene selection [7]. However, the results obtained by using the hybrid method are less meaningful since the application of tabu approaches in PSO is unable to search a near-optimal solution in search spaces. Next, Li *et al.* have introduced a hybrid of PSO and genetic algorithms (GA) for the same purpose [4]. Unfortunately, the accuracy result is still not high and many genes are selected for cancer classification since there are no direct probability relations between GA and PSO.

Next, Chuang *et al.* proposed an improved binary PSO [8]. 100% classification accuracy in many data sets had been yielded by using the proposed method, but it utilized a large number of selected genes (large gene subset) to obtain the high accuracy. This method used a large number of genes because the global best particle was reset to the zero position when its fitness values did not change after three consecutive iterations. Chuang *et al.* [9],[10] introduced a combination of tabu search and PSO for gene selection [9], and currently they proposed a hybrid of BPSO and a combat GA for the same purpose [10]. However, both proposed approaches still need a high number of selected to result high classification accuracy. A significant weakness was found resulting from the combination of PSO and tabu search or a combat GA which did not share probability significance in their processes. Generally, the PSO-based methods are intractable to efficiently produce a small (near-optimal) subset of informative genes for high classification accuracy [4],[7]-[10]. This is mainly because the total number of genes in gene expression data is too large (high-dimensional data).

The diagnostic goal is to develop a medical procedure based on the least number of possible genes that needed to detect diseases. Thus, we introduce an enhancement of binary PSO based on the proposed constraint and rule (CPSO) to select a small (near-optimal) subset of informative genes that is most relevant for the cancer classification. The small subset means that it contains the small number of selected genes. In order to test the effectiveness of our proposed method, we apply CPSO to five gene expression data sets, including binary-classes and multi-classes data sets.

This paper is organized as follows. In Section 2 and Section 3, we briefly describe the conventional version of binary PSO and CPSO, respectively. Section 4 presents data sets used and experimental results. Section 5 summarizes this paper by providing its main conclusions and addresses future developments.

2   The Conventional Version of Binary PSO (BPSO)

BPSO is initialized with a population of particles. At each iteration, all particles move in a problem space to find the optimal solution. A particle represents a potential solution in an n-dimensional space. Each particle has position and velocity vectors for directing its movement. The position vector and velocity vector of the ith particle in the n-dimension can be represented as $X_i = (x_i^1, x_i^2, ..., x_i^n)$ and $V_i = (v_i^1, v_i^2, ..., v_i^n)$, respectively, where $x_i^d \in \{0,1\}$; i=1,2,..m (m is the total number of particles); and d=1,2,..n (n is the dimension of data) [2]. v_i^d represent an element of particle velocity vectors. It is a real number for the d-th dimension of the particle i, where the maximum v_i^d, $V_{max} = (1/3) \times n$.

In gene selection, the vector of particle positions is represented by a binary bit string of length n, where n is the total number of genes. Each position vector (X_i) denotes a gene subset. If the value of the bit is 1, it means that the corresponding gene is selected. Otherwise, the value of 0 means that the corresponding gene is not selected. Each particle in the t-th iteration updates its own position and velocity according to the following equations:

$$v_i^d(t+1) = w(t) \times v_i^d(t) + c_1 r_1^d(t) \times (pbest_i^d(t) - x_i^d(t)) + c_2 r_2^d(t) \times (gbest^d(t) - x_i^d(t)) \tag{1}$$

$$Sig(v_i^d(t+1)) = \frac{1}{1 + e^{-v_i^d(t+1)}} \tag{2}$$

$$\text{if } Sig(v_i^d(t+1)) > r_3^d(t), \text{ then } x_i^d(t+1) = 1; \text{ else } x_i^d(t+1) = 0 \tag{3}$$

where c_1 and c_2 are the acceleration constants in the interval [0,2]. $r_1^d(t), r_2^d(t), r_3^d(t) \sim U(0,1)$ are random values in the range [0,1] that sampled from a uniform distribution. $Pbest_i(t) = (pbest_i^1(t), pbest_i^2(t), ..., pbest_i^n(t))$ and $Gbest(t) = (gbest^1(t), gbest^2(t), ..., gbest^n(t))$ represent the best previous position of the ith particle and the global best position of the swarm (all particles), respectively. They are assessed base on a fitness function. $Sig(v_i^d(t+1))$ is a sigmoid function where $Sig(v_i^d(t+1)) \in [0,1]$. $w(t)$ is an inertia weight and initialized with 1.4. It is updated as follows:

$$w(t+1) = \frac{(w(t) - 0.4) \times (MAXITER - Iter(t))}{(MAXITER + 0.4)} \tag{4}$$

where *MAXITER* is the maximum iteration (generation) and *Iter(t)* is the current iteration.

3   An Enhancement of Binary PSO (CPSO)

Almost all previous works of gene expression data researches have selected a subset of genes to obtain excellent cancer classification. Therefore, in this article, we propose CPSO for selecting a near-optimal (small) subset of genes. It is proposed to overcome the limitations of BPSO and previous PSO-based methods [4],[7]-[10]. CPSO in our work differs from BPSO and the PSO-based methods on two parts: 1) we propose the constraint of elements of particle velocity vectors; 2) we introduce a rule for updating $x_i^d(t+1)$, whereas BPSO and the PSO-based methods have used the original rule (Eq. 3) and no constraint of elements of particle velocity vectors. The constraint and rule are introduced in order to:

1. increase the probability of $x_i^d(t+1)=0$ $(P(x_i^d(t+1)=0))$.
2. reduce the probability of $x_i^d(t+1)=1$ $(P(x_i^d(t+1)=1))$.

The increased and decreased probability values cause a small number of genes are selected and grouped into a gene subset. $x_i^d(t+1)=1$ means that the corresponding gene is selected. Otherwise, $x_i^d(t+1)=0$ represents that the corresponding gene is not selected.

The constraint of elements of particle velocity vectors and the rule are proposed as follows:

$$Sig(v_i^d(t+1)) = \frac{1}{1+e^{-v_i^d(t+1)}}$$
(5)

subject to $v_i^d(t+1) \geq 0$

if $Sig(v_i^d(t+1)) > r_3^d(t)$, then $x_i^d(t+1)=0$; else $x_i^d(t+1)=1$ (6)

Theorem 1. The constraint of elements of particle velocity vectors and the rule increase $P(x_i^d(t)=0)$ because the minimum value for $P(x_i^d(t)=0)$ is 0.5 when $v_i^d(t)=0$ (min $P(x_i^d(t)=0) \geq 0.5$). Mean while, they decrease the maximum value for $P(x_i^d(t)=1)$ to 0.5 (max $P(x_i^d(t)=1) \leq 0.5$). Therefore, if $v_i^d(t)>0$, then $P(x_i^d(t)=0) >> 0.5$ and $P(x_i^d(t)=1) << 0.5$.

Proof. ($\Rightarrow$) Figure 1 shows that a) The constraint of elements of particle velocity vectors and the rule in CPSO increase $P(x_i^d(t)=0)$; b) Equations (1-3) in BPSO yield $P(x_i^d(t)=0) = P(x_i^d(t)=1) = 0.5$. For example, the calculations for $P(x_i^d(t)=0)$ and $P(x_i^d(t)=1)$ in Fig. 2(a) are shown as follows:

if $v_i^d(t)=1$, then $P(x_i^d(t)=0)=0.73$ and $P(x_i^d(t)=1)=1-P(x_i^d(t)=0)=0.27$.
if $v_i^d(t)=2$, then $P(x_i^d(t)=0)=0.88$ and $P(x_i^d(t)=1)=1-P(x_i^d(t)=0)=0.12$.

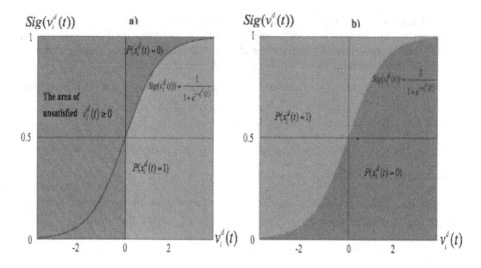

Fig. 1. The areas of $P(x_i^d(t)=0)$ and $P(x_i^d(t)=1)$ based on sigmoid functions in a) CPSO; b) BPSO. The grey and light grey colors show the areas for $P(x_i^d(t)=0)$ and $P(x_i^d(t)=1)$ respectively, and whereas the dark grey color indicates the part of unsatisfied $v_i^d(t) \geq 0$.

The fitness value of a particle (a gene subset) is calculated as follows:

$$fitness(X_i) = w_1 \times A(X_i) + (w_2(n - R(X_i)))/n \qquad (7)$$

in which $A(X_i) \in \lfloor 0,1 \rfloor$ is leave-one-out-cross-validation (LOOCV) classification accuracy that uses the only genes in a gene subset (X_i). This accuracy is provided by support vector machine classifiers (SVM). $R(X_i)$ is the number of selected genes in X_i. n is the total number of genes for each sample. w_1 and w_2 are two priority weights corresponding to the importance of accuracy and the number of selected genes, respectively, where $w_1 \in [0.1, 0.9]$ and $w_2 = 1 - w_1$.

4   Experiments

4.1   Data Sets and Experimental Setup

The gene expression data sets used in this study are summarized in Table 1. They included binary-classes and multi-classes data sets. Experimental results that produced by CPSO are compared with an experimental method (BPSO) for objective comparisons. Additionally, the latest PSO-based methods from previous related works are also considered for comparison with CPSO [4],[7]-[10]. Firstly, we applied the gain ratio technique for pre-processing in order to pre-select 500-top-ranked genes. These genes are then used by CPSO and BPSO. Next, SVM is used to measure LOOCV accuracy on gene subsets that produced by CPSO and BPSO. For LOOCV, one sample in the training set is withheld and the remaining samples are used for building a classifier to classify the class of the withheld sample. By cycling through all the samples, we can get cumulative accuracy rates for classification accuracy of methods. In this research, LOOCV is used for measuring classification accuracy due to the small number of samples in gene expression data. Several experiments are independently conducted 10 times on each data set using CPSO and BPSO. Next, an average result of the 10 independent runs is obtained. High LOOCV accuracy, the small number of selected genes, and low running time are needed to obtain an excellent performance.

Table 1. The summary of gene expression data sets

Data set	No. classes	No. samples	No. genes	Source
Leukemia	2 (ALL and AML)	72 (67 ALL and 25 AML)	7,129	http://www.broad.mit.edu/cgi-bin/cancer/datasets.cgi
Lung	2 (MPM and ADCA)	181 (31 MPM and 150 ADCA)	12,533	http://chestsurg.org/publications/2002-microarray.aspx.
MLL	3 (ALL, MLL, and AML)	72 (24 ALL, 20 MLL, and 28 AML)	12,582	http://www.broad.mit.edu/cgi-bin/cancer/datasets.cgi
SRBCT	4 (EWS, RMS, NB, and BL)	82 (28 EWS, 25 RMS, 18 NB, and 11 BL)	2,308	http://research.nhgri.nih.gov/microarray/Supplement/
Colon	2 (Normal and tumor)	62 (22 normal and 40 tumor)	2,000	http://microarray.princeton.edu/oncology/affydata/index.html

Note:
MPM = malignant pleural mesothelioma.   MLL = mixed-lineage leukemia.
ADCA = adenocarcinoma.   AML = acute myeloid leukemia.
ALL = acute lymphoblastic leukemia.   SRBCT = small round blue cell tumors.

4.2   Experimental Results

Based on the standard deviation of classification accuracies in Table 2, results that produced by CPSO were almost consistent on all data sets. Interestingly, all runs have achieved 100% LOOCV accuracy with less than 50 selected genes on the SRBCT data set. Moreover, over 97% classification accuracies have been obtained on other data sets, except for the colon data set. This means that CPSO has efficiently selected and produced a near-optimal gene subset from high-dimensional data (gene expression data).

Table 2. Experimental results for each run using CPSO on the leukemia, colon, lung, MLL, and SRBCT data sets

Run#	Leukemia		Colon		Lung		MLL		SRBCT	
	#Acc (%)	#Se-lected Genes	#Acc (%)	#Se-lected Genes	#Acc (%)	# Selected Genes	#Acc (%)	#Se-lected Genes	#Acc (%)	#Se-lected Genes
1	100	10	90.32	4	99.45	9	97.22	32	100	20
2	100	5	90.32	6	99.45	9	98.61	113	100	48
3	100	3	88.71	28	99.45	7	97.22	38	100	42
4	98.61	9	91.94	10	99.45	30	97.22	28	100	50
5	98.61	9	88.71	8	99.45	8	97.22	6	100	21
6	100	31	88.71	8	99.45	9	95.83	6	100	37
7	98.61	11	88.71	7	98.90	8	97.22	11	100	32
8	98.61	10	88.71	7	99.45	5	97.22	37	100	27
9	98.61	8	88.71	5	99.45	15	97.22	88	100	21
10	98.61	9	88.71	130	99.45	13	97.22	33	100	50
Average ± S.D.	99.17 ± 0.72	10.50 ± 7.61	89.36 ± 1.13	21.30 ± 38.80	99.39 ± 0.15	11.30 ± 7.17	97.22 ± 0.66	39.20 ± 35.04	100 ± 0	34.80 ± 12.30

Note: Results of the best subsets is shown in shaded cells. A near-optimal subset that produces the highest classification accuracy with the smallest number of genes is selected as the best subset. #Acc and S.D. denote the classification accuracy and the standard deviation, respectively, whereas #Selected Genes and Run# represent the number of selected genes and a run number, respectively.

Figure 2 shows that the averages of fitness values of CPSO increase dramatically after a few generations on all the data sets. A high fitness value is obtained by a combination between a high classification rate and a small number (subset) of selected genes. The condition of the proposed constraint of elements of particle velocity vectors that should always be positive real numbers started in the initialization method, and the new rule for updating particle's positions provoke the early convergence of CPSO. In contrast, the averages of fitness values of BPSO was no improvement until the last generation due to $P(x_i^d(t)=0)=P(x_i^d(t)=1)=0.5$.

For an objective comparison, CPSO is compared with BPSO. According to the Table 3, overall, it is worthwhile to mention that the classification accuracy and the number of selected genes of CPSO are superior to BPSO in terms of the best, average, and standard deviation results on all the data sets. The classification accuracies of BPSO and CPSO were same on the lung and SRBCT data sets. However, the number of selected genes of BPSO was higher than CPSO to achieve the same accuracy.

CPSO also produces smaller numbers of genes and lower running times compared to BPSO on all the data sets. CPSO can reduce its running times because of the following reasons:

- CPSO selects the smaller number of genes compared to BPSO;
- The computation of SVM is fast because it uses the small number of features (genes) that selected by CPSO for classification process.

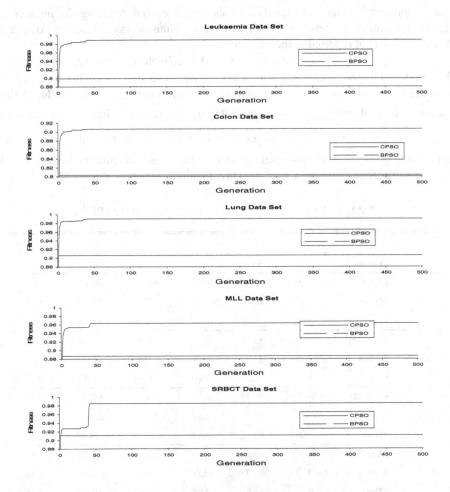

Fig. 2. The relation between the average of fitness values (10 runs on average) and the number of generations for CPSO and BPSO

We also compare our work with previous related works that used PSO-based methods in their proposed methods [4],[7]-[10]. It is shown in Table 4. For all the data sets, the averages of the number of selected genes of our work were smaller than the previous works. Our work also have resulted the higher averages of classification accuracies on the leukemia and SRBCT data sets compared to the previous works. However, experimental results produced by Shen *et al.* were better than our work on the colon data set [7]. This is due to the incorporation of tabu search (TS) as a local improvement procedure enables the algorithm HPSOTS to overleap local optima and show satisfactory performance in classifying cancer classes and reducing the number of genes. Running time between CPSO and the previous works cannot be compared because it was not reported in their articles.

According to Fig. 2 and Tables 2-4, CPSO is reliable for gene selection since it has produced the near-optimal solution from gene expression data. This is due to the proposed constraint of elements of particle velocity vectors and the introduced rule increase the probability $x_i^d(t+1)=0$ $(P(x_i^d(t+1)=0))$. The increased probability value for $x_i^d(t+1)=0$ causes the selection of a small number of informative genes and finally produces a near-optimal subset (a small subset of informative genes with high classification accuracy) for cancer classification.

Table 3. Comparative experimental results of CPSO and BPSO

Data	Method / Evaluation	CPSO			BPSO		
		Best	#Ave	S.D	Best	#Ave	S.D
Leu-kemia	#Acc (%)	100	99.17	0.72	98.61	98.61	0
	#Genes	3	10.50	7.16	216	224.70	5.23
	#Time	5.26	6.13	1.44	13.86	13.94	0.03
Colon	#Acc (%)	91.94	89.36	1.13	87.10	86.94	0.51
	#Genes	10	21.30	38.80	214	231	10.19
	#Time	8.78	9.26	0.70	30.58	30.63	0.27
Lung	#Acc (%)	99.45	99.39	0.18	99.45	99.39	0.18
	#Genes	5	11.30	7.17	219	223.33	4.24
	#Time	63.53	64.40	0.87	110.71	111.07	0.23
MLL	#Acc (%)	98.61	97.22	0.66	97.22	97.22	0
	#Genes	113	39.20	35.04	218	228.11	4.86
	#Time	9.51	11.64	4.98	19.37	19.90	0.35
SRBCT	#Acc (%)	100	100	0	100	100	0
	#Genes	20	34.80	12.30	206	221.30	7.35
	#Time	21.67	21.76	1.32	44.86	44.88	0.01

Note: The best result of each data set is shown in shaded cells. It is selected based on the following priority criteria: 1) the highest classification accuracy; 2) the smallest number of selected genes. #Acc and S.D. denote the classification accuracy and the standard deviation, respectively, whereas #Genes and #Ave represent the number of selected genes and an average, respectively. #Time stands for running time in the hour unit.

Table 4. A Comparison Between Our Method (CPSO) and previous PSO-Based Methods

Data	Method / Evaluation	CPSO	PSOTS [7]	PSOGA [4]	IBPSO [8]	TS-BPSO [9]	BPSO-CGA [10]
Leu-kemia	Average #Acc (%)	(99.17)	(98.61)	(95.10)	-	-	-
	Best #Acc (%)	100	-	-	100	100	100
	Average #Genes	(10.50)	(7)	(21)	-	-	-
	Best #Genes	3	-	-	1034	2577	300
Colon	Average #Acc (%)	(89.36)	(93.55)	(88.7)	-	-	-
	Best #Acc (%)	91.94	-	-	-	-	-
	Average #Genes	(21.30)	(8)	(16.8)	-	-	-
	Best #Genes	10	-	-	-	-	-
Lung	Average #Acc (%)	(99.39)	-	-	-	-	-
	Best #Acc (%)	99.45	-	-	-	-	-
	Average #Genes	(11.30)	-	-	-	-	-
	Best #Genes	5	-	-	-	-	-
MLL	Average #Acc (%)	(97.22)	-	-	-	-	-
	Best #Acc (%)	98.61	-	-	-	-	-
	Average #Genes	(39.20)	-	-	-	-	-
	Best #Genes	113	-	-	-	-	-
SRBCT	Average #Acc (%)	(100)	-	-	-	-	-
	Best #Acc (%)	100	-	-	100	100	100
	Average #Genes	(34.80)	-	-	-	-	-
	Best #Genes	20	-	-	431	1084	880

Note: '-' means that a result is not reported in the related previous work. A result in '( )' denotes an average result.
PSOGA = A hybrid of PSO and GA. PSOTS = A hybrid of PSO and tabu search. IBPSO = An improved binary PSO.
TS-BPSO = A combination of tabu search and BPSO. BPSO-CGA = A hybrid of BPSO and a combat genetic algorithm.

5   Conclusion

Overall, based on the experimental results, the performance of CPSO was superior to BPSO and previous PSO-based methods in terms of classification accuracy and the number of selected genes. CPSO was excellent because the probability $x_i^d(t+1)=0$ has been increased by the proposed constraint of elements of particle velocity vectors and the introduced rule. The constraint and rule have been proposed in order to yield a near-optimal subset of genes for better cancer classification. CPSO also obtains lower running times because it selects the small number of genes compared to BPSO. For future works, a modified representation of particle's positions in PSO will be proposed to reduce the number of genes subsets in solution spaces.

Acknowledgement. We would like to thank Malaysian Ministry of Science, Technology and Innovation for supporting this research by an e-science research grant (Grant number: 06-01-06-SF1029). This research is also supported by a GUP research grant (Grant number: Q.J130000.2507.04H16) that was sponsored by Universiti Teknologi Malaysia.

References

1. Kennedy, J., Eberhart, R.: Particle swarm optimization. In: Proceedings of the 1995 IEEE International Conference on Neural Networks, vol. 4, pp. 1942–1948 (1995)
2. Kennedy, J., Eberhart, R.: A discrete binary version of the particle swarm algorithm. In: Proceedings of the 1997 IEEE International Conference on Systems, Man, and Cybernetics, vol. 5, pp. 4104–4108 (1997)
3. Knudsen, S.: A Biologist's Guide to Analysis of DNA Microarray Data. John Wiley & Sons, New York (2002)
4. Li, S., Wu, X., Tan, M.: Gene selection using hybrid particle swarm optimization and genetic algorithm. Soft Comput. 12, 1039–1048 (2008)
5. Mohamad, M.S., Omatu, S., Deris, S., Misman, M.F., Yoshioka, M.: Selecting informative genes from gene expression data by using hybrid methods for cancer classification. Int. J. Artif. Life & Rob. 13(2), 414–417 (2009)
6. Mohamad, M.S., Omatu, S., Yoshioka, M., Deris, S.: A cyclic hybrid method to select a smaller subset of informative genes for cancer classification. Int. J. Innovative Comput., Inf. & Control 5(8), 2189–2202 (2009)
7. Shen, Q., Shi, W.M., Kong, W.: Hybrid particle swarm optimization and tabu search approach for selecting genes for tumor classification using gene expression data. Comput. Biol. & Chem. 32, 53–60 (2008)
8. Chuang, L.Y., Chang, H.W., Tu, C.J., Yang, C.H.: Improved binary PSO for feature selection using gene expression data. Comput. Biol. & Chem. 32, 29–38 (2009)
9. Chuang, L.Y., Yang, C.H., Yang, C.H.: Tabu search and binary particle swarm optimization for feature selection using microarray data. J. Comput. Biol. 16(12), 1689–1703 (2009)
10. Chuang, L.Y., Yang, C.H., Li, J.C., Yang, C.H.: A hybrid BPSO-CGA approach for gene selection and classification of microarray data. J. Comput. Biol. 18, 1–14 (2011)

Parameter Estimation Using Improved Differential Evolution (IDE) and Bacterial Foraging Algorithm to Model Tyrosine Production in Mus Musculus (Mouse)

Jia Xing Yeoh[1], Chuii Khim Chong[1], Yee Wen Choon[1], Lian En Chai[1], Safaai Deris[1], Rosli Md. Illias[2], and Mohd Saberi Mohamad[1,*]

[1] Artificial Intelligence and Bioinformatics Research Group, Faculty of Computing, Universiti Teknologi Malaysia, Skudai, 81310 Johor, Malaysia
`{jeyeoh3,ckchong2,ywchoon2,lechai}@live.utm.my,`
`{safaai,saberi}@utm.my`
[2] Department of Bioprocess Engineering, Faculty of Chemical Engineering, Universiti Teknologi Malaysia, Skudai, 81310 Johor, Malaysia.
`r-rosli@utm.my`

Abstract. The hybrid of Differential Evolution algorithm with Kalman Filtering and Bacterial Foraging algorithm is a novel global optimization method that is implemented in this research to obtain the best kinetic parameter value. The proposed algorithm is then used to model tyrosine production in *mus musculus* (mouse) by using a dataset, JAK/STAT (Janus Kinase Signal Transducer and Activator of Transcription) signal transduction pathway. Global optimization is a method to identify the optimal kinetic parameter using ordinary differential equation. From the ordinary parameter of biomathematical field, there are many unknown parameters and commonly the parameters are in nonlinear form. Global optimization method includes differential evolution algorithm which will be used in this research. Kalman Filter and Bacterial Foraging algorithm help in handling noise data and faster convergences respectively in the conventional Differential Evolution. The results from this experiment show estimatedly optimal kinetic parameters values, shorter computation time, and better accuracy of simulated results compared with other estimation algorithms.

Keywords: Parameter Estimation, Differential Evolution Algorithm, Bacterial Foraging Algorithm, Kalman Filtering Algorithm, Modeling.

1 Introduction

Metabolic pathway can be described by a combination of processes types including reversible reactions and in some with respects of multi-molecule reactions. Recently, many research have been done in the field of modelling in biology system where most of the pathways can be represented in the ordinary differential equation. Mathematical modelling of biological metabolic pathways is increasingly attracting attention and is

---

[*] Corresponding author.

J. Li et al. (Eds.): PAKDD 2013 Workshops, LNAI 7867, pp. 179–190, 2013.
© Springer-Verlag Berlin Heidelberg 2013

a central theme in system biology to accomplish four goals which are system structure identification, system behaviour analysis system control and system design [1].

In designing the mathematical modelling of biological pathway, parameter estimation is the most challenging part to retrieve optimal parameter values that could obtain the best fit with the experimental data. Parameter estimation is a concept where a sample data is used to estimate the value of a population's parameter such as mean and variance. Usually, the ordinary differential equation is used in modelling biological data in analysis, prediction, and optimizing the biological system itself. For this research, Differential Evolution algorithm with the implementation of Bacterial Foraging algorithm has been design to conduct the parameter estimation on JAK/STAT signal transduction pathway to model the tyrosine production in mus musculus.

Modeling is a process of generating abstract, conceptual, graphical and mathematical models. There are several processes in the biology modeling. In the process of modeling the biological system, the most challenging part is the determination of the model parameter. Furthermore, biological processes and interaction are highly non-linear and complex, hence mathematical analysis is needed to capture the nonlinear of the data. Therefore, parameter estimation plays an important role in modeling the biological system, which however is very difficult. Parameter estimation is used to determine rate constants and kinetic orders so that the dynamic profiles satisfactorily fit the measured observation in the biology system. Basically biological processes are modeled using Ordinary Differential Equations (ODEs) to describe the evolution over time of certain quantities of interest [2]. Generally, equation depends on several parameters and usually the parameters are unknown.

This research focuses on the optimization result of the kinetic parameter estimation. Yao and William [3] used Genetic Algorithm (GA) to solve the parameter estimation for linear and nonlinear digital filters and were applied to both feed forward and recurrent neural network. There was a problem in using the GA stem from its computational complexity and it was trapped in local minimal. Rodolfo *et al.* [4] studied on the optimal tuning of the parameters of a fuzzy controller for a network based control system. In this research, the SA faced a problem of time consumption for the estimation of the parameter estimation. Moonchai *et al.* [5] implemented DE as parameter estimation approach by enhancing the production of lactic acid production, glucose consumption, and bacteriocin production. Differential evolution algorithm (DE) is developed for the purpose to optimize real parameters and real valued functions. Although DE is a good algorithm in estimating kinetic parameter, there are still challenges where the algorithm may be influenced by noisy data during parameter estimation. The problem of noisy data can be solved by using Kalman Filtering algorithm (KF), where the KF can filter the noisy data by updating the population and also improving the performance of parameter estimation. The combination of DE and KF is called Improved Differential Evolution algorithm [6]. Besides that, the performance of parameter estimation can also be improved by implementing Bacterial Foraging algorithm (BF) in the algorithm with DE and KF, where the BF help in faster convergences by implementing the reproduction and chemostatic state into mutation and crossover of the DE. The reproduction state of the BF is implemented in mutation state of DE while the chemostatic state of the BF is modified in the crossover path of DE, where these will help in faster convergence and avoid from being trapped in local minima.

In order to get the best performances of the modeling of tyrosine production, the estimation of the best kinetic parameters should be perform. To get the best value of parameter estimation, DE with KF and BF are used in this research, where the DE is used to find the true global minimum regardless of the initial parameter values, fast convergence, and using few control parameters [7]. This algorithm has not been implemented in modeling the tyrosine production in mus musculus, and the performance of the implementation of this algorithm is believe in improve the performance in parameter estimation [8]. This algorithm is able to produce best result with shortest computational time and improvement on the accuracy of the parameter estimation.

2   Material and Method

The dataset that used in this research is JAK/STAT signal transduction pathway. The mechanism of JAK/STAT will give several of differential equation and their parameters in the equation. This ordinary equation is that will be used in the biological modeling. The mechanism of the JAK/ STAT signal transduction pathway is shown in the figure below. The numbers in the figure indicated the step of the

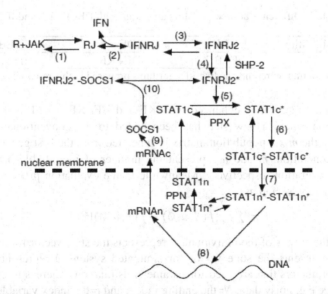

Fig. 1. JAK/STAT signal transduction pathway mechanism. (Source: Control Mechanism of JAK/STAT Signal Transduction Pathway [8]).

mechanism: 1, binding of JAK to the intracellular domain of the IFN-γ receptor (IFNR) and forms the IFNR–JAK complex (designated as RJ). 2, IFN-γ binds to the extracellular domain of the RJ complex and forms the IFN-γ–IFNR–JAK complex (designated as IFNRJ). 3, IFN binding drives the association of two receptor monomers into a receptor dimer (IFNRJ2). 4, The dimerization of the RJ complex leads to the phosphorylation of several tyrosine residues by JAK, yielding a form as IFNRJ2*. 5, The STAT1 binds to IFNRJ2* and is phosphorylated by JAK. 6, The phosphorylated STAT1 forms a homo-dimer. 7,The phosphorylated dimers of STAT1 are translocated to the nucleus. 8, STAT1also work as the transcription factors. 9, SOCS1 is induced by JAK/STAT pathway. 10,the SOCS1 binds to the activated receptor–JAK and inhibits its kinase activity [8].

Based on the previous study, this study proposes the Improved Differential Evolution and Bacterial Foraging algorithm (IDEBF), which is a hybrid of DE, KF, and BF. Table 1 shows the difference between the existing algorithm and IDEBF, where the existing algorithm comprises of only DE, whereas IDEBF is a hybrid of IDE and BF and IDE is a hybrid of DE and KF. Fixed control parameter values used in this study are as follow:

i.   Population size, NP: 10
ii.   Mutation factor, F: 0.5
iii.   Crossover constant, CR: 0.9
iv. B and R matrices identity matrices.
v. H is generated from Jacobian matrix and ODE information.

Table 1. Difference between existing algorithm with DEBF, IDE and IDEBF

Existing Algorithm	DEBF	IDE	IDEBF
DE	DE+BF	DE+KF	IDE+BF

Note: Shaded column represents the hybrid algorithms proposed in this research

The conventional DE is enhanced with KF and BF. KF would help in updating the population where a new step has been added to the conventional DE. In the initialization, the m x n population matrix is generated from the first generation till the maximum generation. m and n represent the number of identifiable parameter and number of generation respectively. Meanwhile in the evaluation process, the fitness function, J is represented as

$$J = \sum_{i=i}^{n} |f(X, u, \emptyset) - f(Y, u, \emptyset)|^2 \tag{1}$$

to evaluate the fitness of the individual. X represents the state vector for measurement system, Y represents the state vector for simulated system, $\emptyset$ represents the set of unknown parameters that are used for parameter estimation, whereas u represents the external force e.g. noisy data, N=the ending index, and i=the index variable.

After that, the updating of the population based on Kalman gain value K is retrieved from Equation 3. KF helps in handing the noisy data and updates the population once again. This is done until the evaluation process meets the stopping criterion. The update population process is carried out by using the formulas below.

$$temp\_population = (temp\_population' + K)' \qquad (2)$$

$$K = P * H' * inv(H * P * H' + R) \qquad (3)$$

H=observation matrix
R=measurement noise covariance
P=covariance of the state vector estimate
H' =inverse of matrix H

The BF is implemented in this mutation and crossover process of the conventional DE where the reproduction and chemostatic state of the BF are implemented into the mutation and crossover of the DE respectively. The BF involved in the mutation step of DE is created by using the following equation:

$$y_j = \begin{cases} \tilde{y}_j + \Delta\left(k, y_j^{(U)} - \tilde{y}_j\right), \tau = 0 \\ \tilde{y}_j - \Delta\left(k, \tilde{y}_j - y_j^{(L)}\right), \tau = 1 \end{cases} \qquad (4)$$

where the random constant τ becomes 0 or 1, $y_j^{(U)}$ and $y_j^{(L)}$ is the lower and upper range of y_j and $\Delta(k, w)$ is given as

$$\Delta(k, w) = w..\left(1 - \frac{k}{z}\right)^A \qquad (5)$$

$\eta = 0$ or 1 randomly and z is the maximum number of the generations as defined by the user. kth is represented as reproduction state.

A modification in simple crossover is used in DE algorithm using

$$_j^u = \lambda \bar{y}_j^v + (1 + \lambda)\bar{y}_j^u \qquad (6)$$

$$_j^v = \lambda \bar{y}_j^u + (1 - \lambda)\bar{y}_j^v \qquad (7)$$

where $\bar{y}_j^u$ and $\bar{y}_j^v$ refer to parent's generations and $_j^u$ and $_j^v$ refer to the offspring's generations and and j is the chromosome of chemotactic step and λ is the multiplier [9].

The complexity of this algorithm is $O(n)$ as the highest order of the formulas involved are two.

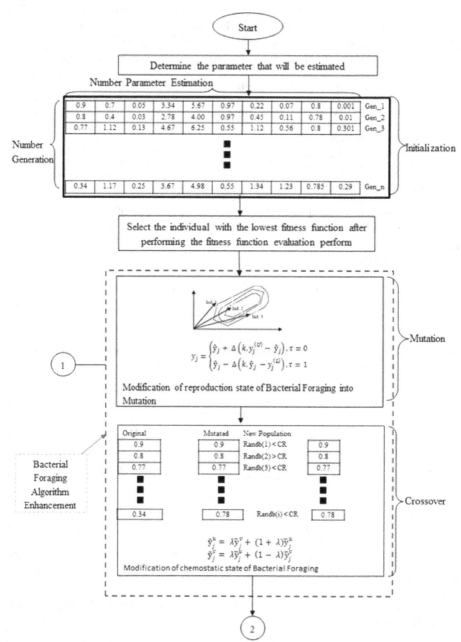

Note: Modification in mutation and crossover by using Bacterial Foraging Algorithm in DE to improve DE performance (highlighted with the dotted box).

Fig. 2(a). Schematic Overview of IDEBF

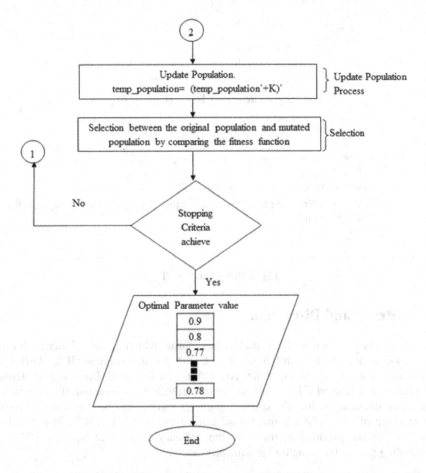

Note: Modification in mutation and crossover by using Bacterial Foraging Algorithm in DE to improve DE performance (highlighted with the dotted box).

Fig. 2(b). Schematic Overview of IDEBF

After the improvement of the DE with KF and BF, the algorithms will be implemented in the SBToolBox in Matlab and run in the Matlab with the dataset to get the best kinetic parameter estimation. Figure 2 and figure 3 shows the overall process of IDEBF and pseudo code for IDEBF in the estimation of the kinetic parameter values repectively.

Initialized and evaluate population, NP
Repeat
   For i := 1 to NP do
      Mutation of parent generation:
$$y_j = \begin{cases} \tilde{y}_j + \Delta\left(k, y_j^{(U)} - \tilde{y}_j\right), \tau = 0 \\ \tilde{y}_j - \Delta\left(k, \tilde{y}_j - y_j^{(L)}\right), \tau = 1 \end{cases}$$
      Create new offspring generation by the crossover of parent generation:
$$\tilde{y}_j^u = \lambda \bar{y}_j^v + (1 + \lambda)\bar{y}_j^u$$
$$\tilde{y}_j^v = \lambda \bar{y}_j^u + (1 - \lambda)\bar{y}_j^v$$

   endfor;
   Update Population;
     temp_population= (temp_population'+K)'
   Selection between original population and mutated population by comparing the
   fitness function
until stopping condition;

Fig. 3. Pseudo code of IDEBF

3   Result and Discussion

Five algorithms have been compared in this journal which include Genetic Algorithm (GA), Differential Evolution (DE), Improve Differential Evolution (IDE) ,Differential Evolution and Bacterial Foraging Algorithm (DEBF) and Improved Differential Evolution and Bacterial Foraging Algorithm (IDEBF). To evaluate the accuracy for each estimation algorithm, the kinetic parameter values have been indicated. From the mechanism of JAK/STAT signal transduction pathway [10], SOCS1 is the activator for the tyrosine production, therefore the ordinary differential equation (ODE) for estimating parameter value for tyrosine production is

$$\frac{d(SOCS1)}{dt} = \frac{v26 - v28 - v29 + v32 + v40 - v42 - v43 - v44}{cytoplasm} \tag{8}$$

Where
v26 = cytoplasm * v26_kf * mRNAc ,
v28 = cytoplasm * v28_kf * SOCS1,
v29 = cytoplasm * (v29_kf * SOCS1 * IFNRJ2_star - v29_kb * IFNRJ2_star_SOCS1
v32 = cytoplasm * v32_kf * IFNRJ2_star_SHP2_SOCS1_STAT1c,
v40 = cytoplasm * v40_kf * IFNRJ2_star_SHP2_SOCS1 ,
v42 = cytoplasm * (v42_kf * SOCS1 * IFNRJ2_star_STAT1c - v42_kb * IFNRJ2_star_SOCS1_STAT1c),
v43 = cytoplasm * (v43_kf * SOCS1 * IFNRJ2_star_SHP2 - v43_kb * IFNRJ2_star_SHP2_SOCS1) ,
v44 = cytoplasm * (v44_kf * SOCS1 * IFNRJ2_star_SHP2_STAT1c - v44_kb * IFNRJ2_star_SHP2_SOCS1_STAT1c) ,
cytoplasm = fixed value of 1.

IFNRJ2_star,   IFNRJ2_star_SHP2_SOCS1_STAT1c,   IFNRJ2_star_SHP2_SOCS1,
   IFNRJ2_star_STAT1c,   IFNRJ2_star_SOCS1_STAT1c,   IFNRJ2_star_SHP2,
   IFNRJ2_star_SHP2_STAT1c show the concentration of different activators.

The estimation of the kinetic parameter values is estimated by implementing the estimation algorithm in the SBToolBox of Matlab. The parameter values that are retrieved from Matlab will be substituted in the Copasi with the simulated kinetic parameter values to evaluate the average error rate and standard deviation for estimating the accuracy of the estimation algorithm. Table 2 shows the parameter estimation values for the estimation algorithms.

Table 2. Kinetic parameter values of DEBF compared with GA and DE.

Kinetic parameters	Measurement kinetic parameter values	Simulated kinetic parameter values				
		GA	DE	DEBF	IDE	IDEBF
v26kf	0.0100	0.2884	0.0073	0.0055	0.0044	0.0046
v28kf	0.0005	0.0007	0.0017	0.0001	0.0007	0.0004
v29kf	0.0200	0.0478	0.0216	0.0084	0.0241	0.3436
v29kb	0.1000	0.0975	0.0839	0.6912	0.102	0.5888
v32kf	0.0030	0.0006	0.006	0.0016	0.0015	0.0025
v40kf	0.0030	0.0347	0.0074	0.0014	0.0025	0.0061
v42kf	0.0200	0.0536	0.0979	0.0321	0.1654	0.0045
v42kb	0.1000	0.1859	0.1112	0.0639	0.1091	0.6518
v43kf	0.0200	0.0149	0.0195	0.0428	0.0194	0.0119
v43kb	0.1000	0.0424	0.3522	0.0994	0.0816	0.1151
v44kf	0.0200	0.0054	0.235	0.0199	0.0145	0.0428
v44kb	0.1000	0.1701	0.0883	0.4386	0.1368	0.0424

The time series data for the concentration of SOCS1 is generated from Equation 8. Measurement result, y, and simulated result yi, are in the time series data for GA, DE, IDE and IDEBF respectively. Equation 9, Equation 10 and Equation 11 show the formula to obtain the Error rate (e), Average error rate (A), and Standard Deviation (STD) values respectively.

$$e = \sum_{i=0}^{n}(y - yi)^2 \qquad (9)$$

$$A = \frac{e}{N} \qquad (10)$$

$$STD = \sqrt{\frac{e}{N}} \qquad (11)$$

Table 3 displays the average error rate and the standard deviation for five estimation algorithms for the tyrosine production in JAK/STAT signal transduction pathway.

Table 3. Average of error rate and STD values for SOCS1

Evaluation criteria	GA	DE	DEBF	IDE	IDEBF
Average of error rate, A	2.201E-07	2.687E-07	1.786E-07	1.763E-07	1.682E-07
Standard Deviation, STD	3.640E-07	4.489E-07	3.155E-07	2.882E-07	2.872E-07

Note: Shaded column represents the best results.

Each algorithm was compared through 50 runs for the JAK/STAT signal transduction pathway dataset to retrieve the standard deviation and the average error rate for the SOCS1. From the result displayed in Table 3, IDEBF shows the lowest average of error rate and standard deviation with values of 1.6820E-07and 2.8718E-07 respectively. DE shows the worst performance of the average error rate and the standard deviation among the three estimation algorithms with values of 2.6867E-07 and 4.4891E-07 respectively. Meanwhile, IDE shows the second lowest average of error rate and standard deviation with values of 1.7627E-07and 2.8816E-07 respectively, followed by DEBF with the average of error rate value of 1.7860E-07 and standard deviation value is 3.1548E-07, while GA has values of 2.2095E-07 and 3.6401E-07 for average error rate and standard deviation respectively. The average error rate and the standard deviation values of IDEBF are close to 0. This shows that the result is more consistent and IDEBF shows the best accuracy compared to the other methods where it has the lowest average error rate and standard deviation among all the comparison methods. The hybrid of KF and BF into conventional BE helps in updating the population and faster convergence to retrieve the best kinetic parameter values.

Besides that, the computational time, the start and the end of the parameter estimation time is record to get the total of execution time for the performance. The computational time is calculated by the end time – start time of the execution. Table 4 below shows the computational time execution for the estimation algorithms using a Core 2 PC with 2GB main memory. According to the result in Table 4, DE shows the worst execution time for the parameter estimation compared to GA, DEBF, IDE and IDEBF algorithms which used 14 minutes and 30 seconds to evaluate the kinetic parameter values. On the hand, IDEBF shows the shortest execution time for the estimation of the kinetic parameter values which only used 6 minutes and 1 second to complete the execution, followed by IDE with execution time of 7 minutes and DEBF with 8 minutes and 13 seconds. The hybrid of KF and BF helps in shortening the computational time of the parameter estimation for the JAK/STAT signal transduction pathway dataset.

Table 4. Execution time of DEBF compared with GA and DE

Computation Usage	GA	DE	DEBF	IDE	IDEBF
Execution time (hh.mm.ss)	00:011:20	00:14:30	00:08:13	00:07:00	00:06:01

Note: Shaded column represents the best results.

Figure 4 below that the line of the simulated IDEBF is the closest to the experimental result, therefore is the most consistent compared to the other methods. The line of IDE is second closest to the experimental result, followed by DEBF and GA where DEBF and GA are less consistent compared to IDEBF. Meanwhile, the line of the simulated DE is farther apart from the estimation parameter values. Therefore, DE is the least inconsistent compared to the other methods. KF helps in handling the noise data by updating the population and the BF updates the mutation and crossover of the DE via implemented reproduction, k^{th} and chemostatic, ^{jth} state where it helps in the convergence where modelling creates the tendency for genetic characteristics of populations to stabilize over time. Besides that, the local minima also can be avoided by modifying DE with bacterial foraging algorithm.

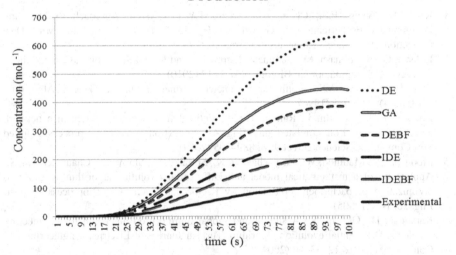

Fig. 4. Comparison of the simulated result with the measurement result of kinetic parameter values

4   Conclusion and Future Work

This research has proven that BF help in faster convergences in the conventional DE and helps in to shorten the computational time and good accuracy of the kinetic parameters values where the average error rate and standard deviation value are close to 0. KF helps in handling the noise data by using the Kalman gain method while the BF helps in faster convergences and avoids being trapped in the local minima in the reproduction state and chemostatic state in the mutation and crossover of DE. Therefore, the hybrid of the KF and BF in the DE has improved the accuracy of the parameter estimation where the hybrid method has the lowest average error rate and standard deviation and IDEBF has been proven to shorten the computational time as well. In future work, the dataset can be pre-processed before utilizing the kinetic parameter estimation where it helps in shortening the computational time. However, there is only one dataset that has been conducted in this study. For future research, other datasets can be experimented to retrieve the optimal parameter values for the biological pathway.

Acknowledgments. We would like to thank Malaysian Ministry of Science, Technology and Innovation for supporting this research by an e-science research grant (Grant number: 06-01-06-SF1029). This research is also supported by a GUP research grant (Grant number: Q.J130000.2507.04H16) that was sponsored by Universiti Teknologi Malaysia.

References

1. Ko, C.L., Wang, F.S., Chao, Y.P., Chen, T.W.: S-system Approach to Modeling Recombinant Escherichia coli Growth by Hybrid Differential Evolution with Data Collection. Biochemical Engineering Journal 3, 174–180 (2006)
2. Lillacci, G., Khammash, M.: Parameter Estimation and Model Selection in Computational Biology. PloS Computational Biology 6(3), 1–17 (2010)
3. Yao, L., William, A.S.: Nonlinear Parameter Estimation via the Genetic Algorithm. IEEE 42(4), 927–935 (1994)
4. Rodolfo, E.H., Agustín, J., Ramón, G.: An optimal fuzzy control system in a network environment based on simulated annealing. An application to a drilling process. Applied Soft Computing. Science Direct 9(3), 889–895 (2009)
5. Moonchai, S., Madlhoo, W., Jariyachavalit, K., Shimizu, H., Shioya, S., Chauvatcharin, S.: Application of a mathematical model and Differential Evolution algorithm approach to optimization of bacteriocin production by Lactococcus lactis C7. Bioprocess Biosyst. Eng. 28, 1–17 (2005)
6. Karaboga, D., Okdem, S.: A simple and global optimization algorithm for engineering problems: Differential evolution algorithm. Turkish Journal of Electrical Engineering and Computer Sciences 12, 53–60 (2004)
7. Chong, C.K., Mohamad, M.S., Deris, S., Shamsir, M.S., Choon, Y.W., Chai, L.E.: Improved Differential Evolution Algorithm for Parameter Estimation to Improve the Production of Biochemical Pathway. International Journal of Interactive Multimedia and Artificial Intelligence 1(5), 22–29 (2012)
8. Yamada, S., Shiono, S., Joo, A., Yoshimura, A.: Control mechanism of JAK/STAT signal transduction pathway. FEBS Lett. 534(1-3), 190–196 (2003)
9. Dong, H.K., Ajith, A., Jae, H.C.: A hybrid genetic algorithm and Bacterial Foraging approach for global optimization. Information Science 177(18), 3918–3937 (2007)
10. Satoshi, Y., Satoru, S., Akiko, J., Akihiko, Y.: Control Mechanism of JAK/ STAT signal Transduction Pathway. Federation of European Biochemical Societies. Elsevier Science 534(1-3), 190–196 (2002)

Threonine Biosynthesis Pathway Simulation Using IBMDE with Parameter Estimation

Chuii Khim Chong[1], Mohd Saberi Mohamad[1,*], Safaai Deris[1], Mohd Shahir Shamsir[2], Yee Wen Choon[1], and Lian En Chai[1]

[1] Artificial Intelligence and Bioinformatics Research Group, Faculty of Computing, Universiti Teknologi Malaysia, Skudai, 81310 Johor, Malaysia
ckchong2@live.utm.my, {saberi,safaai}@utm.my,
{ywchoon2,lechai2}@live.utm.my
[2] Department of Biological Sciences, Faculty of Biosciences and Bioengineering, Universiti Teknologi Malaysia, Skudai, 81310 Johor, Malaysia
shahir@utm.my

Abstract. When analysing a metabolic pathway through mathematical model, it is important that the significant parameters are being correctly estimated. However, this process often comes across problems such aseasily being trapped in local minima, repetitive exposure to worse results during the search process, and occurrence of noisy data. Thus, an improved Bee Memory Differential Evolution algorithm (IBMDE), which is a hybrid of the Differential Evolution algorithm (DE), the Kalman Filter (KF), Artificial Bee Colony algorithm (ABC), and a memory feature is presented this paper. IBMDE is an improved estimation algorithm as previous work only utilised DE. The threonine biosynthesis pathway is the metabolic pathways used in this paper. For metabolite O-Phosphohomoserine production simulation, the IBMDE able to produce the estimated optimal kinetic parameter values with significantly reduced error rate (63.67%) and shows a faster convergence time (71.46%) compared to the Nelder Mead (NM), the Simulated Annealing (SA), the Genetic Algorithm (GA), and DE respectively. In addition, IBMDE demostrates to be a reliable estimation algorithm.

Keywords: Parameter Estimation, Differential Evolution Algorithm, Kalman Filter, Artificial Bee Colony Algorithm, Memory feature.

1 Introduction

Systems biology manifests a biological system by a set of ordinary differential equations (ODEs) in mathematical models [1]. The essential interactions show quantitatively through ODEs with the aim in explaining the behaviour at the system level. Hand-tuning and *in-vitro* biochemical experiments are the main methods to retrieve the values of unknown parameters in the ODEs [2]. Under some conditions, these values are collected through estimation, and therefore, it is important that the

---

* Corresponding author.

J. Li et al. (Eds.): PAKDD 2013 Workshops, LNAI 7867, pp. 191–200, 2013.

estimation methods used in mathematical models are thoroughly studied [1]. Parameter estimation in system biology reduces the variance between experimental data and simulated data. It usually works as a part of a recursive process to develop mathematical models that are able to provide optimal estimated values for biological systems. Nevertheless, increasing number of unknown parameters and noisy experimental data of dynamic biochemical pathways cause most traditional estimation methods to generate inaccurate estimations [3].

Under the category of evolutionary algorithms, the Differential Evolution algorithm (DE) has been found to be the best estimation algorithm. It works to optimize a problem repetitively with the fixed objective function. The major advantages of DE are efficiency, high speed, ease of use, and simplicity [4]. It had been implemented by Moonchai *et al.* [5] to improve the production of bacteriocin by estimating the control parameters which were temperature and pH. Therefore, in this paper, it is implemented as the main estimation algorithm to solve the increasing number of unknown parameters. Kalman gain, K, value is used by the Kalman Filter (KF) in handling the noisy data through normalization. IDE (the Improved Differential Evolution algorithm) is the hybrid of these two algorithms [6].

Easily trapped in the local minimal due to faster convergence speed [4] and attempts to expose to worse results during the search process repeatedly are the disadvantages of DE. Therefore, to solve the mentioned disadvantages, IDE is then further combine with two modifications – the artificial bee colony algorithm (ABC) and a memory feature to generate the improved Bee Memory Differential Evolution algorithm (IBMDE). ABC capable to rise the probability in finding the optimal solutions by the food source possibility and this characteristic avoides the trapped in local minima [7]. The memory feature, however, capable to keep track of the best candidate ever during the search process with the extra memory named *gbest* and this prevents the worse result from being exposed again.

The paper is structured into four sections, where Section 2 introduce the method implemented, IBMDE, and subsequently Section 3 with experimental setup, results, and discussion. Finally, the conclusion and future works is showed in Section 4.

2   Methodology

An improved estimation algorithm, the Improved Bee Memory Differential Evolution algorithm (IBMDE) is presented in this paper. Previous work [5] only used DE while IBMDE uses a hybrid of DE, KF, ABC, and memory feature for parameter estimation. The details of the IBMDE is demostrated in Figure 1. As in conventional DE, a n x m population matrix, P, the initial population is produced in the initialization process. m is the number of unknown parameters and n is the number of generations. Each gene of the individuals in the initial population gained its own value based on Equation (1). Each gene represents a parameter value and individual, (Ind_i), indicates a set of estimated parameter values (possible solution) which i is the index variable where $1 \leq i \leq n$. For initialisation process, g indicates the ones matrix with dimension of n x 1, $I_{initial} = \{I_1, I_2, ..., I_m\}$ where I is the initial values for each parameter, and $rand(n,m)$ indicates a n x m matrix with random values between 0 and 1.

$$P = g * I_{initial} * 10^{0.5*rand\,(n*m)} \tag{1}$$

In the evaluation process, the fitness function, J, as shown:

$$J_i = \sum_{j=1}^{m} |f(D,E_{exp}) - f(D,S_{sim})|^2 \tag{2}$$

is implemented to analyse the fitness of each individual. D are the ordinary differential equations (ODEs) implemented to obtained the time series data values, $E_{exp} = \{E_1, E_2, ..., E_m\}$ where E is the experimental parameter values, $S_{sim} = \{S_1, S_2, ..., S_m\}$ where S is the optimal estimated parameter values, j is the index variable where $1 \leq j \leq m$, and $f(D, z)$ is the function to retrieve time series data values with fixed parameter values, z. The best candidate (candidate with the lowest fitness value) is stored in a memory named *gbest*. Equation (3) is used to calculate the probability of each candidate, $prob(i)$, where $fit(i)$ is the fitness value with index i and max indicates the function to obtain the maximum value. The upper bound and lower bound are altered to individuals with the highest and lowest probability value respectively after obtaining the probability value of each individual as long as the fitness value is not converged.

$$prob(i) = 0.1 * (fit(i) / \max(fit(i))) + 0.9 \tag{3}$$

$$M = P(i_3) + F * (P(i_1) - P(i_2)) \tag{4}$$

Three individuals (i_1, i_2, i_3) are chosen and then are replaced into the formula as presented in Equation (4). M indicates the mutated population matrix and F is the mutation factor. The subsequent crossover process is primarily executed according to the CR and $U(0,1)_i$ values. For mutation population matrix, each individual has its own $U(0,1)$ value. CR indicates the crossover constant value, $U(0,1)_i$ is the uniform random value between 0 and 1 with index i, and C is the crossover population matrix. If the CR value is lower than the $U(0,1)$ value of individual in the mutated population, then the mutation population's individual would become the resultant population's individual for the crossover process and vice versa.

The following is the updating process which is executing based on Equation (5). This step would update the population which is generated by the crossover process and it is performed according to Kalman gain value, K, retrieved from Equation (6). The K value from Equation (6) takes the process and measurement noise covariance into account and UP indicates the updated population matrix. In this study, B and R matrix are identity matrices while H is retrieved from Jacobian matrix and the ODEs information. Besides that, H matrix is invertible but it does not have to be a square matrix and its number of rows must be equivalent with the number of unknown parameters. For *in silico* approaches, Gaussian noise is used to simulate the noisy data so the model is close to the nature of biology. After a small number of trials are performed with the reasonable range of 0 to 1, the noisy data value implements in this study is 0.1. The evaluation process is performed where the results retrieved from the update process are analysed with the initial population's individual after normalizing the noisy data. Individual with lowest fitness value is chosen between initial and updated population. The results generate from the evaluation process would be replaced by *gbest* values and records in solution population matrix, O, if its fitness value is lower than the fitness value of *gbest* and vice versa. Next, the whole process isrepeated until the stopping criterion is met. The stopping criteria are set via predefined maximum loop values or when the fitness function has converge. The modified selection and ABC are highlighted with the dotted box in Figure 1.

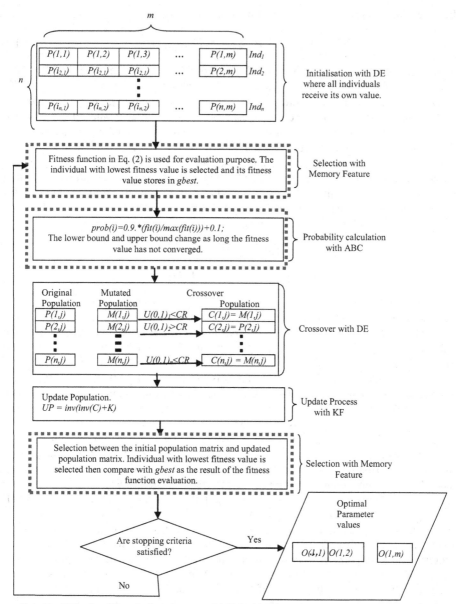

Note: The ABC and modify evaluation processes are highlighted in red.

Fig. 1. Flowchart of IBMDE

$$UP = inv(inv(C) + K)$$ (5)

$$K = P * H' * inv(H * P * H' + R)$$ (6)

where K = Kalman gain value, P = covariance of the state vector estimate, H = observation matrix, R = measurement noise covariance, inv = inverse function, and H' = inverse of matrix H,.

3   Experimental Setup

The optimal values for kinetic parameters that consisted in the threonine biosynthesis pathway model for *E-coli* [8] are gathered then undergo IBMDE. These pathway consists of 11 metabolites, 11 ODEs, seven reactions involved and 46 unknown parameters; but only 1 ODE, two reactions and ten unknown parameters are used for generating time series data of metabolite O-Phospho-homoserine (HSP). HSP is a substrate for threonine biosynthesis while threonine uses as treament for several nervous system disorders.The control parameters' values used in this study are crossover constant, CR=0.9, mutation factor, F=0.5, and population size, NP=10. These parameter values showed better results than the other values after a small number of trials are conducted between the reasonable range of 0 to 10. In this study, the main software used are the Copasi and SBToolbox in Matlab 2008a. An online database, Biomodel, is managed by European Bioinformatics Institute (EMBL-EBI) isused to retrieve the metabolic pathways.

The Nelder Mead (NM), the Simulated Annealing (SA), the Genetic Algorithm (GA), DE, and IBMDE are five estimation algorithms implemented in this study to allow the comparisons to be performed. Table 1 shows the experimental kinetic parameter values collected from previous related work [8] and the simulated kinetic parameters are generated by all the mentioned estimation algorithms. Average of error rates which were produced from the time series data values for the concentration of the metabolite HSP are implemented to assess the accuracy of the algorithm. Moreover, the simulation is repeated 50 times to calculate its standard deviation (*STD*) value and the average of error rates are then tested statistically with the chi square test to evaluate the reliability of the algorithm.

Table 1. Kinetic parameter values of IBMDE compared with NM, SA, GA and DE for metabolite HSP

Kinetic parameters	Measurement kinetic parameter values[8]	Simulated kinetic parameter values				
		NM	SA	GA	DE	IBMDE
vtsy_vm5	0.0434	0.038	0.089	2.849	0.038	0.181
vtsy_k5hsp	0.31	0.461	0.282	0.820	0.144	2.183
vhk_vm4f	0.1	0.204	0.057	16.577	1.690	62.174
vhk_lys	0.46	0.524	2.271	0.0564	0.524	1.750
vhk_k4lys	9.45	7.875	10.351	1.886	0.775	109.980
vhk_k4atp	0.072	0.052	0.026	15.507	0.013	0.110
vhk_k4ihs	4.7	5.952	1.532	3.2988	5.901	2.327
vhk_k4hs	0.11	0.2	0.017	6.6031	4.184	51.068
vhk_k4thr	1.09	1.2100	3.5	0.0224	1.307	4.164
vhk_k4iatp	4.35	3.1638	0.397	4.148	7.7305	248.351

Note: Table shows the kinetic parameter values implemened in the calculation of average of error metabolite HSP in Table 2.

Both experimental and simulated kinetic parameter values are subsituted into the ordinary differential equations (ODEs) for the metabolite HSP, as shown below:

$$\frac{dHSP}{dt} = vtsy + vhk \tag{7}$$

where

$vtsy$ = compartment * vtsy_vm5 * hsp / (hsp + vtsy_k5hsp),

vhk = compartment * (vhk_vm4f * hs * atp / ((1 + vhk_lys / vhk_k4lys) * (atp + vhk_k4atp * (1 + hs / vhk_k4ihs)) * (hs + vhk_k4hs * (1 + thr / vhk_k4thr) * (1 + atp / vhk_k4iatp)))),

compartment = constant value of 1,

adp = concentration for metabolite adenosine diphosphate which is equal to 0,

atp = concentration of metabolite adenosine triphosphate which is equal to 10,

hsp = concentration of metabolite HSP which is equal to 0,

hs = concentration of metabolite homoserine which is equal to 0,

thr = concentration of metabolite threonine which is equal to 2.

Equation (7) is used to retrieve the time series data values for the concentration of metabolite HSP. Experimental results, y, and simulated results y_{sim}, for NM, SA, GA, DE, and IBMDE are consisted in the time series data values respectively. Equation (8), Equation (9), and Equation (10) are used to calculate the error rate (e), average of error rate (A), and standard deviation (STD) value respectively.

$$e = \sum_{w=1}^{Q}(y - y_{sim})^2 \tag{8}$$

$$A = \frac{e}{Q} \tag{9}$$

$$STD = \frac{\sum_{w=1}^{Q}((y - y_{sim})^2 - mu)^2}{Q-1} \tag{10}$$

where w=the index variable, mu= the mean value, and Q= the number of rows of time series data values.

4   Experimental Results and Discussion

The average of error rate for each estimation algorithm is shown in Table 2. The results show that IBMDE has the lowest average of error rate with 0.001764 metabolite HSP. This proved that with the capability to keep tract of the best candidate ever during the search process by the memory named *gbest*, the accuracy of the estimation result has enhanced. This is due to the fact that with the memory, *gbest*, the search process has been prevented from being explored to worse results.

Table 2. Average of error rates for metabolite HSP

Metabolite	NM	SA	GA	DE	IBMDE
HSP	0.002830	0.002699	0.0052727	0.001886	0.001764

Note: Shaded column represents the best results.

Table 3 shows the number of generations needed for each estimation algorithm to converge to its optimal fitness value for metabolite HSP whereas the execution time of each estimation algorithm on a Core i5 PC with 4GB main memory for metabolite HSP is shown in Table 4. Based on the results, SA requires the longest time, 698.2019 seconds with 5009 number of generations to converge to the optimal value for all kinetic parameters. On the contrary, the IBMDE requires the shortest time, 343.4834 seconds with 4 number of generations. Less execution times (less number of seconds recorded) and less number of generations required to converge are two factors that enhance the effiency of the estimation algorithm in identifying the optimal solution. In short, the addition of a memory feature has avoided exposing space with worse results, and the addition of ABC has reduced the search space. Therefore, IBMDE showed higher accuracy and shorter computational time.

Table 3. Number of generations for metabolite HSP

Metabolite	NM	SA	GA	DE	IBMDE
HSP	33	5009	91	86	4

Note: Shaded column represents the best results.

Table 4. Execution times in unit of second (s) for metabolite HSP

Metabolite	NM	SA	GA	DE	IBMDE
HSP	531.1887	698.2019	400.5667	398.3966	343.4834

Note: Shaded column represents the best results.

Figure 2 shows the metabolite production graph for the metabolite HSP based on the kinetic parameters collected from previous related work [8] and produced by the mentioned estimation algorithms. The results illustrate that the kinetic parameters generated by IBMDE have enhanced the production rate as the experimental line is lower than its dotted simulation line. This enhancement is supported by the increase in speed and concentration kinetic parameters for metabolite HSP as compared to previous related work [8]. The speed kinetic parameters named vm5 and vm4f, rise by 0.138 $\mu mol/(l*min)$ and 62.0741 $\mu mol/(l*min)$ respectively while for the concentration kinetic parameters - vtsy_k5hsp, vhk_k4atp, vhk_k4hs, vhk_k4thr, and vhk_k4iatp, the values rise by 1.8733 $mmol/l$, 0.383 $mmol/l$, 50.9584 $mmol/l$,

3.0741 *mmol/l*, and 244.0015 *mmol/l* respectively. *μmol* is micromole, *mmol* is milimole, *l* is liter, *s* is seconds, and *min* is minutes. In Figure 2, ORI indicates the production graph that is generated with the kinetic parameters obtained from previous related work [8] whereas IBMDE indicates the production graphs that are generated by IBMDE. Speed is assumed to be the crucial kinetic parameter which can be increased to enhance the the interested metabolites' production [10]. The reasons that cause the increase in the speed parameter are increase in the surface area, substrate concentration, temperature, and the addition of catalyst. The enzyme and temperature fail to be the reasons to increase the speed parameter under particular conditions. When none of the reaction presents the flux coefficient value is equal to one and the temperature implemented exceeds the optimal temperature of the enzyme, then the addition of temperature and enzyme cause no effect. Other than that, the production of the interested metabolite can be improved by rising the concentration of the reactants. This implies that the product increase as more sources.

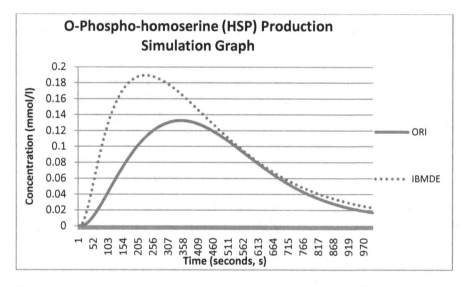

Fig. 2. Production Simulation Graph for IBMDE of metabolite O-Phospho-homoserine (HSP)

Table 5 shows the benckmark functions tested with Particle Swarm Optimisation (PSO), DE, and IBMDE. For these benchmark function tests, control parameters used for PSO are swarm size= 40, inertia weight= 0.7290, particle's best weight= 1.4945, and swarm's best weight= 1.4945 while for DE and IBMDE are NP=20, CR= 0.9, and F=0.5. Based on the results, IBMDE passes four tests out of five tests. Once again, it showed its ability in obtaining the optimal solution but it failed in the Rosenbrock test. This is due to the fact that Rosenbrock's landscape modifies from simple to complex and this implies that the diversity of control parameters is getting lesser. The mentioned problem can be solved by requiring large number of generations.

Table 5. Mean and Standard Deviation of the Best Fitness for PSO, DE, and IBMDE on benchmark functions

Optimisation algorithm	Ackley	Griewank	Rastrigin	Rosenbrock	Sphere
IBMDE	0.407400	0.039567	0.012922	0.143954	0.004890
	(0.461369)	(0.086018)	(0.052491)	(0.237157)	(0.014177)
PSO	12.140694	0.511792	2.138276	0.00558	0.00219
	(9.576828)	(0.288929)	(2.433339)	(0.160866)	(0.090779)
DE	5.175276	0.442472	-0.03718	5.65050	-0.18775
	(4.878749)	(0.196465)	(0.303299)	(8.543702)	(0.051303)

Note: Shaded column represents the best results.

A fitness function is used to reduce the variance between experimental and simulated results in this study. Based the results obtained from this experiment, the *STD* value and mean for the metabolite HSP are 0.001753 and 0.00136 respectively. Standard deviation is a calculation of how widely are the values being distributed from the mean (the average value). The results generated by IBMDE were consistent and the difference between each 50 run was small as the *STD* value for IBMDE was close to the mean value. Chi-square test (X^2 test), a statistical test has to be performed as stated by Lillacci and Khammash [2], in order to assure that the simulated results are statistically consistent with the experimental results. The confidence coefficient, γ, and degree of freedom, s, used in this paper are 0.995 and 1. Interval estimates, σ^2, produced based on s, γ, and the formula found in Lillacci and Khammash [2] are 0.00004 $\leq \sigma^2 \leq$ 9.550. The hypothesis proposed is the simulated results are statistically consistent with the experimental results. The X^2 value for the metabolite HSP is 0.00004 based on the chi-square equation; which implies that the X^2 value is existed in within the range of σ^2. Thus, the hypothesis is accepted as the IBMDE passed the X^2 test. The estimated results demonstrated to be statistically consistent with the experimental results.

5   Conclusion

IBMDE, a hybrid of DE, KF, ABC, and memory feature effectively reduced the search space through the probability value obtained from ABC in the search process and ultimately resulted in faster convergence time while only DE was used in previous work [5]. The exposing of worse search spaces has avoided with the ability to store of the best candidate ever with the *gbest* value during the search process and consequently helped in enhancing the accuracy of the estimated results. Beside that, handle noisy data by KF enhances the estimation's accuracy. In short, IBMDE performed better than SA, NM, GA, and DE in terms of computational time and accuracy. Furthermore, IBMDE also has proved that it is a reliable estimation algorithm as it passed the chi square test and can be used in used the areas that contains noisy data for example in the electrical and electronic engineering field. Besides that, IBMDE can be implemented to other metabolic pathways to improve the interested metabolites which are essential for medical and industrial use.

DE is very sensitive towards its control parameters: mutation factor (F), crossover constant (CR), and population size (NP) [9]. Thus, as future work, the self-adapting approach to these control parameters can be added to improve the performance of the conventional DE as well as the IBMDE.

Acknowledgments. We would like to thank Malaysian Ministry of Science, Technology and Innovation for supporting this research by an e-science research grant (Grant number: 06-01-06-SF1029). This research is also supported by a GUP research grant (Grant number: Q.J130000.2507.04H16) that was sponsored by Universiti Teknologi Malaysia.

References

1. Steuer, R.: Exploring the Dynamics of Large-Scale Biochemical Networks: A Computational Perspective. The Open Bioinformatics Journal 5, 4–15 (2011)
2. Lillacci, G., Khammash, M.: Parameter Estimation and Model Selection in Computational Biology. PLoS Computational Biology 6(3), 1–17 (2010)
3. Zhong, J., Martin, B.: Joint State and Parameter Estimation For Biochemical Dynamic Pathways With Iterative Extended Kalman Filter: Comparison With Dual State and Parameter Estimation. The Open Automation and Control Systems Journal 2, 69–77 (2009)
4. Chiou, J.P., Wang, F.S.: Estimation of Monod model parameters by hybrid differential evolution. Bioprocess and Biosystems Engineering 24, 109–113 (2001)
5. Moonchai, S., Madlhoo, W., Jariyachavalit, K., Shimizu, H., Shioya, S., Chauvatcharin, S.: Application of a mathematical model and Differential Evolution algorithm approach to optimization of bacteriocin production by Lactococcus lactis C7. Bioprocess and Biosystems Engineering 28, 1–17 (2005)
6. Chong, C.K., Mohamad, M.S., Deris, S., Shamsir, M.S., Choon, Y.W., Chai, L.E.: Improved Differential Evolution Algorithm for Parameter Estimation to Improve the Production of Biochemical Pathway. International Journal of Interactive Multimedia and Artificial Intelligence 1(5), 22–29 (2012)
7. Karaboga, D.: An idea based on honey bee swarm for numerical optimization. Technical Report TR06 (2005)
8. Chassagnole, C., Fell, D., Rais, B., Kudla, B., Mazat, J.: Control of the threonine-synthesis pathway in Escherichia coli: a theoretical and experimental approach. Biochem. J. 356(2), 433–444 (2001)
9. Feng, L., Yang, Y.-F., Wang, Y.-X.: A New Approach to Adapting Control Parameters in Differential Evolution Algorithm. In: Li, X., Kirley, M., Zhang, M., Green, D., Ciesielski, V., Abbass, H.A., Michalewicz, Z., Hendtlass, T., Deb, K., Tan, K.C., Branke, J., Shi, Y. (eds.) SEAL 2008. LNCS, vol. 5361, pp. 21–30. Springer, Heidelberg (2008)
10. Ferchichi, M., Crabble, E., Hintz, W., Gil, G.H., Almadidy, A.: Influence of culture parameters on biological hydrogen production by Clostridium saccharoperbutylacetonicum ATCC 27021. World Journal of Microbiology & Biotechnology 21, 855–862 (2005)

A Depression Detection Model
Based on Sentiment Analysis in Micro-blog
Social Network

Xinyu Wang[1], Chunhong Zhang[1], Yang Ji[1], Li Sun[1], Leijia Wu[2],
and Zhana Bao[3]

[1] Beijing University of Posts and Telecommunications (BUPT), Beijing, China
{wxinyu906,zhangch.bupt.001,ji.yang.0001,buptsunli}@gmail.com
[2] University of Technology, Sydney, Australia
leijia.wu@alumni.uts.edu.au
[3] Graduate School of Global Information and Telecommunication Studies,
Waseda University, Japan
znabao@ruri.waseda.jp

Abstract. Datasets originating from social networks are valuable to
many fields such as sociology and psychology. But the supports from
technical perspective are far from enough, and specific approaches are
urgently in need. This paper applies data mining to psychology area for
detecting depressed users in social network services. Firstly, a sentiment
analysis method is proposed utilizing vocabulary and man-made rules to
calculate the depression inclination of each micro-blog. Secondly, a depression detection model is constructed based on the proposed method
and 10 features of depressed users derived from psychological research.
Then 180 users and 3 kinds of classifiers are used to verify the model,
whose precisions are all around 80%. Also, the significance of each feature is analyzed. Lastly, an application is developed within the proposed
model for mental health monitoring online. This study is supported by
some psychologists, and facilitates them in data-centric aspect in turn.

Keywords: data mining, Chinese sentiment analysis, depression.

1 Introduction

The rise of online social network provides unprecedented opportunities for solving problems in a wide variety of fields with information techniques [1]. For example, traditional psychology research is based on questionnaires and academic
interviews, but many psychologists are now turning their sights to web media.
They try to analyze the data of social networks from the view of psychology.
Undoubtedly, this discipline integration injects vigor into psychology, however,
the supports from technical perspective are far from enough. Only some simple
statistic tools are applied in such kind of research, and little attention is paid to
design specific data mining methods, especially in Chinese text processing.

J. Li et al. (Eds.): PAKDD 2013 Workshops, LNAI 7867, pp. 201–213, 2013.
© Springer-Verlag Berlin Heidelberg 2013

This paper applies data mining techniques to psychology, specifically the field of depression, to detect depressed users in social network services (SNS). The expansion of data mining to psychology is of great technical and social significance. It is proved that the proposed model in this paper could effectively help for detecting depressed ones and preventing suicide in online social networks.

"I suffer from depression, thus trial for death. There's no special reason. Please do not care about my departure. Bye, everyone." On March 18th, 2012, a micro-blog posted by Zoufan dropped a bomb in Sina Micro-blog. Then on March 19th, JiangNing Police confirmed that Zoufan had committed suicide. Zoufan, whose real name is MaJie, was a talented university student in Nanjing. Her suicide for depression left us with endless sorrow. Zoufan Tragedy resulted from depression has aroused extensive concern of the whole society in China. The micro-blog contents of Zoufan are like death signals, revealing total despair and depression characteristics. But unfortunately, they did not attract attentions in time, until she resolutely said goodbye to the world with her last micro-blog.

This research is accomplished with the help of psychologists. They detect some depressed users within psychological diagnostic criteria, and observe the online behaviors of them. This paper constructs a depression detection model based on the features of depressed users derived from psychological observations. The result is verified to be efficient, so this model could be used for large-scale mental health monitoring, and avoid the tragedy of Zoufan occurring again.

Definitely, there are some challenges in our study. The complexity of Chinese text processing is one of them. The ambiguity definition relies on almost all the levels of syntactical unit in Chinese linguistics, which brings difficulties for word segmentation and linguistic rules construction [2]. Coupled with the particularity of the micro-blog content of depressed users, it takes great effort to adjust our model to improve its performance. Another challenge is how to distinguish training dataset and select features as criteria in the model. Due to the particularity of depression, this work is not easy for data mining experts, so the help of psychologists is asked as instructions.

To sum up, the contributions of this paper are: (1) From the aspect of methodology, data mining techniques is expanded to depression area. (2) Sentiment analysis algorithm, specifically for Chinese micro-blog is proposed for calculating the depression inclination. (3) An association model is established between features abstracted from Micro-blog system and depression inclination. The model also determines the principle features which affecting depression detection significantly. (4) An application in Sina Micro-blog is developed for monitoring the users' mental health in SNS. The basic idea of this paper could be explicitly extended to other language scenarios.

2   Related Work

2.1   Research of Depression in Psychology

Depression is the world's fourth largest disease and will be in the second place in 2020 according to World Health Organization statistics [3]. The main clinical symptom of depressed patients is lasting depressed state of mood and lack of positive emotions. They prefer to be alone rather than together with others. What's more, most of depressed patients suffer from chronic insomnia.

The research of depression in social network in psychology comes in two types: one is to discover disciplines of a crowd of depressed users [4-5]; the other is to look into a specific case elaborately [6]. Literature [4] observes linguistic markers of depression through collecting posts by depressed and non-depressed individuals from Internet forum. It analyzes the text with LIWC, a computerized word counting tool, and shows that the online depressed writers use more first person singular pronouns but less first person plural pronouns, more negative emotion words but less positive emotion words. Literature [6] discusses the relations between SNS behaviors and depression levels based on Zoufan Event. It is established by questionnaire and statistic tools, and reveals that frequencies of the original posts could indicate micro-bloggers' depressed levels. Also, the period of time users post micro-blogs is a consideration as most depression patients suffer from chronic insomnia.

These researches of depression features in the perspective of psychology provide reliable background knowledge for our study. However, when comes to data analysis problems, only some simple statistic tools are designed for them, which undoubtedly limit their researches. Therefore a specific data mining technique to detect depressed users is designed in this study based on their results.

2.2 Sentiment Analysis Techniques

As the cardinal symptom of depression is severe negative emotions and lack of positive emotions, sentiment analysis is the most important step in depression detection. Sentiment analysis aims at mining users' opinions and sentiment polarity from the texts they posted [7]. Recently many progresses have been made in sentiment analysis on Twitter data. These researches include two aspects:

- Subject-independent analysis, namely judging the polarity of the tweets without considering if it is relevant to a subject [8-10]. The main approaches are based on hashtags, smileys and some abstract features.

- Subject-dependent analysis, namely judging the polarity of the tweets based on the given subject [11-12]. The sentiments of the tweets as positive, negative or neutral in [11], according to not only the abstract features but also the target-dependent features, which refers to the comments on the target itself and the related things, which are defined as extended targets.

Sentiment analysis research on Chinese text is still in its starting stage [13]. The highest accuracy of polarity discrimination on Chinese text is only 59.27% in the latest NTCIR evaluation [14]. Little study has been made for solving problems in a specific field, although analysis strategy differs a lot for different fields. For example, depression sufferers tend to think the topic about "death", so this kind of words should be paid special attention to when constructing the vocabulary. Micro-blogs are often written in a colloquial style, which also bring new challenges when instituting the linguistic rules in the proposed method.

The problem addressed in this paper is subject-dependent sentiment analysis of micro-blogs. Inspired by the work in literature [11], abstract features and target-dependent features are taken into account. This study stresses the particularity of depression and micro-blog content, and the whole model is specifically designed based on them. As shown in Fig.1, a sentiment analysis method is firstly proposed utilizing vocabulary and man-made rules to calculate the depressive inclination of each micro-blog in Fig.1 (A). The vocabulary and man-made rules in sentiment analysis method are constructed based on the Chinese syntax rules, the particularity of depression and micro-blogs (section 3). Then as shown in Fig.1 (B), a depression detection model is constructed based on the proposed method and 10 features of depressed users derived from psychological research (section 4). Lastly, the significance of each feature is analyzed and a simplified model is proposed for the application in Sina Micro-blog.

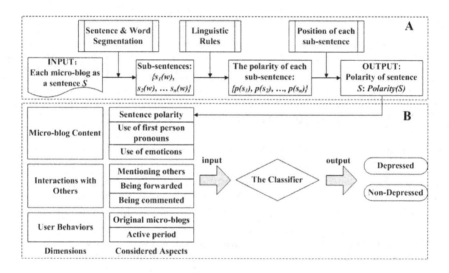

Fig. 1. Framework of the proposed model in this paper

3   Sentiment Analysis of Micro-blog Content

The most direct expression of depressed mood is the users' micro-blog content, so the sentiment analysis method in this section helps to figure out the polarity of each piece of micro-blog, which emphasizes the depression inclination reflected from the content. A vocabulary is constructed based on HowNet [15], and the sentence structure patterns and calculation rules are derived according to Chinese syntax rules. As described above, the particularity of depression and micro-blogs are paid special attention to the whole process.

3.1 Vocabulary Construction

The most essential particularity of depression and micro-blogs is the use of words. A vocabulary fitting for depression detection is constructed based on How-Net, a comprehensive vocabulary of Chinese words, as shown in Table 1.

Table 1. Words in HowNet vocabulary [15]

2 Item		Num.	Example
Emotion Words	Positive	4566	pretty, love, like, happy, good
	Negative	4370	ugly, sad, depressed, unhappy, bad
Degree Modifiers		219	most(2), over(1.75), very(1.5), more(1), -ish(0.75),insufficient(0.5)

HowNet contains most of the popular emotion words and degree modifiers. The weights of degree modifiers are quantified into six levels according to their intensities. HowNet is designed for general sentiment analysis. In order to make it fit for depressed inclination calculation, several adjustments are made as follows:

1. Emotion words, cyberspeaks, modal particles and negative words are added:
   1) Depressed users tend to use more emotion words, especially negative emotion words [4], some of which are even only for them. For example, "bye" is a neutral word for normal people, but it's a typical negative one for depressed users. So these typical emotion words for depression are added.
   2) Considering that cyberspeaks are in prevalent in Internet, they are playing an important role in micro-blogs. Therefore these words are also added, for example, "smilence", which means "smile silently", into the vocabulary.
   3) As micro-blogs are often written in a colloquial style, modal particles often occur in micro-blogs to express feelings directly, such as "ha-ha" and "a-ha", so these modal particles are added into the vocabulary too.
   4) Besides degree modifiers, negative words could also modify the expressions, which do not exist in HowNet. Negative words totally reverse the meaning of the expression, such as "not", "never". The negative words selected from a dictionary are imported as a new item into the vocabulary.
2. The part of speech of each word are recognized:
   The proposed calculation rules is derived from Chinese syntax rules, which are defined by parts of speech. So the part of speech of each word are recognized and also imported as an attribute into the vocabulary.

Finally, the vocabulary is constructed with three items as shown in Table 2. 1210 emotion words and 36 negative words are added. Each word holds its own part of speech and weight. Degree modifiers are inherited from HowNet.

3.2 Linguistic Rules Construction

The meaning of a sentence could not be decided only by the words it uses, but also by the order of words, named the structure of the sentence. For example, "我

Table 2. Words in the proposed vocabulary

3 Items		Num.	Part of speech	Weight	Notation
Emotion	Positive	5127	verb, adjective,	+1	W_EW
Words	Negative	5019	adverb, modal particle	-1	
Degree Modifiers		219	adjective, adverb	Inherited from HowNet	W_DM
Negative Words		36	adverb	-1	W_NW

不很高兴(slightly unhappy)", " 我很不高兴(very unhappy)", the two sentences share the same 5 characters, but have obvious different extent of how happy it is, so the structure of sentence should be taken into account in the process of polarity calculation. The structure of sentences could be described as the linguistic rules, which reflects the complexity of Chinese language in one aspect. In this section, linguistic rules based on the proposed vocabulary is constructed by taking the colloquial style of micro-blog into account.

According to Chinese syntax rules, the proposed linguistic rules are derived as shown in Table 3. In the rules, Sentence structure patterns are recognized with different items of words in the vocabulary, and each pattern has its own calculation rule based on the weight of each word. If the sentence is recognized as "Partial Negative Structure", a coefficient should be multiplied for precise result, which is set as -0.5 in Table 3. How to calculate the polarity of a given sentence according to the rules will be introduced in the next section.

Table 3. Linguisitc rules based on the proposed vocabulary

Chinese syntax rules	Linguistic rules in our method	
	Structure pattern	Calculation rules of each pattern
Single Word Structure:	W_EW	玩/play = +1 = 1
v, adj, modal particles		哈哈/ha-ha = +1 = 1
Adverbial-Modifier Structure	W_DM+W_EM	很高兴/very happy = 1.5×(+1) = 1.5
Verb-Complement Structure	W_EM+W_DM	好得很/awfully well = (+1)×1.5 = 1.5
Negative Structure	W_NW+W_EW	不高兴/not happy = (-1)×1 = -1
Complete Negative Structure	W_DM+W_NW +W_EW	很不高兴/very unhappy = 1.5×(-1)×1 = -1.5
Partial Negative Structure	W_NW+W_DM +W_EW	不很高兴/slightly unhappy = (-0.5)×[(-1)×1.5×1] = 0.75 *: -0.5 is the coefficient in our rule.
Coordinate Structure	W_EW+W_EW	幸福开心/glad and happy = (+1)+(+1) = 2

3.3 Procedure of the Proposed Method

Within the preparation of vocabulary and linguistic rules construction, the proposed method contains 3 main steps as shown in Fig.1 (A).

Sentence Segmentation and Word Segmentation. A piece of micro-blog allows 140 characters at most, so it may contain several sub-sentences. Punctuations are taken as symbols to segment sentences. ICTCLAS Chinese word segmentation systems [16], the most popular one throughout the world, is applied for segmenting word and labeling part of speech of each word.

- Each micro-blog is regarded as a sentence S, and each S is a sequence of N sub-sentences denoted by $S = \{s_1, s_2, \ldots s_n\}$, where s_n is the n_{th} sub-sentence.

- A sub-sentence s_i is a collection of M words denoted by $s_i = \{w_1(sp_1), w_2(sp_2), \ldots, w_M(sp_M)\}$, where $w_m(sp_m)$ is the m_{th} word in the collection, and sp_m refers to its part of speech.

Polarity Calculation of Each Sub-sentence. After being segmented, the polarity of each sub-sentence s_i could be calculated by structure pattern mining and the corresponding calculation rules. The process is implemented as follows:

Algorithm 1. Polarity calculation algorithm

1: **Sub-sentence** s_i: I am extremely happy and very glad today.
2: **Word   segmentation:**   I(noun),   today(noun),   extremely(adverb), happy(adjective), and(adverb), very(adverb), glad(adjective).
3: **Keyword   extraction   in   vocabulary:**   extremely(adverb)#W_DM, happy(adjective)#W_EW, very(adverb)#W_DM, glad(adjective)#W_EW
4: **Structure pattern mining:**
   W_EW+W_EW: happy(adjective)#W_EW+ glad(adjective)#W_EW;
   W_DM+W_EM: extremely(adverb)#W_DM+ happy(adjective)#W_EW;
   W_DM+W_EM: very(adverb)#W_DM + glad(adjective)#W_EW.
5: **Polarity   calculation   of   sub-sentence** s_i: p(s_i)= [weight(extremely)×weight(happy)]   +[weight(very)×weight(glad)]= [2×(+1)]+[1.5×(+1)]= +3.5.

Polarity Calculation of Sentence S. The polarity of sentence S is determined by the polarities and positions of its sub-sentences, as the position of a sub-sentence s_i in S can indicate its importance [17]. This is especially noticeable in micro-blog, because it enables people to record their immediate feelings at any time. If a micro-blog content is long, the beginning and ending sub-sentences often reflect the writer's feelings more directly, thus more important than those in the middle. Therefore, the higher weights are assigned to sub-sentences at the two ends of the micro-blog as (1). With the polarity and position of each sub-sentence, the polarity of S is calculated as (2).

$$\lambda(s_i) = \frac{1}{\min(i, N - i + 1)}, 1 \leq i \leq N \qquad (1)$$

$$Polarity(S) = \sum_{i=1}^{N} [\lambda(s_i) \times p(s_i)] \qquad (2)$$

N is the number of sub-sentences in S, and i is the position of s_i in S. A positive *polarity(S)* means the sentence expresses a positive sentiment of the user, and a negative one means opposite. If the polarity equals to zero, then it is objective. The absolute value $|polarity(S)|$ shows the intensity of the sentiment.

Research in psychology shows that depressed individuals focus more on negative aspects of their lives [4]. So the polarity of users' micro-blog contents is an important feature in depression detection in section 4, which is normalized as (3), where $|S|$ is the total number of micro-blogs during a given period of time.

$$NormalizedSentencePolarity = \sum\nolimits_{|S|} Polarity(S)\big/|S| \qquad (3)$$

4   Depression Detection Model

When it comes to depression detection, many other features need to be considered. In this section, the work of psychologists is firstly introduced, and then the classifier based on their work is designed for depression detection.

4.1   Psychologists' Work

Psychologists observe the online behaviors of depressed users, and discover potential features that could be used to distinguish depressed and non-depressed individuals. All these features mainly come from three dimensions: micro-blog content, interactions and behaviors [4-6]. Table 4 lists the statistical data of ten features of two depressed and two normal samples in two weeks, in which A and B are the anonymized users. It reveals that most features show significant differences. For example, depressed users tend to use more first person singular pronouns but less emoticons. However, some features show little influence on these four users, such as times of being forwarded and commented. The proposed model obtained by training data will further illustrate the significance of each feature for depression detection in section 5.

4.2   Model Construction

Taking the achievement of psychologists as background knowledge, their observations need to be converted to parameters that are easily imported into the model as shown in Fig.1 (B). As the calculation of sentence polarity has been discussed in section 3, how to obtain, process and normalize other features will be introduced in this part.

The Use of First Person Singular and Plural Pronouns. As the result in [4] shows, depressed users tend to focus on themselves and detach from others. They use more first person singular pronouns ("I") but less first person plural pronouns ("We"). So the use of first person pronouns is considered in two aspects:

- The quantity of first person pronouns, reflecting their focuses on themselves.

- The ratio of first person singular pronouns to first person plural pronouns as (4), where Q_{fs} and Q_{fp} represent the quantities of first person singular and plural pronouns respectively.

Table 4. Features of typical depressed and non-depressed samples

		Depressed samples		Non-depressed samples	
		Zoufan	A	Li Kaifu	B
Number of micro-blogs($|S|$)		215	124	1156	621
Micro-blog content	1st person singular	264 (123%)	142 (115%)	404 (34.9%)	97 (15.6%)
	1st person plural	3 (1.4%)	7 (5.6%)	94 (8.1%)	8 (1.3%)
	Positive emoticons	8 (3.7%)	23 (18.5%)	234 (20.2%)	76 (12.2%)
	Negative emoticons	9 (4.2%)	19 (15.3%)	99 (8.6%)	24 (3.9%)
Interactions	Mentioning	22 (10.2%)	10 (8.1%)	574 (49.7%)	621 (100%)
	Being Forwarded	161592 (752%)	7 (5.60%)	3229210 (2793%)	35 (5.6%)
	Being Commented	210902 (981%)	50 (40.30%)	1458263 (1262%)	129 (20.80%)
Behaviors	Original blogs	183 (85.1%)	91 (73.4%)	758 (65.6%)	75 (12.1%)
	Blogs posted between 0 : 00 − 6 : 00 o'clock	57 (26.5%)	67 (54.0%)	30 (2.6%)	12 (1.9%)

$$Ratio\_StoP = \frac{\sum_{|S|} Q_{fs}}{\sum_{|S|} Q_{fp} + 1} \tag{4}$$

For this purpose, all the first person singular and plural pronouns in users' micro-blogs need to be detected. It requires that the first person pronouns must be the subject of the sentence. So besides detecting all the first person words, whether they are the subject of the sentence or not should also be checked. To solve this problem, we choose to check if the word following them could be used as predicate. If they could, this sentence is considered as the first person pronoun. Obviously, this method would meet problems when the sentence structure is too complex, for example, some adverbials are following the subject. But as discussed above, micro-blogs are often written in a colloquial style, and complex structures are not frequent, so the proposed method is effective after being tested.

The Use of Emoticons. As shown in Table 4, depressed individuals use less emoticons, and the result in [4] shows they focus more on negative aspects of their lives. So similar with the consideration of first person pronouns, the use of emoticons is also considered in two aspects: the absolute quantity of emoticons, and the relative ratio of positive emoticons to negative ones. For this purpose, all the emoticons should be detected and distinguished as positive or negative ones. So firstly the common 76 emoticons are divided into 3 categories: 34 positive ones, 32 negative ones and 10 neutral ones. Then all the emoticons in users' micro-blogs detected are matched with the 3 emoticon categories. In this way both the numbers of positive and negative emoticons are obtained.

User Interactions with Others. Micro-blog provides three ways for users to interact with each other: one is to mention others in order to attract them via @*username*; another is to forward, aims to pass along those information to their own followers; and the last one is to make comments, which only appear under the original micro-blog to express their own attitudes. In our model, user interactions are measured with these three common parameters: times of mentioning others, times of being forwarded and times of being commented, which could be collected through Sina Micro-blog open platform API [18]. The features input into the classifier are normalized by $Times/|S|$.

User Behaviors in Micro-blog. As the discovery in [6], frequencies of the posting original blogs could indicate depression levels of the user. So the percentage of original micro-blogs is taken as one of the features in user behaviors, calculated as *(number of original posts)/|S|*.

It is also found in [6] that the period users post micro-blogs is another indicator of depression level. Table 4 reveals depressive ones tending more active between 0:00-6:00a.m. Therefore, the percentage of micro-blogs posted in this period is calculated as *(number of micro-blogs posted during 0:00-6:00a.m.)/|S|*, which is used as another feature in user behaviors.

5   Experiment

5.1   Data Acquisition and Experiment Result

The proposed model is applied to detect depressed users in Sina Micro-blog, a social network service like Twitter. It is one of the most influential SNS in China.

During August 1th -15th, 2012, a group of psychologists made diagnosis on hundreds of volunteers with the means of questionnaire and interviews. They identified 122 depressed sufferers and 346 normal ones. Among them 90 depressed and 90 non-depressed users who use Sina Micro-blog are picked as training dataset. Their information during August 1th -15th are collected through Sina Micro-blog Open Platform API [18]. A total of 6,013 micro-blogs are collected, of which the user who owns the most micro-blogs owns 173, and the least one owns 3 pieces. Over 50,000 sub-sentences are obtained after sentence segmentation. Our experiment is based on these data.

After data processing with methods in section 3&4, ten features are obtained for depression detection. Waikato Environment for Knowledge Analysis (Weka), one of the most useful tools for classification [19], is applied to help classify the users into normal or depressed category. To ensure the result being more reliable, three different kinds of classification approaches are employed: Bayes, Trees and Rules [19-20]. The result is obtained with 10-fold cross validation in Fig.2 (A). ROC Area refers to the area under ROC curve, measuring the quality of a classifier. F-measure is the harmonic mean of precision and recall, denoting the accuracy of a classifier comprehensively.

The result in Fig.2 (A) reveals the precisions of the proposed model with different classifiers are all around 80%, which is considered acceptable by psychologists to detect depressed users in SNS. Among the incorrect cases, the number of individuals incorrectly classified into normal category and incorrectly into depressed category are approximately equal. Most of these individuals own

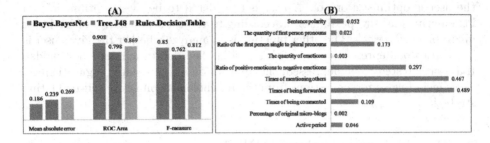

Fig. 2. Classification results of training dataset & Sig. of 10 features in the model

less than 10 pieces of micro-blogs, indicating that lack of data information would bring error to the proposed model.

According to the psychological research, only 3 out of 1000 users online are depressed, so it's very difficult to conduct experiments on large data. However, more than 100 non-depressed familiar friends in Micro-blog are tested with the application in section 6, and more than 85% of them are correctly classified.

5.2 Model Simplification

Besides verifying the effectiveness of the 10 features in the proposed model, the significance of each feature is also studied. Binary logistic regression analysis with Statistical Product and Service Solution (SPSS) is applied to evaluate the significance of each feature in the model [19]. The result is shown in Fig.2 (B). A lower Sig. represents that it is more important. The threshold for Sig. is set as 0.1 and five features are selected for simplifying the model. Experiments show that the precision of the simplified model is declined by less than 5%, however, the bytes of data needed to collect and computing time are significantly reduced. So the application in section 6 is developed with the simplified model.

Furthermore, as Fig.2 (B) shows, the total number of emoticons and original micro-blogs are the most important features, and times of mentioning others and being forwarded are the least important ones. This is a little different from the observation of psychologists in Table 4, which shows times of mentioning others could easily distinguish depressed and non-depressed individuals. It may enlighten psychologists about some further research.

6   Application

Since mental health problem has become the most serious one for modern urban people, the proposed method of sentiment analysis and depression detection model in this paper can be applied in social network services for user mental health state assessment and monitoring. For this purpose, an application in Sina Micro-blog is developed named "Mental Health Testing".

The application provides two functions. One is to calculate the polarity of each piece of micro-blog with the sentiment analysis method, which reflects whether the user is optimistic or not. A user is considered to be "very optimistic", "a little optimistic" or "pessimistic" according to the total popularity of his latest micro-blogs in a week. The other function is to analyze whether the given user is inclined to be depressed or not with the simplified depression detection model. If a user is tested to be depressed, the application also provides diagnostic messages including some suggestions from the psychologists on active self-regulating strategies.

7   Conclusions and Future Work

A model for detecting depressed users in social network based on sentiment analysis is proposed in this paper. The sentiment analysis method pays special attention to the characteristics of depression and Chinese micro-blog content, and ten features are applied in the depression detection model. The precisions obtained from training dataset are all around 80%, and the significance of each feature in the model is also analyzed for model simplification. An application in Sina Micro-blog is developed to test the polarity of micro-blog and the mental state of users, which has helped psychologists detect several potential depressed users in Sina Micro-blog. Although the depression detection model is proposal based on Chinese vocabulary, the basic idea of the frame especially the sentence structure pattern mining and principle micro-blog features related to depression could be explicitly extended to other language scenarios.

In this work, the training data detected by psychologists are widely scattered in social network. It is hard to analyze the relationship between them, so user interaction is paid little attention and simply three parameters are considered. However, homophily is manifest in the group of depression users, which means, the friends of the depression are more likely to be depressive, and different kinds of interactions indicate different results. Thus the influence of ties between users is contemplated to be studied in the future and a deeper understanding about depression in SNS will be provided.

Acknowledgement. This work is supported by Project on the Architecture, Key technology research and Demonstration of Web-based wireless ubiquitous business environment (No.2012ZX03005008-001) and China-Finland Cooperation Project on The Development and Demonstration of Intelligent Design Platform Driven by Living Lab Methodology (No.2010DFA12780). The authors would like to thank Xiaofeng Qiu, Cheng Cheng and Xinning Zhu for insightful discussions.

References

1. Aggarwal, C.C.: Social Network Data Analytics. Springer, New York (2011)
2. Hsieh, Y., Bolan, J.E.: Predicting Processing Difficulty in Chineses Syntactic Ambiguity Resolution: A Parallel Approach. Poster, The 84th Annual Meeting of the Linguistic Society of America, Baltimore, MD (2010)

3. World Health Organization, http://www.who.int/en/
4. Ramirez-Esparza, N., Chung, C.K., Kacewicz, E., Pennebaker, J.W.: The Psychology of Word Use in Depression Forums in English and in Spanish: Testing Two Text Analytic Approaches. In: Proceedings of the International Conference on Weblogs and Social Media, pp. 102–108. AAAI Press, Menlo Park (2008)
5. Moreno, M., Jelenchick, L., Egan, K., Cox, E., Young, H., Gannon, K., et al.: Feeling Bad on Facebook: Depression Disclosures by College Students on Social Networking Site. Depression and Anxiety 28, 447–455 (2011)
6. Ji, Y.: Social Displacement, Homophily and Depression Levels: The Case of Zoufan on a Chinese Social Network Site. Cyberpsychology, Behavior, and Social Networking. For Peer Review (2012)
7. Pang, B., Lee, L.: Opinion Mining and Sentiment Analysis. Now Publisher Inc. (2008)
8. Davidiv, D., Tsur, O., Rappoport, A.: Enhanced Sentiment Learning Using Twitter Hash-tags and Smileys. In: Proceedings of the 23rd International Conference on Computational in Linguistics, pp. 241–249. Coling 2010 Organizing Committee, Beijing (2010)
9. Barbosa, L., Feng, J.L.: Robust Sentiment Detection on Twitter from Biased and Noisy Data. In: Proceedings of the 23rd International Conference on Computational in Linguistics, pp. 36–44. Coling 2010 Organizing Committee, Beijing (2010)
10. Go, A., Huang, L., Bhayani, R.: Twitter Sentiment Classification using Distant Supervision. Project Report, CS224N (2009)
11. Jiang, L., Yu, M., Zhou, M., Liu, X., Zhao, T.: Target-dependent Twitter Sentiment Classification. In: Proceeding of 49th Annual Meeting of the Association for Computational Linguistics: Human Language Technologies, vol. 1, pp. 151–160 (2011)
12. Parikh, R., Movassate, M.: Sentiment Analysis of User-Generated Twitter Updates using Various Classification Techniques. Final Report, CS224N (2009)
13. Tan, S.B., Zhang, J.: An Empirical Study of Sentiment Analysis for Chinese Documents. Expert Systems with Applications 34, 2262–2269 (2008)
14. NII Test Collection for IR Systems, http://research.nii.ac.jp/ntcir/
15. Dong, Z., Dong, Q.: HowNet—A Hybrid Language and Knowledge Resource. In: Proceedings of International Conference on Natural Language Processing and Knowledge Engineering, pp. 820–824. IEEE Press, Los Alamitos (2003)
16. Institute of Computing Technology, Chinese Lexical Analysis System, http://ictclas.org/
17. Zhang, C.L., Zeng, D., Li, J.X., Wang, F.Y., Zuo, W.L.: Sentiment Analysis of Chinese Documents: From Sentence to Document Level. Journal of the American Society for Information Science and Technology 60, 2474–2487 (2009)
18. Sina Micro-blog Open Platform, http://open.weibo.com
19. Han, J.W., Kamber, M.: Data Mining Concepts and Techniques. Morgan Kaufmann, San Francisco (2006)
20. Witten, I.H., Frank, E.: Data Mining: Pratical Machine Learning Tools and Techniques, 2nd edn. Morgan Kaufmann, San Francisco (2005)

Modelling Gene Networks by a Dynamic Bayesian Network-Based Model with Time Lag Estimation

Lian En Chai, Mohd Saberi Mohamad[*], Safaai Deris, Chuii Khim Chong, and Yee Wen Choon

Artificial Intelligence and Bioinformatics Group,
Faculty of Computing, Universiti Teknologi Malaysia, 81310, Skudai, Johor, Malaysia
lechai2@live.utm.my, {saberi,safaai}@utm.my,
{ckchong2,ywchoon2}@live.utm.my

Abstract. Due to the needs to discover the immense information and understand the underlying mechanism of gene regulations, modelling gene regulatory networks (GRNs) from gene expression data has attracted the interests of numerous researchers. To this end, the dynamic Bayesian network (DBN) has emerged as a popular method in GRNs modelling as it is able to model time-series gene expression data and feedback loops. Nevertheless, the commonly found missing values in gene expression data, the inability to take account of the transcriptional time lag, and the redundant computation time caused by the large search space, frequently inhibits the effectiveness of DBN in modelling GRNs from gene expression data. This paper proposes a DBN-based model (IST-DBN) with missing values imputation, potential regulators selection, and time lag estimation to tackle the aforementioned problems. To evaluate the performance of IST-DBN, we applied the model on the *S. cerevisiae* cell cycle time-series expression data. The experimental results revealed IST-DBN has decreased computation time and better accuracy in identifying gene-gene relationships when compared with existing DBN-based model and conventional DBN. Furthermore, we expect the resultant networks from IST-DBN to be applied as a general framework for potential gene intervention research.

Keywords: Dynamic Bayesian network, missing values imputation, time-series gene expression data, gene regulatory networks, network inference.

1 Introduction

In recent years, the advent of DNA microarray technology has permitted researchers to develop novel experimental approaches for probing into the complicated system of gene regulation. The ensuing output, known as gene expression data, brings forth valuable information such as the robustness, behaviours or anomalies demonstrated by the cellular system under different circumstances [1].

---

[*] Corresponding author.

J. Li et al. (Eds.): PAKDD 2013 Workshops, LNAI 7867, pp. 214–222, 2013.

Over the years, different computational approaches have been established to automate GRNs modelling. Particularly, Bayesian network (BN), which relies on probabilistic measure to recognize causal interactions between a set of variables, was widely used to model GRNs. BN has several advantages: ability to work on local components, prevent data overfitting by assimilation of other mathematical models, and capable of merging prior knowledge to reinforce the causal links. However, BN also has two limitations: it cannot model feedback loops and handle time-series gene expression data. In biological perspective, feedback loops signify the homeostasis process in living organisms. Therefore, the dynamic Bayesian network (DBN) has been introduced as an alternative to counter BN's drawbacks. DBN was first proposed by Friedman et al. [2] in GRNs inference and Ong et al. [3] extended the approach with prior biological knowledge in modelling of the tryptophan metabolism in E. coli. Additionally, Kim et al. [4] devised a non-parametric regression DBN model based on B-splines to handle the linear dependencies found in gene expression datasets.

However, missing values distributed across gene expression data might influence up to 90% of the genes and consequently affecting downstream analysis and modelling methods [5]. Also, in predicting gene-gene relationships, conventional DBN normally includes all genes into the subsets of potential regulators and their target genes, and in turn triggers the large search space and the redundant computational cost which obstructs the usefulness of DBN modelling [6]. In light of these problems, Chai et al. [7] proposed a DBN-based model (ISDBN) with missing values imputation and potential regulators selection.

The disadvantage of ISDBN and conventional DBN is that they do not have the capability to tackle transcriptional time lag effectively, whereby the target genes are provided a time delay by their regulators before their expressions in the system. This drawback hinders the accuracy of DBN-based methods in modelling GRNs. To address this problem, we proposed to further enhance the aforementioned model with time lag estimation (IST-DBN) which uses the time difference between the initial changes of expression level of potential regulators against their target genes as an appropriate transcriptional time lag.

2   Methods

In essence, IST-DBN consists of four steps: missing values imputation, potential regulators selection, time lag estimation and DBN modelling. Fig. 1 illustrates the schematic overview of IST-DBN.

2.1   Missing Values Imputation

Missing values in gene expression data happen for various factors. Tiny impurities would corrupt the microarray slides at a number of spots as they are very small and crammed. After scanning and digitalising the array, the problematic spots are labelled as missing. Numerous imputation algorithms have been developed to handle missing values by exploiting the underlying expression data structure and pattern. Particularly, LLSimpute extracts information from local similarity structures by creating a linear combination of similar genes and target genes with missing values via a similarity measure [8]. This algorithm consists of two steps. Firstly, k genes are selected by the L_2-norm, where k is a positive integer that defines the number of coherent genes to the target gene. For instance, to impute a missing value g located at x_{11} in a $m \times n$ matrix X, the k-nearest neighbour gene vectors for x_1,

$$v_{s_i}^{\mathrm{T}} \in X^{1 \times n} \quad 1 \leq i \leq k \tag{1}$$

are first computed, whereby the gene expression data is described as a $m \times n$ matrix X (m is the number of genes, n is the number of observations), and x_1 represents the row of the first gene with n observations. s_i is a list of k-nearest neighbour genes vectors, which in turn corresponds to the i-th row of the transpose vector v^{T}. The second step involves regression and estimation of the missing values. A matrix, $A \in X^{k \times (n-1)}$ whereby the k rows of the matrix contains vector v, and two vectors, $b \in X^{k \times 1}$ and $w \in X^{(n-1) \times 1}$, are subsequently formed. The vector b contains the first element of k vectors v^{T}, while vector w contains $n - 1$ elements of vector x_1. A k-dimensional coefficient vector y is then computed such that the least square problem is minimised as

$$\min_y |A^{\mathrm{T}} y - w|^2 \tag{2}$$

Let y^* to denote the vector whereby the square is minimised such that

$$w \simeq A^{\mathrm{T}} y^* = y_1^* a_1 + y_2^* a_2 + \cdots + y_k^* a_k \tag{3}$$

where $a_i \in A^{k \times 1}$, and therefore, the missing value g can be imputed as a linear combination of coherent genes such that

$$g = b^{\mathrm{T}} y = b^{\mathrm{T}} (A^{\mathrm{T}})' w \tag{4}$$

where $(A^{\mathrm{T}})'$ exists as the pseudoinverse of A^{T} [5].

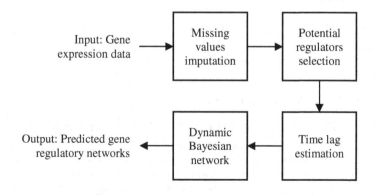

Fig. 1. Schematic overview of IST-DBN

2.2   Potential Regulators Selection

In most cases, the expression level of transcriptional factors (TFs) would fluctuate prior to or simultaneously with their target genes [9]. Based on this characteristic, we conceived an algorithm which would decrease the search space by restricting the number of potential regulators for each target genes. The first step is to determine a threshold, either experimentally or fixed as the average expression level of the genes. In this paper, the threshold for up-regulation and down-regulation are determined based on the baseline cut-off of the gene expression values. As such, for the *S. cerevisiae* dataset used in this paper, the threshold is decided as ≥ 1.2 for up-regulation and ≤ 0.7 for down-regulation. The gene expression values are then classified into three states: up-, down- and normal regulation. The three states denote whether the expression value is greater than, lower than or similar to the threshold.

After that, the exact time units of initial up-regulation and down-regulation of each gene are determined, and genes with prior changes in expression level are included into the subset of potential regulators against genes with later expression changes. As genes with late expression changes might comprise a large number of potential regulators, we have limited the maximum time gap for prior expression changes to five time units to prevent choosing potential regulators for a target gene from the whole gene expression dataset. To further illustrate this idea, let us first assume two hypothetical genes: gene 1 and gene 2. Gene 1 experienced an initial expression change at time t_1 before gene 2's initial expression change at time t_2, and so gene 1 is included into the subset of potential regulators for gene 2 (See Fig. 2). The same process applies to other up- or down-regulated genes which fulfil the criteria.

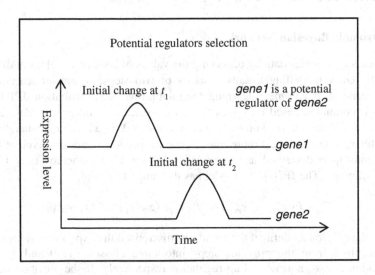

Fig. 2. Schematic overview of potential regulators selection

2.3   Time Lag Estimation

Transcriptional time lag is defined as the time delay between the expression of regulators and the expression of their target genes to protein products. Using the two hypothetical genes, 1 and 2, and that gene 1 regulates gene 2. Gene 1 initiates expression fluctuation at time t_x and gene 2 has an expression change at t_y. The time difference between t_x and t_y is considered as the transcriptional time lag. In DBN modelling of GRNs, potential regulators are paired up with target genes based on the statistical analysis of their causal strength between time units. However, even though the actual transcriptional time lag might be across several time units, DBN typically aligns regulator-gene pairs by only one time unit. IST-DBN takes into account of the actual transcriptional time lag by pairing up target genes and their potential regulators based on the time difference between their pre-determined initial changes in expression level. The previous step, potential regulators selection, lay paths for this step by indicating the initial expression changes between target genes and regulators. To illustrate this idea, let us assume another hypothetical gene 3 and gene 4 which are both potential regulators for gene 2. The transcriptional time lag between gene 1 and gene 2 is one time unit, gene 3 and gene 2 is two time units, while gene 4 and gene 2 is one time unit. For a target gene, potential regulators are divided into separate groups based on the time lag (e.g. one or two time units), mainly due to the fact that a target gene may have several regulators acting upon it in different or within same time unit. In this example, gene 1 and gene 4 would be filtered into one group because they have one time unit of transcription time lag against gene 2. On the other hand, gene 3 would be placed in another group since it has a transcription time lag of two time units against gene 2, which is dissimilar to gene 1 and gene 4.

2.4   Dynamic Bayesian Network

DBN models time-series data by observing the values of a set of variables at different time units. DBN modelling usually consists of two steps: parameter learning and structure learning. In parameter learning, the joint probability distribution (JPD) of the variables is computed based on Bayes theorem. Assuming a microarray dataset with m genes and n observations, known as a $m \times n$ matrix $X = (x_1, \ldots, x_m)$ whereby each row, vector $x_m = (x_{m1}, \ldots, x_{mn})$ represents a gene expression vector observed at time t. The relationship is described as a *first-order Markov chain* whereby only forward edges are allowed. The JPD of the model has the general form of:

$$P(x_{11}, \ldots, x_{mn}) = P(x_1)P(x_2|x_1) \ldots P(x_i|x_{i-1}) \tag{5}$$

Based on the previously defined threshold, we discretised the expression values of the results acquired from the previous steps into three classes: -1, 0 and 1, which correspond to down-, normal and up-regulation respectively. In the previous step, we have already divided the potential regulators into groups based on their transcriptional time lag against the target gene. Using the previous example which comprises gene 1 – 4, two groups exist – gene 1 and 4 as a group, and gene 3 as a group. These groups of potential regulators are then further divided in subsets due to the necessity of examining all possible sets of regulators or co-regulators against target gene. In this example, in the group of potential regulators consisting gene 1 and gene 4, the subsets would be {1}, {4} and {1, 4}; the group of gene 3 would have only one subset, which is {3}. Based on the transcriptional time lag, each of the subset and the target gene are subsequently organised into a data matrix with their discretised expression values. The conditional probabilities of each subset of potential regulators against their target genes are then computed. The next step is to search for the optimal network structure via a scoring function based on the Bayesian Dirichlet equivalence (BDe). The final results are imported into GraphViz (*http://www.graphviz.org*) for network visualisation and analysis.

3   Result and Discussion

3.1   Experimental Data and Setup

The *S. cerevisiae* cell cycle time-series gene expression data [10] encloses 6178 genes which were observed at four medium time series (alpha, CDC15, CDC28 and elu; 18, 24, 17 and 14 time points) and two short time series (CLN3, CLB2; both 2 time points). It also consists of 5.912% missing values (28,127 out of 475,706 observations).

The DBN modelling portion of IST-DBN is implemented under the framework of BNFinder [11], whereas the missing values imputation, potential regulators selection and the time lag estimation are implemented in MATLAB environment. For performance evaluation, we compared the accuracy and computation time of the proposed IST-DBN against ISDBN and DBN (typified by BNFinder). The accuracy is measured by comparing the results from the three models to the established *S. cerevisiae* cell cycle pathway at KEGG (*http://www.kegg.jp*). The computation time of the models are compared on a 3.2GHz Intel Core i3 computer with 2GB main memory. The results are summarised in Table 1, in which the first row represents the network modelled by IST-DBN, the second row represents the network modelled by ISDBN, and the third row represents the network modelled by DBN. An edge indicates a relationship between the two connected genes. 'Correctly predicted relationships' denotes the number of relationships found in the established networks and also in the modelled results, 'sensitivity' is the percentage of correctly predicted relationships out of all predicted relationships, and 'specificity' correspond to the percentage of correct prediction that no relationship exists between two genes.

3.2   Experiment Results

Out of the established 35 gene-gene relationships, IST-DBN managed to identify 32 relationships (Fig. 3.) while ISDBN identified 30 – it failed to detect CLN1-CDC28 and FUS3-CDC28. CLN1 and FUS3 were assigned as the potential regulators of CDC28, however both of them have a transcription time lag exceeding 2 time units, and this caused ISDBN to erroneously dismiss them in the final group of potential regulators for CDC28. IST-DBN took into account of the transcriptional time lag and realigned them accordingly, which in turn increased the strength of their causal relationships with CDC28. Furthermore, by pairing up regulators and genes with a biologically relevant transcriptional time lag, IST-DBN was able to limit down the false positives to two while ISDBN erroneously detected six false positives. Both models were able to identify the feedback loop of the cell cycle pathway, for example, the sub-network of CDC28-SWI4/6-YOX1-MCM1-CLN3-CDC28 which signifies the transcription regulation during G1 phase of the cell cycle. On the other hand, DBN only identified 27 relationships. It missed out YHP1-MCM1, SWI4-CLN1 and CDC28-WHI5. This is more or less attributed to the fact that many missing values were found in the original expression profiles of the six genes, and the lack of an efficient imputation method caused DBN to lose its accuracy. IST-DBN reported 91.43% sensitivity and 98.08% specificity compared to ISDBN's 85.71% sensitivity and 94.06% specificity. DBN performed the worst among the three models, registering 77.14% sensitivity and 93.22% specificity.

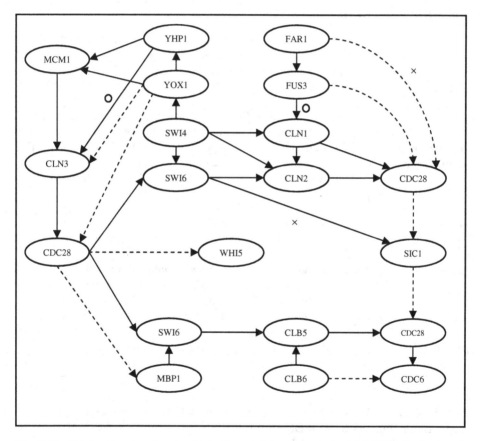

Fig. 3. Predicted cell cycle sub-network for *S. cerevisiae* dataset using IST-DBN. Dash edges (---) denote down-regulations and straight-lined edges (—) denote up-regulations. A cross represents an incorrect prediction; a circle represents an incorrect regulation type; an edge without any attachment is a correct prediction.

While an edge denotes the existence of a relationship between two genes, there are four possible situations: correct direction and regulation type, correct direction but incorrect regulation type, misdirected but correct regulation type, and misdirected and wrong regulation type. One misdirected relationship and two regulation types in ISDBN were correctly reversed in IST-DBN. Also, the search space for both models is relatively small as the number of potential regulators is limited to those which experienced prior expression changes against targeted genes. Hence both models registered similar computation time in which IST-DBN has a slightly faster computation time of 24 minutes and 33 seconds compared to ISDBN's 25 minutes and 9 seconds. In contrast, DBN reported a computation time of 1 hour 8 minutes and 23 seconds, mostly due to the large search space where it includes all genes as potential regulators against target genes.

Table 1. The results of experiment study

Model	Correctly predicted relationships	Sensitivity	Specificity	Computation time (HH:MM:SS)
IST-DBN	32	91.43%	98.02%	00:24:33
ISDBN	30	85.71%	94.06%	00:25:09
DBN	27	77.14%	93.22%	01:08:23

4   Conclusion

Conventional DBN has been hampered by three problems: the missing values in gene expression data, the relatively large search space caused by comprising all genes into the subset of potential regulators against target genes, and the lack of a way to handle transcriptional time lag. ISDBN was proposed by Chai *et al.* [7] to address the first two problems: Missing values are imputed based on linear combination of similar genes, and the search space is reduced by limiting the subset of potential regulators based on particular criteria. However, this model does not take into account of the transcription time lag. Therefore, in this paper, we proposed an enhanced ISDBN with time lag estimation (known as IST-DBN) to tackle the third problem. Instead of aligning by the default one time unit, IST-DBN uses the time difference between expression changes to pair up regulators and target genes. In this way, IST-DBN is able to capture most of the statistical correlation between genes that have a longer transcriptional time lag. Based on the *S. cerevisiae* cell cycle pathway dataset, IST-DBN showed promising results in terms of accuracy and computation time when compared to ISDBN and conventional DBN. It would be of our upmost interest to apply IST-DBN to other datasets, for instance, *E. coli* and *D. melanogaster*, as the resultant GRNs might be very useful for future gene intervention experiments or hypotheses testing purposes.

Acknowledgments. We would like to thank the Malaysian Ministry of Science, Technology and Innovation for supporting this research by an e-science research grant (Grant number: 06-01-06-SF1029). This research is also supported by a GUP research grant (Grant number: Q.J130000.2507.04H16) that was sponsored by Universiti Teknologi Malaysia.

References

1. Karlebach, G., Shamir, R.: Modelling and analysis of gene regulatory networks. Nat. Rev. Mol. Cell Bio. 9(10), 770–780 (2008)
2. Friedman, N., Murphy, K., Russell, S.: Learning the structure of dynamic probabilistic networks. In: Proc. 14th Conference on the Uncertainty in Artificial Intelligence, San Mateo, pp. 139–147 (1998)
3. Ong, I.M., Glasner, J.D., Page, D.: Modelling regulatory pathways in E. coli from time series expression profiles. Bioinformatics 18, S241–S248 (2002)
4. Kim, S.Y., Imoto, S., Miyano, S.: Dynamic bayesian network and nonparametric regression for nonlinear modeling of gene networks from time series gene expression data. In: Priami, C. (ed.) CMSB 2003. LNCS, vol. 2602, pp. 104–113. Springer, Heidelberg (2003)
5. Ouyang, M., Welsh, W.J., Geogopoulos, P.: Gaussian mixture clustering and imputation of microarray data. Bioinformatics 20(6), 917–923 (2004)
6. Jia, Y., Huan, J.: Constructing non-stationary dynamic Bayesian networks with a flexible lag choosing mechanism. BMC Bioinformatics 2010(11), S27 (2010)
7. Chai, L.E., Mohamad, M.S., Deris, S., Chong, C.K., Choon, Y.W., Ibrahim, Z., Omatu, S.: Inferring gene regulatory networks from gene expression data by a dynamic Bayesian network-based model. In: Omatu, S., Paz Santana, J.F., González, S.R., Molina, J.M., Bernardos, A.M., Rodríguez, J.M.C. (eds.) DCAI. AISC, vol. 151, pp. 379–386. Springer, Heidelberg (2012)
8. Kim, H., Golub, G., Park, H.: Missing value estimation for DNA microarray gene expression data: local least squares imputation. Bioinformatics 21(2), 187–198 (2005)
9. Yu, H., Luscombe, N.M., Qian, J., Gerstein, M.: Genomic analysis of gene expression relationships in transcriptional regulatory networks. Trends Genet. 19, 422–427 (2003)
10. Spellman, P.T., Sherlock, G., Zhang, M.Q., Iyer, V.R., Anders, K., Eisen, M.B., Brown, P.O., Botstein, D., Futcher, B.: Comprehensive identification of cell cycle regulated genes of the yeast Saccharomyces cerevisiae by microarray hybridization. Mol. Biol. Cell 9, 3273–3297 (1998)
11. Wilczynski, B., Dojer, N.: BNFinder: exact and efficient method for learning Bayesian networks. Bioinformatics 25(2), 286–287 (2009)

Identifying Gene Knockout Strategy Using Bees Hill Flux Balance Analysis (BHFBA) for Improving the Production of Succinic Acid and Glycerol in *Saccharomyces cerevisiae*

Yee Wen Choon[1], Mohd Saberi Mohamad[1,*], Safaai Deris[1], Rosli Md. Illias[2],
Lian En Chai[1], Chuii Khim Chong[1]

[1] Artificial Intelligence and Bioinformatics Research Group, Faculty of Computing,
Universiti Teknologi Malaysia, Skudai, 81310 Johor, Malaysia
ywchoon2@live.utm.my, {saberi,safaai}@utm.my,
{lechai2,ckchong2}@live.utm.my
[2] Department of Bioprocess Engineering, Faculty of Chemical Engineering,
Universiti Teknologi Malaysia, Skudai, 81310 Johor, Malaysia
r-rosli@utm.my

Abstract. Strains of *Saccharomyces cerevisiae* can be manipulated to improve product yield and growth characteristics. Optimization algorithms are developed to identify the effects of gene knockout on the results. However, this process is often faced the problem of being trapped in local minima and slow convergence due to repetitive iterations of algorithm. In this paper, we proposed Bees Hill Flux Balance Analysis (BHFBA) which is a hybrid of Bees Algorithm, Hill Climbing Algorithm and Flux Balance Analysis to solve the problems and improve the performance in predicting optimal sets of gene deletion for maximizing the growth rate and production yield of desired metabolite. *Saccharomyces cerevisiae* is the model organism in this paper. The list of knockout genes, growth rate and production yield after the deletion are the results from the experiments. BHFBA performed better in term of computational time, stability and production yield.

Keywords: Bees Algorithm, Hill Climbing, Flux Balance Analysis, Microbial Strains, Optimization.

1 Introduction

Microbial strains optimization has become popular in genome-scale metabolic networks reconstructions recently as microbial strains can be manipulated to improve product yield on desired metabolites and also improve growth characteristics [1]. Reconstructions of the metabolic networks are found to be very useful in health, environmental and energy issues [2]. The development of computational models for simulating the actual processes inside the cell is growing rapidly due to vast numbers of high-throughput experimental data. The main goal of the development is to

---

* Corresponding author.

J. Li et al. (Eds.): PAKDD 2013 Workshops, LNAI 7867, pp. 223–233, 2013.

construct efficient and accurate pathway models that are useful in predicting cellular responses and providing better understanding of complex biological functions. However, data ambiguity due to the complexities of the metabolic networks has made the effects of genetic modification on the desirable phenotypes hard to predict. Furthermore, a vast number of reactions in cellular metabolism lead to combinatorial problem in obtaining optimal gene deletion strategy. The computational time will increase exponentially as the size of the problem increases. In later years, rational design strategies, based on genetic engineering, are implemented to retrofit microbial metabolism. It is widely known as metabolic engineering.

Many algorithms were developed in order to identify the gene knockout strategies for obtaining improved phenotypes. The first rational modeling framework (named OptKnock) for introducing gene knockout leading to the overproduction of a desired metabolite was developed by Burgard et al., 2003 [3]. OptKnock identifies a set of gene (reaction) deletions to maximize the flux of a desired metabolite with the internal flux distribution is still operating such that growth is optimized.

OptKnock is implemented by using mixed integer linear programming (MILP) to formulate a bi-level linear optimization that is very promising to find the global optimal solution. OptGene is an extended approach of OptKnock which formulates the *in silico* design problem by using Genetic Algorithm (GA) [4]. Meta-heuristic methods are capable in producing near-optimal solutions with reasonable computation time, furthermore the objective function that can be optimized is flexible. SA is then implemented to allow the automatic finding of the best number of gene deletions for achieving a given productivity goal [5]. However, the results are not yet satisfactory.

A hybrid of BA and FBA was proposed by Choon et al., 2012 [6], it showed a better performance in predicting optimal gene knockout strategies in term of growth rate and production yield. Pham et al., 2006 [7] introduced Bees Algorithm (BA), is a typical meta-heuristic optimization approach which has been applied to various problems, such as controller formation [8], image analysis [9], and job multi-objective optimization [10]. BA is based on the intelligent behaviours of honeybees. It locates the most promising solutions, and selectively explores their neighbourhoods looking for the global maximum of the objective function. BA is efficient in solving optimization problems according to the previous studies [7, 10]. However, due to the dependency of BA on random search, it is relatively weak in local search activities [11]. Hence, BHFBA is proposed to improve the performance of BAFBA as Hill climbing algorithm is a promising algorithm in finding local optimum. This paper shows that BHFBA is not only capable in solving larger size problems in shorter computational time but also improves the performance in predicting optimal gene knockout strategy than previous works. In this work, we present the results obtained by BHFBA in two case studies where *S.cerevisiae (Saccharomyces cerevisiae)* iFF708 model is the target microorganisms [12]. In addition, we also conduct a benchmarking to test performance of the hybrid of Bee algorithm and Hill climbing algorithm.

2   Bees-Hill Flux Balance Analysis (BHFBA)

In this paper, we proposed BHFBA in which BAFBA is only applied to identify optimal gene knockout strategies recently. Fig. 1 shows the flow of BAFBA while Fig. 2 shows our proposed BHFBA. The important steps are explained in the following subsections.

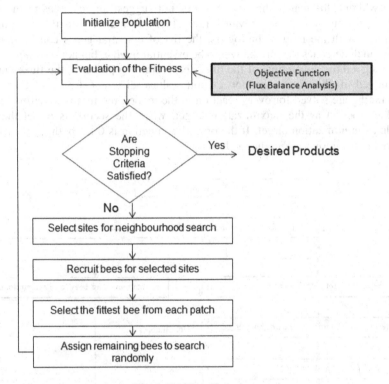

Fig. 1. BAFBA Flowchart

2.1   Model Pre-processing

The model is pre-processed through several steps based on biology assumptions as well as computational approaches to reduce the search space as while as increase the accuracy. Lethal reactions such as the genes that are found to be lethal *in vivo*, but not *in silico*, should be removed to improve the quality of the results. The results are invalid if a lethal reaction is deleted. The following are the details of computational pre-processing steps to the model [5].

a.   Fluxes that are not associated with any genes, such as the fluxes related to external metabolites and exchange fluxes that represent transport reaction should not be involved in the process. These fluxes do not have a biological meaning thus they should not be knocked out.

b.   Essential genes that cannot be deleted from the microorganism's genome need to be removed. The search space for optimization is reduced due to that these genes should not be considered as targets for deletion. A linear programming problem is defined by setting the corresponding flux to 0, while maximizing the biomass flux for each gene in the microorganism's genome. If the biomass flux result from the Linear Programming algorithm is zero (or near zero) then the gene is marked as essential. This biological meaning of this fact is that the microorganism is unable to survive without this gene. This process does not suggest any changes to the model like the previous one, but provides favorable information for the optimization algorithms. With the help of biologists, the list of essential genes can be manually edited to include genes that are known to be essential *in vivo*, but not *in silico*.

c.   Given the constraints of the linear programming problem, the fluxes need to be removed if the fluxes cannot exhibit values different from 0. Two linear programming are solved for every reaction in the model: the first is to define the flux over that reaction as the maximization target, while the second is to set the same variable as minimization target. If the objective function is 0 for both problems, then the variable is removed from the model.

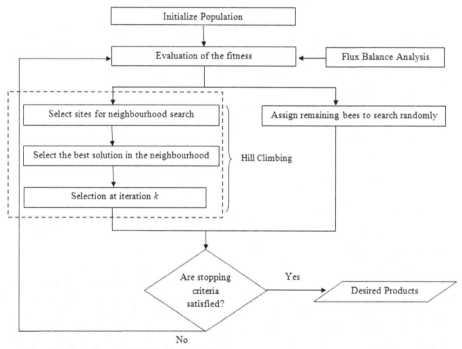

Note: Red-dotted box is Hill Climbing algorithm.

Fig. 2. BHFBA Flowchart

2.2 Bee Representation of Metabolic Genotype

One or more genes can be discovered in each reaction in a metabolic model. In this paper, each of those genes is represented by a binary variable indicating its absence or presence (0 or 1), these variables form a 'bee' representing a specific mutant that lacks some metabolic reactions when compared with the wild type (Fig. 3.)

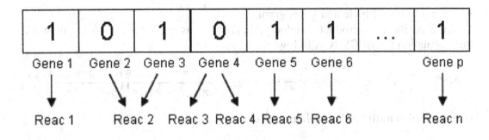

Note: Reac represents reaction.

Fig. 3. Bee representation of metabolic genotype

2.3 Initialization of the Population

The algorithm starts with an initial population of n scout bees. Each bee is initialized as follows: assume that a reaction with n genes. Bees in the population are initialized by setting present or absent status to each gene randomly. Initialization of the population is done randomly so that all bees in the population have an equal chance of being selected. The result might not truly reflect the population if it is done with bias setting.

2.4 Scoring Fitness of Individuals

Each site is given a fitness score that determines whether to recruit more bees or should be abandoned. In this work, we used FBA to calculate the fitness score for each site and the equation is as follow:

Maximize Z, where

$$Z = \sum_i c_i v_i = \mathbf{c} \cdot \mathbf{v} \tag{1}$$

where c = a vector that defines the weights for of each flux.

Cellular growth is defined as the objective function Z, vector c is used to select a linear combination of metabolic fluxes to include in the objective function, v is the flux map and i is the index variable $(1, 2, 3, ..., n)$. After optimizing the cellular growth, mutant with growth rate more than 0.1 continues the process by minimizing and maximizing the desired product flux at fixed optimal cellular growth value.

Hence, we can enhance yield of our desired products at fixed optimal cellular growth. Production yield is the maximum amount of product that can be generated per unit of substrate. The following shows the calculation for production yield:

$$Production\ yield\ = \frac{production\ rate_{production}}{consumption\ rate_{substrate}}\ \left(\frac{mmol}{mmol}\right)\left(\frac{gm}{gm}\right) \qquad (2)$$

where mmol = millimole and gm is gram.

We used Biomass-product coupled yield (BPCY) as the fitness score in this work, the calculation for BPCY is as follow:

$$BPCY\ =\ production\ yield\ \times growth\ rate\ \left(\frac{mmol}{mmol \times hour}\right)\left(\frac{gm}{gm \times hour}\right) \qquad (3)$$

where mmol is millimole, hr is hour and gm is gram.

2.5   Neighbourhood Search (Hill Climbing Algorithm)

The algorithm carries out neighbourhood searches in the favored sites (m) by using Hill climbing algorithm. Hill climbing is an iterative algorithm that starts with an arbitrary solution to a problem, then attempts to find a better solution by incrementally changing a single element of the solution. In this paper, the initial solution is the m favored sites from the population initialized by BA. The algorithm starts with the solution and makes small improvements to it by adding or reducing a bee to the sites. User defined the value of initial size of patches (ngh) and uses the value to update site (m) which is declared in the previous step to search in neighbourhood area. In this paper, m is equal to 15 and ngh is equal to 30, the values are obtained by conducting a small number of trials with the range of 10 to 25 and 20 to 35 respectively. This step is important as there might be better solutions than the original solution in the neighbourhood area.

2.6   Randomly Assigned and Termination

The remaining bees in the population are sent randomly around the search space to scout for new feasible solutions. This step is done randomly to avoid overlooking the potential results that are not in the range. These steps are repeated until either the maximum loop value is met or the fitness function has converged. At the end, the colony generates two parts to its new population – representatives from each selected patch and other scout bees assigned to perform random searches.

3   Results and Discussion

In this paper, *S.cerevisiae* iFF708 model is used to test on the operation of BHFBA [12]. The model contains 1175 reactions and 584 metabolites. However, the SBML model shows a total of 1382 reactions which includes the pseudo-exchange reactions. The model is pre-processed through several steps based on biology assumptions and computational approaches before BHFBA is applied. This resulted in the size of the model is reduced to 631 reactions. Lethal reactions such as the genes that are found to be lethal *in vivo*, but not *in silico*, are not included as the possible targets in BHFBA. The reason to remove lethal reaction is that the microorganism is unable to survive without this reaction. Even though the data is reduced to 631 reactions, this number can still be large for solving quadruple deletion problem; the number of possible combinations of quadruple deletions in a model with 631 reactions is more than 6.5 x 10^9. The *S.cerevisiae* simulations are performed for aerobic minimal media conditions. The glucose uptake rate are fixed to 10 mmol/gDW/hr while a set non-growth associated maintenance of 7.6 mmol ATP/gDW/hr. The experiments are carried out by using a 2.3 GHz Intel Core i7 processor and 8 GB DDR3 RAM computer.

Table 1 and Table 2 summarize the results obtained from BHFBA for succinic acid and glycerol production from *S.cerevisiae*. Succinic acid is one of the intermediates of the TCA cycle and is a chemical to be used as a feedstock for the synthesis of a wide range of other chemical with several industrial applications. Besides, as a metabolite from the central carbon metabolism, succinic acid represents a good case study for identifying metabolic engineering strategies. Glycerol is naturally produced by *S.cerevisiae* in small quantities during anaerobic fermentation or under osmotic stress. It is interesting to study the effects of gene deletions on yield and productivity of glycerol as it plays an important role in maintaining the cytosolic redox balance under anaerobic conditions. As shown from the results, this method has produced better results to the previous works in term of growth rate and BPCY meanwhile potential genes which can be removed are identified [5][10].

Table 1. Comparison between different methods for production of Succinic acid in *S.cerevisiae*

Method	BPCY	List of knockout genes
BHFBA	0.097323	ADH4**, FUM1_1,SDH3_2*
BAFBA [10]	0.089	MAE1, SDH3_2*, TPI1, MET3**
SA + FBA [5]	0.05398	PGII_I, PGII_2, FBPI, PDC6, ADH4**, SDH3_2*, AAHI_I, URHI_I, U30_, MET3**, ALD4_2, GSHI, UI03_, YER053C, CTPI_I

Note: The shaded column represents the best result. N/A – Not Applicable. * Common genes for all methods. ** Common genes in either 2 methods. BPCY is in gram (gram-glucose.hour)$^{-1}$.

Table 1 and Figure 4 show that BHFBA performed better than the previous works with BPCY 0.0973. Knocking out succinate dehydrogenase (SDH3_2) interrupts the formation from succinic acid to fumarate. Without the conversion from succinic acid to fumarate, production yield of succinic is improved. Next, by knocking out fumarase (FUM1_1) interrupts the TCA cycle, which resulted in the concentration of fumarate increases which entails an increase in the concentration of succinic acid [13]. In addition, alcohol dehydrogenase (ADH4) is suggested to knockout. This knockout eliminated the production of ethanol which is known as competing product.

Table 2 shows the results of BHFBA and previous works. BHFBA obtained a slightly better BPCY that is 0.0973. The deletion of aldehyde dehydrogenase (ALD2) inhibits the formation of ethanol which is a competing product. Due to the deletion the competing by-products are eliminated which resulted in the increment of the glycerol production. In addition, the deletion of pyruvate dehydrogenase (PDA1) inhibits the formation of acetyl-CoA which leads to deactivation of citric acid cycle. Due to the deletion the competing by-products are eliminated which resulted in the increment of the glycerol production. From the knockout lists, it can be concluded that all the mutants are suggested to deactivate or inhibit the citric acid cycle.

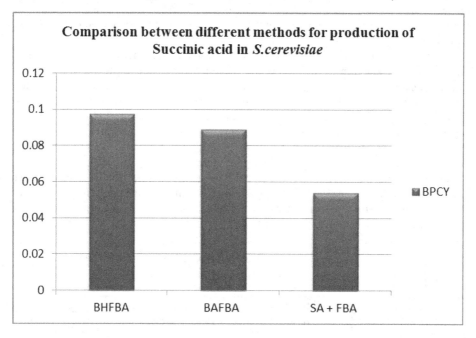

Fig. 4. Comparison between different methods for production of Succinic acid in *S.cerevisiae*

Table 3 shows the computational time comparison between BHFBA and BAFBA for 1000 iterations. The methods are tested with iteration value 500 to 2000 and 1000 iterations produce a better result. Hence, we set the iteration value to 1000 for both cases. The average computational time of BHFBA improved 36% of the BAFBA result for 1000 iterations.

Table 2. Comparison between different methods for production of glycerol in *S.cerevisiae*

Method	BPCY	List of knockout genes
BHFBA	0.0973	ALD2, PDA1*, SDH3_2*, ZWF1
BAFBA [10]	0.0972	U43_, ICL1, PDA1*, RPE1, SDH3_2*

Note: The shaded column represents the best result. N/A – Not Applicable. * Common genes for all methods. ** Common genes in either 2 methods. BPCY is in gram (gram-glucose.hour)$^{-1}$.

Table 3. Comparison between average computational time of BHFBA and BAFBA for 1000 iterations

Method	Computation Time (s)
BHFBA	3696
BAFBA [10]	5774

In addition, since BA and Hill Climbing algorithm is a new hybrid algorithm. Hence, we conducted a benchmarking to test performance of a hybrid of BA and Hill Climbing algorithm (BH). As BA is looking for the maximum, the functions are inverted before the algorithm is applied. The De Jong, Martin & Gaddy, and Schwefel functions are used in this paper. Table 4 shows the mathematical representation of the functions. Table 5 shows mean and standard deviation (STD) of the three functions, De Jong, Martin & Gaddy, and Schwefel, tested on both original BA and BH.

Table 4. Mathematical representation of De Jong and Beale functions

Name	Mathematical representation
De Jong	$maxF = (3905.93) - 100(x_1^2 - x_2)^2 - (1 - x_1)^2$
Martin & Gaddy	$minF = (x_1 - x_2)^2 + ((x_1 + x_2 - 10) / 3)^2$
Schwefel	$minF = 418.9829*n + sum(-x(i)*sin(sqrt(abs(x(i)))))$

Table 5. Obtained fitness value of both De Jong and Beale functions

Function	Mean		STD	
	BA	BH	BA	BH
De Jong	3.91e+03	3.90e+03	0.000504	4.79e-13
Martin & Gaddy	11.1083	11.1111	0.002797	0
Schwefel	8.38e+02	8.38e+-2	2.205e-05	0

As seen from the results, both BHFBA and BH performed better than other algorithms. It can be concluded that the capability of Hill Climbing algorithm in finding local optimum improved the performance of the original BA. The original BA with the problem of repetitive iterations of the algorithm in local search where each bee keep searching until the best possible answer is reached. Our proposed BHFBA solved the problem by implementing Hill Climbing algorithm into the local search part. Hill Climbing algorithm is a powerful local search algorithm which attempts to find a better solution by incrementally changing a single element of the solution until no further improvements can be found, the search process is recorded so the process is not repeated. Furthermore, one of the advantages of Hill Climbing algorithm is it can return a valid solution even if it is interrupted at any time before it ends.

4   Conclusion and Future Works

In this paper, BHFBA is proposed to predict optimal sets of gene deletion to maximize the production of desired metabolite. Experimental results on *S.cerevisiae* iFF708 model obtained from literature showed that BHFBA is effective in generating optimal solutions to the gene knockout prediction, and is therefore a useful tool in Metabolic Engineering [12]. We are interested in applying other fitness functions in BHFBA such as minimization of metabolic adjustment (MOMA) and regulatory on/off minimization (ROOM) to further improve the performance of BHFBA. Besides that, BA employs many tunable parameters which are difficult for the users to determine so it is important to find ways to help the users choose suitable parameters.

Acknowledgement. Institutional Scholarship MyPhD provided by the Ministry of Higher Education of Malaysia finances this work. We would like to thank Malaysian Ministry of Science, Technology and Innovation for supporting this research by an e-science research grant (Grant number: 06-01-06-SF1029). This research is also supported by a GUP research grant (Grant number: Q.J130000.2507.04H16) that was sponsored by Universiti Teknologi Malaysia.

References

1. Feist, A.M., Herrgård, M.J., Thiele, I., Reed, J.L., Palsson, B.Ø.: Reconstruction of biochemical networks in microorganisms. Nat. Rev. Microbiol. 72, 129–143 (2009)
2. Chandran, D., Copeland, W.B., Sleight, S.C., Sauro, H.M.: Mathematical modeling and synthetic biology. Drug Discovery Today Disease Models 5(4), 299–309 (2008)
3. Burgard, A.P., Pharkya, P., Maranas, C.D.: OptKnock: A bilevel programming framework for identifying gene knockout strategies for microbial strains optimization. Biotechnol. Bioeng. 84, 647–657 (2003)
4. Patil, K.R., Rocha, I., Förster, J., Nielsen, J.: Evolutionary programming as a platform for in silico metabolic engineering. BMC Bioinformatics 6, 308 (2005)
5. Rocha, M., Maia, P., Mendes, R., Pinto, J.P., Ferreira, E.C., Nielsen, J., Patil, K.R., Rocha, I.: Natural computation meta-heuristics for the in silico optimization of microbial strains. BMC Bioinformatics 9, 499 (2008)
6. Pham, D.T., Ghanbarzadeh, A., Koç, E., Otri, S., Zaidi, M.: The bees algorithm – a novel tool for complex optimization problems. In: Proceedings of the Second International Virtual Conference on Intelligent Production Machines and Systems, July 3-14 (2006)
7. Choon, Y.W., Mohamad, M.S., Deris, S., Chong, C.K., Chai, L.E., Ibrahim, Z., Omatu, S.: Identifying Gene Knockout Strategies Using a Hybrid of Bees Algorithm and Flux Balance Analysis For in silico Optimization of Microbial Strains. In: Omatu, S., Paz Santana, J.F., González, S.R., Molina, J.M., Bernardos, A.M., Rodríguez, J.M.C. (eds.) DCAI. AISC, vol. 151, pp. 371–378. Springer, Heidelberg (2012)
8. Pham, D.T., Darwish, A.H., Eldukhri, E.E.: Optimisation of a fuzzy logic controller using the bees algorithm. International Journal of Computer Aided Engineering and Technology 1(2), 250–264 (2006)
9. Olague, G., Puente, C.: The honeybee search algorithm for three-dimensional reconstruction. In: Rothlauf, F., et al. (eds.) EvoWorkshops 2006. LNCS, vol. 3907, pp. 427–437. Springer, Heidelberg (2006)

10. Pham, D.T., Ghanbarzadeh, A.: Multi-objective optimisation using the bees algorithm. Paper in Proceedings of the Third International Virtual Conference on Intelligent Production Machines and Systems, July 2-13 (2007)
11. Cheng, M.Y., Lien, L.C.: A Hybrid Swarm Intelligence Based Particle Bee Algorithm For Benchmark Functions and Construction Site Layout Optimization. In: Proceedings of the 28th ISARC, Seou, pp. 898–904 (2011)
12. Forster, J., Famili, I., Fu, P., Palsson, B.Ø., Nielsen, J.: Genome-scale reconstruction of the Saccharomyces cerevisiae metabolic network. Genome Res. 13, 244–253 (2003)
13. Bohl, K., de Figueiredo, L.F., Hadicke, O., Klamt, S., Kost, C., Schuster, S., Kaleta, C.: CASOP GS: Computing intervention strategies targeted at production improvement in genome-scale metabolic networks. In: The 5th German Conference on Bioinformatics 2010, September 20-22 (2010)

Mining Clinical Process in Order Histories Using Sequential Pattern Mining Approach

Shusaku Tsumoto and Hidenao Abe[*]

Department of Medical Informatics, School of Medicine,
Faculty of Medicine
Shimane University
89-1 Enya-cho Izumo 693-8501 Japan
tsumoto@med.shimane-u.ac.jp

Abstract. In hospital information system, order-entry system is used to transfer the orders from doctors or nurses to other medical stuffs. Thus, since order histories will store the clinincal process of each doctors in a sequential way, reuse of such data will capture the process of each clinician. This paper applied two types of sequential pattern mining approaches to analysis of a sequential process for each care process. The empirical results show the methods enable us to capture the temporal characteristics of behavior of clinicians, which will give a subset of decision making process in clinical environments.

Keywords: Process Mining, Sequential Pattern Mining, Rule Mining, CPOE Error Analysis.

1 Introduction

In recent years, almost all large-scale hospitals have introduced a hosptial information system (HIS) for management of all clinical activities. One of the main components is a computerized physician order entry (CPOE) system that transpors the orders from a physician or a nurse to other medical staffs.

One of the main advantage which has not been discussed before is that CPOE system can store all the order histories, which can be viewed as data of behavior of clinincal process. Thus, analysis of the stored data will give knowledge about characteristic of each clinician's decision process. Furthermore, the history may store sudden order revisions which are signs of medical error [1] and medical error risks [2]. However, as pointed out in conventional studies [3,4], application of mining methods to such data has not been achieved yet in the literature.

This paper introduces two sequential pattern mining algorithms for analysis of order histories and applied to the task for evaluation of order change of prescription, which may induced risk of medical errors. The empirical results

---

[*] The present affiliation of Hidenao Abe is Bunkyo University, 1100 Namegaya, Chigasaki-shi, Kanagawa 253-8850 JAPAN.

J. Li et al. (Eds.): PAKDD 2013 Workshops, LNAI 7867, pp. 234–246, 2013.

showed the methods enable us to capture the temporal characteristics of behavior of clinicians, which will give a subset of decision making process in clinical environments.

The paper is organized as follows. Setion 2 explains two preprocessing methods: one extracts the characteristic order entry subsequences without gaps between order entries as used in [5]. The other one obtains the subsequences allowing gaps between the order entries. By assuming the obtained subsequences as the features for order histories, the classification learning models are obtained for the dataset by algorithms shown in Section 3. Section 4 evaluated the efficiency of the two sets of characteristic order entry subsequences by comparing the accuracies of classification learning algorithms. By regarding the result, the differences of the classification rules are discussed. Finally, Section 5 concludes this paper.

2   Preprocessing

In order to analyze some processes that consist of sequenced events, quantitative aspect and qualitative aspects of processes should be considered. As for the quantitative aspect, the total number of the included events and the frequencies of each event represent their features for distinguishing each process. On the other hand, the qualitative aspect has mainly featured each event based on their frequencies as the characteristics of the processes. In this paper, both qualitative features and the features based on the subsequences are used for analyzing the characteristics of clinical care processes.

2.1   Processes as Data of Event Sequences

A hospital information system stores the histories of their clinical process through the issuance of orders and their execution in a sequential way: the system records the events from the beginning to the end of the process as an instance of the data. The data consisting of one sequence of carried out events in one process is called sequence data with keeping the orders between the events as shown in Figure 1.

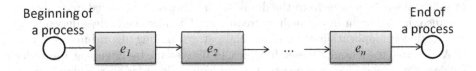

Fig. 1. Process as one sequential data S_i

Suppose e_j represents one events in a process, the whole of process including m events is defined as one sequence of the events $S_i =< e_1, e_2, ..., e_m >$. The set of the process is obtained as the dataset $D = \{S_1, S_2, ..., S_n\}$, including n sequences. The elements of each process can be assumed as items for the sequential pattern mining approach.

2.2   Quantitative Features of the Processes

In order to characterize the sequences of events, the quantitative features that are various statistics of each sequence are useful to distinguish each sequence by using real numbers. Such quantitative features are based on the length of the sequences and the counts of the included events of each sequence.

On the COPE systems, physicians can enter the orders for the patient's treatment such as the following orders.

- Medication order (Med)
- Laboratory test order (LabTest)
- Physiological function test order (PhyTest)
- Injection order (Inj)
- Rehabilitation order (Reha)
- Blood translation order (Trans)
- Hospital control order (HospCtrl)

By assuming the orders for each patient in a reasonable sequence on the treatment, the total number of the orders included in the order entry sequences corresponds to the length of the sequence. At the same time, the frequencies of each order included in the sequences are counted as the quantitative features of the sequences.

2.3   Qualitative Features of the Processes

For the set of sequential data, we can apply a sequential pattern mining approach [6], instead of identifying characteristic groups of the events in the set of the processes manually.

Sequential pattern mining is a unsupervised mining approach for extracting meaningful subsequences from the dataset, that consists of ordered items as one instance, by using an index such as frequency. The meaningfulness depends on the context in application of an sequential pattern mining algorithm.

As for the sequential dataset from a CPOE system, by assuming the order entries in a period as one sequence, the characteristic order entry subsequences can be extracted by using the following sequential pattern mining approaches: one extracts subsequences without gaps between each event; the other allows gaps between each event in its extracted subsequences.

In order to construct the features of the characteristic order entry subsequences, the following steps is performed:

1. Gathering sequences of the processes annotated by the reasonable beginning and ending of them
2. Applying a sequential pattern mining algorithm for extracting characteristic order entry subsequences from the overall sequences
3. Selecting top N characteristic order entry subsequences according to the scores in each sequential mining algorithm

Extracting Subsequences by FLR-score. For extracting subsequences without gaps between items, sequential pattern mining algorithms have developed and used in various fields such as n-gram [7] and LCS [8].

In the following experiments, we applied an automatic term extraction method [9] that ware developed for extracting meaningful words and phrases in the set of documents. For extracting characteristic partial order sequences in the set of order entry sequences, we assume the order entry sequences as the documents for this method. This method involves the detection of meaningful subsequences by using the following score for each candidate C:

$$FLR(C) = f(C) \times (\prod_{j=1}^{m}(FL(e_j)+1)(FR(e_j)+1))^{\frac{1}{2m}}$$

where $f(C)$ means frequency of a candidate subsequence C appeared isolated, and $FL(e_j)$ and $FR(e_j)$ indicate the frequencies of the orders before and after each order entry e_j in bi-grams including each C. Each candidate C consists of m events corresponding to the order entries e_j. FLR score of C calculate in each set of sequences D, gathered for a given period such as monthly, yearly, and so forth.

An example for calculating the FLR score is shown in Figure 2. The four CPOE sequences are in the database. By counting $(m+1)$-grams for each candidate C, the system counts $f(C)$, $FL(e_j)$, and $FR(e_j)$. In the figure, the system assumes one medication order entry Med as the candidate C. The candidate has only one element $e_1 = Med$. The calculation of FLR score applies for the all of the candidates with the lengths from $m = 1$ to $m = 3$. Then, we select the top N candidates as the characteristic subsequences.

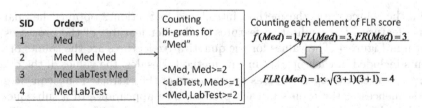

Fig. 2. Example of the sequential pattern extraction for the CPOE sequences by using the FLR score

Extracting Subsequences by PrefixSpan. The approach for extracting the subsequences with gaps between items have developed recent decade such as PrefixSpan [10] and other frequent sequential pattern mining algorithms [6]. Although the degree of comprehensiveness is lower than the subsequences without gaps, the algorithms can extract the subsequences rapidly than the former algorithms.

By taking PrefixSpan for extracting order entry subsequences, we gathered the set of sequences S_i of the processes by assuming each order entry as an item e_i. The support of $Supp(S_i)$ counted for the sequential dataset D as same as the FLR score calculation. For example, there are four order entry sequences as shown in Figure 3. The method counts the numbers of records including each order entry e_j as the items. Then, it projects the original sequence database by using the items that are included more records than the given minimum support $MinSupp$ as the prefixes. This process iterates while the items are included more than the given minimum support. When the iteration stops, the method output the subsequences that appears more than the minimum support, traversing the tree structure of the projections from the root to the leaves.

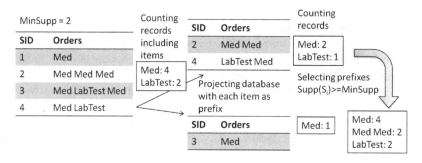

Fig. 3. Example of the sequential pattern extraction for the CPOE sequences by using PrefixSpan

3   Classification

From the source data, the method introduced in Section 2 obtains the quantitative features, the qualitative features, and other features of the processes as shown in Figure 4. The values for the quantitative features are the counts of the events included in each process in this method. Besides, the values of the qualitative features are represented as appearances of the extracted subsequences in the sequences of the events in each process. The appearance of a subsequence is judged by considering the gaps in the subsequences for each sequence. Then, the value for the subsequences represent as 0/1 for each feature.

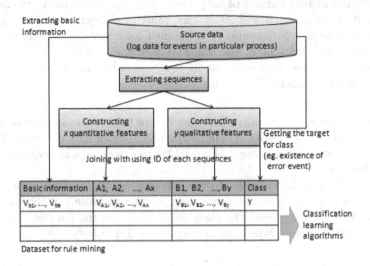

Fig. 4. Overview the process for obtaining a dataset for rule mining

For a hospital information system, it commonly holds patient IDs and their basic information. As for such basic information of patients we can gather their sex, age, and number of disease by identifying ID numbers. The basic features of the patients are appended to the counts of the orders in each process, the appearances of characteristic order entry subsequences, and the class values.

4 Empirical Comparison of Two Sequential Pattern Mining Algorithms

This section applied two proposed algorithms to actual order histories stored in Shimane University Hospital that has 616 beds and more than 1000 outpatients a day. According to the pre-processing process as described in Section 2, we obtained datasets for rule mining algorithms, containing basic information of the patients, counts of the orders, and the appearances of extracted characteristic order entry subsequences. Then, by applying a sub-sequence extraction method, two sequential pattern mining methods, introduced in Section 3 were applied to capture the temporal patterns of clincians' behavior. The relationships are described by if-then rules in the followings.

4.1 Analysis

4.2 Inpatient and Outpatient

In this case study, the two monthly order entry history data for June 2008 and June 2009 is used as source data for the rule mining based on the quantitative and qualitative features of each order entry sequence. The processed dataset were split into history dataset of outpatients and inpatients due to the following reasons. As for the outpatient situations, most of patients visit each sector at once a day. The care for inpatients is planned for every day according to their therapeutical schedule. Thus, the annotation of the beginning and the end for daily sequence of the orders is one of the reasonable annotations for ordinal inpatient and outpatient clinical care processes.

Target: Medication Change. The experiment focuses the medication changes to capture the characteristics of clinincal behavior which may be a sign of a rapid change in the status of a patient. The change may lead to a medication error or other clinical risks.

Based on the numbers of order entries, the class for the medication order entry changes is set up by using the corrections and the deletions of the medication order on the CPOE system. The class distributions of the datasets for the two months, June 2008 and June 2009, are shown in Table 1.

Table 1. Class distributions about the medication order changes on June 2008 and June 2009

	Jun. 2008		Jun. 2009	
	In.	Out.	In.	Out.
Without Med. Change	6607	9863	6864	10096
With Med. Chenge(s)	529	338	562	413
TOTAL	7136	10201	7426	10509

In order to avoid tautological rules from the datasets, the features directly counting the class for the following analysis were removed; corrections of the medication order and deletions of the medication order.

4.3   Quantitative Features of the Clinical Care Processes on the CPOE System

In order to obtain qualitative features of each process sequence, the numbers of the order entries and their changes in inpatient and outpatient situations were counted respectively. The statistics of the numbers of the 22 order entries, which include the five kinds of orders and their total on overall, correction, and deletion, as shown in Table 2.

The averaged numbers of the medication orders shows more than four. This indicate that most of the patients in the hospital are medicated four or five kindsof drugs in each visit for outpatient or daily care for inpatient situations. Excepting the total number of the daily order entries, the minimum number of these order entries is 0.

Table 2. The maximum and averaged numbers of daily counts of the five order entries

| | June 2008 | | | | June 2009 | | | |
| | Inpatient | | Outpatient | | Inpatient | | Outpatient | |
Att.	max	avg.	max	avg.	max	avg.	max	avg.
Total	47	4.24	47	3.89	58	4.32	63	3.94
Med	44	2.54	47	3.05	48	2.65	62	3.09
LabTest	19	0.56	11	0.54	19	0.50	10	0.54
PhyTest	8	0.07	8	0.11	7	0.08	8	0.10
Inj	29	1.00	22	0.15	39	0.96	17	0.17
Reha	5	0.09	14	0.04	14	0.11	9	0.04
MedCrr	25	0.20	21	0.08	32	0.22	13	0.09
LabTestCrr	13	0.08	7	0.02	10	0.05	5	0.01
PhyTestCrr	3	0.01	2	0.01	4	0.01	1	0.01
InjCrr	8	0.09	7	0.03	10	0.10	12	0.02
RehaCrr	2	0.00	12	0.00	3	0.00	3	0.00
MedDel	20	0.06	20	0.02	14	0.05	27	0.01
LabTestDel	3	0.02	3	0.01	4	0.02	2	0.02
PhyTestDel	2	0.00	2	0.00	2	0.00	2	0.00
InjDel	5	0.01	5	0.00	21	0.01	4	0.00
RehaDel	3	0.00	2	0.00	6	0.00	3	0.00
TotalSub	31	3.75	30	3.72	37	3.84	36	3.77
MedSub	29	2.28	29	2.95	36	2.39	35	2.99
LabTestSub	13	0.47	11	0.51	13	0.42	8	0.51
PhyTestSub	7	0.06	8	0.10	7	0.06	6	0.09
InjSub	21	0.85	15	0.13	27	0.85	13	0.14
RehaSub	5	0.09	5	0.03	8	0.10	6	0.04

4.4   Preprocessing: Extraction of Subsequences

In the experiments, a set characteristic order entry subsequences C was selected when the FLR score was larger than 1, $FLR(C) > 1.0$. As for the PrefixSpan, the minimum support for obtaining the subsequences was set up as $MinSupp(s_i) > 1$. Table 3 shows the obtained subsequences by using the two sequential pattern mining approach.

Table 3. Numbers of obtained subsequences by using the FLR term extraction method and PrefixSpan

| | Jun. 2008 | | Jun. 2009 | |
	In.	Out.	In.	Out.
FLR	2194	1251	2288	1315
PrefixSpan	346	413	365	389

According to the scores of each sequential pattern mining algorithm, top 20 subsequences of each dataset were selected as the characteristic order entry subsequences. Table 4 shows the top 10 subsequences extracted by the FLR score and PrefixSpan.

Table 4. Top 10 characteristic partial order sequences based on the FLR scores and PrefixSpan method: (a) on June 2008, (b) on June 2009

(a) June 2008

Rank	Inpatient		Outpatient	
	Subsequences (FLR)	Subsequences (PrefixSpan)	Subsequences (FLR)	Subsequences (PrefixSpan)
1	Med	Med	Med	Med
2	Med Med	Med Med	Med Med	Med Med
3	HospCtrl Med	HosCtrl Med	LabTest Med	Med Med Med
4	Med HospCtrl	Med HosCtrl	Med LabTest Med	LabTest Med Med
5	Med LabTest	Med Med Med	LabTest Med Med	Med LabTest
6	LabTest Med	LabTest Med	Med LabTest	Med Med Med Med
7	Med Med Med	Med LabTest	Med Med Med Med	LabTest Med Med Med
8	Med Reha	Med Reha	LabTest Med Med Med	Med Med Med Med Med
9	HospCtrl Med Med	HospCtrl Med Med	Med Med Med Med Med	HospCtrl Med
10	Reha Med	Med HospCtrlCrr	HospCtrl Med	Med Med Med Med Med Med

(b) June 2009

Rank	Inpatient		Outpatient	
	Subsequences (FLR)	Subsequences (PrefixSpan)	Subsequences (FLR)	Subsequences (PrefixSpan)
1	Med	Med	Med	Med
2	Med Med	Med Med	Med Med	Med Med
3	HospCtrl Med	HosCtrl Med	LabTest Med	LabTest Med
4	Med HospCtrl	Med HospCtrl	Med Med Med	Med Med Med
5	Med LabTest	Med Med Med	Med LabTest	LabTest Med Med
6	Med Med Med	Med Reha	LabTest Med Med	Med LabTest
7	LabTest Med	HospCtrl Med Med	Med Med Med Med	Med Med Med Med
8	Med Reha	Med LabTest	Med Med Med Med Med	Med Med Med Med Med
9	Reha Med	Reha Med	LabTest Med Med Med	LabTest Med Med Med
10	HospCtrl Med Med	LabTest Med	HospCtrl Med	HospCtrl Med

As shown in Table 4, most of the subsequences of the two algorithms are the same. However, the ranks are slightly different because of the difference of the scoring indexes.

In the following rule mining phase, we used the top 20 characteristic subsequences from each set of subsequences with/without gaps between order entries. The values of the features are 0/1 for representing appearances of each subsequence in one order sequence.

4.5 Empirical Comparison of Classification Algorithms

In order to compare the efficiency of the two sets of extracted subsequences as the features of the clinical care processes, the following three feature sets were set up as shown in Table 5 for the five classification learning algorithms.

Table 5. Setting of the three feature sets for rule mining

	Feature Set		
	I	II	III
Basic information	X	X	X
Quant. Features	X	X	X
Subsequences by FLR		X	
Subsequences by PrefixSpan			X
# of Attributes	34	54	54

As for the representative classification learning algorithms, NaiveBayes(NB), k-NN($k = 5$), C4.5 [11], OneR [12], and PART [13] [1] in this comparison.

The averaged error rates obtained by 50 times repeated 10-fold cross validation of the five learning algorithm for the three different feature sets are shown in Table 6 for inpatient and Table 7 for outpatient.

Table 6. Error rates(%) for classifying the three dataset with/without the features based on the two sequential pattern mining algorithms for inpatient order sequences

| | 2008 (baseline=7.41) | | | 2009 (baseline=7.57) | | |
| | Feature Set | | | Feature Set | | |
	I	II	III	I	II	III
NB	12.66	12.55	9.79	13.66	7.60	8.90
k-NN	9.55	5.08	2.78•	12.26	2.21•	2.70
C4.5	0.87	0.71•	1.23	0.74	0.34•	1.18
OneR	4.77	4.77	2.03	4.67	1.72•	1.72•
PART	0.59•	0.81	0.82	0.50•	0.63	0.59

Table 7. Error rates(%) for classifying the three dataset with/without the features based on the two sequential pattern mining algorithms for outpatient order sequences

| | 2008 (baseline=3.31) | | | 2009 (baseline=3.93) | | |
| | Feature Set | | | Feature Set | | |
	I	II	III	I	II	III
NB	9.25	9.34	10.89	9.58	11.92	12.73
k-NN	5.68	2.81	2.80•	6.25	2.91	2.87•
C4.5	1.44•	1.44•	1.44•	0.52	0.48•	0.52•
OneR	3.30•	3.30•	3.30•	2.72•	2.72•	2.72•
PART	1.50	1.37•	1.50	0.78	0.52•	0.71

As shown in the tables, Table 6 and Table 7, by using the datasets with the three feature sets, the decision tree and the two rule mining algorithms achieve higher accuracies, that are emphasized, just predicting the majority class; no medication order change. Especially, the datasets of Feature Set II achieved the highest accuracies with lowest error rates with marked • for most of the learning algorithms even in both of the inpatient datasets and the outpatient datasets. This indicates that the FLR score that combines the frequency of the subsequence and the authority degree in the sequence has more meanings rather than just using the frequencies of the subsequences.

---

[1] All of the algorithms are Weka [14] implementation.

4.6 Comparison of Obtained Rules

In order to compare the availability of the partial order entry sequences for detecting medication order changes, the contents of the representative rules obtained for each dataset were examined. Here, the classification rules obtained by PART were selected because PART achieved the best performance.

Figure 5 shows the rules obtained for the datasets that PART rules achieve highest including both the quantitative features and the subsequences.

```
2008 Outpatient:

IF      # of total order entries <=17
    and # of Medication order > 3
    and # of Biophysican Test order = 0
    and "Med Med Med"
  and Disease (DPC) != null
THEN Medication Order Change="NO"
(coverage 45, incorrect 4)
```

```
2009Outpatient:

IF      # of Medication order <=9
    and # of Medication order without changes > 3
    and "Med Med Med"
    and Disease (DPC) != null
THEN Medication Order Change="NO"
(coverage 50, incorrect 2)
```

Fig. 5. The rules of PART describing the relationship between some characteristic order entry subsequences and the medication order changes with the highest coverage on each dataset

The rules containing the characteristic order partial sequences are shown in Figure 5. Although these rules represent the relationships between the order entry subsequences and the no order change, the coverage and the correctness of these rules are high. Although the rules with the characteristic order entry subsequences cover only few instances, their accuracies are higher than the rules that are constructed with the numbers of order entries. Based on this result, the order partial sequences distinguish the result without the medication order changes more concretely.

5   Conclusion

This paper conducted empirical comparison of characteristic order entry subsequences related to the medication order entry changes by using rule mining approach. The sets of characteristic order entry subsequences were obtained by the two sequential pattern mining algorithms. The one obtains the characteristic order entry subsequences without gaps between order entries by using FLR score. The other obtains the subsequences allowing gaps between the order entries by using PrefixSpan. By assuming the obtained subsequences as the features for each medication order entry change, the classification learning models are obtained for the datasets.

The obtained classification rules on the two sets of qualitative features of each sequence were more accurate than that of just using the quantitative features of each sequences consisting of the counts of five kinds of order entries. The obtained rules described the relationship between the subsequences and the medication order changes such as the combination of the number of the order entries and the three continued medication order entry subsequence ("Med Med Med"). In spite of the traditional method for extracting the subsequences without gaps between the order entries, the subsequences obtained by it provided more accurate and comprehensive sequences of order entries than that with the gaps between the order entries. However, we just used the frequency of the subsequences in later approach. The index for ranking the subsequences remains rooms for more improvement.

Future work will analyze the position of order changes such as the beginning of order entries, the end of order entries, and other position in the sequences. Then, by using more detailed systematic logs of the CPOE system, this analysis method will be applied for analyzing the relationship between detailed operation and the order changes, which are directly corresponding to the operations on the physicians' screens.

Acknowledgements. This research is supported by Grant-in-Aid for Scientific Research (B) 24300058 from Japan Society for the Promotion of Science(JSPS).

References

1. Currie, L.M., Desjardins, K.S., Stone, P.W., Lai, T.Y., Schwartz, E., Schnall, R., Bakken, S.: Near-miss and hazard reporting: promoting mindfulness in patient safety education. Studies in Health Technology and Informatics 129(pt. 1), 285–290 (2007)
2. Magrabi, F., McDonnell, G., Westbrook, J., Coiera, E.: Using an accident model to design safe electronic medication management systems. Stud. Health Technol. Inform. 129, 948–952 (2007)
3. Bates, D.W.: Computerized physician order entry and medication errors: finding a balance. J. of Biomedical Informatics 38, 259–261 (2005)
4. Koppel, R., Metlay, J.P., Cohen, A., Abaluck, B., Localio, A.R., Kimmel, S.E., Strom, B.L.: Role of computerized physician order entry systems in facilitating medication errors. J. Am. Med. Assoc. 293(10), 1197–1203 (2005)

5. Abe, H., Tsumoto, S.: Mining classification rules for detecting medication order changes by using characteristic cpoe subsequences. In: Kryszkiewicz, M., Rybinski, H., Skowron, A., Raś, Z.W. (eds.) ISMIS 2011. LNCS, vol. 6804, pp. 80–89. Springer, Heidelberg (2011)
6. Mabroukeh, N.R., Ezeife, C.I.: A taxonomy of sequential pattern mining algorithms. ACM Comput. Surv. 43, 3:1–3:41 (2010)
7. Shannon, C.E.: A mathematical theory of communication. The Bell System Technical Journal 27, 379–423, 623–656 (1948)
8. Hirschberg, D.S.: Algorithms for the longest common subsequence problem. J. ACM 24, 664–675 (1977)
9. Nakagawa, H.: Automatic term recognition based on statistics of compound nouns. Terminology 6(2), 195–210 (2000)
10. Pei, J., Han, J., Mortazavi-Asl, B., Pinto, H., Chen, Q., Dayal, U., Hsu, M.C.: Prefixspan: Mining sequential patterns efficiently by prefix-projected pattern growth. In: Proc. of the 17th International Conference on Data Engineering, pp. 215–224. IEEE Computer Society, Los Alamitos (2001)
11. Quinlan, J.R.: Programs for Machine Learning. Morgan Kaufmann Publishers (1993)
12. Holte, R.C.: Very simple classification rules perform well on most commonly used datasets. Machine Learning 11, 63–91 (1993)
13. Frank, E., Wang, Y., Inglis, S., Holmes, G., Witten, I.H.: Using model trees for classification. Machine Learning 32(1), 63–76 (1998)
14. Witten, I.H., Frank, E.: Data Mining: Practical Machine Learning Tools and Techniques with Java Implementations. Morgan Kaufmann (2000)

Multiclass Prediction for Cancer Microarray Data Using Various Variables Range Selection Based on Random Forest

Kohbalan Moorthy, Mohd Saberi Mohamad[*], and Safaai Deris

Artificial Intelligence and Bioinformatics Research Group, Faculty of Computing,
Universiti Teknologi Malaysia, 81310, Skudai, Johor, Malaysia
kohbalan2@live.utm.my, {saberi,safaai}@utm.my

Abstract. Continuous data mining has led to the generation of multi class datasets through microarray technology. New improved algorithms are then required to process and interpret these data. Cancer prediction tailored with variable selection process has shown to improve the overall prediction accuracy. Through variable selection process, the amount of informative genes gathered are much lesser than the initial data, yet the selective subset present in other methods cannot be fine-tuned to suit the necessity for particular number of variables. Hence, an improved technique of various variable range selection based on Random Forest method is proposed to allow selective variable subsets for cancer prediction. Our results indicate improvement in the overall prediction accuracy of cancer data based on the improved various variable range selection technique which allows selective variable selection to create best subset of genes. Moreover, this technique can assist in variable interaction analysis, gene network analysis, gene-ranking analysis and many other related fields.

Keywords: Variable Selection, Cancer Prediction, Random Forest, Gene Expression, Microarray Data.

1   Introduction

Microarray technology allows continuous analysis and interpretation of the expression levels present in the observed variables from microarray data. Analysing microarray data is a challenging task, as the high dimensionality of the data requires large processing power with sufficient amount of memory resources. Furthermore, microarray technology allows the expansion of information of the sample itself, where detailed insights of the data can be used for gene regulation and identification based on gene expression data [1]. In addition, it has been used in studies related to cancer prediction, identification of relevant variables for diagnosis or therapy and investigation of drug effects on cancer prognosis [2]. Biologists require accurate predictive tools as well as group of relevant variables for biomarkers in cancer

---

[*] Corresponding author.

J. Li et al. (Eds.): PAKDD 2013 Workshops, LNAI 7867, pp. 247–257, 2013.

identification [3]. Cancer informatics has been expected to be a part of the advancement in the identification and validation of biomarkers through the combine interdisciplinary fields, which expands from the bioinformatics [4].

In this article, we begin with describing the research keywords in this introduction section followed by describing the methodology section where the proposed technique is briefly explained; followed by the result and discussion section, where the main characteristics of the datasets are explained, and the complete analysis of the findings is presented. Comparisons with previous similar research papers are also presented to further justify the improvement achieved using the proposed technique. Lastly, the future works and conclusion of this article are presented.

Prior to cancer prediction, performing variable selection allows grouping of relevant variables into a subset. Some of the main reasons for performing variable selection are to avoid over fitting for improved model performance, to gain faster and less costly models and lastly to dig deeper into the data generation processes. Variable selection approach is grouped into three main categories, which are filter based approach, wrapper based approach and embedded based approach [5].

Filter based approach is defined as when the variable selection process is carried out independently of the cancer prediction algorithms. If the classifier is being used to evaluate every selected subset of the variable selection process throughout the entire prediction process, then it is known as a wrapper based approach [6]. Embedded approach uses the same classifier dependent selection as the wrapper based approach, except that it has better computational complexity. According to Wong, Leckie and Kowalczyk [7], filter based approach performs variable selection without any dependence on the classifier being chosen, which may not be sufficient enough to generate higher accuracy in cancer prediction as those of wrapper and embedded approaches, which have certain degree of dependencies with the classifier algorithm being used. In spite of that, wrapper based approach is not preferred in sample prediction due to huge combination of variable subset required to be examined. Moreover, the wrapper method requires high computation time and it is much slower in determining the best subset of variables [8].

Accurately categorizing the selected variables into their respective class as into normal or tumour is known as the process of binary prediction. Classifier can be defined as an artificial intelligence device, which has the potential to make prediction. In usual cancer prediction scenario, most developed algorithms focus on maximizing the overall correct classifiers in order to gain higher prediction accuracy even though there is an imbalance in the different class size [9]. Some examples of classifiers are support vector machines (SVM), neural network (NN), k-nearest neighbor (kNN) and classification tree.

In genetic associated studies, Random Forest has been used widely for both prediction and variable selection [10]. Random Forest was first developed by Breiman [11] for the purpose of classification, regression, clustering and also survival analysis. In this field, the practice and application of variable ranking are according to the variables contribution towards a disease. Random forest has been one of the favoured methods used in variable importance measurement for variable ranking and selection. Diaz-Uriarte and Alvarez de Andres [12] had proposed a variable selection and classification based on Random Forest for the first time as an embedded approach. Besides that, Random Forest algorithm is effective in predicting samples, as well as revealing interactions among the variables. Additionally, a limiting value is achieved as the number of trees set in the Random Forest is increased continuously, making it an ideal error classifier with no over fitting occurrence of the data. In Random Forest, trees are grown, and from the training sample, each tree grows without pruning from the actual data based on random variable selection.

For the creation of gene expression profiles, many researchers are continuously seeking for state of the art prediction algorithms that can provide better accuracy. Variable selection has played a vital role in increasing the prediction accuracy for cancer related disease but most of the variable selection techniques available are unrelated to the prediction algorithm [12]. Moreover, the amount of variables selected in variable sub-sets are dependent on the variable selection technique used and cannot be fine-tuned to suit the requirement for particular number of variables. Hence, we propose a technique known as various variables range selection based on a Random Forest method for selective subset, leading to better prediction of cancer datasets.

2   Methodology

Diaz-Uriarte and Alvarez de Andres [12] first proposed the variable selection through Random Forest algorithm. Moorthy and Mohamad [13] then proposed an improved version of the variable selection. In this research, we propose an improvement on the variable selection technique based on the Random Forest method, which are various variables range selection. Most existing techniques and methods used for variable selection do not reveal the amount of variables selected for training the classifier [14]. Moreover, the selected subset of variables is very dependent on the variable selection technique and does not have the capability to tune and finalize the amount of the selected variables for extended usage in other related fields, such as gene network analysis, gene-gene interaction analysis, and gene annotations. Besides that, most of the variable selection techniques produce constant output of variables for the use of the prediction algorithms. Therefore, there are no possibilities of tweaking that particular variable selection technique to evaluate the different output performance of the classifier [15].

Through this research, an enhancement to the variable selection technique is introduced to provide the flexibility and options to generate different variable sets with better accuracy, as well as the ability to control the amount of variables required on each variable subset. The idea of this improvement focuses on allowing the variable selection algorithm to test and evaluate a certain range of variables from the overall dataset and evaluate the final prediction accuracy. Furthermore, it allows analysis and comparison of different variable subsets towards the prediction accuracy. The main reason for introducing this improved variable selection technique is to provide various variables range selection in any particular selected variable subset for better prediction of cancer. Apart from that, it is also to allow other researchers to further modify and set their desire range of required variables in any particular subset, which can provide better analysis capability in similar research areas.

In order to achieve the proposed various variable range technique, modification to the steps in the backward elimination process were carried out to accept inputs of selective range of variables, which were taken as minimum value (MinVar) and maximum value (MaxVar). Prior to that, the cancer dataset were represented in two different forms of dataset information (Data) and to class the dataset to (Class). While performing the backward elimination process, a new subset was generated and evaluated where the previous error rates obtained (p.mean) were compared with the current error rates obtained (c.mean), and if there was a lower error rates, then the previous best would be replaced with the current best. Once the best subset of variables was determined and the required number of variables was satisfied, we then used the variable subset (bestSub) for the prediction process. A complete flow of the various variable range selection technique is been presented in Figure 1, where the dotted line represents the changes made to achieve the range selection.

Various Variables Range Selection Technique
1: **Input:** Data, Class, MinVar and MaxVar
2: **Output:** Selected variables and error rates
3: **while** backward elimination process = true **do**
4:     removes fraction of variables;
5:     test and evaluate remaining variables;
6:     c.mean = current error rates;
7:     p.mean = previous error rates;
8:     **if** c.mean <= p.mean
9:         p.mean = c.mean;
10:         selVar = current subset of variables;
11:         **if** selVar <= MaxVar and selVar >= MinVar
12:             bestSub = selVar;
13:         **end if**
14:     **end if**
15:     **if** selVar < MinVar
16:         break;
17:     **end if**
18: **end while**

Fig. 1. Pseudo code for the various variables range selection technique developed for controlled amount of selected variables in a particular subset

3   Results and Discussion

In this research, we used cancer related datasets, which were gene expression dataset obtained through the microarray technology. The datasets involved in this research could be grouped into various cancer types, which include breast cancer (Breast), blood cancer (Lymphoma), small round blue cell tumours (SRBCT), brain cancer (Brain) and a set of 60 human tumour cell lines derived from various tissues of origin (NCI60). These cancer datasets were multiclass cancer datasets where various cancer types are considered simultaneously in the microarray experiments.

The cancer datasets used for this research were in text file format and had been pre-formatted to suit the software. For each of the cancer dataset, they have two main text files, which were class file and data file. The class file contained the information to identify the data file according to normal or tumour samples. The data file consists of numerical values, where the rows represent the total number of variables in any particular cancer dataset and the columns represent the total number of patients. The detailed description of the cancer dataset is presented in the Table 1, where the number of variables, patients and the main reference of the data are listed.

Table 1. Main characteristics of the cancer dataset used in this research

Dataset Name	Variables	Patients	Class	Reference
Breast	4869	95	3	[16]
Lymphoma	4026	62	3	[17]
SRBCT	2308	63	4	[18]
Brain	5597	42	5	[19]
NCI60	5244	61	8	[20]

The experimental setup for this research involves R-programming language and the development platform is based on Linux environment. The R script is implemented with *RandomForest* and *varSelRF* package for the execution of this experiment in R console. This experiment is conducted using high performance computing (HPC) based on SUN Cluster which has 48 numbers of CPU with a 2.3GHz processing power each, a total memory size of 64GB and a total storage size of 11TB.

The complete analysis for the selected cancer datasets had been tabulated according to selected various variables range selection, and both the number of variables in a subset and error rates were obtained. The results obtained are an averaged from multiple runs with total iteration of 2000 runs per selected variable range for each dataset. The selected various variables range had been set to into four different partitions as to 2 to 10 variables for the first range, 10 to 50 variables for the second range, 50 to 250 variables for the third range and the final range from 250 variables to the maximum number of variables present in any particular dataset.

The selected various variables range selection settings executed were used to determine the local optimum variables subset for the entire dataset and each subset could be selected to be further used into the prediction process. In terms of the error rates calculation, the .632+ Bootstrap error rates from Efron and Tibshirani [21] had been applied. The complete result is presented in Table 2.

From the results gathered, we can see that the best subset of variables for Breast dataset consists of 214 variables that make up the lowest error rates obtained compared to other various variables range selection, but the recommended subset would be 6 variables which resulted in an error rates of 0.349810. This is because the difference in the total selected variables differs from 6 variables to 214 variables

Table 2. Prediction error rates based on various variables range selection technique where the shaded area represents lowest error rates

Various Variable Range Selection	Breast		Lymphoma		SRBCT		Brain		NCI60	
	*No of Variables	Error Rates	*No of Variables	Error Rates	*No of Variables	Error Rates	*No of Variables	Error Rates	*No of Variables	Error Rates
2 – 10	6	0.349810	2	0.039340	9	0.041312	9	0.205099	10	0.331037
10 – 50	45	0.357240	30	0.041338	22	0.044975	18	0.227755	30	0.338226
50 – 250	70	0.347039	73	0.038521	52	0.041826	42	0.211870	60	0.320460
250 – max**	214	0.342566	222	0.043340	248	0.044492	246	0.218365	230	0.335289

* Total variables present in any particular selected subset.
** All variables in the dataset.

which is an increase of 36 folds higher whereas the differences in the error rates were merely 2%. This 2% differences could not compensate to the improvement in accuracy compared to the ratio of the variables. Apart from that, the Lymphoma and NCI60 dataset showed a similar variables range category as both the datasets has a best subset between 50 to 250 variables range.

The best subset for Lymphoma dataset consists of 73 variables where the error rates obtained is 0.038521 whereas for NCI60 dataset, the best subset is 60 variables with error rates of 0.320460. Larger number of variables is required to achieve higher prediction accuracy since the dataset is a multiclass dataset and certain minimum informative variables is required to identify and train the classifier to predict the different number of class present in those datasets, especially for NCI60 dataset where there are 8 different types of tumours present in that dataset.

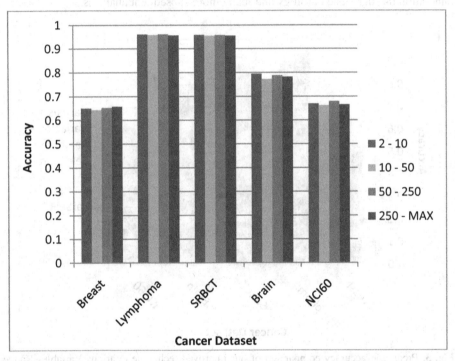

Fig. 2. Comparison of various variables range selection towards the overall prediction accuracy of the cancer datasets

SRBCT and Brain cancer dataset requires lesser variables in the subset to achieve lowest error rates in its various variables range selection category compared to other multiclass dataset. These both datasets has the best subset of 9 variables which is the most minimum number of variables required to achieve the high accuracy in the prediction. The error rates obtained are 0.041312 and 0.205099 for SRBCT and Brain cancer dataset respectively. Most probably, both this datasets had much lesser informative variables in overall compared to other datasets. Therefore, higher number of variables would only affect the prediction accuracy and increased the error rates. With the various variables range selection, the best subset from each range partition had been used for the random forest classifier to obtain the highest possible accuracy, which is presented in the Figure 2.

From our analysis, we could deduce that the suitable range for informative variables was at 5 – 75 variables, as most of the dataset shown better or higher accuracy in this range. Even though the difference was not intermittent in terms of accuracy, but the amount of variables were either too less or too many for other selected ranges. However, other researchers may use the variance of the variables amount for subsequent analysis as well as a variable filtration for large datasets. Besides that, the various variables range selection can be altered to suit other requirements such as for the construction of gene network analysis, genes functional annotation through gene ontology and many more subsequent analyses.

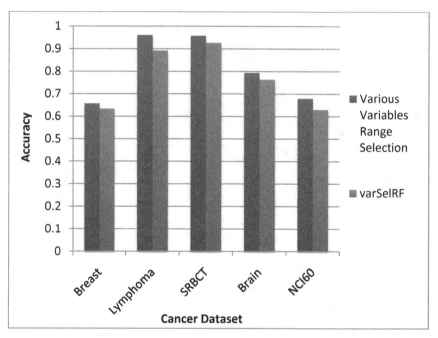

Fig. 3. Prediction accuracy comparison of our improved technique (Various Variables Range Selection) with previous works (varSelRF) from Diaz-Uriarte and Alvarez de Andres [12]

In order to justify the improvement achieved using this improved variable selection technique, a comparison with a previous work was done and the accuracy achieved is shown in Figure 3. Based on the comparison, we can see that our improved technique has increased the prediction accuracy for all the datasets used. The average improvement between our results and previous work prediction accuracy for all datasets is 5.29%, where there is a 3.69% increase in prediction accuracy for Breast cancer dataset, a huge 7.64% increase for Lymphoma dataset, 3.39% increase for SRBCT dataset, 3.97% increase for Brain dataset and finally a 7.75% increase in prediction for NCI60 dataset. This is due to the fact that the selected variables in the variable selection process have more significant variables compared to the previous work.

4   Future Works

Cancer detection through Single nucleotide polymorphism (SNP) is a crucial stage in the prediction of cancer patients and it would be another step of advancement if the Random Forest method can be altered to accept feeds from the SNP type microarray data in future. Besides that, the annotation of the selected variables and cross-referencing with genes databases could provide better understanding and validation of future predicted variables subsets.

5   Conclusion

The various variables range selection technique has been tested with five different multiclass cancer datasets and the outcome of the prediction has been presented in the result and discussion section. With the wide possibilities of variables subset selection, the accuracy of the prediction based on the selected subsets has shown similar or better accuracy with no such fluctuation on the overall accuracy. This allows different range of variables to be selected from the entire datasets without deteriorating the prediction accuracy.

Most variable selection techniques do not provide the actual number of variables in the selected subset, nor the flexibility to tune the amount of variables to be chosen in any particular variable subset prior to prediction. We have shown a method of solution with the proposed various variables range selection technique, which allows fine-tuning of the amount of variables selected in any particular variable subset without degrading the prediction accuracy. Through the development of the various variables range technique for the Random Forest variable selection, different subsets of variables with better prediction accuracy have been listed for various use of gene expression analysis. The possibility for further analysis through gene network analysis, gene – gene interaction analysis and other related analysis is also made available, for the researchers may have their own preference of range of selection to obtain various sets of variables. This will not only allow controlling the amount of variables to be obtained but also provide accuracy of estimation based on the comparison of the selected variables.

Acknowledgement. We would like to thank Malaysian Ministry of Science, Technology and Innovation for supporting this research by an e-science research grant (Grant number: 06-01-06-SF1029). This research is also supported by a GUP research grant (Grant number: Q.J130000.2507.04H16) that was sponsored by Universiti Teknologi Malaysia and we would like to thank Center for Information and Communication Technology (CICT) in Universiti Teknologi Malaysia for supporting and providing facilities and services of high performance computing.

References

1. Paz, J.L., Seeberger, P.H.: Recent Advances and Future Challenges in Glycan Microarray Technology Carbohydrate Microarrays. In: Chevolot, Y. (ed.), vol. 808, pp. 1–12. Humana Press (2012)
2. Liew, A.W.-C., Law, N.-F., Yan, H.: Missing value imputation for gene expression data: computational techniques to recover missing data from available information. Briefings in Bioinformatics 12, 498–513 (2011)
3. Duval, B., Hao, J.-K.: Advances in metaheuristics for gene selection and classification of microarray data. Briefings in Bioinformatics 11, 127–141 (2010)
4. Wu, D., Rice, C., Wang, X.: Cancer bioinformatics: A new approach to systems clinical medicine. BMC Bioinformatics 13, 71 (2012)
5. Van Steen, K.: Travelling the world of gene–gene interactions. Briefings in Bioinformatics 13, 1–19 (2012)
6. Hua, J., Tembe, W.D., Dougherty, E.R.: Performance of feature-selection methods in the classification of high-dimension data. Pattern Recogn. 42, 409–424 (2009)
7. Wong, G., Leckie, C., Kowalczyk, A.: FSR: feature set reduction for scalable and accurate multi-class cancer subtype classification based on copy number. Bioinformatics 28, 151–159 (2012)
8. Nanni, L., Brahnam, S., Lumini, A.: Combining multiple approaches for gene microarray classification. Bioinformatics 28, 1151–1157 (2012)
9. Lin, W.-J., Chen, J.J.: Class-imbalanced classifiers for high-dimensional data. Briefings in Bioinformatics (2012)
10. Boulesteix, A.-L., Bender, A., Lorenzo Bermejo, J., Strobl, C.: Random forest Gini importance favours SNPs with large minor allele frequency: impact, sources and recommendations. Briefings in Bioinformatics 304, 292–304 (2012)
11. Breiman, L.: Random Forests. Mach. Learn. 45, 5–32 (2001)
12. Diaz-Uriarte, R., Alvarez de Andres, S.: Gene selection and classification of microarray data using random forest. BMC Bioinformatics 7, 3 (2006)
13. Moorthy, K., Mohamad, M.S.: Random forest for gene selection and microarray data classification. Bioinformation 7, 142–146 (2011)
14. Koukouvinos, C., Parpoula, C.: Variable Selection and Computation of the Prior Probability of a Model via ROC Curves Methodology. Journal of Data Science 10, 653–672 (2012)
15. Wang, H., Lo, S.-H., Zheng, T., Hu, I.: Interaction-based feature selection and classification for high-dimensional biological data. Bioinformatics 28, 2834–2842 (2012)
16. van 't Veer, L.J., Dai, H., van de Vijver, M.J., He, Y.D., Hart, A.A., Mao, M., Peterse, H.L., van der Kooy, K., Marton, M.J., Witteveen, A.T., Schreiber, G.J., Kerkhoven, R.M., Roberts, C., Linsley, P.S., Bernards, R., Friend, S.H.: Gene expression profiling predicts clinical outcome of breast cancer. Nature 415, 530–536 (2002)
17. Alizadeh, A.A., Eisen, M.B., Davis, R.E., Ma, C., Lossos, I.S., Rosenwald, A., Boldrick, J.C., Sabet, H., Tran, T., Yu, X., Powell, J.I., Yang, L., Marti, G.E., Moore, T., Hudson, J., Lu, L., Lewis, D.B., Tibshirani, R., Sherlock, G., Chan, W.C., Greiner, T.C., Weisenburger, D.D., Armitage, J.O., Warnke, R., Levy, R., Wilson, W., Grever, M.R., Byrd, J.C., Botstein, D., Brown, P.O., Staudt, L.M.: Distinct types of diffuse large B-cell lymphoma identified by gene expression profiling. Nature 403, 503–511 (2000)

18. Khan, J., Wei, J.S., Ringner, M., Saal, L.H., Ladanyi, M., Westermann, F., Berthold, F., Schwab, M., Antonescu, C.R., Peterson, C., Meltzer, P.S.: Classification and diagnostic prediction of cancers using gene expression profiling and artificial neural networks. Nat. Med. 7, 673–679 (2001)
19. Pomeroy, S.L., Tamayo, P., Gaasenbeek, M., Sturla, L.M., Angelo, M., McLaughlin, M.E., Kim, J.Y., Goumnerova, L.C., Black, P.M., Lau, C., Allen, J.C., Zagzag, D., Olson, J.M., Curran, T., Wetmore, C., Biegel, J.A., Poggio, T., Mukherjee, S., Rifkin, R., Califano, A., Stolovitzky, G., Louis, D.N., Mesirov, J.P., Lander, E.S., Golub, T.R.: Prediction of central nervous system embryonal tumour outcome based on gene expression. Nature 415, 436–442 (2002)
20. Ross, D.T., Scherf, U., Eisen, M.B., Perou, C.M., Rees, C., Spellman, P., Iyer, V., Jeffrey, S.S., Van de Rijn, M., Waltham, M., Pergamenschikov, A., Lee, J.C., Lashkari, D., Shalon, D., Myers, T.G., Weinstein, J.N., Botstein, D., Brown, P.O.: Systematic variation in gene expression patterns in human cancer cell lines. Nat. Genet. 24, 227–235 (2000)
21. Efron, B., Tibshirani, R.: Improvements on Cross-Validation: The.632+ Bootstrap Method. Journal of the American Statistical Association 92, 548–560 (1997)

A Hybrid of SVM and SCAD with Group-Specific Tuning Parameters in Identification of Informative Genes and Biological Pathways

Muhammad Faiz Misman, Weng Howe Chan, Mohd Saberi Mohamad[*], and Safaai Deris

Artificial Intelligence and Bioinformatics Research Group, Faculty of Computing, Universiti Teknologi Malaysia, 81310, Skudai, Johor, Malaysia
faizmisman@gmail.com, whchan2@live.utm.my, {saberi,safaai}@utm.my

Abstract. Advancements in pathway-based microarray classification approach leads to a new era of genomic research. However, it is limited by issues regarding the quality of the pathway data as these data are usually curated from biological literatures and in specific biological experiment (e.g. lung cancer experiment), context free pathway information collection process lead to the presence of uninformative genes in the pathways. Many methods in this approach neglect these limitations by treating all genes in a pathway as significant. In this paper, we propose a hybrid of support vector machine and smoothly clipped absolute deviation with group-specific tuning parameters (gSVM-SCAD) to select informative genes within pathways before the pathway evaluation process. Experiments conducted on gender and lung cancer datasets shows that gSVM-SCAD obtains significant results in identifying significant genes and pathways, and in classification accuracy.

Keywords: Pathway analysis, smoothly clipped absolute deviation, support vector machines, gene selection.

1   Introduction

Incorporation of prior pathway data into microarray analysis has become a popular research area in bioinformatics due to the advantages in providing further biological interpretation compare to single gene microarray analysis. Such advantages further spurred the development of various approaches to identify informative genes and pathways that contribute to the certain cellular processes. The goal of the pathway-based microarray analysis is to identify significant pathways and also genes within the pathways that contribute to the phenotypes of interest. This is in contrast to single gene microarray analysis that identifies only the significant genes. Two most common approaches in pathway-based microarray analysis are enrichment analysis approaches (EA) and machine learning approaches (ML) [1].

---

[*] Corresponding author.

J. Li et al. (Eds.): PAKDD 2013 Workshops, LNAI 7867, pp. 258–269, 2013.

However, there are some challenges in pathway-based microarray analysis such as the quality of pathway data where some of the uninformative genes maybe included into pathways while informative genes being excluded [2]. In order to deal with this challenge, researchers attempt to make improvement by removing unaltered genes in pathways [1] and include additional functional interpretation in EA approaches [3]. While for ML approaches, gene selection methods have been included to select informative genes within a pathway before the classification model building instead of including all the genes within a pathway into the model building [2, 4, 5].

However, EA approaches considered all genes within pathways as equally important [1]. Alternatively, ML can select the only important genes within a pathway by including the gene selection method. In contrast to EA, ML aim to identify both relevant genes and pathways that related to the phenotypes of interest. Therefore, ML can bring more insight in a biological perspective. ML is used in this research due to its advantages. However, there are arguments against incorporating gene selection methods in ML where informative genes may be discarded [1]. This is due to the nature of microarray data where it can impose sparseness and biasness on the penalty function that act as the gene selection method in evaluating the informative genes [6]. Therefore, the efficient and robust gene selection technique is needed in order to deal effectively with the problems arise in pathway-based microarray analysis.

Following the good results obtained from support vector machines (SVM) in classifying gene expression data, hybrid of SVM with smoothly clipped absolute deviation (SCAD) penalty was produced, named as SVM-SCAD [7]. SCAD provides nearly unbiased coefficient estimation and select the important genes consistently compared to other popular penalty function such as least absolute shrinkage and selection operator (LASSO) [8]. SVM-SCAD had proved its ability in selecting the informative genes and the method is comparable to LASSO penalty function. Hence, in order to identify both significant genes and pathways that related to phenotypes of interests, this paper proposed an improved of SVM-SCAD with group-specific tuning parameters, termed as gSVM-SCAD.

2   Proposed Method (gSVM-SCAD) and Experimental Data

2.1   SVM-SCAD

Given a data set $\{(xi,yi)\}$, $yi \in \{-1,1\}$ is the sample tissue with possible two classes $y_i = -1$ and $y_i = 1$ for each data set used in this paper, while $x_i = (x_{i1},\dots,x_{id}) \in R^d$ represents the input vector of expression levels of d genes of the i-th sample tissue. SVM is a large margin classifier which separates classes of interest by maximizing the margin between them using the kernel function [7, 9]. This has been widely used especially in microarray classification area [10]. SVM distinguish input variables into its classes by a margin of

$$min_{\beta,c} \sum [1 - y_i f(x_i)]_+ + pen_\lambda(\beta) \tag{1}$$

$[1-y_i f(x_i)]+$ is the SVM convex hinge loss function where

$$[1 - y_i f(x_i)]_+ \leq \lambda f(x_i) + (1 - \lambda) f(y_i)$$

while pen$\lambda(\beta)$ is the penalty function with parameters λ, where $\beta = (\beta 1, ..., \beta i)$ are the coefficients of the hyperplane, while c is the intercept of the hyperplane. Hinge loss function is a commonly used loss function in SVM in order to keep the fidelity of the resulting model to the data set [11]. However, the standard SVM can suffer from irrelevant data, since all the variables are used for constructing the classifier [7]. This is due to the usage of the L2 penalty in a soft-thresholding function for the common SVM. The detailed applications of L2 penalty in a soft-thresholding function and its drawbacks in identifying noises can be obtained from [7].

A penalty function is usually used as a variable selection in the statistics, and in bioinformatics it is called as gene selection. SCAD is different from other popular penalty functions such as LASSO, also called the L1 penalty [8], this is because SCAD provides nearly unbiased coefficient estimation when dealing with large coefficients. This is contrary to other penalty functions that usually increase the penalty linearly as the coefficient increases [6]. SCAD penalty has the form of

$$pen_\lambda(\beta) = \Sigma_{j=1}^d P_\lambda(\beta_j) \tag{2}$$

where $P_\lambda(\beta_j)$ is a penalty function with tuning parameter λ for β_j. For providing nearly unbiased, sparsity, and continuity estimate of β [7], the continuous differentiable penalty function is defined as

$$pen_\lambda(\beta_j) = \begin{cases} \lambda|\beta|, & if \ |\beta| \leq \lambda \\ -(|\beta|^2 - 2a\lambda|\beta| + \lambda^2)/(2(a-1)), & if \ \lambda < |\beta| \leq a\lambda \\ ((a+1)\lambda)/2, & if \ |\beta| > a\lambda \end{cases} \tag{3}$$

where a and λ are tuning parameters with a > 2 and λ > 0 [6]. For a tuning parameter a, previous research suggested the parameter a = 3.7 due to the minimal achievement in a Bayes risk [6]. Therefore, in this research a = 3.7 is used while λ is a tuning parameter obtained using generalized approximate cross validation (GACV) tuning parameter selection methods (as discussed latter).

In order to surmount the limitations of the SVM due to its inability to distinguish between noise and informative data, SVM-SCAD was proposed by replacing the L2 penalty in function (1) with (2), which takes the form

$$min_{\beta,c} \frac{1}{n} \Sigma[1 - y_i f(x_i)]_+ + \Sigma_{j=1}^d P_\lambda(\beta_j) \tag{4}$$

In order to select the informative genes, SVM-SCAD have to minimize the function (4) using the successive quadratic algorithm (SQA) and repeated for kth times until convergence, where k = 1,...,n. During the procedure, if $\beta_j^k < \epsilon$, the gene is considered as uninformative. Where β is the coefficient for the gene j in the kth iteration and ϵ is a preselected small positive thresholding value with ϵ = yi - f(xi).

2.2 Tuning Parameter Selection Method

In SCAD there are two tuning parameters namely a and λ that play an important role in determining an effective predictive model. The tuning parameter selection in SVM-SCAD is used to estimate the nearly optimal λ in order to identify the effective predictive model for SCAD. In this paper, the generalized approximate cross validation (GACV) [12] is used to select the nearly optimal λ. The formula as given below:

$$GACV_\lambda = \frac{1}{n}\sum_{i=1}^{n}[1 - y_i f(x_i)]_+ + DF_\lambda \tag{5}$$

where n is a total number of samples, DF_λ is a degree of freedom where

$$DF_\lambda = \frac{1}{n}\left[\sum_{y_if(x_{i\lambda})<--1} 2\frac{a_{\lambda i}}{2n\lambda}\cdot\|K(.,x_i)\|_{Hk}^2 + \sum_{y_if(x_{i\lambda})\epsilon[-1,1]}\frac{a_{\lambda i}}{2n\lambda}\cdot\|K(.,x_i)\|_{Hk}^2\right]$$

where $\frac{a_{\lambda i}}{2n\lambda} = \frac{f(x_{i\lambda})[y_i]-f(x_{i\lambda})[x]}{y_i-x}$ and $\|K(.,x_i)\|_{Hk}^2$ is the reproducing kernel hilbert space (RKHS) with SVM reproducing kernel K. If all samples in microarray data are correctly classified, then $y_if(x_{i\lambda}) > 0$ and sum following 2 in DF_λ does not appear and $DF_\lambda = K(0,0)/n\gamma^2$ where γ is the hard margin of an SVM [12]. The nearly optimal tuning parameter λ is obtained by minimizing the error rate from the GACV.

2.3 The Proposed Method (gSVM-SCAD)

In SVM-SCAD, the magnitude of penalization of β is determined by two tuning parameters a and λ. Since a has been setup as 3.7 [6], there is only one parameter λ left that play an important role. In order to incorporate pathway or set of gene data, the gSVM-SCAD used group-specific parameters λ_j estimation. In this paper, there are k groups of genes where $k = 1...n$, each gene able to be in one or more pathways. We grouped the genes based on their pathway information from the pathway data. In order to provide the group-specific tuning parameters, we modified (2) to the form of

$$pen_{\lambda k}(\beta_j) = \sum_{j=1}^{d} P\lambda_k(\beta_j) \tag{6}$$

where by allowing each pathway to have its own parameter λ_k as in (6) instead of general λ in (2), the genes within pathways can be selected and classified more accurately.

Table 1 illustrates the procedure of gSVM-SCAD. The procedure consisted of 3 main steps. In the first step, the genes in microarray data are selected and grouped based on their prior pathway information from the pathway data. This process repeated for each pathway in the pathway data and there is a possibility that some genes are not involved in any pathways. From this step, the new sets of gene expression data are produced to be evaluated by the SVM-SCAD. In step 2, each pathway is evaluated using the SVM-SCAD. This procedure is started with the tuning parameter selection (step 2.1) where in this research, the grid search is applied. According to previous research, the best λ can be obtained in the range of $0 < \lambda < 2$, therefore the grid search ranges from 0.001 to 0.009, 0.01 to 0.09, and 0.1 to 1 are used. The GACV is used to estimate the error for each tuning parameter value from the grid search. The nearly optimal tuning parameter produces the minimum GACV error. In step 2.2, the genes in the pathway are evaluated using SVM-SCAD and the informative genes within pathway is selected and selected while the non-informative genes are excluded from the pathway. In step 2.3, the informative genes obtained are classified between phenotypes of interests using an SVM. The classification error from the selected genes for each pathway is calculated using 10-fold CV in step 3. Biological validation for top pathways is conducted using the information from the biological research databases.

Table 1. The gSVM-SCAD procedure

Input: GE: Gene expression data , PD: Pathway data , TP : Tuning parameter, λ
Output: SP: Significant pathways , IG: Informative genes
Begin
Step 1: Grouping genes based on their pathway information
        For $j=1$ to max number of pathways in PD **do**
           Find genes from GE that related to the pathway
           Select and assign the related genes as a one group
      End-for
Step 2: Evaluate the pathways
    For $j=1$ to max number of pathways in PD **do**
        Step 2.1: Estimation of TP using a GACV
        For TP = 0.001 to 0.009 ,0.01 to 0.09 and 0.1 to 1 **do**

$$GACV_\lambda = \frac{1}{n} \sum_{i=1}^{n} [1 - y_i f(x_i)_\lambda]_+ + DF_\lambda$$

      End-for
$\lambda = argmin_\lambda\{GACV(\lambda)\}$ // best TP produces minimum GACV error
    Step 2.2: **Select the informative genes using the SVM-SCAD**
        Let β^k as the estimate of β at step k where $k = 0, \dots ,$ n
        The value of β^0 set by an SVM
    While β^k not converge **do**
           Minimizing the $\frac{1}{n}\Sigma[1-y_if(x_i)]_+ + \Sigma^d_{j=1} P\lambda_k(\beta_j)$
           $k = k + 1$
    If $\beta^k_j \leq \epsilon$ **then**
        The gene j considered as non-informative and discarded
      End-if
      End-while
    Step 2.3: Classify the selected genes using an SVM
    Step 3: Calculate the classification error using a 10-fold CV
  End-for
End

There are several main differences between gSVM-SCAD and other current methods in ML approaches. Firstly, it provides the genes selection method to identify and select the informative genes that are related to the pathway and the phenotype of interest which provides more in biological aspect. Secondly, the penalty function SCAD is more robust when dealing with a high number of genes, and it selects important genes more consistently than other popular LASSO (L1) penalty function [13]. And lastly, with group-specific tuning parameters, the gSVM-SCAD provides more flexibility in choosing the best λ for each pathway so that each pathway can be assessed more accurately. Therefore, by selecting the informative genes within pathway, the gSVM-SCAD can be seen as the best method in dealing with pathway data quality problems in pathway-based microarray analysis.

2.4   Experimental Data Sets

The performance of the gSVM-SCAD is tested using two types of data, gene expression and biological pathway data. The role of biological pathway data is as a metadata or prior biological knowledge. Both gene expression and pathway data are the same as those used in previous research done by Pang and colleagues [14].

In gene expression data, it consists of m samples and n gene expression levels. The first column of the data represents the name of genes while the next column represents the gene expression levels. The data set forming a matrix of $E = \left\{ e_{i,j} \right\}_{m \times n}$ where $e_{i,j}$ represents the expression level of the gene j in the tissue sample i. In this paper, two gene expression data sets are used: lung cancer, and gender. The information of the data sets is shown in Table 2.

Table 2. Gene expression data sets

Name	No. of samples	No. of genes	Class	Reference
Lung	86	7129	2(normal and tumor)	[15]
Gender	32	22283	2(male and female cells)	unpublished

Total 480 pathways are used in this research. 168 pathways were taken from KEGG and 312 pathways were taken Biocarta pathway database. In a pathway data set, the first column represents the pathway name while the second column represents the gene name.

3   Experimental Results and Discussion

In this paper, to evaluate the performance of the gSVM-SCAD, we used a 10-fold cross validation (10-fold CV) classification accuracy. The results obtained from the gSVM-SCAD are validated with the biological literatures and databases. Since the limited pages for this paper, we only chose the top five pathways with highest 10-fold CV accuracy from both data sets for biological validation (commonly applied with several authors such as Pang et al. (2006) and Wang et al. (2008)).

3.1   Performance Evaluation

For the performance evaluation of the SCAD penalty function, the SCAD was compared with the popular L_1 penalty function by hybridizing it with an SVM classifier (L_1 SVM), obtained from R package named penalizedSVM [16]. The L_1 SVM also applied with group-specific tuning parameters to determine λ. This experiment was done intentionally to test the robustness of the SCAD penalty in identifying informative genes when dealing with large coefficients compare to the L1 method. Then the gSVM-SCAD was compared with the current SVM-SCAD with respect to one general parameter tuning for all pathways, the tuning parameters $\lambda = 0.4$ as used in previous research [7]. For comparison with other classification methods without any gene selection process, the gSVM-SCAD was compared with four classifiers that are without any penalty function or gene selection method. The classifiers are PathwayRF [14], neural networks, k-nearest neighbour with one neighbours (kNN), and linear discriminant analysis (LDA). The purpose of this comparisons is to show that not all genes in a pathway contribute to a certain cellular process. The results of the experiment are shown in Table 3.

Table 3. A comparison of averages of 10-fold CV accuracy from the top ten pathways with other methods

Method	Lung Cancer (%)	Gender (%)
gSVM-SCAD	**73.77**	**87.33**
L$_1$-SVM	55.14	80.76
SVM-SCAD	53.5	77.96
Neural Networks	70.39	81.54
kNN	61.73	82.44
LDA	63.24	75.81
PathwayRF	71.00	81.75

As shown in Table 3, in comparing the gSVM-SCAD with L1-SVM and SVM-SCAD, it is interesting to note that the gSVM-SCAD outperforms the other two penalized classifiers in both datasets with gSVM-SCAD is 18.63% higher than L1-SVM for lung cancer data set, and 6.57% higher in gender data set. This is due to the SCAD as a non-convex penalty function is more robust to biasness when dealing with a large number of coefficients β in selecting informative genes compared to the L1 penalty function [6]. Therefore the proposed method with SCAD penalty function is more efficient in selecting informative genes within a pathway compare to LASSO penalty. Table 3 further shows that the gSVM-SCAD had better results than SVM-SCAD, with 20.27% and 9.37% higher in lung cancer and gender data sets respectively. It is demonstrated that group specific tuning parameters in gSVM-SCAD provides flexibility in determining the λ for each pathway compared to the use of general λ for every pathway. This is because genes within pathway usually have a different prior distribution.

In order to show that not all genes in a pathway contributed to the development of specific cellular processes, the gSVM-SCAD is compared with four classifiers. The results are also shown in Table 3. For lung cancer data, gSVM-SCAD outperformed all the classifiers, with 2.77% higher than PathwayRF, 3.8% higher than neural networks, 10.53% higher than LDA, and lastly 12.04% higher than kNN. For gender data, result obtained by gSVM-SCAD is 5.58% higher than PathwayRF, 5.79% higher than neural networks, 4.89% higher than kNN one neighbor and 11.52% higher than LDA.

From the results in Table 2, the gSVM-SCAD shows a better performance when compared to almost four classifiers for both data sets. This is because the standard classifiers built a classification model using all genes within the pathways. If there are uninformative genes inside the pathways, it reduced the classification performance. In contrast, the gSVM-SCAD does not include all genes in the pathways into development of a classification model, as not all genes in a pathway contribute to cellular processes, due to the quality of pathway data.

3.2   Biological Validation

The gSVM-SCAD has been tested using the lung cancer data set that has two possible output classes: tumor and normal. The selected genes and the top five pathways presented in Table 4. For lung cancer data set, we used HLungDB [17] and genecards version 3.06 (www.genecards.org) to validate the selected genes within pathways.

Table 4. Selected genes from the top five pathways in the lung cancer data set

Pathways	No. of genes	Selected gene(s)
WNT Signaling Pathway	24	**APC , MYC, AXIN1, GSK3B, CTNNB1** [18], **HNF1A** [22], **CREBBP** [23], **HDAC1** [24], **WNT1** [25], **CSNK1A1** [26], **CSNK2A1** [15], **TLE1** [27] *PPARD, PPP2CA, TAB1, DVL1*
AKAP95 role in mitosis and chromosome dynamics	10	**DDX5** [28], **PRKACB** [15], **CDK1** [29], **CCNB1** [30], *PPP2CA, PRKAR2B, PRKAR2A*
Induction of apoptosis	36	**FADD** [31], **TNFSF10** [32], **CASP3, CASP6, CASP7, CASP8, CASP9, CASP10** [20], **BCL2** [33], **BIRC3** [34], **TRAF** [35], **BIRC** [36], **TNFRSF25** [37] , **RARA** [38], *TRADD, RELA, DFFA, RIPK1*
Tyrosine metabolism	45	**AOC3, NAT6, ADH7, MAOA, MAOB** [15], **DDC** [39], **ADH1C** [40], **GHR** [41], **TPO** [42], **ALDH3A1** [43], *ADH5, PNMT, TAT, ARD1A, DBT, AOC2, ALDH1A3, AOX1, PRMT2, FAH, ALDH3B2, KAT2A, ADH6, ADH4, GOT2*
Activation of Csk	30	**PRKACB, HLA-DQB1** [15], **CREBBP** [21] *CD247, IL23A, PRKAR1B, GNGT1, CD3D, CD3E*

* Genes in *italic* text are uninformative genes while gene in **bold** text are genes with direct relationship to the disease.

For the WNT signaling pathway, it is reported that the pathway plays a significant role in the development of lung and other colorectal cancers [18]. From 24 genes inside the pathways, 16 genes selected by the gSVM-SCAD where twelve genes were validated as related to the lung cancer development while other remaining genes are not contributing to the lung cancer. With respect to the second pathway, it also contributes to the development of lung cancer, since the AKAP95 protein plays an important role in cell mitosis [19], the gSVM-SCAD identifies seven out of 10 genes included in the pathway with four genes such as DDX5, PRKACB, CDK1, and CCNB1 playing an important role in lung cancer development, while others have no evidence in lung cancer development.

The gSVM-SCAD identifies that induction of apoptosis pathway as one of the lung cancer related pathway, where this pathway has been reported by Lee et al. [20] as one of the contributor to the lung cancer development. Thirteen out of eighteen genes in the induction of apoptosis have been selected by the gSVM-SCAD as the significant genes, with thirteen genes being related to the lung cancer. For the Tyrosine metabolism pathway, there are no references showing that this pathway is related to the lung cancer development. However, the gSVM-SCAD has selected several genes within this pathway that play an important role in the development of lung cancer, such as AOC3, DDC, GHR, TPO, NAT6, ALDH3A1, ADH7, MAOA, MAOB and ADH1C. This makes it possible that this pathway may relate to the development of lung cancer and thus prompting biologists to conduct further research on this pathway. While for the Activation of Csk pathway, Masaki et al. [21] have reported that the activation of this pathway plays an important role in the development of lung cancer, with three genes marked as lung cancer genes.

For the gender dataset, we used 480 pathways. For this data set, we were looking the genes within pathways that existed in the lymphoblastoid cell lines for both male and female [14]. The top 5 pathways with highest 10-fold CV accuracy are shown in Table 5. Our gSVM-SCAD had selected 11 genes out of total 726 genes within top 5 pathways. From the 11 genes, 8 genes are proved to be related in lymphoblastoid cell lines for both male and female gender.

Table 5. Selected genes from the top five pathways in gender dataset

Pathways	No. of genes	Selected gene(s)
Testis genes from xhx and netaffx	111	**RPS4Y1** [44]
GNF female genes	116	**XIST**
RAP down	434	**DDX3X, HDHD1A** [44] **NDUFS3** [45]
XINACT	34	*RSP4X*, **DDX3X, PRKX** [44]
Willard inact	31	*RPS4X*, **STS** [44], *RPS4P17*

* Genes in *italic* text are uninformative genes while gene in **bold** text are genes with direct relationship to the disease.

4   Conclusion

This paper focuses to identify the significant genes and pathways that relate to phenotypes of interest by proposing the gSVM-SCAD. From the experiments and analyses, the gSVM-SCAD is shown to outperform the other ML methods in both data sets. In comparison of penalty function, gSVM-SCAD has shown its superiority in selecting the informative genes within pathways compare to L_1 SVM. By providing group-specific tuning parameters, gSVM-SCAD had shown a better performance compare to an SVM-SCAD that provides a general penalty term for all pathways. Furthermore, majority of the genes selected by gSVM-SCAD from both data lung cancer and gender data sets are proved as biologically relevance.

Despite the good performance based on the comparisons done in this paper, gSVM-SCAD still possesses a limitation because SCAD penalty is a parametric method that relies on the parameter λ to balance the trade-off between data fitting and model parsimony [7] and the results will be affected if improper selection by the GACV. This can be seen in Table 4 where there are still a lot false positives. When λ is too small, it can lead to the overfitting of the training model and give too little sparse to the produced classifier; and if λ is too big, it can lead to the underfitting to the training model, which again can give very sparse to the classifier [7]. Therefore, further research regard this matter shall be done to surmount the limitation in gSVM-SCAD.

Acknowledgement. We would like to thank Malaysian Ministry of Science, Technology and Innovation for supporting this research by an e-science research grant (Grant number: 06-01-06-SF1029). This research is also supported by a GUP research grant (Grant number: Q.J130000.2507.04H16) that was sponsored by Universiti Teknologi Malaysia.

References

1. Wang, X., Dalkic, E., Wu, M., Chan, C.: Gene Module Level Analysis: Identification to Networks and Dynamics. Curr. Opin. Biotechnol. 19, 482–491 (2008)
2. Chen, X., Wang, L., Smith, J.D., Zhang, B.: Supervised principle component analysis for gene set enrichment of microarray data with continuous or survival outcome. Bioinformatics 24, 2474–2481 (2008)
3. Hummel, M., Meister, R., Mansmann, U.: GlobalANCOVA: Exploration and Assessment of Gene Group Effects. Bioinformatics 24, 78–85 (2008)
4. Tai, F., Pan, W.: Incorporating Prior Knowledge of Predictors into Penalized Classifiers with Multiple Penalty Terms. Bioinformatics 23, 1775–1782 (2007)
5. Tai, F., Pan, W.: Incorporating Prior Knowledge of Gene Functional Groups into Regularized Discriminant Analysis of Microarray Data. Bioinformatics 23, 3170–3177 (2007)
6. Fan, J., Li, R.: Variable selection via nonconcave penalized likelihood and its oracle properties. JASA 96, 1348–1360 (2001)
7. Zhang, H.H., Ahn, J., Lin, X., Park, C.: Gene selection using support vector machines with non-convex penalty. Bioinformatics 22, 88–95 (2006)
8. Tibshirani, R.: Regression shrinkage and selection via the lasso. J. R. Stat. Soc. Series B (Statistical Methodology) 58, 267–288 (1996)

9. Wang, J.T., Wu, X.: Kernel design for RNA classification using Support Vector Machines. Int. J. Data Min. Bioinform. 1, 57–76 (2006)

10. Guyon, I., Weston, J., Barnhill, S., Vapnik, V.: Gene selection for cancer classification using support vector machines. Machine Learning 46, 389–422 (2002)

11. Wu, Y., Liu, Y.: Robust Truncated Hinge Loss Support Vector Machines. JASA 102, 974–983 (2007)

12. Wahba, G., Lin, Y., Zhang, H.: GACV for support vector machines, or, another way to look at margin-like quantities. In: Smola, A.J., Bartlett, P., Schoelkopf, B., Schurmans, D. (eds.) Advances in Large Margin Classifiers, pp. 297–309. MIT Press (2000)

13. Wang, H., Li, R., Tsai, C.L.: Tuning parameters selectors for the smoothly clipped absolute deviation method. Biometrika 94, 553–568 (2007)

14. Pang, H., Lin, A., Holford, M., Enerson, B.E., Lu, B., Lawton, M.P., Floyd, E., Zhao, H.: Pathway analysis using random forest classification and regression. Bioinformatics 16, 2028–2036 (2006)

15. Battacharjee, A., Richards, W.G., Satunton, J., et al.: Classification of human lung carcinomas by mRNA expression profiling reveals distinct adenocarcinoma subclasses. PNAS 98, 13790–13795 (2001)

16. Becker, N., Werft, W., Toedt, G., Lichter, P., Benner, A.: PenalizedSVM: A R-package for feature selection SVM classification. Bioinformatics 25, 1711–1712 (2009)

17. Wang, L., Xiong, Y., Sun, Y., Fang, Z., Li, L., Ji, H., Shi, T.: HLungDB: an integrated database of human lung cancer research. Nucleic Acids Res. 38, D665–D669 (2010)

18. Mazieres, J., He, B., You, L., Xu, Z., Jablons, D.M.: Wnt signaling in lung cancer. Cancer Letters 222, 1–10 (2005)

19. Collas, P., Le Guellec, K., Taskén, K.: The A-kinase-anchoring protein AKAP95 is a multivalent protein with a key role in chromatin condensation at mitosis. J. Cell Biol. 147, 1167–1179 (1999)

20. Lee, S.Y., Choi, Y.Y., Choi, J.E., et al.: Polymorphisms in the caspase genes and the risk of lung cancer. J. Thorac. Oncol. 5, 1152–1158 (2010)

21. Masaki, T., Igarashi, K., Tokuda, M., et al.: $pp60^{c-src}$ activation in lung adenocarcinoma. Eur. J. Cancer 39, 1447–1455 (2003)

22. Lanzafame, S., Caltabiano, R., Puzzo, L., Immè, A.: Expression of thyroid transcription factor 1 (TTF-1) in extra thyroidal sites: papillary thyroid carcinoma of branchial cleft cysts and thyroglossal duct cysts and struma ovarii. Pathologica 98, 640–644 (2006)

23. Tillinghast, G.W., Partee, J., Albert, P., Kelly, J.M., Burtow, K.H., Kelly, K.: Analysis of genetic stability at the EP300 and CREBBP loci in a panel of cancer cell lines. Genes Chromosomes and Cancer 37, 121–131 (2003)

24. Sasaki, H., Moriyama, S., Nakashima, Y., Kobayashi, Y., Kiriyama, M., Fukai, I., Yamakawa, Y., Fujii, Y.: Histone deacetylase 1 mRNA expression in lung cancer. Lung Cancer 46, 171–178 (2004)

25. Huang, C.L., Liu, D., Ishikawa, S., Nakashima, T., Nakashima, N., Yokomise, H., Kadota, K., Ueno, M.: Wnt1 overexpression promotes tumour progression in non-small cell lung cancer. Eur. J. Cancer 44, 2680–2688 (2008)

26. Wrage, M., Ruosaari, S., Eijk, P.P., et al.: Genomic profiles associated with early micrometastasis in lung cancer: relevance of 4q deletion. Clin. Cancer Res. 15, 1566–1574 (2009)

27. Jagdis, A., Rubin, B.P., Tubbs, R.R., Pacheco, M., Nielsen, T.O.: Prospective evaluation of TLE1 as a diagnostic immunohistochemical marker in synovial sarcoma. Am. J. Surg. Pathol. 33, 1743–1751 (2009)

28. Su, L.J., Chang, C.W., Wu, Y.C., et al.: Selection of DDX5 as a novel internal control for Q-RT-PCR from microarray data using a block bootstrap re-sampling scheme. BMC Genomics 8, 140 (2007)

29. Hsu, T.S., Chen, C., Lee, P.T., et al.: 7-Chloro-6-piperidin-1-yl-quinoline-5,8-dione (PT-262), a novel synthetic compound induces lung carcinoma cell death associated with inhibiting ERK and CDC2 phosphorylation via a p53-independent pathway. Cancer Chemother. Pharmacol. 62, 799–808 (2008)

30. Kosacka, M., Korzeniewska, A., Jankowska, R.: The evaluation of prognostic value of cyclin B1 expression in patients with resected non-small-cell lung cancer stage I-IIIA—preliminary report. Pol. Merkur. Lekarski 28, 117–121 (2010)

31. Bhojani, M.S., Chen, G., Ross, B.D., Beer, D.G., Rehemtulla, A.: Nuclear localized phosphorylated FADD induces cell proliferation and is associated with aggressive lung cancer. Cell Cycle 4, 1478–1481 (2005)

32. Sun, W., Zhang, K., Zhang, X., et al.: Identification of differentially expressed genes in human lung squamous cell carcinoma using suppression substractive hybridization. Cancer Lett. 212, 83–93 (2004)

33. Nhung, N.V., Mirejovsky, T., Mirejovsky, P., Melinova, L.: Expression of p53, p21 and bcl-2 in prognosis of lung carcinomas. Cesk. Patol. 35, 117–121 (1999)

34. Ekedahl, J., Joseph, B., Grigoriev, M.Y., et al.: Expression of inhibitor of apoptosis proteins in small- and non-small-cell lung carcinoma cells. Exp. Cell Res. 279, 277–290 (2002)

35. Li, X., Yang, Y., Ashwell, J.D.: TNF-RII and c-IAPI mediate ubiquitination and degradation of TRAF2. Nature 416, 345–347 (2002)

36. Kang, H.G., Lee, S.J., Chae, M.H., et al.: Identification of polymorphisms in the XIAP gene and analysis of association with lung cancer risk in a Korean population. Cancer Genet. Cytogenet. 180, 6–13 (2008)

37. Anglim, P.P., Galler, J.S., Koss, M.N., et al.: Identification of a panel of sensitive and specific DNA methylation markers for squamous cell lung cancer. Mol. Cancer. 7, 62 (2008)

38. Wan, H., Hong, W.K., Lotan, R.: Increased retinoic acid responsiveness in lung carcinoma cells that are nonresponsive despite the presence of endogenous retinoic acid receptor (RAR) beta by expression of exogenous retinoid receptors retinoid X receptor alpha, RAR alpha, and RAR gamma. Cancer Res. 61, 556–564 (2001)

39. Vos, M.D., Scott, F.M., Iwai, N., Treston, A.M.: Expression in human lung cancer cell lines of genes of prohormone processing and the neuroendocrine phenotype. J. Cell Biochem. Suppl. 24, 257–268 (1996)

40. Freudenheim, J.L., Ram, M., Nie, J., et al.: Lung cancer in humans is not associated with lifetime total alcohol consumption or with genetic variation in alcohol dehydrogenase 3 (ADH3). J. Nutr. 133, 3619–3624 (2003)

41. Cao, G., Lu, H., Feng, J., Shu, J., Zheng, D., Hou, Y.: Lung cancer risk associated with Thr495Pro polymorphism of GHR in Chinese population. Jpn. J. Clin. Oncol. 38, 308–316 (2008)

42. Werynska, B., Ramlau, R., Podolak-Dawidziak, M., et al.: Serum thrombopoietin levels in patients with reactive thrombocytosis due to lung cancer and in patients with essential thrombocythemia. Neoplasma 50, 447–451 (2003)

43. Muzio, G., Trombetta, A., Maggiora, M., et al.: Arachidonic acid suppresses growth of human lung tumor A549 cells through down-regulation of ALDH3A1 expression. Free Radic. Biol. Med. 40, 1929–1938 (2006)

44. Johnston, C.M., Lovell, F.L., Leongamornlert, D.A., Stranger, B.E., Dermitzakis, E.T., Ross, M.T.: Large-scale population study of human cell lines indicates that dosage compensation is virtually complete. PLoS Genetics 4, e9 (2008)

45. Zhu, X., Peng, X., Guan, M.X., Yan, Q.: Pathogenic mutations of nuclear genes associated with mitochondrial disorders. Acta Biochim. Biophys. Sinica 41, 179–187 (2009)

Structured Feature Extraction
Using Association Rules

Nan Tian[1], Yue Xu[1], Yuefeng Li[1], and Gabriella Pasi[2]

[1] Faculty of Science and Engineering, Queensland University of Technology,
Brisbane, Australia
{n.tian,yue.xu,y2.li}@qut.edu.au
[2] Department of Informatics, Systems and Communication
University of Milano Bicocca
Milano, Italy
pasi@disco.unimib.it

Abstract. As of today, opinion mining has been widely used to identify the strength and weakness of products (e.g., cameras) or services
(e.g., services in medical clinics or hospitals) based upon people's feedback such as user reviews. Feature extraction is a crucial step for opinion
mining which has been used to collect useful information from user reviews. Most existing approaches only find individual features of a product
without the structural relationships between the features which usually
exists. In this paper, we propose an approach to extract features and
feature relationship, represented as tree structure called a feature hierarchy, based on frequent patterns and associations between patterns
derived from user reviews. The generated feature hierarchy profiles the
product at multiple levels and provides more detailed information about
the product. Our experiment results based on some popularly used review datasets show that the proposed feature extraction approach can
identify more correct features than the baseline model. Even though the
datasets used in the experiment are about cameras, our work can be applied to generate features about a service such as the services in hospitals
or clinics.

Keywords: Feature Extraction, Opinion Mining, Association Rules,
Feature Hierarchy, User Reviews.

1 Introduction

The advent of Web 2.0 has changed the way people use the Internet profoundly. It
promotes and emphasizes user involvement such as viewpoint and opinion sharing. Compared to the former view of the Web as an enormous reading repository,
the Web 2.0 is considered a big leap. In recent years, due to the rapid development of Web 2.0, the information left by online users on Internet exploded. Such
overwhelming user generated contents like reviews, comments, discussion forums
and blogs contain people's thoughts, feelings and attitudes. For instance, people
write reviews to explain how they enjoy or dislike a product they purchased.

J. Li et al. (Eds.): PAKDD 2013 Workshops, LNAI 7867, pp. 270–282, 2013.

Yet, there are also reviews or comments to the services provided by medical doctors in hospitals or clinics. This helps to identify features or characteristics of the reviewed object (i.e., product or service) from users' point of view, which is an important addition to the given specification or introduction. As a result, users can make their purchase decision by referring to this extracted information [9]. However, to detect and identify the relevant features from review data is extremely challenging.

In recent years, feature-based opinion mining has become a hot research area. A significant amount of research has been done to improve the accuracy and effectiveness of feature generation for products [4,9,8,6,5]. However, most techniques only extract features; the structural relationship between product features has been omitted. For example, *"picture resolution"* is a common feature of digital camera in which *"resolution"* expresses the specific feature concept to describe the general feature *"picture"*. Yet, existing approaches treat *"resolution"* and *"picture"* as two individual features instead of finding the relationship between them. Thus, the information derived by existing feature extraction approaches is not sufficient for generating a precise product model since all features are allocated in the same level and independent from each other.

Association rule mining is a popular and well explored method in data mining [7]. Based on association rules, we can discover relations. However, making use of association rules is challenging [12]; for instance, the number of association rules could be huge for large datasets. To address this problem, we generate a list of potential features and select useful association rules based upon these features. The selected rules are used to identify relationship information between the generated features.

Our approach takes advantage of existing feature extraction approaches, and it makes two contributions. First, we present a method to make use of association rules to find the relations between generated features. In addition, we create a product feature hierarchy that profiles the object which has been reviewed more accurately by identifying the concrete relationship between general features and their specific features.

2   Related Work

Our research aims to extract useful product information based on user generated information to create a product model. This work is closely related to feature-level opinion mining which has drawn many researchers' attention in recent years.

In [4], Hu and Liu firstly proposed a feature-based opinion mining approach that is able to identify product features and corresponding opinions from customer reviews. According to the observation that features are generally nouns, they used pattern mining to generate a list of frequent items which are nouns and noun phrases. Then, to extract correct features from the list, they used compactness pruning to eliminate invalid noun phrases and redundancy pruning to remove nouns which appeared in other noun phrases. After the pruning, a list of frequent features is derived. For those infrequent product features that cannot be found by frequent items, they extract infrequent nouns that are closed to opinion words (adjectives) extracted from reviews based on frequent features.

Popescu and Etzioni proposed a Web-based domain-independent information extraction system named OPINE [8]. This system improves the accuracy of existing feature extraction approaches by filter extracted noun phrases by examining the point-wise mutual information value between the phrase and meronymy discriminators associated with the product class.

Scaffidi et.al presented a search system called Red Opal which is able to identify product features and score the product on each feature by examining prior customer reviews in [9]. This automatic system enables users to locate products rapidly based on features. To improve the performance of product feature extraction, they made use of a language model to find features by comparing the frequency of nouns in the review and in generic English. The comparison results indicate Red Opal has higher and constant precision compared to [4].

In [5], Hu et.al also proposed a new method to improve the existing feature based opinion mining. They utilized SentiWordNet to identify all sentences that contain noun, verb, adjectives, adverb phrases that may indicate users' opinions. The identified opinion sentences are then used to generate explicit features. As to implicit feature extraction, a mapping database has been created for detect certain adjectives that indicate features such as (expensive, price) and (heavy, weight). They derived better recall and precision results on extracting opinion sentences compared to [4].

Lau et.al presented an ontology-based method to profile the product in order to improve the performance of opinion mining [6]. Specifically, a number of ontology levels have been constructed such as feature level that contains predefined or identified features for a certain product and sentiment level in which all sentiment words from reviews that modified a feature are stored. This ontology model simplified and improved the accuracy of opinion mining task.

However, none of aforementioned approaches is able to identify the relationships between the extracted product features, whereas the structural relationships between product features are crucial for profiling the product precisely.

3   The Proposed Approach

This section provides a deep insight of our product feature extraction approach. We would like to construct a product model based on information generated from user reviews. Finding correct product features is just one concern of our work. In addition, we are interested in identifying the relationship between the extracted features. Thus, we propose a feature hierarchy based method to extract features from user review dataset.

The whole process consists of two main steps: product hierarchy construction using Min-Max association rules and hierarchy expansion based on reference features. The input of our system is a collection of user reviews for a certain product. The output is a product feature hierarchy which contains not only all generated

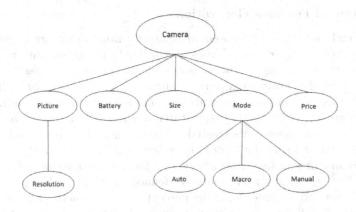

Fig. 1. An Example Feature Hierarchy

features but also the relationship information between them. A simple example of our product feature hierarchy for product camera is shown in Figure 1.

3.1   Pre-processing and Transaction File Generation

First of all, from a collection of reviews, we construct a single document called an *aggregated review document* which combines all the reviews in the collection, keeping each sentence in an original review as a sentence in the constructed aggregated review document. To extract useful information from the aggregated review document, three steps are undertaken to process the text of user reviews.

First, part-of-speech (POS) tagging is the fundamental and crucial step. In this step, we used a POS tagger (Stanford POSTagger) to generate a POS tag for each word in the aggregated review document to indicate whether the word is a noun, adjective or adverb etc. For instance, after the POS tagging, *"The flash is very weak."* would be transformed to *"The/DT flash/NN is/VBZ very/RB weak/JJ ./.",* where *DT, NN, VBZ, RB,* and *JJ* represent Determiner, Noun, Verb, Adverb and Adjective, respectively.

According to the assumption that most product features are nouns or noun phrases, which has been a thumb rule applied in most existing opinion mining approaches [3], we process each sentence in the aggregated review document to only keep words that are nouns. All the remaining nouns are also pre-processed by stemming and spelling correction. Each sentence in the aggregated review document consists of all identified nouns of a sentence in an original review.

Then, a transactional dataset is generated from the aggregated review document. Each sentence which consists of a sequence of nouns in the aggregated review document is treated as a transaction in the transactional dataset.

3.2   Potential Features Generation

Our first task is to generate potential product features that are expressed by those identified nouns or noun phrases. According to [3], significant product features are discussed extensively by users in reviews. For instance, *"battery"* which is a hot feature of the camera appears frequently in user reviews for digital cameras. Upon this, for most existing feature extraction approaches, pattern mining techniques are used to generate frequent itemsets from the transactional dataset and these frequent itemsets are treated as the potential features. Specifically, an itemset is a set of items (i.e., words in review text in this paper) that appear together in one or multiple transactions in a transactional dataset. Given a set of items, $I = \{i_1, i_2, ... i_n\}$, an itemset is defined as $X \subseteq I$. The support of an itemset X, denoted as *Supp(X)*, is the percentage of transactions in the dataset that contain X. All frequent itemsets from a set of transactions that satisfy a user-specified minimum support will be extracted as the potential features.

However, not all frequent itemsets are genuine since some of them may be just frequent but meaningless. For example, *"camera, year"* is a frequent phrase which has been identified from the aggregated review document but is not a correct feature. Hu and Liu proposed a method to check the compactness of itemsets in order to remove those meaningless frequent itemsets [3]. An itemset is considered 'compact' if for any two adjacent words in the itemset, the distance between the two words in their original review text is less than 3. Thus, if a frequent itemset appears in compact form in the transactional dataset, it is considered a valid potential feature; otherwise, it is not considered a potential feature and will be removed. For example, the itemset *"auto, mode"* is considered as a potential feature since it is compact and appears frequently in the aggregated review document.

After the compactness pruning, we can get a list of frequent itemsets, denoted as FP. These frequent itemsets are the potential features for further use.

3.3   Product Feature Hierarchy Construction

This step aims at constructing a feature hierarchy by identifying the relationship between the discovered potential features. To achieve this, we propose to utilize association rules generated from the discovered potential product features.

Association rule mining can be described as follows: Let $I = \{i_1, i_2, ... i_n\}$, be a set of items, and the dataset consists of a set of transactions $D = \{t_1, t_2, ... t_m\}$. Each transaction t contains a subset of items from I. Therefore, an association rule r represents an implication relationship between two itemsets which can be defined as the form $X \rightarrow Y$ where $X, Y \subseteq I$ and $X \cap Y = \emptyset$. The itemsets X and Y are called antecedent and consequent of the association rule, respectively. Usually, to assist selecting useful rules, two measures can be used:

1. The support of the association rule r $Supp(X \cup Y)$ indicates the proportion of transactions in the dataset which contain both X and Y;
2. The confidence of association rule r is denoted as $Conf(X \rightarrow Y)$ which shows the dependency between X and Y by calculating the percentage of

transactions that contain X in the dataset which also contain Y. In short, $Conf(X \rightarrow Y) = Supp(X \cup Y)/Supp(X)$.

For easily describing our approach, we define some useful and important concepts as follows:

Definition 1. (Feature hierarchy): A feature hierarchy consists of a set of features and their relationships, denoted as $FH = \{F, L\}$, F is a set of features where $F = \{f_1, f_2, ...f_n\}$ and L is a set of relations. The feature hierarchy has the following constraints:

(1) The relationship between a pair of features is the sub-feature relationship. For $f_i, f_j \in F$, if f_j is a sub-feature of f_i, then (f_i, f_j) is a link in the hierarchy and $(f_i, f_j) \in L$, which indicates that f_j is more specific than f_i. f_i is called the parent feature of f_j denoted as $P(f_j)$.

(2) Except for the root, each feature has only one parent feature. This means that the hierarchy is structured as a tree.

(3) The root of the hierarchy represents the product itself.

Definition 2. (Feature Existence): For a given feature hierarchy $FH = \{F, L\}$, let $W(g)$ represent a set of words that appear in a potential feature g, let $ES(g) = \{a_i | a_i \in 2^{w(g)}, a_i \in F\}$ contain all subsets of g which exist in the feature hierarchy called the existing subsets of g, if $\bigcup\limits_{a_i \in ES(g)} W(a_i) = W(g)$, then g considered existence in FH, denoted as $exist(g)$, otherwise $\neg exist(g)$. For instance, for the itemset *"camera, battery"*, if both *"camera"* and *"battery"* that are subsets of *"camera, battery"* are in the feature hierarchy, *"camera, battery"* is considered existence within the hierarchy.

Opinion mining is also referred as sentiment analysis [1,11,10]. Adjectives or adverbs that appear together with product features are considered as the sentiment words. The following definition defines the sentiment words that are related to a product feature.

Definition 3. (Related sentiments): For a feature $f \in F$, let $RS(f)$ denote a set of sentiment words which appear in the same sentences as f in user reviews, $RS(f)$ is defined as the related sentiments of f. For instance, both *"good"* and *"detailed"* are considered related sentiments of *"picture quality"* in the sentence *"I have found that picture quality is extremely good and detailed."*.

Definition 4. (Sentiment Sharing): For features $f_1, f_2 \in F$, the sentiment sharing between f_1 and f_2 is defined as $SS(f_1, f_2) = |RS(f_1) \cap RS(f_2)|$.

For deriving sub features using association rules, we need to select a set of useful rules rather than to try all the rules. In the next two subsections, we will first propose a method to select rules, then some strategies to update the feature hierarchy by adding sub features using the selected rules.

3.3.1 Rule Selection

Let $R = \{r_1, r_2, ...r_n\}$ be a set of Min-Max rules generated from the frequent itemsets FP, each rule r in R has the form $X_r \to Y_r$, X_r and Y_r are the antecedent and consequent of r, respectively.

Assuming that f_e is a feature which has already been in the current feature hierarchy FH, to generate the sub features for f_e, we first select a set of candidate rules, denoted as $R^c_{f_e}$, which could be used to generate the sub features:

$$R^c_{f_e} = \{X \to Y | X \to Y \in R, X = f_e, Supp(X) > (Y)\} \qquad (1)$$

As defined in Equation (1), the rules in $R^c_{f_e}$ should satisfy two constraints. The first constraint, $X = f_e$, specifies that the antecedent of a selected rule must be the same as the feature f_e. Sub features represent specific cases of a feature, they are more specific compared to the feature. The second constraint is based on the assumption that more frequent itemsets usually represent more general concepts, and less frequent itemsets usually represent more specific concepts. For instance, *"picture"*, which is a more general feature concept according to common knowledge, appears much more frequently than its specific features such as *"resolution" (of picture)* and *"color" (of picture)*. This constraint specifies that only the rules which can derive more specific features will be selected. These selected rules will be used to construct a feature hierarchy which will be discussed in next section. The feature hierarchy represents the relationships between features. The hierarchical relationship represented in the feature hierarchy is the *"is-a"* relation which means a feature in the hierarchy is a more specific feature of its parent feature. By using the selected rules which satisfy the second constraint, the hierarchical relationship in the hierarchy can be established. For example, suppose that *camera → battery* is a selected rule, based on this rule, *"battery"* will be added to the feature hierarchy as a sub feature (i.e., a child) of *"camera"*.

For example, the rule *mode → macro* generated from user reviews to camera and $Supp(mode) > Supp(macro)$ which means *"mode"* was more frequently mentioned than *"macro"* in user reviews. According to the definition in Equation (1), *mode → macro* would be chosen to generate sub features for the feature *"mode"*.

Not all selected rules represent correct sub-feature relationship. For instance, compared to the rule: *camera → auto*, *mode → auto* is more appropriate for describing a sub-feature relationship according to common knowledge. Therefore, the rule *camera → auto* should not be considered when we generate the sub features for *"camera"*. Upon this, we aim to prune the unnecessary rules before generating sub features for each hierarchy feature. In detail, traditional opinion mining in sentiment analysis has been at document level assuming the polarities of sentiments are the same for all features of a product [3]. However, sentiment words are often context-dependent [2,6]. The same sentiment word may not have the same polarity for different features. For example, the word *"big"* may have a positive meaning for memory volume, but may be not a positive sentiment for the size of a laptop computer. On the other hand, different features may have different sentiment words to describe them. For example, *"heavy"* is not a proper sentiment to describe the size of screen. A feature and its sub features should share similar sentiment words since they describe the same aspect of a product at different abstract levels. Therefore, for selecting rules to derive sub features for a given feature, we should select rules whose antecedent (representing the feature) and consequent (representing a possible sub feature) share as many sentiment words as possible because the more the sentiment words they share, the more possible they are about the same aspect of the product. Based on this view, we propose the following equation to calculate a score for each candidate rule $X \rightarrow Y$ in $R_{f_e}^c$:

$$Weigh(X \rightarrow Y) = \alpha \times \frac{SS(X,Y)}{|RS(X) \cup RS(Y)|} + \beta(Supp(Y) \times Conf(X \rightarrow Y)) \quad (2)$$

$0 \leq \alpha, \beta \leq 1$. There are two parts in Equation (2). The first part is the percentage of the shared sentiment words given by $SS(X,Y)$ over all the sentiment words used for either X or Y. The higher the percentage, the more possible that X and Y are related features. The second part is used to measure the belief to the consequent Y by using this rule since $Conf(X \rightarrow Y)$ measures the confidence to the association between X and Y and $Supp(Y)$ measures the popularity of Y. Given a threshold σ, we propose to use the following equation to select the rules from the candidate rules in $R_{f_e}^c$. The rules in R_{f_e} will be used to derive sub features for the features in FP. R_{f_e} is called the rule set of f_e.

$$R_{f_e} = \{X \rightarrow Y | X \rightarrow Y \in R_{f_e}^c, Weigh(X \rightarrow Y) > \sigma\} \quad (3)$$

3.3.2 Feature Hierarchy Construction

Let $FH = \{F, L\}$ be a feature hierarchy which could be an empty tree, FP be a set of frequent itemsets generated from user reviews which are potential features, and R be a set of rules generated from user reviews. This task is to construct a feature hierarchy if F is empty or update the feature hierarchy if F is not empty by using the rules in R. Let UF be a set of features on the tree which need to be processed in order to construct or update the tree. If F is empty, the itemset in FP which has the highest support will be chosen as the root of FH, it will be the only item in UF at the beginning. If F is not empty, UF will be F, i.e., $UF = F$.

Without losing generality, assuming that F is not empty and the set of features currently on the tree (e.g., we may build the feature hierarchy based on an existing simple model such as a digital camera model derived from Amazon which indicates that a digital camera consists of a number of specific features: *"price"*, *"size"*, *"battery"*, *"ease of use"*), UF is the set of features which need to be processed to update or construct the tree, for each feature in UF, let f_e be a feature in UF, i.e., $f_e \in UF$ and $X \rightarrow Y \in R_{f_e}$ be a rule with $X = f_e$, the next step is to decide whether or not Y should be added to the feature hierarchy as a sub feature of f_e. There are two possible situations: Y does not exist in the feature hierarchy, i.e., $\neg exist(Y)$ and Y does exist in the hierarchy, i.e., $exist(Y)$. In the first situation, the feature hierarchy will be updated by adding Y as a sub feature of f_e, i.e., $F = F \cup \{Y\}$, $L = L \cup (f_e, Y)$, and Y should be added to UF for further checking.

In the second situation, i.e., Y already exists in the hierarchy, i.e., according to Definition 2, there are two cases, $Y \notin ES(Y)$ (i.e., Y is not in the tree) or $Y \in ES(Y)$ (i.e., Y is in the tree). In the first case, Y is not considered a sub feature of f_e and no change to the tree. In the second case, $\exists f_y \in F$, f_y is the parent feature of Y, i.e., $P(Y) = f_y$ and $(f_y, Y) \in L$. Now, we need to determine whether to keep f_y as the parent feature of Y or change the parent feature of Y to f_e. That is, we need to examine f_y and f_e to see which of them is more suitable to be the parent feature of Y. The basic strategy is to compare f_y and f_e to see which of them share more sentiment words with Y, the more sentiment words they share, the more likely they represent similar aspect of the product. That is, if $SS(f_y, Y) < SS(f_e, Y)$, the link (f_y, Y) will be removed from the hierarchy tree, (f_e, Y) will be added to the tree, and $UF = UF \cup \{Y\}$, otherwise, no change to the tree and f_y is still the parent feature of Y.

3.3.3   Algorithms

In this section, we will describe the algorithms to construct the feature hierarchy. As mentioned above, if the tree is empty, the feature with the highest support will be chosen as the root. So, at the very beginning, F and UF contain at least one item which is the root.

Algorithm 1. Feature Hierarchy Construction

Input:
    R, $FH = \{F, L\}$, FP.

Output:
    FH, RF //RF is the remaining features which are not added to FH after the construction

1: if $F = \emptyset$, then $root := argmax_{f \in FP}\{supp(f)\}$, $F := UF := \{root\}$;
2: else $UF := F$;
3: for each feature $f_e \in UF$
4:     if $R_{f_e} \neq \emptyset$ //R_{f_e} is the rule set of f_e, it is not empty
5:         for each rule $X \rightarrow Y \in R_{f_e}$
6:             if $\neg exist(Y)$ //Y does not exist on the tree
7:                 $F := F \cup \{Y\}$, $L := L \cup (f_e, Y)$, $UF := UF \cup \{Y\}$, $FP = FP - \{Y\}$;
8:             else //Y exists on the tree
9:                 if $Y \in ES(Y)$ and $SS(f_y, Y) < SS(f_e, Y)$ //f_y is P_s parent feature
10:                     $L := L \cup (f_e, Y)$, $L := L - (f_y, Y)$; //add (f_e, Y) to and remove (f_y, Y)

11:                else //$Y \notin ES(Y)$, Y is not on the tree
12:                   $FP = FP - \{Y\}$;
13:         endfor
14:     endif
15:     $UF := UF - \{f_e\}$; //remove f_e from UF
16: endfor
17: $RF := FP$;

After the hierarchy construction, some potential features may be left over in RF and have not been added to the hierarchy. The main reason is because these itemsets may not frequently occur in the reviews together with the features that have been added in the hierarchy. In order to prevent valid features from being missed out, we check those remaining itemsets in RF by examining the shared sentiment words between the remaining itemsets and the features on the hierarchy. If a remaining itemset in RF has some sentiment words and also shares certain number of sentiment words with a feature in the hierarchy, this itemset could be a feature. Let $FH = \{F, L\}$ be the constructed feature hierarchy, RF be the set of remaining potential features, for a potential feature g in RF and $RS(g) > \alpha$ (i.e., g has some related sentiment words), the basic strategy to determine whether g is a feature or not is to check whether or not there is a feature on the current hierarchy which shares some common sentiment words with g. Let $F_g = \{f|f \in F, SS(f, g) > 0\}$ be a set of features which share some sentiment words with g, if $F_g \neq \emptyset$, g is considered a feature. Furthermore, we can determine the most related feature for g based on the sentiment sharing, the most related feature is defined as $f_m = argmax_{f \in F_g}\{SS(f, g)\}$. g will be added to the hierarchy with f_m as its parent feature. If there are multiple such features f_m which have the highest sentiment sharing with g, the one with the highest support will be chosen as the parent feature of g.

The following algorithm formally describes the method mentioned above to expand the hierarchy by adding the remaining features.

Algorithm 2. Feature Hierarchy Expansion

Input:
    $FH = \{F, L\}$, RF, α.
Output:
    FH
1: for each feature $g \in RF$
2:     if $RS(g) > \alpha$ and $(F_g := \{f|f \in F, SS(f, g) > 0\}) \neq \emptyset$
3:        $M := \{a|a \in F_g \text{ and } SS(a, g) = max_{f \in F_g}\{SS(f, g)\}\}$
4:        $f_m := argmax_{f \in M}\{supp(f)\}$
5:        $F := F \cup \{g\}$, $L := L \cup (f_m, g)$
6:        $RF := RF - \{g\}$;

After the expansion, the features left over in RF are not considered as features for this product.

4   Experiment

Our feature extraction approach generates a feature hierarchy based on the useful information extracted from user reviews. To evaluate the effectiveness of the proposed approach, we examined the generated feature hierarchy to check how many accurate features in user reviews have been extracted.

We conducted our experiment by using user reviews of four types of digital cameras. Two digital cameras' review datasets are used in [4] and the other two are published by Liu in 2008 [13]. Each review in the review datasets has been manually annotated. In detail, each sentence of the review was read by an examiner, all possible features that are modified by sentiments are annotated by the examiner. In addition, the polarity strength of the opinion towards a certain feature is annotated as well. For example, "*flash* [−2] ## *The flash is very weak.*" is an annotated review sentence which indicates that the user holds a negative attitude towards feature "*flash*" with a polarity score 2. We take these manually tagged features as the correct features to evaluate the proposed method, called Feature Hierarchy in the following tables.

To further illustrate the effectiveness of our approach, we chose the feature extraction method Feature-Based Summarization (FBS) proposed in [4] as the baseline for comparison.

Table 1. Precision Comparison Between FBS Frequent Feature Extraction and Feature Hierarchy

	Digital Camera 1	Digital Camera 2	Digital Camera 3	Digital Camera 4
Feature Hierarchy	0.62	0.46	0.63	0.58
FBS	0.45	0.44	0.51	0.42

Table 2. Recall Comparison Between FBS Frequent Feature Extraction and Feature Hierarchy

	Digital Camera 1	Digital Camera 2	Digital Camera 3	Digital Camera 4
Feature Hierarchy	0.56	0.59	0.58	0.65
FBS	0.57	0.58	0.57	0.63

Table 3. F1 Score Comparison Between FBS Frequent Feature Extraction and Feature Hierarchy

	Digital Camera 1	Digital Camera 2	Digital Camera 3	Digital Camera 4
Feature Hierarchy	0.59	0.51	0.60	0.61
FBS	0.51	0.50	0.54	0.51

Table 1, 2, 3 illustrate the precision, recall, and F1 score results produced by the proposed approach and the baseline model using the datasets for four cameras, respectively. From the results, we can see that both the precision and F1 score results produced by the proposed approach are significantly better than the baseline model. In addition, the recall of the proposed method is also better than the baseline model in most cases.

Overall, the experiment results are promising which shows that the use of associations between features can improve the performance of feature extraction.

Figure 1 which is part of feature hierarchy generated from our proposed approach illustrates the relationships between camera features. In detail, the structure consists of three levels which contains a number of features. Based on common knowledge, this model is correct. The camera has a number of sub features such as battery and price. In addition, some sub feature of camera also have their own sub features. e.g., *auto mode*, *manual mode*, and *macro mode*; each of them is a specific option of *mode*.

5   Conclusion

In this paper, we introduced a new feature extraction approach based on frequent patterns and association rules to generate features of a product and also the product's feature hierarchy. The objective is to not only extract product features mentioned in user reviews but also identify the relationship between the generated features. The results of our experiment indicate that the proposed approach can identify more correct features than the baseline model and the generated feature hierarchy is effective in extracting product features. Additionally, the feature relationships captured in the feature hierarchy provide more detailed information about products which is one step further towards profiling products at a multi-level rather than at a single level as what most existing feature generation methods produced. Most existing feature generation methods only generate a list of features. Since our work is based on user reviews, it can be easily applied to other domains such as generating features of services in hospitals or clinics. For instance, based on the customer reviews for a hospital, a hierarchy which contains service features such as *value, triage, radiology* can be generated.

References

1. Abbasi, A., Chen, H., Salem, A.: Sentiment analysis in multiple languages: Feature selection for opinion classification in Web forums. ACM Transactions on Information Systems 26(3) (2008)
2. Ding, X., Liu, B., Yu, P.S.: A Holistic Lexicon-Based Approach to Opinion Mining. In: International Conference on Web Search and Web Data Mining, pp. 231–240 (2008)
3. Hu, M., Liu, B.: Mining Opinion Features in Customer Reviews. In: 19th National Conference on Artifical Intelligence, pp. 755–760 (2004)
4. Hu, M., Liu, B.: Mining and Summarizing Customer Reviews. In: 10th ACM SIGKDD International Conference on Knowledge discovery and Data Mining, pp. 168–177. ACM, New York (2004)
5. Hu, W., Gong, Z., Guo, J.: Mining Product Features from Online Reviews. In: IEEE 7th International Conference on E-Business Engineering, pp. 24–29 (2010)
6. Lau, R.Y.K., Lai, C.C.L., Ma, J., Li, Y.: Automatic Domain Ontology Extraction for Context-Sensitive Opinion Mining. In: Thirtieth International Conference on Information Systems (2009)
7. Pasquier, N., Bastide, Y., Taouil, R., Lakhal, L.: Efficient mining of association rules using closed itemset lattices. Information Systems 24(1), 25–46 (1999)

8. Popescu, A.-M., Etzioni, O.: Extracting Product Features and Opinions from Reviews. In: Human Language Technology Conference and Conference on Empirical Methods in Natural Language Processing, pp. 339–346. Association for Computational Linguistics Stroudsburg, PA (2005)

9. Scaffidi, C., Bierhoff, K., Chang, E., Felker, M., Ng, H., Jin, C.: Red Opal: Product-Feature Scoring from Reviews. In: 8th ACM Conference on Electronic Commerce, pp. 182–191. ACM, New York (2007)

10. Subrahmanian, V., Reforgiato, D.: AVA: Adjective-Verb-Adverb Combinations for Sentiment Analysis. In: IEEE Intelligent Systems, pp. 43–50 (2008)

11. Wright, A.: Our sentiments, exactly. Communications of the ACM 52(4), 14–15 (2009)

12. Xu, Y., Li, Y., Shaw, G.: Reliable Representations for Association Rules. Data and Knowledge Engineering 70(6), 237–256 (2011)

13. Opinion Mining, Sentiment Analysis, and Opinion Spam Detection, http://www.cs.uic.edu/~liub/FBS/sentiment-analysis.html

Evaluation of Error-Sensitive Attributes

William Wu and Shichao Zhang

Faculty of Engineering and Information Technology, University of Technology, Sydney
{william.wu,shichao.zhang}@uts.edu.au

Abstract. Numerous attribute selection frameworks have been developed to improve performance and results in the research field of machine learning and data classification (Guyon & Elisseeff 2003; Saeys, Inza & Larranaga 2007), majority of the effort has focused on the performance and cost factors, with a primary aim to examine and enhance the logic and sophistication of the underlying components and methods of specific classification models, such as a variety of wrapper, filter and cluster algorithms for feature selection, to work as a data pre-process step or embedded as an integral part of a specific classification process. Taking a different approach, our research is to study the relationship between classification errors and data attributes not before, not during, but after the fact, to evaluate risk levels of attributes and identify the ones that may be more prone to errors based on such a post-classification analysis and a proposed attribute-risk evaluation routine. Possible benefits from this research can be to help develop error reduction measures and to investigate specific relationship between attributes and errors in a more efficient and effective way. Initial experiments have shown some supportive results, and the unsupportive results can also be explained by a hypothesis extended from this evaluation proposal.

Keywords: ambiguous value range, error-sensitive attribute, attribute-error evaluation, attribute selection, post-classification analysis.

1 Introduction

A practical scenario to introduce this research work is, a data classification was carried out for a dataset of 10,000 sample instances with 50 data attributes, the result showed 100 misclassification errors. Our research question is, which attribute, or which three attributes, may be considered the most error-sensitive attributes amongst the 50 attributes? One possible benefit from identifying such error-sensitive attributes can be to help develop error reduction measures in a more specific and attribute-oriented way; another possible benefit can be to raise stake holders' awareness of those specific attributes, to help further investigate possible special relationship between attributes and errors in a more effective way.

Three specific terms, "ambiguous value range", "attribute-error counter" and "error-sensitive attribute", are used frequently in this research discussion, and they all refer to binary classification scenarios within the context of this research at this early stage. The term "ambiguous value range" describes the attribute values of Negative and Positive samples co-exist in one or more value ranges, highlighting special "grey

J. Li et al. (Eds.): PAKDD 2013 Workshops, LNAI 7867, pp. 283–294, 2013.

area" of values in which one value range of some Negative instances overlaps the value range of some Positive instances, therefore ambiguity may arise because one cannot determine a sample instance's class label by using its attribute's value within such an ambiguous value range. The term "attribute-error counter" describes the number of misclassified sample instances of a particular attribute with its attribute values being within one ambiguous value range. The term "error-sensitive attribute" describes an attribute that is considered to be more prone and risky to cause or associate with errors during a data classification process, and the risk assessment is initially based on the counting and ranking of "attribute-error counters" amongst the attributes of a targeted dataset. More details about these terms are to be discussed in the next few sections.

The rest of this paper is organized as follows. Section-2 explains some initial thoughts that lead to this evaluation idea, section-3 reviews some early influential research works that helped establish the foundation for this evaluation proposal, section-4 describes more details about the proposed evaluation, section-5 summarises experiments on five datasets, section-6 discusses the experiment results and the evolvement of related ideas, and finally, section-7 concludes the current evaluation development and outlines a possible plan for future study.

2   Initial Groundwork and Assumptions

At this early stage of the research, only attributes with numeric values are considered, and no missing value is expected. Such a simplified scope will keep the formulation of value ranges consistent amongst the available test datasets and throughout this discussion.

Continuing the brief scenario described in section-1, for the 9,900 samples that have been correctly classified, values of an attribute can be grouped into two possible types, the Unambiguous type, in which Negative instances have a different attribute value range from Positive instances, as shown in the left diagram of Figure 1, hence a classifier can label sample instances according to such distinguishable value ranges without ambiguity; and the Ambiguous type, in which some attribute values being inside an ambiguous overlap range which is shared by both Negative and Positive instances, as shown in the **blue** overlap area of the right diagram of Figure 1, therefore classification errors may occur due to such ambiguity as a part of the possible cause for errors.

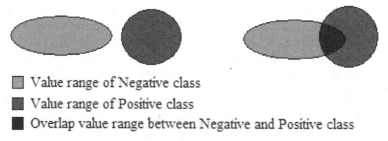

■ Value range of Negative class
■ Value range of Positive class
■ Overlap value range between Negative and Positive class

Fig. 1. Left diagram shows two distinct value ranges, and right diagram shows an overlap area between the two value ranges

A misclassification error with its one or more attribute values being inside one or more ambiguous ranges may not necessarily be the sole reason causing the error, but such ambiguity may potentially increase the risk of being misclassified. Based on this presumption, if such an attribute whose ambiguous values are associated with a higher count of misclassification errors, this attribute can be considered more risky and more sensitive to errors, or, more error-sensitive than other attributes which are associated with lower counts of errors. Other possible factors can be, for example, the correlation effect when multiple attributes simultaneously involved, the propagation of errors from other attributes or factors, the overshadowing effect from other critical elements, and the possibility of sample data contamination, "noisy" data, or misreading values, etc (Taylor 1996; Yoon 1989).

3   Related Work

Decision trees have a reputation of being efficient and illustrative in machine learning and data classification, one prominent decision tree model is Quinlan's C4.5 model (Alpaydin 2004; Han & Kamber 2006; Quinlan 1993; Witten & Frank 2005), therefore, C4.5 decision tree has been adapted as the primary classification model in this research for investigation and experiment purposes.

One key step in conducting decision tree classification is the attribute selection process when constructing the tree from root to leaves, and Quinlan's C4.5 model has adopted a selection method known as gain ratio. This gain ratio method originated from the information gain concept described in Shannon's information theory (Shannon 1948). When using information gain as the attribute selection and partition criterion, it has a strong bias for selecting attributes with many outcomes, for example, the trivial attribute of "Record ID" or "Patient ID", which is not supposed to be related with the classification process itself but a unique ID value to identify each record by the stakeholders. To address this deficiency, information gain ratio was introduced as the attribute selection criterion in C4.5, to apply "a kind of normalization in which the apparent gain attributable to tests with many outcomes is adjusted", which means such information gain is to be divided into as many as its possible partitions or outcomes for an attribute or a node, so it "represents the proportion of information generated by the split that is useful, i.e., that appears helpful for classification" (Quinlan 1993).

A variety of other attribute selection methodologies have also been developed, such as the Gini index method that was built into the CART decision tree model (Breiman et al. 1984), the RELIEF algorithm (Kira & Rendell 1992), the Sequential Forward Selection (SFS) method and the Sequential Backward Elimination (SBE) method (Kittler 1978). A number of major categories have been defined to group and organize various attribute selection algorithms (Guyon & Elisseeff 2003; Saeys, Inza & Larranaga 2007), such as the Wrapper type, which is to build or "wrap" a search and evaluation routine around the data classification model and as a part of the classification process, e.g. SFS and SBE; the Filter type, which works like a pre-process routine and to evaluate the relevance of attributes first then to select a subset of attributes with higher relevance, e.g. information gain and gain ratio method; and the Embedded type, which works interactively with the classification model in searching and selecting a subset of the attributes during the training process, e.g. the application of Gini index in the CART model.

Conventional feature selection frameworks typically aim to generate a prioritized attribute list as the first phase, then to conduct classification process based on the selected and ranked attribute in an attempt to achieve better performance in the second phase (Liu H et al. 2010). Many works by other researchers are also connected to this proposed evaluation idea at various degrees, we have only mentioned some of the highlights in this limited section.

4   Evaluation Process Description

Our current approach in this evaluation process may seem sharing some similarity with the Filter type feature selection process, however, one main difference is our approach can be considered as a post-classification routine - a new third phase process, to evaluate the resulted errors from the classification process from the second phase which may have already incorporated its pre-determined feature selection routine, with the aim to explore attribute-error relationship and error-reduction measures, as illustrated in Figure 2:

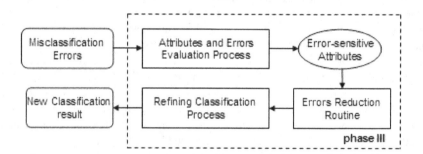

Fig. 2. Proposed attribute-evaluation process in a three-phase model

This evaluation begins as a post-classification analysis. For each attribute used in the data classification, the lower and upper bound values of the correctly classified Negative and Positive instances are to be identified, so are the mean values of these two correctly classified groups of samples. By comparing the lower and upper bound value of each class group, the boundaries of each attribute's ambiguous value range can be determined. If an overlap range can be found, this overlap range can then be claimed the "ambiguous value range", because possible ambiguity may arise from the fact that both Negative and Positive instances have attribute values inside this same value range.

For each attribute contains such an ambiguous value range, a check on the attribute value of all misclassified instances is conducted. If a misclassified instance's attribute value is within this ambiguous value range, then add one to the attribute-error counter of this attribute. After calculating the attribute-error counters for all involved attributes, the attribute with the highest counter value can be considered as the most error-sensitive attribute. That is because its higher count of errors indicates this attribute may have a higher level of risk to be misclassified than other attributes, therefore it may be more prone and more sensitive to errors than others. Alternatively, the ratio of the attribute-error counter to the number of instances having ambiguous values may also be used to measure such an error-sensitivity level. This latter approach may seem similar to the progression path from info gain to gain ratio; however, additional work will be required to examine this expansion further.

Another way to illustrate this evaluation model is through a basic scenario and its process summary in a pseudo code style demonstration:

Input: A dataset of $(m + n)$ sample instances containing t attributes with their pre-determined class labels and the newly classified labels; m samples correctly classified and n samples misclassified during the classification process

Output: A ranking list of the t attributes sorted by their attribute-error counter values from high to low; initial error-reduction measure could be introduced based on the result, followed by a re-run of the classification process to compare and verify

Evaluation process in three steps:

step-1: work out ambiguous value ranges and attribute-error counter values
   for 1 to t attributes
      for 1 to m correctly classified Negative and Positive instances
         find Negative instances' min & max value and their mean value;
         find Positive instances' min & max value and their mean value;
         compare these min/max values to determine the ambiguous value range;
      for 1 to n misclassified instances
         if the attribute value is within its attribute's ambiguous value range
         then add one to its attribute's attribute-error counter;
   end;

step-2: sort the attribute-error counter values from high to low to highlight the most error-sensitive attributes at the top positions

step-3: compare this error-sensitive attribute ranking list with other attributes ranking lists, such as info-gain and gain-ratio ranking list, to evaluate the most error-sensitive attributes and possible error-reduction measures

---

One critical issue in this evaluation process is how to determine the lower and upper bound of the ambiguous value range for each attribute. In this early stage of the research and due to the page number constraint of this paper, only two simplified overlap situations from three value range scenarios are discussed here, as shown in the following three diagrams in Figure 3:

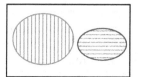 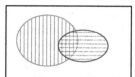 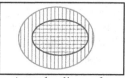

| Two distinct value ranges for Negative and Positive class | An identifiable overlap area of two value ranges | A total eclipse of two value ranges |

Fig. 3. Three value range scenarios and two in overlap situation

For the first overlap situation when the overlap area is small and distinguishable as shown in the middle diagram, the ambiguous value range can be determined by working out the min/max attribute value of the Negative/Positive class and using them as the lower and upper boundary. For the second overlap situation when it is less distinguishable as shown in the right diagram, the ambiguous value range can be determined by using the mean value of the Negative and the Positive instances' attribute values as the lower and upper boundary instead.

One hypothesis arises from this evaluation idea is, if the most error-sensitive attribute is not the most significant attribute that has been used by the underlying classification model, then the removal or weighting down one or two most error-sensitive attributes may help reduce the classification's error-rate. To test whether our proposed evaluation process can actually identify the most error-sensitive attributes, experiments have been carried out on a number of real world datasets. These experiments and their analysis are discussed in the next two sections.

5   Experiments

Initial experiments were carried out using Quinlan's C4.5 algorithm-based J48 classifier and with 10-fold cross validation mode in WEKA (Hall et al. 2009). Five datasets from the UCI Machine Learning Repository (Frank & Asuncion 2010) have been used to test this evaluation idea, and the initial error reduction measure was to filter out the most error sensitive attributes in a re-run of the classification process. Two datasets, the Wisconsin and Liver Disorders dataset, appeared to show supportive results at various levels, one test scenario on the Liver Disorders dataset resulted in the error rate reduced by almost 3%. One dataset, the Pima diabetes dataset, showed some unsupportive results, and the worse result was the error rate actually increased by almost 7%; however, the unsupportive results for this dataset could be explained by a good reason and could potentially turn itself into the supportive group. Results from the other two datasets, the   Page Blocks and Ecoli dataset, appeared to be rather neutral on the surface; yet further analysis showed they could be considered as supporting evidence when taking into account of the intricate value patterns of some key attributes and the correlation amongst them. Some of the experiment results are highlighted as follows.[1]

5.1   Error-Sensitivity Ranking vs. Gain Ratio and Info Gain Ranking

One key contribution from this research intends to be the possible identification of the most error-sensitive attributes, and it may help raise the data stakeholders and domain experts' awareness of those specific error-prone attributes, and help develop error-corrective and preventative measures in a more effective way. C4.5's underlying attribute selection and ranking process is based on gain ratio, by comparing the attributes' error-sensitivity ranking against the gain ratio and info gain ranking, it may provide a miniature knowledge-base to help understand what attributes are the most

Table 1. Comparing attribute-error counter, gain ratio and info gain rankings

Rank	by Attribute-error counter	by GainRatio	by InfoGain
Wisconsin breast cancer dataset			
1	Uni Cell Size (35)	Normal Nucleoli (0.399)	Uni Cell Size (0.675)
2	Uni Cell Shape (35)	Sing Ep Cell Size (0.395)	Uni Cell Shape (0.66)
3	Clump Thickness (30)	Uni Cell Size (0.386)	Bare Nuclei (0.564)
Liver Disorders dataset			
1	sgot (22)	gammagt (0.097 +- 0.065)	gammagt (0.051 +- 0.013)
2	mcv (16)	alkphos (0 +- 0)	alkphos (0 +- 0)
3	alkphos (10)	mcv (0 +- 0)	mcv (0 +- 0)
Page Blocks classification dataset			
1	mean_tr (89)	length (0.2993)	height (0.2357)
2	p_black (43)	height (0.1494)	mean_tr (0.1828)
3	eccen (29)	mean_tr (0.143)	wb_trans (0.1537)
Ecoli dataset			
1	chg (17)	alm1 (0.3999)	alm1 (0.627)
2	alm1 (15)	alm2 (0.3683)	alm2 (0.563)
3	lip (14)	lip (0.1977)	aac (0.26)
Pima Indians diabetes dataset			
1	plas (83)	plas (0.0986)	plas (0.1901)
2	mass (70)	mass (0.0863)	mass (0.0749)
3	age (31)	age (0.0726)	age (0.0725)

---

[1] The information provided in section-5&6 is in a much simplified version due to page number constraint. Details on result combinations using min/max and mean values of binary class groups as ambiguous value range boundaries, as well as test combinations from filtering one to multiple most error-sensitive attributes, and the subsequent result analysis, can be provided if required, and they may be included in future papers for in-depth discussion if this evaluation idea is to be accepted as a starting point.

informative, what attributes are the most error-sensitive, and how attributes may be related to each other in terms of relevant ranking positions by the classifier and the classification result, so further more specific relationship between attributes and classification errors could be revealed by utilizing such information.

Due to the page number constraint, the following table only highlights the comparison of the top three ranked attributes resulted from our evaluation process and the gain ratio and info gain algorithm performed on the five UCI datasets.

5.2   Performance Comparison Based on Evaluation Results

One possible way to verify the above evaluation results is, to filter out one or more attributes evaluated to be the most error-sensitive ones, and then re-run the data classification on the updated dataset. Hypothetically, it may produce more accurate results with lower error-rate, if and only if the filtering has no significant impact on the classifier's underlying attribute selection process. This preliminary error-reduction method has produced a number of attribute filter combinations for each dataset, varying from using the single most error-sensitive attribute to a combination of multiple most error-sensitive attributes.

The reason for testing with different filter combination is, during experiments, it was found that simply filtering out the single most error-sensitive attribute or two did not necessarily produce the most desirable results, and a slightly different filter combination might result with a better result with lower error-rate. A possible cause of this could be the internal correlation between the most error-sensitive attributes and other attributes used by the classifier. These heuristic experiments were an attempt to inspire new thoughts from the data's stakeholders and domain experts, so they can look closer at the relationship between errors and attributes. The following table only highlights a few of the interesting results from a large array of combinations:

Table 2. Performance comparison amongst the datasets

Wisconsin cancer dataset	Re-run C4.5 classification without top 2 most error-sensitive attributes - Uni Cell Size and Shape
Original C4.5 classification with 9 attributes	
=== Stratified cross-validation ===	=== Stratified cross-validation ===
Correctly Classified Instances 654 93.562%	Correctly Classified Instances 667 95.422%
Incorrectly Classified Instances 45 6.438%	Incorrectly Classified Instances 32 4.578%
Liver Disorders dataset	Re-run C4.5 classification without top 2 most error-sensitive attribute – sgot and mcv
Original C4.5 classification with 6 attributes	=== Stratified cross-validation ===
=== Stratified cross-validation ===	Correctly Classified Instances 243
Correctly Classified Instances 233 67.536%	70.435%
Incorrectly Classified Instances 112	Incorrectly Classified Instances 102
32.464%	29.565%

Table 2. (*Continued*)

Page Blocks classification dataset	Re-run C4.5 classification without top most error-sensitive attribute – mean_tr
Original C4.5 classification with 10 attributes === Stratified cross-validation === Correctly Classified Instances 5321 97.223% Incorrectly Classified Instances 152 2.777%	=== Stratified cross-validation === Correctly Classified Instances 5320 97.205% Incorrectly Classified Instances 153 2.795%

Ecoli dataset	Re-run C4.5 classification without top most error-sensitive attribute – chg
Original C4.5 classification with 7 attributes === Stratified cross-validation === Correctly Classified Instances 318 94.643% Incorrectly Classified Instances 18 5.357%	=== Stratified cross-validation === Correctly Classified Instances 318 94.643% Incorrectly Classified Instances 18 5.357%

Pima Indians diabetes dataset	Re-run C4.5 classification without top 2 most error-sensitive attributes – plas and mass
Original C4.5 classification with 8 attributes === Stratified cross-validation === Correctly Classified Instances 568 73.958% Incorrectly Classified Instances 200 26.042%	=== Stratified cross-validation === Correctly Classified Instances 515 67.057% Incorrectly Classified Instances 253 32.943%

6   Experiment Analysis

Experiments have shown that the calculation method of using the min/max value of the Negative and Positive samples as the ambiguous value range boundaries cannot reliably distinguish attributes with different error-sensitivity levels, as most attributes in the five datasets appeared to have their two class-label value ranges in an almost total eclipse situation. The key reason for this situation can be because this first method does not exclude the outlier values in either the Negative or Positive class, especially when those outlier values are likely the min/max values.

Therefore, the alternative method – using the mean attribute value of Negative and Positive samples as the boundaries of ambiguous value range, has been used for the experiments. Some of result analysis has been summarised in the following two parts.

6.1   Comparing the Three Ranking Methods and the Mixed Results

The calculation method of both gain ratio and info gain is based on the available training samples, in comparison, our error-sensitive attribute evaluation method is primarily based on classification error samples generated by the classifier, and the current stage of our research, the classifier is C4.5.

Part of this evaluation's hypothesis is, when one or more attributes were identified as the most error-sensitive attributes but not as the top ranked gain ratio attributes, and later they were filtered out as a preliminary error-reduction measure in a re-run of the classification process, the error-rate may reduce. Experiment results from the Wisconsin dataset and Liver Disorders dataset had shown their error-rate reduced between 2~3%, these results appeared to be supporting the proposed hypothesis.

On the other hand, the significant increase in error-rate from one Pima diabetes dataset result could be explained by the unison of the top three attributes in all three ranking methods, that is because when the most error-sensitive attributes were filtered out, that also filtered out the most informative attributes being used by the gain ratio algorithm behind the C4.5 classifier because they were the same attributes, and that could have seriously reduced the accuracy and reliability of the classifier, therefore resulted in significant increase in error-rate.

What remained to be explained are the results from the Page Blocks and Ecoli dataset. The filtering out the most error-sensitive attribute had little impact on the error-rate in the re-run of classification process, and adding the second and third most error-sensitive attribute to the filter had only increased the error-rate by a small margin, that was in contrast with the significant increase in error-rate when testing the Pima diabetes dataset with three of its most error-sensitive attributes filtered out. Further examination into the attribute values revealed some intricate value patterns and possible correlation between key attributes, so that might have led to such interesting results. More information on such intricacy may be detailed in a longer version of paper.

One may argue that the use of mean attribute value of the Negative and Positive class instances as the boundary of the ambiguous value range is unsophisticated, and, more datasets should be used, multi-class scenarios should be considered, etc. All these are valid points, and they are the issues to be worked on in the next stage of the research.

6.2   Comparing with Experiments by Other Researchers

Another way to analyse our experiments is to compare them with the ones performed by other researchers using the same datasets, to check for any special mentioning about the identification of error-sensitive attributes, to seek supporting evidence from direct or implicit references recognized by other researchers which might shed light on similar attribute/risk evaluation ideas.

Such supporting references are not easy to find. In the first relevant research paper mentioned in the Pima data file (Smith et al. 1988), its focus was on the theoretical background and implementation of the ADAP neural network model, no specific analysis on classification errors and their possible relationship with specific attributes. A good number of other data classification models were developed and experimented using the Pima data file, for example, the ARTMAP-Instance Counting algorithm (Carpenter & Markuzon 1998), the hybrid Bayes classifier and evolutionary algorithm (Raymer et al. 2001), the automated comparative disease profile generation and diagnosis system (Wei & Altman 2004), and the general regression neural networks model (Kayaer & Yyldyrym 2003). They have also primarily emphasised on individual classification algorithms and their potential for classification enhancement, but no suggestion or mention about the possible causes of classification errors and their association with data attributes.

Similarly, when discussing the use of the Wisconsin cancer dataset, amongst the data classification models that have been studied so far, such as the multi-surface pattern separation model (Wolberg & Mangasarian 1990), the two parametric bilinear programming methods for feature minimization models, and the cancer image analysis application based on other linear methods (Mangasarian, Street & Wolberg 1994), the main focus of these experiments was primarily on the classification performance and the comparison between their models and other benchmark models, such as CART and C4.5, no specific discussion on the possible role/impact of certain attributes and certain value ranges with higher risk level towards their classification errors.

7 Conclusion

Our research into this error-sensitive attribute evaluation is still in its early stage and still evolving; only some rudimentary methods of calculation and five datasets have been used to test this evaluation model. Building on some encouraging research results so far, one possible direction for further study would be to examine the correlation nature between the most error-sensitive attributes and their high misclassification counts, to search for more relevant datasets to test the evaluation process and error-reduction measures. If this evaluation model can be proven to be a valid model in a more systematic way and by a wider range of datasets, it may lead to a more effective development of error-reduction measures, and may help contribute to the enhancement of data classification process.

References

Alpaydin, E.: Introduction to Machine Learning. The MIT Press, London (2004)

Bredensteiner, E.J., Bennett, K.P.: Feature Minimization within Decision Trees. Computational Optimization and Applications 10(2), 111–126 (1998)

Breiman, L., Friedman, J.H., Olshen, R.A., Stone, C.J.: Classification and Regression Trees. Wadsworth International Group, Belmont (1984)

Carpenter, G.A., Markuzon, N.: ARTMAP-IC and medical diagnosis: Instance counting and inconsistent cases. Neural Networks 11, 323–336 (1998)

Frank, A., Asuncion, A.: UCI Machine Learning Repository. University of California, Irvine (2010), http://archive.ics.uci.edu/ml

Guyon, I., Elisseeff, A.: An introduction to variable and feature selection. The Journal of Machine Learning Research 3, 1157–1182 (2003)

Hall, M., Frank, E., Holmes, G., Pfahringer, B., Reutemann, P., Witten, I.H.: The WEKA Data Mining Software: An Update. SIGKDD Explorations 11(1) (2009)

Han, J., Kamber, M.: Data mining: concepts and techniques, 2nd edn. Morgan Kaufmann, San Francisco (2006)

Kayaer, K., Yyldyrym, T.: Medical diagnosis on pima indian diabetes using General Regression Neural Networks. Paper presented to the International Conference on Artificial Neural Networks/International Conference on Neural Information Processing, Istanbul, Turkey (2003)

Kira, K., Rendell, L.A.: A practical approach to feature selection. In: Proceedings of the Ninth International Workshop on Machine Learning, pp. 249–256. Morgan Kaufmann Publishers Inc. (1992)

Kittler, J.: Feature set search algorithms. Pattern recognition and signal processing 41, 60 (1978)

Liu, H., Motoda, H., Setiono, R.: Feature Selection: An Ever Evolving Frontier in Data Mining. Journal of Machine Learning Research: Workshop and Conference Proceedings 10, 10 (2010)

Mangasarian, O.L., Street, W.N., Wolberg, W.H.: Breast Cancer Diagnosis and Prognosis via Linear Programming, Mathematical Programming Technical Report (1994)

Quinlan, J.R.: C4. 5: programs for machine learning. Morgan Kaufmann (1993)

Raymer, M.L., Doom, T.E., Kuhn, L.A., Punch, W.L.: Knowledge Discovery in Medical and Biological Datasets Using a Hybrid Bayes Classifier/Evolutionary Algorithm. In: Proceedings of the IEEE 2nd International Symposium on Bioinformatics and Bioengineering Conference, pp. 236–245 (2001)

Saeys, Y., Inza, I., Larranaga, P.: A review of feature selection techniques in bioinformatics. Bioinformatics 23(19), 2507–2517 (2007)

Shannon, C.E.: A Mathematical Theory of Communication. The Bell System Technical Journal 27, 379–423, 623–656 (1948)

Smith, J.W., Everhart, J.E., Dickson, W.C., Knowler, W.C., Johannes, R.S.: Using the ADAP Learning Algorithm to Forecast the Onset of Diabetes Mellitus. In: Proc. Annu. Symp. Comput. Appl. Med. Care., vol. 9, pp. 261–265 (1988)

Taylor, J.R.: An Introduction to error analysis: The Study of uncertainties in physical measurements, 2nd edn. University Science Books, Sausalito (1996)

Wei, L., Altman, R.B.: An Automated System for Generating Comparative Disease Profiles and Making Diagnoses. IEEE Transactions on Neural Networks 15 (2004)

Witten, I.H., Frank, E.: Data Mining: Practical machine learning tools and techniques, 2nd edn. Morgan Kaufmann, San Francisco (2005)

Wolberg, W.H., Mangasarian, O.L.: Multisurface method of pattern separation for medical diagnosis applied to breast cytology. Proceedings of the National Academy of Sciences 87, 9193–9196 (1990)

Yoon, K.: The propagation of errors in multiple-attribute decision analysis: A practical approach. Journal of the Operational Research Society 40(7), 681–686 (1989)

Mining Correlated Patterns with Multiple Minimum All-Confidence Thresholds

R. Uday Kiran and Masaru Kitsuregawa

Institute of Industrial Science, The University of Tokyo, Komaba-ku, Tokyo, Japan
{uday_rage,kitsure}@tkl.iis.u-tokyo.ac.jp

Abstract. Correlated patterns are an important class of regularities that exist in a database. The *all-confidence* measure has been widely used to discover the patterns in real-world applications. This paper theoretically analyzes the all-confidence measure, and shows that, although the measure satisfies the null-invariant property, mining correlated patterns involving both frequent and rare items with a single minimum all-confidence (*minAllConf*) threshold value causes the "rare item problem" if the items' frequencies in a database vary widely. The problem involves either finding very short length correlated patterns involving rare items at a high *minAllConf* threshold, or generating a huge number of patterns at a low *minAllConf* threshold. The cause for the problem is that the single *minAllConf* threshold was not sufficient to capture the items' frequencies in a database effectively. The paper also introduces an alternative model of correlated patterns using the concept of multiple *minAllConf* thresholds. The proposed model facilitates the user to specify a different *minAllConf* threshold for each pattern to reflect the varied frequencies of items within it. Experiment results show that the proposed model is very effective.

Keywords: Knowledge discovery, frequent patterns, correlated patterns and *rare item problem*.

1 Introduction

1.1 Background and Related Work

Mining frequent patterns (or itemsets) [1] from transactional databases has been actively and widely studied in data mining. In the basic model, a pattern is said to be frequent if it satisfies the user-defined minimum support (*minSup*) threshold. The *minSup* threshold controls the minimum number of transactions that a pattern must cover in a transactional database. Since only a single *minSup* threshold is used for the entire database, the model implicitly assumes that all items within a database have uniform frequencies. However, this is often not the case in many real-world applications. In many applications, some items appear very frequently in the data, while others rarely appear. If the items' frequencies vary a great deal, mining frequent patterns with a single *minSup* threshold leads to the dilemma known as the *rare item problem* [2]. It involves either completely missing of frequent patterns involving rare items at a high *minSup* threshold or generating too many patterns at a low *minSup* threshold.

J. Li et al. (Eds.): PAKDD 2013 Workshops, LNAI 7867, pp. 295–306, 2013.

To confront the rare item problem in applications, alternative interestingness measures have been discussed in the literature [3,4]. Each measure has a selection bias that justifies the significance of a knowledge pattern. As a result, there exists no universally acceptable best measure to judge the interestingness of a pattern for any given dataset or application. Researchers are making efforts to suggest a right measure depending upon the user and/or application requirements [5,6,7].

Recently, *all-confidence* is emerging as a measure that can disclose true correlation relationships among the items within a pattern [8,9]. The two key reasons for its popular adoption are *anti-monotonic* and *null-invariant properties*. The former property facilitates in the reduction of search space as all non-empty subsets of a correlated pattern must also be correlated. The latter property facilitates to disclose genuine correlation relationships without being influenced by the object co-absence in a database. The basic model of correlated patterns is as follows [10].

Let $I = \{i_1, i_2, \cdots, i_n\}$ be a set of items, and DB be a database that consists of a set of transactions. Each transaction T contains a set of items such that $T \subseteq I$. Each transaction is associated with an identifier, called TID. Let $X \subseteq I$ be a set of items, referred as an itemset or a *pattern*. A pattern that contains k items is a k-pattern. A transaction T is said to contain X if and only if $X \subseteq T$. The support of a pattern X in DB, denoted as $S(X)$, is the number of transactions in DB containing X. The pattern X is said to be **frequent** if it occurs no less frequent than the user-defined minimum support (*minSup*) threshold, i.e., $S(X) \geq minSup$. The *all-confidence* of a pattern X, denoted as *all-conf(X)*, can be expressed as the ratio of its support to the maximum support of an item within it. That is, $all\text{-}conf(X) = \dfrac{S(X)}{max\{S(i_j)|\forall\, i_j \in X\}}$.

Definition 1. *(The correlated pattern X.) The pattern X is said to be* **all-confident** *or* associated *or* correlated *if*

$$S(X) \geq minSup$$

$$and$$

$$\frac{S(X)}{max(S(i_j)|\forall i_j \in X)} \geq minAllConf. \tag{1}$$

Where, *minAllConf* is the user-defined minimum all-confidence threshold value. The *minSup* threshold controls the minimum number of transactions a pattern must cover in a database. The *minAllConf* threshold controls the minimum number of transactions a pattern must cover with respect to its items' frequencies in a database.

Table 1. Transactional database

TID	ITEMS	TID	ITEMS	TID	ITEMS	TID	ITEMS	TID	ITEMS
1	a, b	5	c, d	9	c, d, g	13	a, b, e	17	c, d
2	a, b, e	6	a, c	10	a, b	14	b, e, f, g	18	a, c
3	c, d	7	a, b	11	a, b	15	c, d	19	a, b, h
4	e, f	8	e, f	12	a, c, f	16	a, b	20	c, d, f

Example 1. Consider the transactional database of 20 transactions shown in Table 1. The set of items $I = \{a, b, c, d, e, f, g, h\}$. The set of items a and b, i.e., $\{a, b\}$ is a pattern. It is a 2-pattern. For simplicity, we write this pattern as "ab". It occurs in 8 transactions (*tids* of $1, 2, 7, 10, 11, 13, 16$ and 19). Therefore, the support of "ab," i.e., $S(ab) = 8$. If the user-specified $minSup = 3$, then "ab" is a frequent pattern because $S(ab) \geq minSup$. The *all-confidence* of "ab", i.e., $all\text{-}conf(ab) = \frac{8}{max(11,9)} = 0.72$. If the user-specified $minAllConf = 0.63$, then "ab" is a correlated pattern because $S(ab) \geq minSup$ and $all\text{-}conf(ab) \geq minAllConf$.

1.2 Motivation

A pattern-growth algorithm known as CoMine has been proposed in [10] to discover the complete set of correlated patterns. We introduced the concept of items' support intervals and proposed an improved CoMine algorithm known as CoMine++ [11]. While testing the performance of our algorithm on various datasets, we have observed that although the null-invariant property of all-confidence facilitates the effective discovery of correlated patterns involving both frequent and rare items, the usage of a single $minAllConf$ threshold for the entire database confines the effective discovery of correlated patterns involving both frequent and rare items to the databases in which the items' frequencies do not vary widely. If the items' frequencies in the database vary widely, then mining correlated patterns with a single $minAllConf$ threshold can lead to the following problems:

– At a high $minAllConf$ threshold, many discovered correlated patterns involving rare items can have very short length. Most of them were singleton patterns as they always have $all\text{-}conf = 1$.
– In order to discover long correlated patterns involving rare items, we have to set low $minAllConf$ threshold. However, it causes combinatorial explosion producing too many correlated patterns.

We call this dilemma as the "rare item problem". In this paper, we analyze the all-confidence measure, introduce concepts to describe the problem and propose a generalized correlated pattern model to address the problem.

1.3 Contributions of This Paper

i. In this paper, we theoretically analyze the all-confidence measure and show that mining correlated patterns involving both frequent and rare items with a single $minAllConf$ leads to the *rare item problem*.
ii. We describe the reason for the problem by using the concepts known as *items' support intervals* and *cutoff-item-supports*.
iii. We also propose a technique to confront the problem. The technique is based on the notion of multiple constraints, where each pattern can satisfy a different $minAllConf$ value depending upon the frequencies of items within itself.
iv. By conducting experiments on various datasets, we show that the proposed technique can discover interesting correlated patterns involving both frequent and rare items without generating a huge number of meaningless correlated patterns.

1.4 Paper Organization

The rest of this paper is organized as follows. Section 2 introduces the rare item problem in the correlated pattern model. Section 3 describes the proposed model. Section 4 presents the experimental evaluations of basic and proposed models. Finally, Section 5 concludes the paper with future research directions.

2   The Rare Item Problem in Correlated Pattern Mining

In this section, we first introduce the concepts "items' support intervals" and "cutoff-item-support." These two concepts facilitate us to understand the problem, which is discussed subsequently.

2.1 Items' Support Intervals

The concept of *items' support intervals* was introduced in [11]. It says that every item can generate correlated patterns of higher-order by combining with only those items that have support within a specific interval. For the user-defined *minAllConf* and *minSup* thresholds, the support interval of an item $i_j \in I$ is

$$\left[max \left(\frac{S(i_j) \times minAllConf,}{minSup} \right), \ max \left(\frac{S(i_j)}{minAllConf}, \frac{}{minSup} \right) \right].$$ The correctness is given in

[11]. The support interval width of items plays a key role in correlated pattern mining. It defines the range of items' frequencies with which an item can combine to generate correlated patterns of higher-order.

Example 2. The support of f in Table 1 is 5. If $minAllConf = 0.63$ and $minSup = 3$, then the item 'f' can generate correlated patterns of higher order by combining with only those items that have support in the range of [3, 8] ($= [max(5 \times 0.63, 3), max(\frac{5}{0.63}, 3)]$).

If the support interval width of an item is large, then it can combine with wide range of items' supports to generate correlated patterns of higher order. If the support interval width of an item is relatively small, then it can combine with only a small range of items' supports to generate correlated patterns of higher order.

2.2 Cutoff-Item-Support

The concept of items' support intervals alone is not sufficient to describe the rare item problem. Therefore, we introduce another concept, called *cutoff-item-support*, to describe the problem. It is as follows.

From the definition of correlated pattern (see Equation 1), it turns out that if X is a correlated pattern, then

$$S(X) \geq max(max(S(i_j)|\forall i_j \in X) \times minAllConf, minSup) \tag{2}$$

Based on Equation 2, we introduce the following definition.

Definition 2. *(Cutoff-item-Support of an item.) The* cutoff-item-support *(CIS) for an item* $i_j \in I$, *denoted as* $CIS(i_j)$, *is the minimum support a pattern* $X \ni i_j$ *must have to be a correlated pattern. It is equal to the maximum of minSup and product between its support and minAllConf. That is,* $CIS(i_j) = max(minSup, S(i_j) \times minAllConf)$.

Example 3. The support of 'a' in Table 1 is 11. If the user-specified $minSup = 3$ and $minAllConf = 0.63$, then the CIS of 'a', denoted as $CIS(a) = 7$ ($\simeq max(3, 0.63 \times 11)$). It means any pattern containing 'a' must have support no less than 7 to be a correlated pattern. Similarly, the CIS values of 'b', 'c', 'd', 'e', 'f', 'g' and 'h' are 6, 6, 4, 3, 3, 3 and 3, respectively.

The CIS of an item plays a key role in correlated pattern mining. If the items have their CIS values very close to their supports, then it is difficult to expect long patterns containing those items (due to the apriori property [1]). If the items have their CIS values very far away from their supports, then it is possible to discover long patterns involving those items. However, this can cause combinatorial explosion, producing too many patterns as the items can combine with one another in all possible ways. Thus, while specifying the $minAllConf$ and $minSup$ thresholds, we have to take care that items' CIS values are neither too close nor too far away from their respective supports.

Definition 3. *(Redefinition of a correlated pattern using items' CIS values.) A pattern* X *is said to be correlated if its support is no less than the maximum CIS value of all its items. That is, if* X *is a correlated pattern satisfying the user-defined minSup and minAllConf thresholds, then* $S(X) \geq max(CIS(i_j)|\forall i_j \in X)$.

Since the CIS of an item $i_j \in X$, i.e., $CIS(i_j) = max(S(i_j) \times minAllConf, minSup)$, the correctness of the above definition is straight forward to prove from Equation 2.

2.3 The Problem

When we use a single $minAllConf$ threshold value to mine correlated patterns, then:

- The support interval width of items do not remain uniform. Instead it decreases from frequent items to (less frequent or) rare items (see Property 1). It is illustrated in Example 4.

  Example 4. In Table 1, the item 'a' appears more frequently than the item 'd'. If the user-defined $minSup = 3$ and $minAllConf = 0.63$, then the support intervals for 'a' and 'd' are $[7, 17]$ and $[6, 14]$, respectively. It can be observed that the support interval width of 'a' is 10, while for 'f' is only 8. Thus, the support interval decreases from frequent to rare items.

  Thus, the usage of a single $minAllConf$ threshold facilitates only the frequent items to combine with wide range of items' supports.

- The difference (or gap) between the items' support and corresponding CIS values do not remain uniform. Instead, it decreases from frequent to rare items (see Property 2).

Example 5. Continuing with Example 3, it can be observed that the difference between the *support* and corresponding *CIS* values of '*a*' and '*d*' are 4 and 2, respectively. Thus, the gap between the items' support and corresponding *CIS* values decreases from frequent to rare items.

Property 1. Let i_j and i_k, $1 \leq j \leq n$, $1 \leq k \leq n$ and $j \neq k$, be the items such that $S(i_j) \geq S(i_k)$. For the user-defined *minAllConf* and *minSup* thresholds, it turns out that the support interval width of i_j will be no less than the support interval width of i_k. That is,

$$max \left(\begin{array}{c} S(i_j) \times minAllConf, \\ minSup \end{array} \right) - max \left(\begin{array}{c} \dfrac{S(i_j)}{minAllConf}, \\ minSup \end{array} \right) \geq$$

$$max \left(\begin{array}{c} S(i_k) \times minAllConf, \\ minSup \end{array} \right) - max \left(\begin{array}{c} \dfrac{S(i_k)}{minAllConf}, \\ minSup \end{array} \right) \tag{3}$$

Property 2. Let i_p and i_q be the items having supports such that $S(i_p) \geq S(i_q)$. For the user-specified *minAllConf* and *minSup* thresholds, it turns out that $S(i_p) - CIS(i_p) \geq S(i_q) - CIS(i_q)$.

The non-uniform width of items' support intervals and the non-uniform gap between the items' support and corresponding *CIS* values causes the following problems while mining correlated patterns with a single *minAllConf* threshold:

   i. At a high *minAllConf* value, rare items will have *CIS* values very close (or almost equivalent) to their respective supports. In addition, the support interval width for rare items will be very small allowing only rare items to combine with one another. Since it is difficult for the rare items to combine with one another and have support which is almost equivalent to their actual support, many discovered rare correlated patterns may have very short length. We have observed that many correlated patterns involving rare items discovered at a high *minAllConf* threshold value were singleton patterns as they always have *all-conf* $= 1$.

  ii. To discover long correlated patterns involving rare items, we must specify a low *minAllConf* threshold value. However, a low *minAllConf* causes frequent items to have their *CIS* values far away from their respective supports causing combinatorial explosion and producing too many correlated patterns.

We call this dilemma as the *rare item problem*. In the next section, we discuss the technique to address the problem.

3   Proposed Model

To address the *rare item problem*, it is necessary for the correlated pattern model to simultaneously set high *minAllConf* threshold for a pattern containing frequent items and low *minAllConf* threshold for a pattern containing rare items. To do so, we exploit the notion of "multiple constraints" and introduce the model of mining correlated patterns using multiple minimum all-confidence thresholds. The idea is to specify *minAllConf* threshold for each item depending upon its frequency (or occurrence behavior in the database) and specify the *minAllConf* for a pattern accordingly. We inherit this approach from the multiple *minSups*-based frequent pattern mining, where each pattern can satisfy a different *minSup* depending upon the items' frequencies within itself [12].

In our proposed model, the definition of correlated pattern remains the same. However, the definition of *minAllConf* is changed to address the problem. In the proposed model, each item in the database is specified with a *minAllConf* constraint, called *minimum item all-confidence (MIAC)*. Next, *minAllConf* of the pattern $X = \{i_1, i_2, \cdots, i_k\}$, $1 \leq k \leq n$, is represented as maximum *MIAC* value among all its items. That is,

$$minAllConf(X) = max \begin{pmatrix} MIAC(i_1), \ MIAC(i_2), \\ \cdots, \qquad MIAC(i_k) \end{pmatrix} \qquad (4)$$

where, $MIAC(i_j)$ is the user-specified *MIAC* threshold for the item $i_j \in X$. Thus, the definition of correlated pattern is as follows.

Definition 4. *(Correlated pattern.) The pattern* $X = \{i_1, i_2, \cdots, i_k\}$, $1 \leq k \leq n$, *is said to be correlated if*

$$S(X) \geq minSup$$
$$and \qquad\qquad\qquad\qquad\qquad\qquad (5)$$
$$all\text{-}conf(X) \geq max \begin{pmatrix} MIAC(i_1), \ MIAC(i_2), \\ \cdots, \qquad MIAC(i_k) \end{pmatrix}$$

Please note that the correctness of *all-confidence* measure will be lost if *minAllConf* of a pattern is represented with the *minimal* *MIAC* of all the items within itself. In particular, if the items' *MIAC* values are converted into corresponding *CIS* values, then the above definition still preserves the definition of correlated pattern given in Definition 3.

Definition 5. *(Problem Definition.) Given the transactional database (DB), the minimum support (minSup) threshold and the items' minimum item all-confidence (MIAC) threshold values, discover the complete set of correlated patterns that satisfy the minSup and maximum MIAC value of all items within itself.*

The proposed model facilitates the user to specify the all-confidence thresholds such that the support interval width of items can be uniform and the gap between the items' supports and corresponding *CIS* values can also be uniform. In addition, it also allows the user to dynamically set high *minAllConf* value for the patterns containing frequent items and low *minAllConf* value for the patterns containing only rare items. As a result, this model can efficiently address the *rare item problem*. Moreover, the proposed model is the generalization of basic model to discover the patterns with all-confidence and support measures. If all items are specified with a same *MIAC* value, then the proposed model is same as the basic model of correlated pattern.

The correlated patterns discovered with the proposed model satisfy the *downward closure property*. That is, all non-empty subsets of a correlated pattern must also be correlated patterns. The correctness is based on Property 3 and shown in Lemma 1.

Property 3. If $Y \supset X$, then $minAllConf(Y) \geq minAllConf(X)$ as $max(MIAC(i_j)|\forall i_j \in Y) \geq max(MIAC(i_j)|\forall i_j \in X)$.

Lemma 1. *The correlated patterns discovered with the proposed model satisfy the downward closure property.*

Proof. Let X and Y be the two patterns in a transactional database such that $X \subset Y$. From the *apriori property* [1], it turns out that $S(X) \geq S(Y)$ and *all-conf*$(X) \geq$ *all-conf*(Y). Further, $minAllConf(Y) \geq minAllConf(X)$ (see, Property 3). Therefore, if *all-conf*$(Y) \geq minAllConf(Y)$, then *all-conf*$(X) \geq minAllConf(X)$.

Pei et al. [13] have proposed a generalized pattern-growth algorithm known as FIC^A (Mining frequent itemsets with convertible anti-monotone constraint) to discover patterns if they satisfy downward closure property. Since the patterns discovered with the proposed model satisfy the downward closure property, FIC^A algorithm can be extended to mine correlated patterns with the proposed model.

4 Experimental Results

In this section, we evaluate the basic and proposed models of correlated patterns. We show that proposed model allows us to find correlated patterns involving rare items without generating a huge number of meaningless correlated patterns with frequent items.

Since the FIC^A algorithm discussed in [13] can discover the complete set of patterns for any measure that satisfies the downward closure property, we extend it to discover correlated patterns with either single *minAllConf* or multiple *minAllConf* thresholds. We do not report the performance of FIC^A algorithm. They are available at [13].

4.1 Experimental Setup

The FIC^A algorithm was written in GNU C++ and run with Ubuntu 10.04 operating system on a 2.66 GHz machine with 1GB memory. The runtime specifies the total execution time, i.e., CPU and I/Os. We pursued experiments on synthetic (T10I4D100K) and real-world (Retail [14] and BMS-WebView-2 [15]) datasets. The T10I4D100K dataset contains 100,000 transactions with 870 items. The Retail dataset contains 88,162 transactions with 16,470 items. The BMS-WebView-2 dataset contains 77,512 transactions with 33,401 items. All of these datasets are sparse datasets with widely varying items' frequencies.

4.2 A Method to Specify Items' *MIAC* Values

For our experiments, we need a method to assign *MIAC* values to items in a dataset. Since the non-uniform difference (or gap) between the items' support and *CIS* values is cause of *rare item problem*, we employ a method that specifies items' *MIAC* values such that there exists a uniform gap between the items' *support* and *CIS* values. It is as follows.

Let δ be the representative (e.g. mean, median, mode) support of all items in the database. Choosing a *minAllConf* value, calculate the gap between support and corresponding *CIS* values (see Equation 6). We call the gap as "support difference" and is denoted as *SD*.

$$SD = \delta - \delta \times minAllConf$$
$$= \delta \times (1 - minAllConf) \qquad (6)$$

Next, we specify *MIAC* values for other items such that the gap (or *SD*) remains constant. The methodology to specify *MIAC* values to the items $i_j \in I$ is shown in Equation 7.

$$MIAC(i_j) = max\left(\left(1 - \frac{SD}{S(i_j)}\right), LMAC\right) \qquad (7)$$

Where, *LMAC* is the user-defined lowest *MIAC* value an item can have. It is particularly necessary as $\left(1 - \frac{SD}{S(i_j)}\right)$ can give negative *MIAC* value for an item i_j if $SD > S(i_j)$.

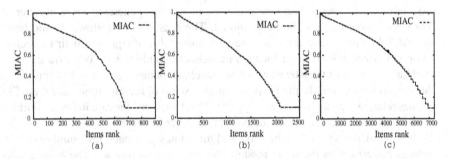

Fig. 1. The items' *MIAC* values in different datasets. (a) T10I4D100k dataset (b) BMS-WebView-2 dataset and (c) Retail dataset.

Fig. 1(a), (b) and (c) respectively shows the *MIAC* values specified by the proposed model in *T10I4D100K*, *BMS-WebView-2* and *Retail* datasets with *minAllConf* = 0.9, *LMAC* = 0.1 and δ representing the mean support of frequent items. The X-axis represents the rank of items provided in the descending order of their support values. The Y-axis represents the *MIAC* values of items. It can be observed that the *MIAC* values decreases as we move from frequent to less frequent (or rare) items. The low *MIAC* values for rare items facilitate them to combine with other items and generate correlated patterns. The high *MIAC* values of frequent items will prevent them from combining with one another in all possible ways and generating huge number of uninteresting patterns.

4.3   Performance Results

Fig. 2(a), (b) and (c) respectively shows the number of correlated patterns generated in the basic model and proposed model of correlated patterns in T10I4D100K, BMS-WebView-2 and Retail datasets. The X-axis represents the *minAllConf* values that are varied from

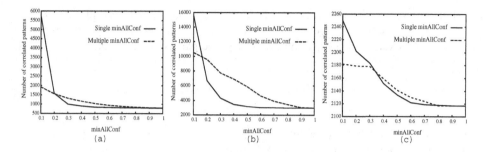

Fig. 2. Generation of Correlated patterns in different datasets. (a) T10I4D100k dataset (b) BMS-WebView-2 dataset and (c) Retail datasets.

0.1 to 1. The Y-axis represents the number of correlated patterns discovered at different *minAllConf* values. Too many correlated patterns were discovered in both models when *minAllConf* = 0. For convenience, we are not showing the correlated patterns discovered at *minAllConf* = 0. The following observations can be drawn from these two graphs:

i. At high *minAllConf* values, the proposed model has generated more number of correlated patterns than the basic model. The reason is as follows. In the basic model, *CIS* values of rare items were very close (almost equal) to their respective supports. Since it is difficult for the rare items to combine with other (rare) items and have support as their own, very few correlated patterns pertaining to rare items have been discovered. In the proposed model, some of the rare items had their *CIS* values relatively away from their supports. This facilitated the rare items to combine with other rare items and generate correlated patterns.

ii. At low *minAllConf* values, the proposed model has generated less number of correlated patterns than the basic model. The reason is as follows. The basic model has specified low *CIS* values for the frequent items at low *minAllConf*. The low *CIS* values of the frequent items facilitated them to combine with one another in all possible ways and generate too many correlated patterns. In the proposed model, the *CIS* values for the frequent items were not very far away from their respective supports (as compared with basic model). As a result, the proposed model was able to prevent frequent items to combine with one another in all possible ways and generate too many correlated patterns.

4.4 A Case Study Using BMS-WebView-2 Dataset

In this study, we show how the proposed model allows the user to find correlated patterns containing rare items without generating a huge number of meaningless correlated patterns with frequent items. Due to page limitations, we confine our discussion only to BMS-WebView-2 dataset. Similar observations were also drawn from the other datasets.

Fig. 3 (a) shows the *CIS* values specified for the items by the basic model. The following observations can be drawn from this figure. (*i*) The gap between the support and CIS values of items decreases as we move from frequent to rare items, irrespective of the *minAllConf* threshold value. (*ii*) At a high *minAllConf* value, rare items have the

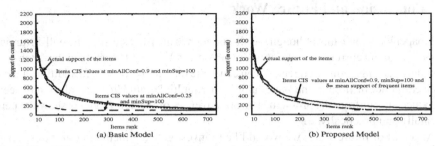

Fig. 3. The *CIS* values specified for the items by both the models. The *minSup* is expressed in support count.

CIS values very close (or almost equivalent) to their respective supports. (*iii*) Choosing a low *minAllConf* value facilitates rare items to have *CIS* values relatively away from their supports. However, it causes frequent items to have their *CIS* values far away from their supports, which can cause combinatorial explosion.

Fig. 3 (b) shows the *CIS* values specified for items by the proposed model. It can be observed that by using item specific *minAllConf* values, appropriate gap between the *support* and *CIS* values of items can be maintained irrespective of their frequencies.

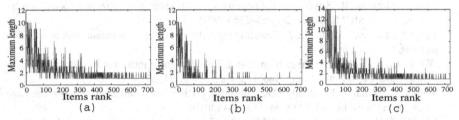

Fig. 4. Maximum length of the items in BMS-WebView-2 dataset. (a) Proposed model with high all-confidence threshold value. (b) Basic model with high all-confidence threshold value. (c) Basic model with low all-confidence threshold value.

Fig. 4(a) shows the maximum length of a correlated patten formed for each frequent item in the proposed model with $minSup = 100$ (in support count), $minAllConf = 0.9$ and δ representing the mean of frequent items. Fig. 4(b) provides the same information for the basic model with $minSup = 100$ and $minAllConf = 0.9$. In the basic model, majority of the rare items (i.e., items having rank greater than 400) had the maximal length of 1. In other words, correlated patterns involving rare items were only singleton patterns. In our proposed model, maximal length of correlated patterns involving rare items ranged from 1 to 4. This shows that the proposed model has facilitated the generation of correlated patterns containing both frequent and rare items at high *minAllConf* value.

At $minAllConf = 0.4$, the basic model has also facilitated the generation of correlated patterns containing rare items. However, the usage of low *minAllConf* threshold has caused combinatorial explosion producing too many correlated patterns. In Fig. 4(c), the increased maximal length of frequent items (i.e., items having rank from 1 to 100) from 10 (at $minAllConf = 0.9$) to 14 (at $minAllConf = 0.4$) signifies the combinatorial explosion in which frequent items have combined with one another in many possible ways.

5 Conclusion and Future Work

This paper has shown that although the all-confidence measure satisfies the null-invariant property, mining correlated patterns with a single *minAllConf* threshold in the databases of widely varying items' frequencies can cause the rare item problem. In addition, a generalized model of mining the patterns with the multiple *minAllConf* values has been introduced to confront the problem. The effectiveness of the new model is shown experimentally and practically.

As a part of future work, we would like to investigate the methodologies to specify items *MIAC* values. It is also interesting to investigate efficient mining of closed and maximal correlated patterns with the proposed model.

References

1. Agrawal, R., Imieliński, T., Swami, A.: Mining association rules between sets of items in large databases. In: SIGMOD, pp. 207–216 (1993)
2. Weiss, G.M.: Mining with rarity: a unifying framework. ACM SIGKDD Explorations Newsletter 6(1), 7–19 (2004)
3. Omiecinski, E.R.: Alternative interest measures for mining associations in databases. IEEE Trans. on Knowl. and Data Eng. 15, 57–69 (2003)
4. Brin, S., Motwani, R., Silverstein, C.: Beyond market baskets: generalizing association rules to correlations. SIGMOD Rec. 26, 265–276 (1997)
5. Tan, P.N., Kumar, V., Srivasta, J.: Selecting the right interestingness measure for association patterns. In: KDD, pp. 32–41 (2002)
6. Wu, T., Chen, Y., Han, J.: Re-examination of interestingness measures in pattern mining: a unified framework. Data Mining Knolwedge Discovery 21, 371–397 (2010)
7. Surana, A., Kiran, R.U., Reddy, P.K.: Selecting a Right Interestingness Measure for Rare Association Rules. In: COMAD, pp. 115–124 (2010)
8. Kim, W.-Y., Lee, Y.-K., Han, J.: CCMine: Efficient mining of confidence-closed correlated patterns. In: Dai, H., Srikant, R., Zhang, C. (eds.) PAKDD 2004. LNCS (LNAI), vol. 3056, pp. 569–579. Springer, Heidelberg (2004)
9. Kim, S., Barsky, M., Han, J.: Efficient mining of top correlated patterns based on null-invariant measures. In: Gunopulos, D., Hofmann, T., Malerba, D., Vazirgiannis, M. (eds.) ECML PKDD 2011, Part II. LNCS, vol. 6912, pp. 177–192. Springer, Heidelberg (2011)
10. Lee, Y.K., Kim, W.Y., Cao, D., Han, J.: CoMine: efficient mining of correlated patterns. In: ICDM, pp. 581–584 (2003)
11. Uday Kiran, R., Kitsuregawa, M.: Efficient Discovery of Correlated Patterns in Transactional Databases Using Items' Support Intervals. In: Liddle, S.W., Schewe, K.-D., Tjoa, A.M., Zhou, X. (eds.) DEXA 2012, Part I. LNCS, vol. 7446, pp. 234–248. Springer, Heidelberg (2012)
12. Liu, B., Hsu, W., Ma, Y.: Mining association rules with multiple minimum supports. In: KDD, pp. 337–341 (1999)
13. Pei, J., Han, J., Lakshmanan, L.V.: Pushing convertible constraints in frequent itemset mining. Data Mining and Knowledge Discovery 8, 227–251 (2004)
14. Brijs, T., Goethals, B., Swinnen, G., Vanhoof, K., Wets, G.: A data mining framework for optimal product selection in retail supermarket data: the generalized PROFSET model. In: KDD, pp. 300–304 (2000)
15. Zheng, Z., Kohavi, R., Mason, L.: Real world performance of association rule algorithms. In: KDD, pp. 401–406 (2001)

A Novel Proposal for Outlier Detection in High Dimensional Space

Zhana Bao and Wataru Kameyama

Graduate School of Global Information and Telecommunication Studies,
Waseda University, Japan

Abstract. Finding rare information behind big data is important and meaningful for outlier detection. However, to find such rare information is extremely difficult when the notorious curse of dimensionality exists in high dimensional space. Most of existing methods fail to obtain good result since the Euclidean distance cannot work well in high dimensional space. In this paper, we first perform a grid division of data for each attribute, and compare the density ratio for every point in each dimension. We then project the points of the same area to other dimensions, and then we calculate the disperse extent with defined cluster density value. At last, we sum up all weight values for each point in two-step calculations. After the process, outliers are those points scoring the largest weight. The experimental results show that the proposed algorithm can achieve high precision and recall on the synthetic datasets with the dimension varying from 100 to 10000.

Keywords: Outlier score, High dimension, Dimensional projection.

1 Introduction

With the advent of the Internet and social networks in the last decades, the enormous volumes of data are emerging. The ever-increasing data have drawn a great challenge on mining the valuable information, especially for some data that are scarcely appearing but contain extremely important knowledge. One of the major tasks is how to detect outliers in high dimensional data space. On this issue, many researchers have given various definitions on outlier based on supervised learning, clustering, particular pattern, etc. Most cited definition is Hawkins: an outlier is an observation that deviates so much from other observations as to arouse suspicion that it was generated by a different mechanism [1]. This definition is also applied in high dimensional space by detecting the suspicious points which deviate farther from the rest of points based on some measures such as distance, density in some subspaces. The ever-proposed outlier detection methods focus on low dimensional space and make great achievements. But these methods do not work effectively in high dimensional space since it is difficult to evaluate the data distribution when the dimension is very high.

In this paper, we present a new algorithm, which calculates points density ratio in each dimension, and evaluate the disperse extent of the points when they are

J. Li et al. (Eds.): PAKDD 2013 Workshops, LNAI 7867, pp. 307–318, 2013.
© Springer-Verlag Berlin Heidelberg 2013

projected to other dimensions iteratively. The major features and achievements of this algorithm are summarized as follows:

- We construct the subspace with equal-width grid, which is similar with ever-proposed subspace-based methods. We improved it with verification in different crossing dimensions. So our proposal can detect the outliers that cannot be found in low dimensional subspaces.

- We take the points in the same area as reference objects, then project these points from its dimension to other dimensions, and then measure the disperse extent of those points. Each point is denoted by its weight values, which gets m weights in the first projected-dimensional subspace and gets m×(m-1) weights in the second projected-dimensional space. The points scoring the highest weight are most likely outliers.

In our proposal, every calculation process is limited to two dimensions, so it avoids the calculation with high dimensions. Therefore, the curse of dimensionality problem does not happen. Unlike ever-proposed algorithms such as the dimension reduction and the subspace detection, the data information does not lose in our algorithm.

This paper is organized as follows. In section 2, we give a brief overview of related works on high dimensional outlier detection. In section 3, we introduce our concept, calculation method and describe the algorithm. In section 4, we evaluate the proposed method by experiments of different dimensional data. And we conclude in section 5.

2   Related Works

For the past ten years, many studies on outlier detection have been conducted for large datasets. We categorize them into the following four groups.

The methods in the first group are based on the measurement of distance or density as used in the traditional outlier detections in low dimension. The most used method is based on local density-LOF [2]. It cites the MinPts-nearest neighbor concept to detect outliers. The normal points values are approximately to the mean value of neighbor's and the ratio is to 1. Therefore, the points whose ratio are obviously larger than 1 or some top largest-value points are outliers. The LOF works well in a low dimensions and is still practical in high dimensions.

The second group is based on the subspace clustering method. Some high dimensional outliers also seem to deviate from others in low dimensions. The outlier points can be regarded as byproducts of clustering methods. The Aggarwals method [3] belongs to this group. He uses the equi-depth ranges in each dimension, with expected fraction and deviation of points in k-dimensional cube D given by $N \times f^k$ and $\sqrt{N \times f^k \times (1 - f^k)}$. This method detects outliers by calculating the sparsity of coefficient S(D).

The third group is the outlier detection with dimension deduction, such as SOM(Self-Organizing Map) [9], mapping high dimensions to two dimensions,

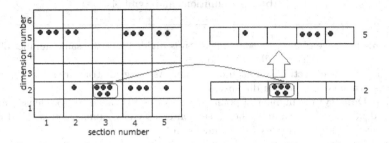

Fig. 1. Space Division and Dimension Projection

then detecting the outliers in two dimensional space. This method may cause information lost when the dimension deducts. Thus, it is only used in some special dataset.

The forth group includes other methods. ABOD (Angel-Based Outlier Detection) [4] is an algorithm with globe method. It is based on the concept of angle vector product and scalar product. The outliers have the small angles since they are far from other points. Another algorithm is called RIC (Robust Information-theoretic Clustering) [5], which uses integer coding points in each dimension, then detects cluster with MDL (Minimum Description Length). Other algorithms such as kernel-based [10] and direct density ratio[5] are also presented to solve this issue.

From above, it can be said that the most measurements on outlier detection are based on distance or density. The good aspect is that the concept is easy to realize. The bad aspect is the occurrence of high dimensional curse. The most of the methods try to mitigate the curse of dimensional effects by subspace clustering. But the main trap into which we fall is to blindly apply concepts that are valid in normal two or three dimensional space to high dimensional one. One example is the use of the Euclidean distance which behaves poorly in high dimension. Therefore, we need to find a novel approach in different view in order to avoid the curse of high dimensions.

3   Proposed Mehtod

3.1   General Idea

For the purpose of data analysis in an intuitive way, the dataset is always mapped to a set of points in a certain dimensional space. Each observation is considered as a data point and each attribute associated with it is considered as a dimension. Thus the set of attributes of the dataset constitutes a dimensional space. Our proposed method is also based on a data points space.

After reviewing the ever-proposed methods, we have found that the key question is to utilize the dimensions as more as possible and to avoid the high dimensional problem at same time. By contrasting the distribution between normal

Table 1. Definitions and Symbols

Section: the range of data in each dimension is divided into the same number of equi-width parts, which is called a section.

scn: the number of sections for each dimension. As the grid structure shown in Fig. 1, scn is defined equal in each dimension.

Section Density: the number of points in one section is called section density and **Sec** or **d** in short. For example, the jth section density of ith dimension is called $\mathbf{d}_{i,j}$.

$\mathbf{d}_i$: the average section density in i^{th} dimension.

asd: the assumed average section density in each dimension. It is given as parameter and is decided by number of total points and **scn**.

Section Cluster: the continuous sections, which have points in, are called a section cluster, a cluster in short.

CluLen: the length of a **section cluster**. It is measured by the number of sections in a section cluster, see Equation (2).

SecDR: the ratio of section density against the average section density in one dimension. SecDR is defined by Equation(1). SecCDR is defined by Equation(2).

PtDR: the points value is equal to **SecDR** which the point belongs. The points in a section share the same **SecDR**. **PtDR** corresponds to **SecDR**. **PtCDR** corresponds to **SecCDR**.

SI: the statistic information of each point defined by Eqution(3).

---

points and outliers, it is found that normal points are frequently clustered together in all dimensions, while outliers seem deviated from normal points in some dimensions or clustered with different points in respective dimensions. Inspired by this feature, we design an approach to detect outliers under different cases through two-step dimensions projections.

Since the data distributions vary in different dimensions, it is difficult to compare all points distributions in general data space. In this paper, we take the points of a small region in one dimension for analysis, and evaluate their distribution changes in other dimensions. For this purpose, the data ranges are divided into the same amount of equal width parts in each dimension. The each part is called a section that contains data points. The data space looks like a big cube with lots of small cubes inside in the case of three-dimensional space. What the real data space looks like can be ignored in this method. We focus on the points in each projected dimensions and distribution change of those points between different dimensions. The new data space is similar to a grid as shown in Fig. 1. In this example, the ten points have different distributions in dimension 2 and dimension 5, it is hard to find which point is outlier. We observe the distribution change of five points in the 3rd section of dimension 2. After the projection from dimension 2 to dimension 5, a point in the 2nd section of dimension 5 is far from other points in the 4th and the 5th sections. In this case, the hidden outlier in dimension 2 can be detected. To sum up, the conventional relationship between points and dimensions are replaced with the new relationship between points, dimensions and sections. The original data is decomposed into the point information and the section information.

3.2   Definitions and Data Structures

To clarify the proposed method, we introduce some definitions and symbols, as shown in Table 1.

The section definition is similar to Aggarwals fraction [3], it is also called cell [7] or grid [8]. The difference is that the points of section are not only used for density ratio calculation, but also are used for dimension projection. It is also different from ever-proposed two-four dimensional cell subspace; the section only divides the range in one-dimensional subspace.

Next, the *scn* is same in each dimension. Since the data ranges are different in different dimensions, it is difficult to compare densities for different dimensions. Then we decided to use the same *scn* in each dimension. The range in each dimension is a product of section width and *scn*, and *asd* is only decided by total points and *scn*. Therefore, the density of points in different dimensions has the same standard evaluation.

3.3   Projected Section Density

Different from the ever-proposed methods whose calculations focus on the points, all the calculations are based on the sections instead of points in our proposal. Then, points become a connection between different dimensions. Therefore, hereafter we refer our proposed method to Projected Section Density method, or PSD in short.

Our proposal divides into three parts: calculate *PtDR* with section density ratio in each dimension, calculate *PtCDR* with cluster-section density ratio in projected dimensions, and sum up all related weights of each point to one score.

Step 1: Detecting Outliers in Each Dimension. Detecting outliers in each dimension is similar with ever-proposed subspace algorithms. Here, we use *PtDR* to detect whether the points are sparse in each dimension. The *PtDR* is the ratio of section density against average section density in one dimension, defined as below:

$$PtDR(p_{i,j}) \Leftarrow SecDR(p_{i,j}) = \frac{d_{i,j}}{d_i} . \tag{1}$$

Where d_i refers to the average density of sections in i^{th} dimension, whose value is obtained from the total number of points divided by the number of sections. $d_{i,j}$ refers to the jth section density where the points $p_{i,j}$ is.

The d_i is different in each dimension. We considered the special case, most of points are only clustered in several sections and have not points in other sections in some dimensions. The average density becomes very low when taking all the sections with points and without points. In that case, the outliers density is close to average low density and get higher density ratio in these dimensions. This high ratio will affect the weight in each dimension and even cover the outliers in worst case. Therefore, we only count the sections with points regardless the sections without points. The *SecDR* result denote to *PtDR*. Then, the point with small *PtDR* is more likely to be an outlier.

Step 2: Detecting Outliers in Crossing Dimensions. When outliers are mixed with normal points in some dimension, they seem normal too. The subspace-based detection methods are hard to detect such outliers. To solve this issue, the dimension projection is proposed.

We project one section's points from its dimension to other dimensions, and compare the points disperse extent in the projected dimension. The points of a section usually do not clustered into one section after projecting them to other dimensions. Nevertheless, normal points are still distributed in nearby continuous sections. Therefore, section-cluster concept is introduced to express these normal cluster points. The outliers are the points far from the normal cluster points or on the edge of very big cluster. Therefore, the outliers are always sparser than other points after projected to other dimensions. The sparse calculations of each point in crossing dimensions is defined as below:

$$PtCDR(p_{i \to k,j}) \Leftarrow SecCDR(p_{i,j}, k) = \frac{Sec(p_{k,j}) \times CluLen_j}{\frac{1}{s} \sum_{f=1}^{s} Sec(p_{k,f}) \times CluLen_f} . \qquad (2)$$

Where CluLen is the cluster length, i.e. range of continuous sections, $Sec(p_{k,j})$ is the density that the points of jth section are projected in k^{th} dimension, and the product of Sec and $CluLen$ with average denote cluster-section density. Then $SecCDR$ is calculated and denote $PtCDR$ of corresponding points. Then outlier's $PtCDR$ are always small.

Step 3: Statistic Information for Each Points Weights. After two steps above, we have total $m+m \times (m-1)$ weight values for each point. Then a statistic formula is used to summarize the point's weights by Equation (3).

$$SI(p_j) = \frac{2 \times m}{\sum_{i=1}^{m} (PtDR[i,j]^2 + \frac{1}{m-1} \times \sum_{k=1}^{m-1} PtCDR[k,j]^2)} . \qquad (3)$$

Where m is the number of dimensions, $PtDR$ is the points weight that is corresponding to $SecDR$ in Equation (1), $PtCDR$ is the points weight correspoding to $SecCDR$ in Equation (2) and $SI(p_j)$ is the statistic information value of p_j. The points whose SI values are much larger than other points are regarded as outliers.

3.4   Algorithm

The detail algorithm is is written in pseudo R code, where the dataset contains n points with m dimensions; and K is the number of outliers . As input parameter, either scn or asd is feasible. In our experiment, asd is choosed as input parameter, and the scn is calculated by the total points divided by asd. we construct the matrix $PointInfo$ and the matrix $SectionInfo$ to record information about point, dimension and section during the calculation. When the projected dimension is processing, the $Ptsecid$ is cited to record the temporary section ID of point in order to build section connection between the points dimension and the projected dimension.

Projected Section Density

```
Input: data[n,m], scn or asd
Output: top K largest SI values from n points
Initialize(PointInfo, SectionInfo)
for i =1 to m do
  di =n/length(SectionInfo[i,]!=0)
  for j =1 to n do
    Get PtDR[i,j] with Equation (1)
  end for
endfor
for k =1 to m do
  Random dimension order
  for i =1 to m do
  for j =1 to n do
    Ptsecid= PointInfo[i,j]
    SecID = PointInfo[i+1, PointInfo[i,]=Ptsecid]
    Get CluLen by counting continuous sections Get SecCDR with Equation(2)
    Get PtCDR from SecCDR
  end for
  end for
end for
Get SI value with Equation(3) for each point
```

From the three-step calculation formulation and the algortihms, the Time complexity of the algorithm is calculated as $O(n \times m^2)$, and the Space complexity is $O(3 \times m \times n)$.

4 Evaluation

In this section, we investigate whether our proposed algotithms can provide a good performance in experiments. We firstly perform experiments on two dimensional data set in Section 4.1, and then we evaluate the performance on high dimensional data set in Section 4.2. Finally, in Section 4.3 we present our analysis on the experimental results. All the experiments were performed on Mac Book Pro with 2.53GHz Intel core 2 CPU and 4G memory. The algorithm is implemented with R language on Mac OS.

We usually need some data such as experimental data or real data to evaluate the proposed method. However, it is difficult to know which data are exact outliers and how the noise data affect the result when real data are used, especially in more than 100 dimensional data. Therefore, we generate a series of synthetic data to evaluate our proposed algorithm. The synthetic data which include outliers and normal points are generated according to Hawkins definition: the outliers belong to a different mechanism other than majority points.

The data are generated respectively in two distributions in Section 4.1 and Section 4.2. Precision, recall and F-measure are used to evaluate and compare the proposed method with others.

4.1   Two-Dimensional Data Experiment

In the two-dimensional experiment, we generate 43 points, which include 40 normal points and 3 outliers, as shown in Figure 2. Among these normal points, 20 points are randomly distributed in a cluster, and 20 points are randomly distributed in another cluster. The 3 points are defined as outliers since they do not belong to any clusters. The data is designed to test our method in two different cases. Two kinds of outliers are shown in Fig. 2, two points are only separated in one cluster in one dimension, they are still far from normal points in 2 dimensional spaces. The last point is far from normal points in all 2 dimensions.

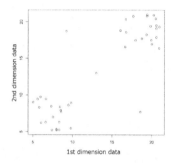

Fig. 2. 2-Dimensional Data Sample

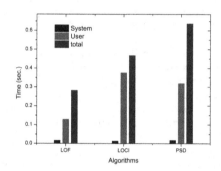

Fig. 3. Three Algorithms's Running Time

For better evaluating experimental result, we compared our proposal with the state-of-the-art algorithm LOF [2] and LOCI [6]. In this experiment, all the three algorithms got the perfect result with 100% precision and 100% recall. We also compare the processing time. R enviroment shows three processing time: system time, user time and total time. The user time is main index. From the Fig. 3, the LOF is the fastest algorithm; LOCI's user time expenses more than our proposal. But the total time is shorter than our proposal. In the experiment, our proposal method can detect the two kinds of outliers, and the accuracy is as same as conventional methods.

4.2   High Dimension Experiment

We generate 8 experimental data sets with 10-10000 dimensions, where data size is 500 or 1000. The generated experimental datasets refer to Hawkinsoutlier definition [1] and Kriegels dataset model [4]. The experimental data set includes normal data with a Gaussian mixture model consisting of five equally weighted Normal distributions, whose mean are randomly ranged from 20 to 80 and whose variance values are randomly ranged from 5 to 20. The experimental data set also includes 10 outliers with random distribution inside normal points, whose range are randomly from 20 to 80.

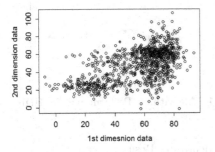
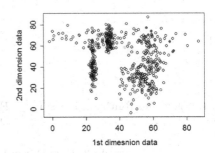

Fig. 4. Dimension Distribution of 500 Points with 10 Dimension

Fig. 5. Dimension Distribution of 1000 Points with 10000 Dimension

Fig. 4 and Fig. 5 show the two samples of high dimensional datasets. Fig. 4 shows the two-dimensional distribution of dataset No.1 having 500 points with 10 dimensions. Fig. 5 shows the two-dimensional distribution of dataset No.8 having 1000 points with 10000 dimensions. After examining points in the two figures, outliers that are labelled red can not be found in two dimensions, while some normal points appear more deviated than real outliers.

In the next step, we also choose the LOF and LOCI algorithms to detect outliers and compare our proposed algorithm to evaluate the efficiency. Nevertheless, LOCI has not got good results in the experiments. The best result is shown with LOCI in 1000 points and 100 dimensions dataset, which the Precision is 20% and Recall is 25%. In other datasets experiment, the LOCI got no outliers or false outliers. Therefore, we only compare our proposal with LOF algorithm. First, we set the parameters for both algorithms. In our proposed algorithm, we set *asd* 20 to 500 points and *asd* 30 to 1000 points; in LOF algorithm, we set *MinPts* 5-10 to the number of k nearest neighbours. Next, we compare the time expense with LOF. As shown in Fig. 6, the LOF algorithm is faster than our algorithm, because the LOF algorithm only considers the distance between points, regardless dimensions; while our proposal considers the both dimension and points. Therefore, our proposal spends more time on projected dimension computation.

Next important part, the Precision, Recall and F-measure are recorded to compare with LOF algorithm in eight experiment results. In Table 2, only the highest F-measures values are selected to contrast. In order to separates outliers from normal points, the suitable value is chosen as a threshold between normal points and outliers. LOF algorithm can find outliers around 100 dimensions, though the precision is only 95.24%. When the dimensions increase to 500, LOF almost gets no outliers. As a contrast, our proposed algorithm performs

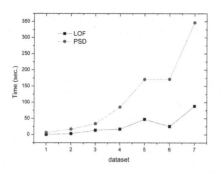
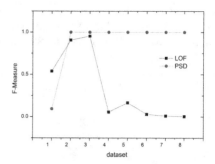

Fig. 6. Algorithms Run Time in High Dimensions

Fig. 7. Algorithms Performance in High Dimensions

Table 2. High Dimension Algorithms Result

ID	Dimension	Point	LOF				PSD			
			Threshold	Precision	Recall	F-measure	Threshold	Precision	Recall	F-measure
1	10	500	1.5100	0.7	0.5000	0.5833	0.7	0.7000	0.0496	0.0927152
2	100	500	1.2200	0.8	0.8889	0.8421	0.4	0.8000	1.0000	0.8888889
3	100	1000	1.2100	1.0	0.9091	0.9524	0.34	1.0000	1.0000	1
4	500	500	1.1200	0.1	1.0000	0.1818	0.49	1.0000	1.0000	1
5	500	1000	1.2700	0.1	1.0000	0.1818	0.4	1.0000	1.0000	1
6	1000	500	0.9964	0.1	1.0000	0.1818	0.5	1.0000	1.0000	1
7	1000	1000	1.0000	1.0	0.0105	0.0208	0.4	1.0000	1.0000	1
8	10000	1000	0.9993	0.8	0.0976	0.1740	0.4	1.0000	1.0000	1

well when the dimension is increasing. Once the dimensions are up to 100, the precision is almost 100%. For both algorithms, their precisions raise when the number of points increases. As a conclusion, our proposed algorithm performs better than LOF in high dimensional space, not only in the precision and the recall, but also more stable when the dimension increases.

The results are clearly shown in Fig. 7. The LOF algorithm produces poorer result in all dimensional data sets. Though the LOF get better result in10 dimensions compared with PSD, the F-measure value is still below 55%. In fact, both algorithms perform badly in 10 dimensions. The reason why our proposal fails to find outliers in 10 dimensions is our strict definition about the outliers. While with the dimension increasing, our algorithm performs better and keep 100% F-measure above 100 dimensions. The results conclusively indicate that our proposal succeeds in detecting the outliers only if they have different distribution with normal points.

4.3   Real Data Set

In this subsection, we compare these algorithms with a real world dataset publicly available at the UCI machine learning repository [11]. We use Arcene dataset that is provided by ARCENE group. The task of the group is to distinguish cancer versus normal patterns from mass-spectrometric data. This is a two-class classification problem with continuous input variables.

The original dataset includes total 900 instances with 10000 attributes. Each subdataset is labelled with positive and negative except for test dataset. The test dataset contains 700 instances, 310 positive and 390 negative instances. The best_SVM_result is available at [12]. The 308 instances are labelled with positive, and the 392 instances are labelled with negative.

In the experiment, we retrieved 392 negative instances, and we apply three algorithms to detect two true positive instances miss-clarified by SVM. As seen in Table 3 showing the results, point IDs of 29 and 182 are the most probably outliers by the intersection of LOF and PSD results. It is noted that the both points appear in the top three detected points of the both results. If we consider the LOCI result, the intersections point ID is 153 and 175, which is entirely different from PSD. Nevertheless, contrast with former results, the first conclusion seems more reasonable.

Table 3. Top 5 Points Detected in Arcane Data

No.	LOF		PSD		LOCI
	SI	PtID	SI	PtID	PtID
1	1.477314	182	0.05711392	29	153
2	1.364228	175	0.05643270	318	175
3	1.347864	29	0.0540054	182	195
4	1.321561	153	0.05281425	215	
5	1.317432	360	0.05047134	234	

5   Conclusion

In this paper, we propose a new algorithm for outlier detection in high dimensional space. The proposed algorithm not only works smoothly in low dimension, but also runs more effectively than LOF in high dimensions, e.g. 10000 dimensions. In another word, the high dimension curse problem has been avoided in our proposed algorithm. Moreover, our proposed solution has provided a general framework to solve the similar high dimension problems. So many existed methods or new methods can be applied under this framework.

Note that our proposed algorithm is composed of the two steps to detect outliers, in each dimension and in each projected dimension respectively. We apply the equal weight to the two steps. However, the best weighting values to these steps needs to be clarified as one of the future works. Another issue is the time expense of the huge cycle calculation. The calculations in the projected dimension are independent for each dimension. The projected dimensions are irrelevant for each other. Therefore, the parallel computing could give some benefit to our proposal to reduce the run time. Another issue is to seek the possibility to other areas like clustering, classification, etc. because the high dimensional curse is also a big issue to such areas.

References

1. Hawkins, D.: Identification of Outliers. Chapman and Hall, London (1980)
2. Breunig, M.M., Kriegel, H.P., Ng, R.T., Sander, J.: LOF: Indentify density based local outliers. In: The Proceedings of the ACM SIGMOD International Conference on Management of Data (2000)
3. Aggarwal, C.C., Yu, P.S.: Outlier detection for high dimensional data. In: Proceedings of the 2001 ACM SIGMOD International Conference on Management of Data, pp. 37–46. ACM, New York (2001)
4. Kriegel, H.P., Schubert, M., Zimek, A.: Angle-based outlier detection in high dimensional data. In: Proceedings of the 14th ACM SIGKDD International Conference on Knowledge Discovery and Data Mining, pp. 444–452. ACM (2008)
5. Hido, S., Tsuboi, Y., Kashima, H., Sugiyama, M., Kanamori, T.: Statistical outlier detection using direct density ratio estimation. Knowledge and Information Systems 26(2), 309–336 (2011)
6. Papadimitriou, S., Kitagawa, H.: B.Gibbons, P.: LOCI: fast outlier detection using the local correlation integral. In: IEEE 19th International Conference on Data Engineering (2003)
7. Hinneburg, A., Keim, D.A.: Optimal grid-clustering: Towards breaking the curse of dimensionality in high dimensional clustering. In: Proceedings of the 25th International Conference on Very Large Data Bases (1999)
8. Ceglar, A., Roddick, J.F., Powers, D.M.W.: CURIO: A fast outlier and outlier cluster detection algorithm for larger datasets. In: Proceedings of the 2nd International Workshop on Integrating Artificial Intelligence and Data Mining, Australia, vol. 84 (2007)
9. Nag, A.K., Mitra, A.: Multiple outelier detection in multivariate data using self-organizing maps title. Computational Statistics 20, 245–264 (2005)
10. Kriegel, H.-P., Kröger, P., Schubert, E., Zimek, A.: Outlier Detection in Axis-Parallel Subspaces of High Dimensional Data. In: Theeramunkong, T., Kijsirikul, B., Cercone, N., Ho, T.-B. (eds.) PAKDD 2009. LNCS, vol. 5476, pp. 831–838. Springer, Heidelberg (2009)
11. Arcene data, http://archive.ics.uci.edu/ml/datasets/Arcene
12. NIPS result, http://clopinet.com/isabelle/Projects/ NIPS2003/analysis.html#svm-resu

CPPG: Efficient Mining of Coverage Patterns Using Projected Pattern Growth Technique

P. Gowtham Srinivas, P. Krishna Reddy, and A.V. Trinath

International Institute of Information Technology Hyderabad, India
gowtham.srinivas@research.iiit.ac.in, pkreddy@iiit.ac.in,
venkatatrinath.atmakuri@students.iiit.ac.in

Abstract. The knowledge of coverage patterns extracted from the transactional data sets is useful in efficient placement of banner advertisements. The existing algorithm to extract coverage patterns is an apriori-like approach. In this paper, we propose an improved coverage pattern mining method by exploiting the notion of "non-overlap pattern projection". The proposed approach improves the performance by efficiently pruning the search space and extracting the complete set of coverage patterns. The performance results show that the proposed approach significantly improves the performance over the existing approach.

Keywords: coverage patterns, online advertising, projected pattern growth.

1 Introduction

The process of coverage pattern mining extracts the knowledge of coverage patterns from transactional databases. Such a knowledge can be employed in improving the performance of several applications such as banner advertisement placement.

The coverage pattern mining problem was introduced in [10] [9]. For a given transactional database D and a set of items, the problem is to extract the coverage patterns based on the threshold values specified by the user for the following parameters: relative frequency, coverage support and overlap ratio. Through experiments it was shown that the knowledge of coverage patterns can be used for efficient banner advertisement placement.

Extracting the complete set of coverage patterns is a challenging task, because the measure *coverage support* doesn't satisfy the downward closure property. An algorithm called *CMine* is proposed in [9] to discover the complete set of coverage patterns which uses the sorted closure property [7]. The apriori-like [3] approach was proposed. As per apriori property, any super pattern (or set) of a non-frequent pattern (or a set) cannot be frequent. Based on this heuristic, the *CMine* approach adopts a multiple-pass, candidate generation and test approach for extracting coverage patterns.

In this paper we have proposed an improved approach over *CMine* to substantially reduce the complexity of candidate generation process. In the literature, following researches [6], [1], [5], [8] explore the technique of *projection of the database* to achieve high performance in frequent pattern mining and frequent sequence mining approaches. In this paper we propose an improved approach which is called as coverage pattern projected growth (CPPG) by exploiting the notion of "non-overlap pattern projection".

J. Li et al. (Eds.): PAKDD 2013 Workshops, LNAI 7867, pp. 319–329, 2013.

The basic idea is to examine only the non-overlap patterns and project only their corresponding non-overlap transactions into the projected databases. The proposed approach improves the performance by efficiently pruning the search space and extracting the complete set of coverage patterns. The performance results show that the proposed approach significantly improves the performance over the existing approach.

The rest of the paper is organized as follows. In the next section, we give an overview of the coverage pattern mining problem *CMine*. In Section 3, we explain the proposed approach. The experimental results are presented in Section 4. The last section contains summary and conclusions.

2   Overview of Coverage Patterns

The model of coverage patterns is as follows [9]. We consider the banner advertisement scenario and the transactions generated from click stream data of a web site to present the model. However, the model can be extended to any transactional data set. Let $W = \{w_1, w_2, \cdots, w_n\}$ be a set of identifiers of web pages and D be a set of transactions, where each transaction T is a set of web pages such that $T \subseteq W$. Associated with each transaction is a unique transactional identifier called TID. Let T^{w_i}, $w_i \in W$ be the set of all $TIDs$ in D that contain the web page w_i. A set of web pages $X \subseteq W$ i.e., $X = \{w_p, \cdots, w_q, w_r\}$, $1 \leq p \leq q \leq r \leq n$, is called the pattern.

Table 1. Transactional database. Each transaction contains the identifiers of the web pages.

TID	1	2	3	4	5	6	7	8	9	10
Web pages	a, b, c	a, c, e	a, c, e	a, c, d	b, d, f	b, d	b, d	b, e	b, e	a, b

The percentage of transactions in D that contain the web page $w_i \in W$ is known as the "relative frequency of a web page $w_i \in W$" and denoted as $RF(w_i)$. A web page is called frequent if its relative frequency is no less than the user-specified threshold value, called minimum relative frequency.

Coverage set of a pattern $X = \{w_p, \cdots, w_q, w_r\}$, $1 \leq p \leq q \leq r \leq n$ is defined as the set of distinct $TIDs$ containing at least one web page of X and is denoted as $CSet(X)$. Therefore, $CSet(X) = T^{w_p} \cup \cdots \cup T^{w_q} \cup T^{w_r}$. The ratio of the size of the coverage set of X to D is called the coverage-support of pattern X and is denoted as $CS(X)$.

Overlap ratio of a pattern $X = \{w_p, \cdots, w_q, w_r\}$, where $1 \leq p \leq q \leq r \leq n$ and $|T^{w_p}| \geq \cdots \geq |T^{w_q}| \geq |T^{w_r}|$, is the ratio of the number of transactions contain $X - \{w_r\}$ and $\{w_r\}$ to the number of transactions in w_r. It is denoted as $OR(X)$ and is measured as follows.

$$OR(X) = \frac{|(Cset(X - \{w_r\})) \cap (Cset\{w_r\})|}{|Cset\{w_r\}|} \tag{1}$$

Note that a coverage pattern is interesting if it has high coverage support and low overlap ratio. For example, in case of banner advertisement scenario, an advertisement is exposed to more number of users due to high coverage support and repetitive display could be reduced due to low overlap ratio. A pattern X is said to be a coverage pattern if $CS(X) \geq minCS$, $OR(X) \leq maxOR$ and $RF(w_i) \geq minRF$, $\forall w_i \in X$. The variables, $minCS$ and $maxOR$ represent user-specified minimum coverage support and maximum overlap ratio, respectively. A coverage pattern X having $CS(X) = a\%$ and $OR(X) = b\%$ is expressed as

$$X \; [CS = a\%, \; OR = b\%] \tag{2}$$

Example 1. *Consider the transactional database shown in Table 1, the relative frequency of 'a' i.e., $RF(a) = \frac{|T^a|}{|D|} = \frac{5}{10} = 0.5$. If the user-specified $minRF = 0.5$, then 'a' is called a frequent web page because $RF(a) \geq minRF$. The set of web pages 'a' and 'b' i.e., $\{a, b\}$ is a pattern. The set of tids containing the web page 'a' i.e., $T^a = \{1, 2, 3, 4, 10\}$. Similarly, $T^b = \{1, 5, 6, 7, 8, 9, 10\}$. The coverage set of $\{a, b\}$ i.e., $CSet(\{a, b\}) = \{1, 2, 3, 4, 5, 6, 7, 8, 9, 10\}$. Therefore, coverage support of $\{a, b\}$ i.e., $CS(\{a, b\}) = \frac{|CSet(\{a,b\})|}{|D|} = \frac{10}{10} = 1$. The $OR(\{a, b\}) = \frac{|CSet(b) \cap CSet(a)|}{|CSet(a)|} = \frac{2}{5} = 0.4$. If $minRF = 0.4$, $minCS = 0.7$ and $maxOR = 0.5$, then the pattern $\{a, b\}$ is a coverage pattern. It is because $RF(a) \geq minRF$, $RF(b) \geq minRF$, $CS(\{a, b\}) \geq minCS$ and $OR(\{a, b\}) \leq maxOR$. This pattern is written as follows:*

$$\{a, b\} \; [CS = 1 \, (= 100\%), \; OR = 0.4 \, (= 40\%)]$$

A pattern X, with $OR(X)$ no greater than $maxOR$ is called as a non-overlap pattern. An item a is said to be a non-overlap item with respect to a pattern X if $OR(\{X, a\})$ is no greater than $maxOR$.

The problem statement of mining coverage patterns is as follows. Given a transactional database D, set of web pages W (or items), and user-specified minimum relative frequency ($minRF$), minimum coverage support ($minCS$) and maximum overlap ratio ($maxOR$), discover the complete set of coverage patterns in the database.

Extracting complete set of coverage patterns for a given $minRF$, $minCS$ and $maxOR$ is a challenging task, because the measure coverage support doesn't satisfy downward closure property. That is, although a pattern satisfies $minCS$, it is not necessary that all its non-empty subsets will also satisfy $minCS$ value.

An efficient algorithm called *CMine* is proposed in [9] to discover the complete set of coverage patterns which uses the sorted closure property [7] of overlap ratio parameter, by considering the fact that every coverage pattern is a non-overlap pattern.

The method *CMine* is Apriori-like, i.e., based on the Apriori property proposed in association rule mining [3], which states the fact that any super pattern of a non frequent pattern cannot be frequent. Based on this heuristic *CMine* adopts a multiple-pass, candidate generation and test approach in coverage pattern mining. We now explain the working of *CMine* algorithm using the transactional database, D, shown in Table 1 for the user-specified $minRF$, $minCS$ and $maxOR$ as 0.4, 0.7 and 0.5, respectively. We use Figure 1 to illustrate the CMine algorithm for finding coverage patterns in D. Here C_k, L_k, NO_k represents the candidate k-non-overlap patterns, coverage k-patterns, Non-Overlap k-patterns respectively.

The algorithm *CMine* scans all the transactions to find the relative frequencies (RF) of each web page w_i. Each web page, $w_i \in T$ which has a relative frequency no less than

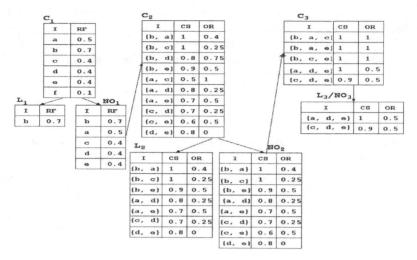

Fig. 1. Working of CMine algorithm. The term 'I' is an acronym for the item set (or web pages).

0.4 is a member of the set of candidate 1-pattern, C_1. From C_1, the set of coverage 1-patterns, L_1, are discovered if their frequencies are greater than or equal to $minCS$. Simultaneously, set of non overlap 1-patterns, NO_1, are discovered if candidate 1-patterns have relative support greater than or equal to $minRF$ and finally the web pages in NO_1 are sorted in the decreasing order of their frequencies. To discover the set of coverage 2-patterns, L_2, the algorithm computes the join of $NO_1 \bowtie NO_1$ to generate a candidate set of 2-patterns, C_2. Next, *overlap ratio* and *coverage ratio* for each candidate pattern is computed. For example, OR(b,a) = 0.4 and CS(b,a) = 1. The columns titled 'CS' and 'OR' respectively show the *coverage support* and *overlap ratio* for the patterns in C_2. The set of candidate 2-patterns that satisfy $maxOR$ are discovered as non-overlap 2-patterns, denoted as NO_2. Simultaneously, the set of candidate 2-patterns that satisfy both $minCS$ and $maxOR$ are discovered as coverage 2-patterns. Next, C_3 is generated by $NO_2 \bowtie NO_2$. We discover non-overlap 3-patterns, NO_3, and coverage 3-patterns, L_3 in the same manner that is stated above. The algorithm stops as no more candidate 4-patterns can be generated from non-overlap 3-patterns. We now analyse the issues with the *CMine* algorithm in the next subsection.

3   Coverage Pattern Projected Growth Method (CPPG)

3.1   Basic Idea

Similar to Apriori [3], the issues of $CMine$ approach are as follows: It generates potentially huge set of candidate non-overlap patterns and requires multiple scans of database. Also, it takes several iterations to mine long non-overlap patterns. It can be observed that the complexity *CMine* method is due to its step-wise candidate non-overlap pattern generation and test. Improving the performance of *CMine* is an issue.

In the literature, efforts are being made to propose improved approaches [6], [1], [5], [8] for extracting frequent patterns by exploring the idea of *projection databases*.

We have made an effort to extend the notion of *projection database* to improve the performance of *CMine* approach. We have proposed a new projection technique called *non-overlap projection* and developed the proposed approach called Coverage Patterns with Pattern Growth (CPPG). The basic idea is to exploit the sorted closure property of *overlap ratio* parameter and retain the spirit of Apriori by using non-overlap items to recursively project the transaction databases into a set of smaller projected databases and extract subsequent non-overlap patterns in each projected database. The process partitions both the data set and the set of non-overlap patterns to be tested, and confines each test being conducted to the corresponding smaller projected database.

3.2   The CPPG Approach

Definition 1. *(Prefix and postfix) Given a pattern* $X = \{i_1, i_2, ..., i_n\}$, *a pattern* $Y = \{i_1', i_2', ..., i_m'\}$ *is called a prefix of* X *if and only if* $i_j' = i_j \; \forall j \leq m$. *Here, we call the pattern* $Z = \{i_{m+1}, i_{m+2}, ..., i_n\}$ *as postfix of the pattern* X *with respect to the pattern* Y.

Example 2. *Consider the pattern* $X = \{b, a, c\}$, *here the patterns* $\{b\}$ *and* $\{b, a\}$ *are the prefixes of pattern* X. *The pattern* $\{a, c\}$ *is the postfix of pattern* X *with respect to the prefix* $\{b\}$ *and* $\{c\}$ *is the postfix of pattern* X *with respect to the prefix* $\{b, a\}$.

Definition 2. *Given a transaction database* D, f-list *is the list of all items in the database with decreasing order of their frequencies.*

Example 3. *Consider the transactional database shown in Table 1. The items it contains are* a, b, c, d, e *and* f. *Frequencies of the items in the database are as follows:* $\{a : 5, b : 7, c : 4, d : 4, e : 4, f : 1\}$. *So, the f-list for this database is:* $\{b, a, c, d, e, f\}$.

Definition 3. *Non-overlap transaction: A transaction* T, *in a database* D, *is said to be a non-overlap transaction with respect to a pattern* $X = \{w_p, \cdots, w_q, w_r\}$, *where* $1 \leq p \leq q \leq r \leq n$ *and* $|T^{w_p}| \geq \cdots \geq |T^{w_q}| \geq |T^{w_r}|$ *if and only if* T *doesn't have any of the web page belonging to* X.

Example 4. *Consider the transaction,* $T = \{a, b, c\}$ *with TID = 1 from the transactional database shown in Table 1 and let* $X = \{d, e\}$. *Here* T *is a non-overlap transaction with respect to* X *because* T *doesn't have any of the item belonging to* X. *Suppose if* $X = \{a, e\}$, *then* T *is not a non-overlap pattern with respect to* X *because* T *contains* $'a'$ *which belongs to* X.

Definition 4. *Non-overlap projection: A non-overlap projection of a transaction* T, *with respect to a pattern* $X = \{w_p, \cdots, w_q, w_r\}$, *where* $1 \leq p \leq q \leq r \leq n$ *and* $|T^{w_p}| \geq \cdots \geq |T^{w_q}| \geq |T^{w_r}|$ *is non-empty if* T *doesn't have any item belonging to* X. *Also the non-overlap projection of* T *with respect to* X *doesn't have any item* w_i *occurring before* w_r *in the f-list. Finally the items in the non-overlap projection are ordered with respect to the f-list.*

Example 5. *Consider the transaction, $T = \{b, d, f\}$ with TID = 5, from the transactional database shown in Table 1. Now non-overlap projection of T with respect to $X = \{a, c\}$ is $Y = \{d, f\}$. Here non-overlap projection of T is not empty because T doesn't have either a or c in it. Also in the non-overlap projection of T with respect to X we doesn't have b in Y because b occurs before c in the f-list.*

Definition 5. *Non-overlap projected database. A non-overlap projected database of a pattern X, with respect to a transaction database D contains the non-overlap projections of all the transactions in D with respect to the pattern X.*

Example 6. *Consider the transactional database, D, shown in Table 1. Now non-overlap projected database of pattern $X = \{a\}$ with respect to D is shown in Table 2.*

Table 2. Projected database with respect to X={a}

TID	Pages	TID	Pages	TID	Pages	TID	Pages	TID	Pages
5	d	6	d	7	d	8	e	9	e

CPPG Method with an Example

For the transactional database D, shown in Table 1, with minRF=0.4, minCS=0.7 and maxOR=0.5, the complete set of coverage patterns in D can be mined by CPPG method in the following steps.

1. Find length-1 frequent patterns and construct the f-list. Scan D once to find all frequent items in the transactions. Each of these frequent items is a length-1 non-overlap pattern. They are $\{a:5\}$, $\{b:7\}$, $\{c:4\}$, $\{d:4\}$, $\{e:4\}$. Where $\{pattern:count\}$ represents the pattern and its associated count. Now construct the f-list = (b, a, c, d, e).

2. Arrange the transactional database D, in the f-list order, at the same time remove the items that doesn't satisfy minRF from D. The transactional database of Table 1 arranged in the f-list order is given in Table 3.

3. Now we partition the complete set of non-overlap patterns into the following subsets according to the five prefixes in the f-list. They are the ones having prefix b, prefix a, prefix c, prefix d and prefix e.

4. For each item in the f-list construct its corresponding non-overlap projected database on D. Also, check for its coverage support, if it is no less than minCS report it as a coverage pattern. Now recursively mine the non-overlap projected databases as follows. Find the support count of each item in the projected database. Using this count find the non-overlap patterns. For each non-overlap pattern find the coverage support and report if it is a coverage pattern. Now recursively project the non-overlap pattern on its corresponding projected database and continue the mining process until the projected database size is empty. The non-overlap projected databases as well as the non-overlap and coverage patterns found in them are listed in Table 4, while the mining process is explained as follows.

Table 3. f-list of transactional database

TID	1	2	3	4	5	6	7	8	9	10
Pages	b, a, c	a, c, e	a, c, e	a, c, d	b, d	b, d	b, d	b, e	b, e	b, a

Table 4. Projected databases, non-overlap and coverage patterns

Prefix	Non-overlap projected database	Non-overlap patterns	Coverage patterns
b	{{a,c,e}, {a,c,e}, {a,c,d}}	{{b}, {b,a}, {b,c}, {b,e}}	{{b}, {b,a}, {b,c}, {b,e}}
a	{{d}, {d}, {d}, {e}, {e}}	{{a}, {a,d}, {a,e}, {a,d,e}}	{{a,d}, {a,e}, {a,d,e}}
c	{{d}, {d}, {d}, {e}, {e}}	{{c}, {c,d}, {c,e}, {c,d,e}}	{{c,d}, {c,d,e}}
d	{{e}, {e}, {e}, {e}}	{{d}, {d,e}}	{{d,e}}
e	-	{{e}}	-

First let us find the non-overlap patterns having prefix a. So, D is projected with respect to a to form the a's non-overlap projected database, which consists of five non-overlap projections: {5:{d}}, {6:{d}}, {7:{d}}, {8:{e}}, {9:{e}}. Here {TID:Projection} denotes the TID of the projection in the original database D. By scanning a's non-overlap projected database once, all the length-2 non-overlap patterns having prefix a can be found they are {a, d}:{0.25, 0.8} and {a, e}:{0.5, 0.7}. Here {patten}:{OR, CS} represents the pattern along with its overlap ratio and coverage support respectively.

Recursively all the non-overlap patterns having prefix a can be partitioned into two subsets: 1. those having prefix {a, d} and 2. those having prefix {a, e}. These subsets can be mined by constructing respective non-overlap projected databases and mining each recursively as follows.

The {a, d} non-overlap projected database consists of only two non-overlap projections {{e}, {e}}. By scanning {a, d}'s non-overlap projected database once, all the length-3 non-overlap patterns having prefix {a, d} can be found they are {a, d, e}:{0.5, 1}. Recursively all the non-overlap patterns having prefix {a, d} can be partitioned into only one subset those having prefix {a, d, e}. As the non-overlap projection database of {a, d, e} doesn't have any non-overlap projections in it the mining process for patterns having prefix {a, d, e} will stop here.

The {a, e} non-overlap projected database consists of zero non-overlap projections so the mining process for patterns having prefix {a, e} will stop here.

Similarly, we can find the non-overlap patterns having prefix {b}, {c}, {d} and {e}, respectively, by constructing {b}-, {c}-, {d}- and {e}-non-overlap projected databases and mining them respectively. The non-overlap projected databases as well as the non-overlap patterns and the coverage patterns found by CPPG method are shown in Table 4. During the mining process for each non-overlap pattern found we compute the coverage support and store the pattern in the coverage pattern set if it satisfies minCS constraint.

The set of non-overlap and coverage patterns is the collection of non-overlap and coverage patterns found in the above recursive mining process. From Figure 1 and Table 4 one can verify that *CPPG* returns exactly the same set of non-overlap and coverage patterns as what CMine method returns. Also one can observe from Figure 1 and Table 4 that *CPPG* doesn't generate the candidate non-overlap patterns {a, c}, {b, d}, {b, a, c}, {b, a, e}, {b, c, e} during the mining process because it uses only non-overlap projections to find the coverage patterns, where as *CMine* generates them during the mining process because the *CMine* algorithm is based on candidate generation and test approach.

3.3 *CPPG*: Algorithm and Analysis

The algorithm of CPPG method is given in Algorithm 1.

Algorithm 1. CPPG

Input: A transactional database D, and the user-specified minimum relative frequency ($minRF$), minimum coverage support ($minCS$) and maximum overlap ratio ($maxOR$)

Output: The complete set of coverage patterns.

Method:

Scan database D and find all the frequent 1-items. For each frequent 1 item 'x' construct its non-overlap projected database $NOP(D)\mid_x$ and call CPPGRec(x, 1, $NOP(D)\mid_x$). Also output 'x' if $RF(x) \geq minCS$.

Subroutine $CPPGRec(\alpha, l, NOP(D)\mid_\alpha)$

Parameters: α : a non-overlap pattern; l: the length of α; $NOP(D)\mid_\alpha$: the non-overlap projected database of α with respect to D.

Method:

1. Scan $NOP(D)\mid_\alpha$ once, find the set of non-overlap items $'i'$.

2. For each non-overlap item $'i'$, append it to α to form a non-overlap pattern α', and output α' if it satisfies $minCS$ constraint.

3. For each α', construct non-overlap projected database of α', $NOP(D)\mid_{\alpha'}$ and call $CPPGRec(\alpha', l+1, NOP(D)\mid_{\alpha'})$

Analysis. The completeness of CPPG method can be justified as follows: let α be a length-l non-overlap pattern and $\{\beta_1, \beta_2, ..., \beta_m\}$ be the set of all length $l+1$ non-overlap patterns having prefix α. The complete set of the non-overlap patterns having prefix α, except for α can be divided into m disjoint subsets. The jth subset ($1 \leq j \leq m$) is the set of non-overlap patterns having prefix β_j. From this we can say CPPG partitions the problem recursively. That is, each subset of non-overlap pattern can be further divided when necessary. This forms a divide and conquer framework. Using this framework it mines all non-overlap patterns that exists in the transactional database using all the frequent items in the transactional database as non-overlap 1-patterns and grows the non-overlap patterns recursively.

Also the CPPG method correctly identifies the non-overlap patterns. Let α and β be two non-overlap patterns in a database D such that α is a prefix of β. We can easily see that $NOP(D)\mid_\beta = (NOP(D)\mid_\alpha)\mid_\beta$. From this we can say that CPPG mines the set of non-overlap patterns correctly by largely reducing the search space. Now we analyse the efficiency of the algorithm as follows.

- **No candidate non-overlap pattern need to be generated** by CPPG. Unlike CMine CPPG only grows longer non-overlap patterns from the shorter non-overlap ones. It does not generate or test any candidate non-overlap pattern non existent in a non-overlap projected database. CPPG searches a much smaller space compared to CMine, which generates and test a substantial number of candidate non-overlap patterns.
- **The non-overlap projected databases keep shrinking.** The non-overlap projected database is smaller than the original database because only the non-overlap projections of a particular non-overlap pattern are projected into the non-overlap projected database.
- **The major cost of the CPPG is the construction of non-overlap projected databases.** To reduce the cost of constructing the projected databases we used a pseudo-projection technique. This technique reduces the cost of projection substantially when the projected database can be held in main memory. The method goes as follows. When the database can be held in main memory, instead of constructing a physical projection, one can use pointers referring to the sequences in the database as a pseudo projection. Every projection consists of two pieces of information: pointer to the transaction in the database and the index of the first element in the non-overlap projection. For example, suppose the transaction database D in Table 1 can be held in the main memory. When constructing a's non-overlap projected database, the non-overlap projection of the transaction with TID equal to 5 = {b, d} consists of two pieces: a pointer to TID = 5 and the index 2, indicating the non-overlap projection starts from the second index of the transaction with TID equals to 5. The pseudo projection avoids the copying of non-overlap projections physically. Thus, it is efficient both in terms of running time and space. However, it is not beneficial to use pseudo projection if the original database doesn't fit in the main memory.

4   Experimental Results

For experimental purposes we have chosen both real world and synthetic datasets. The details of the datasets are as follows:

i. Mushroom dataset is a dense dataset containing 8,124 transactions and 119 distinct items [4].
ii. BMS-POS dataset contains click stream data of a dotcom company [4]. The dataset contains 515,597 number of transactions and 1656 distinct items.
iii. The synthetic dataset T40I10D100K is generated by the dataset generator [2]. The dataset contains 100,000 transactions and 941 distinct items.

The CPPG algorithm was written in Java and run with Windows 7 on a 2.66 GHz machine with 2GB memory.

4.1   Performance of CPPG Algorithm with Respect to CMine Algorithm

Figure 2 shows the performance of CPPG and CMine algorithms at different minCS and maxOR values for the datasets BMS-POS, Mushroom and T40I10D100K. From

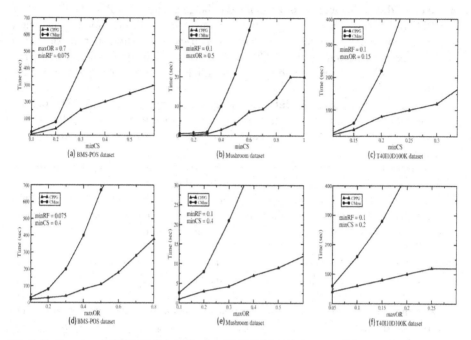

Fig. 2. Performance of CPPG and CMine on BMS-POS, Mushroom, T40I10D100K datasets at different minCS and maxOR values

the experiments one can observe that CPPG outperforms CMine by huge margin on all the datasets. From Figure 2(a) we can observe that for both algorithms CPPG and CMine as minCS is increased for a fixed maxOR and minRF the runtime is increased, this is because as minCS is increased more number of non-overlap patterns are required to generate a coverage pattern which satisfy a particular minCS. This makes the algorithm to generate more number of non-overlap patterns which eventually increases the runtime of the algorithms. The behaviour which was apparent in Figure 2(a) is also observed for Figure 2(b) and Figure 2(c).

Figure 2(d) evaluates the performance of CPPG and CMine with respect to maxOR for minRF=0.75 and minCS=0.4. From this figure we can observe that as maxOR is increased the runtime increases. This is because as maxOR is increased more number of non-overlap patterns are generated which eventually increases the runtime of the algorithm. The behaviour which was apparent in Figure 2(d) is also observed for Figure 2(e) and Figure 2(f).

5   Conclusions and Future Work

In this paper we have proposed an improved coverage pattern mining method, called CPPG. The proposed approach largely reduces the search space and does not generate or test any candidate patterns. CPPG examines only non-overlap patterns and project their corresponding non-overlap transactions into the projected databases. In each projected database, non-overlap patterns are grown by exploring only local non-overlap projections. Our performance results show that CPPG mines the complete set of coverage patterns and is faster than CMine algorithm.

As a part of the future work we want to integrate the topical relevance of web pages with the algorithm for finding coverage patterns of a website to make the results of the coverage patterns applicable in the real scenario of banner advertisement placement.

References

1. Agarwal, R., Aggarwal, C., Prasad, V.: A tree projection algorithm for generation of frequent item sets. Journal of Parallel and Distributed Computing 61(3), 350–371 (2001)
2. Agrawal, R., Imieliński, T., Swami, A.: Mining association rules between sets of items in large databases. In: ACM SIGMOD 1973, pp. 207–216. ACM (1993)
3. Agrawal, R., Srikant, R.: Fast algorithms for mining association rules in large databases. In: VLDB, pp. 487–499. Morgan Kaufmann Publishers Inc., San Francisco (1994)
4. Fimi: Frequent itemset mining implementations repository (July 2010),
   http://fimi.cs.helsinki.fi/
5. Han, J., Pei, J., Mortazavi-Asl, B., Chen, Q., Dayal, U., Hsu, M.: Freespan: frequent pattern-projected sequential pattern mining. In: ACM SIGKDD, pp. 355–359. ACM (2000)
6. Han, J., Pei, J., Yin, Y.: Mining frequent patterns without candidate generation. ACM SIGMOD Record 29, 1–12 (2000)
7. Liu, B., Hsu, W., Ma, Y.: Mining association rules with multiple minimum supports. In: KDD, pp. 337–341. ACM, New York (1999)
8. Pei, J., Han, J., Mortazavi-Asl, B., Wang, J., Pinto, H., Chen, Q., Dayal, U., Hsu, M.: Mining sequential patterns by pattern-growth: The prefixspan approach. IEEE Transactions on Knowledge and Data Engineering 16(11), 1424–1440 (2004)
9. Srinivas, P.G., Reddy, P.K., Bhargav, S., Kiran, R.U., Kumar, D.S.: Discovering coverage patterns for banner advertisement placement. In: Tan, P.-N., Chawla, S., Ho, C.K., Bailey, J. (eds.) PAKDD 2012, Part II. LNCS, vol. 7302, pp. 133–144. Springer, Heidelberg (2012)
10. Sripada, B., Polepalli, K., Rage, U.: Coverage patterns for efficient banner advertisement placement. In: WWW, pp. 131–132. ACM (2011)

A Two-Stage Dual Space Reduction Framework for Multi-label Classification

Eakasit Pacharawongsakda and Thanaruk Theeramunkong

School of Information, Computer, and Communication Technology
Sirindhorn International Institute of Technology
Thammasat University, Thailand

Abstract. Multi-label classification has been increasingly recognized since it can classify objects into multiple classes, simultaneously. However, its effectiveness might be sacrificed due to high dimensionality problem in feature space and sparseness problem in label space. To address these issues, this paper proposes a Two-Stage Dual Space Reduction (2SDSR) framework that transforms both feature space and label space into the lower-dimensional spaces. In our framework, the label space is transformed into reduced label space and then supervised dimensionality reduction method is applied to find a small number of features that maximizing dependency between features and that reduced labels. Using these reduced features and labels, a set of classification models are built. In this framework, we employ two well-known feature reduction methods such as MDDM and CCA, and two widely used label reduction methods i.e., PLST and BMD. However, it is possible to apply various dimensionality reduction methods into the framework. By a set of experiments on five real world datasets, the results indicated that our proposed framework can improve the classification performance, compared to the traditional dimensionality reduction approaches which reduce feature space or label space only.

Keywords: multi-label classification, dimensionality reduction, Singular Value Decomposition, Boolean Matrix Decomposition, Canonical Correlation Analysis.

1 Introduction

In the past, most traditional classification techniques usually assumed a single category for each object to be classified by means of minimum distance. However, in some tasks it is natural to assign more than one categories to an object. For examples, some news articles can be categorized into both *politic* and *crime*, or some movies can be labeled as *action* and *comedy*, simultaneously. As a special type of task, multi-label classification was initially studied by Schapire and Singer (2000) [9] in text categorization. Later many techniques in multi-label classification have been proposed for various applications. However, these methods can be grouped into two main approaches: *Algorithm Adaptation* (AA) and

J. Li et al. (Eds.): PAKDD 2013 Workshops, LNAI 7867, pp. 330–341, 2013.

Problem Transformation (PT) as suggested in [11]. The former approach modifies existing classification methods to handle multi-label data [9]. On the other hand, the latter approach transforms a multi-label classification task into several single classification tasks and then applies traditional classification method on each task [8]. However, these two main approaches might suffer from the high-dimensionality problem in feature space and sparseness problem in label space. To solve these issues, many techniques have been proposed, e.g., sparse regularization, feature selection and dimensionality reduction. Among these methods, the dimensionality reduction which transforms data in a high-dimensional space to those in the lower-dimensional space, has been focused on multi-label classification problem. In general, the dimensionality reduction for multi-label classification can be categorized into three groups: (1) feature space reduction, (2) label space reduction and (3) both feature and label spaces reduction.

The dimensionality reduction in feature space was formerly studied by Yu et al. [13]. In their work, Multi-label Latent Semantic Indexing (MLSI) was proposed to project the original feature space into a reduced feature space. This reduced feature space is constructed by a supervised LSI since the method considers a minimum error in both feature and label spaces. As an optimization problem with SVM as the base classifier, the results showed that classification accuracy could be improved over the method using the original feature space and the traditional LSI. In MLSI, although labels were concerned, the method reduced the feature space but still used the original label space. Motivated by MLSI, Multi-label Dimensionality reduction via Dependence Maximization (MDDM) was proposed by Zhang and Zhou in [14]. In their work, Hilbert-Schmidt Independence Criterion (HSIC) was applied rather than LSI and its aim was to identify reduced feature space that maximizes dependency between the original feature space and the label space. Using MDDM with Multi-label K-Nearest Neighbors (ML-KNN) as a base classifier, this method obtained more accuracy than MLSI. Such methods mainly focused on how to project the original feature space into a smaller one, but still suffered with high-dimensionality in the label space. For this reason, these methods usually have high time complexity in the classification task.

On the other hand, for the label space reduction, to improve efficiency of multi-label classification, Hsu et al. [5] posed a sparseness problem that mostly occurred in the label space and then applied Compressive Sensing (CS) technique, widely used in the image processing field, to encode and decode the label space. In encoding step, the CS technique was used to create a small number of linear random projections while decoding step needs to solve an optimization problem to reconstruct the labels with respect to the sparsity error. It seems that the encoding step of this CS method seems efficient but the decoding step does not. Toward this issue, Tai and Lin [10] proposed Principle Label Space Transformation (PLST) to transform the label space into a smaller linear label space using Singular Value Decomposition (SVD) [2]. With the properties of orthorgonal matrix derived from SVD, this matrix can be used to transform the reduced label space back to the original space. By a number of experiments, PLST was shown to improve classification performance in both accuracy and computational time, compared to BR and CS approaches. Recently, Wicker et al. [12] presented an alternative method to reduce the label space using Boolean Matrix Decomposition (BMD) [6]. While SVD transforms high-dimensional binary labels to lower-dimensional numeric values, BMD still preserves the label information in boolean format. With this property, this work shown better performance, compared to the PLST and BR. While these methods addressed the sparseness problem in the label space, they do not consider the high-dimensionality problem in the feature space. Hence, the classification accuracy might be reduced.

To address high dimensionality problem and sparseness problem in multi-label data, the dual space reduction methods were proposed to reduce dimensions in the feature and label spaces. In our previous work, we proposed Dependent Dual Space Reduction (DDSR) [7]. In that work, a dependency matrix was constructed from feature matrix and label matrix after that both of them were projected into a single reduced space, and then performed prediction on the reduced space. From a set of experiments, DDSR showed better performance comparing to traditional multi-label classification techniques. Motivated by DDSR, this work introduces an alternative dual space reduction framework namely, Two-Stage Dual Space Reduction (2SDSR). In the first stage, a high-dimensional label space is projected to a lower-dimensional label space. With respect to that reduced labels, a high-dimensional feature space is transformed to a reduced feature space as the second stage. With this framework, four widely used dimensionality reduction methods, i.e., MDDM, CCA, PLST and BMD, can be exploited.

In the rest of this paper, Section 2 gives notations for the multi-label classification task and literature review to the dimensionality reduction methods. Section 3 presents an alternative dual space reduction approach, namely Two-Stage Dual Space Reduction (2SDSR). The multi-label benchmark datasets and experimental settings are described in Section 4. In Section 5, the experimental results using five datasets are given and finally Section 6 provides conclusion of this work.

2   Preliminaries

2.1   Definition of Multi-label Classification Task

Let $\mathcal{X} = \mathbb{R}^M$ and $\mathcal{Y} = \{0,1\}^L$ be an M-dimensional feature space and L-dimensional binary label space, where M is the number of features and L is a number of possible labels, i.e. classes. Let $\mathcal{D} = \{\langle \mathbf{x}_1, \mathbf{y}_1 \rangle, \langle \mathbf{x}_2, \mathbf{y}_2 \rangle, ..., \langle \mathbf{x}_N, \mathbf{y}_N \rangle\}$ is a set of N objects (e.g., documents, images, etc.) in a training dataset, where $\mathbf{x}_i \in \mathcal{X}$ is a feature vector that represents an i-th object and $\mathbf{y}_i \in \mathcal{Y}$ is a label vector with the length of L, $[y_{i1}, y_{i2}, ..., y_{iL}]$. Here, y_{ij} indicates whether the i-th object belongs (1) or not (0) to the j-th class (the j-th label or not i.e., whether it is given).

In general, two main phases are exploited in a multi-label classification problem: (1) *model training* phase and (2) *classification* phase. The goal of the *model training* phase is to build a classification model that can predict the label vector $\mathbf{y}_t$ for a new object with the feature vector $\mathbf{x}_t$. This classification model is a mapping function $\mathcal{H} : \mathbb{R}^M \rightarrow \{0,1\}^L$ which can predict a target value closest to its actual value in total. The *classification* phase uses this classification model to assign labels. For convenience, $\mathbf{X}_{N \times M} = [\mathbf{x}_1, ..., \mathbf{x}_N]^T$ denotes the *feature matrix* with N rows and M columns and $\mathbf{Y}_{N \times L} = [\mathbf{y}_1, ..., \mathbf{y}_N]^T$ represents the *label matrix* with N rows and L columns , where $[\cdot]^T$ denotes matrix transpose.

2.2   Singular Value Decomposition (SVD)

This subsection gives a brief introduction to SVD, which was developed as a method for dimensionality reduction using a least-squared technique. The SVD transforms a feature matrix $\mathbf{X}$ to a lower-dimensional matrix $\mathbf{X}'$ such that the distance between the original matrix and a matrix in a lower-dimensional space (i.e., the 2-norm $\| \mathbf{X} - \mathbf{X}' \|_2$) are minimum.

Generally, a feature matrix $\mathbf{X}$ can be decomposed into the product of three matrices as shown in Eq. (1).

$$\mathbf{X}_{N \times M} = \mathbf{U}_{N \times M} \times \mathbf{\Sigma}_{M \times M} \times \mathbf{V}^T_{M \times M}, \tag{1}$$

where N is a number of objects, M is a number of features and $M < N$. The matrices $\mathbf{U}$ and $\mathbf{V}$ are two orthogonal matrices, where $\mathbf{U}^T \times \mathbf{U} = \mathbf{I}$ and $\mathbf{V}^T \times \mathbf{V} = \mathbf{I}$. The columns in the matrix $\mathbf{U}$ are called the *left singular vectors* while as the columns in matrix $\mathbf{V}$ are called the *right singular vectors*. The matrix $\mathbf{\Sigma}$ is a diagonal matrix, where $\mathbf{\Sigma}_{i,j} = 0$ for $i \neq j$, and the diagonal elements of $\mathbf{\Sigma}$ are the singular values of matrix $\mathbf{X}$. The singular values in the matrix $\mathbf{\Sigma}$ are sorted by descending order such that $\mathbf{\Sigma}_{1,1} \geq \mathbf{\Sigma}_{2,2} \geq ... \geq \mathbf{\Sigma}_{M,M}$. To discard noise, it is possible to ignore singular values less than $\mathbf{\Sigma}_{K,K}$, where $K \ll M$. By this ignorance the three matrices are reduced to Eq. (2).

$$\mathbf{X}'_{N \times M} = \mathbf{U}'_{N \times K} \times \mathbf{\Sigma}'_{K \times K} \times \mathbf{V}'^T_{M \times K}, \tag{2}$$

where $\mathbf{X}'_{N \times M}$ is expected to be close $\mathbf{X}_{N \times M}$, i.e. $\| \mathbf{X} - \mathbf{X}' \|_2 < \delta$, $\mathbf{U}'_{N \times K}$ is a reduced matrix of $\mathbf{U}_{N \times M}$, $\mathbf{\Sigma}'_{K \times K}$ is the reduced version of $\mathbf{\Sigma}_{M \times M}$ from M to K dimensions and $\mathbf{V}'_{M \times K}$ is a reduced matrix of $\mathbf{V}_{M \times M}$. While PLST used SVD to transform high-dimensional label space to lower-dimensional feature space, DDSR applied SVD to dependency matrix to transform both feature and label spaces to a single reduced space.

2.3   Canonical Correlation Analysis (CCA)

This subsection summarizes concept of CCA proposed by Hotelling in 1935 [4]. While SVD can decompose only one set of variables, CCA is widely used to measure linear correlation between two sets of variables i.e., feature matrix ($\mathbf{X}$) and label matrix ($\mathbf{Y}$). As more detail, CCA finds a pair of projection vectors $\mathbf{u} \in \mathbb{R}^M$ and $\mathbf{v} \in \mathbb{R}^L$ that maximize correlation between matrix $\mathbf{X}_{N \times M}$ and

$\mathbf{Y}_{N \times L}$, where N is a number of objects, M is a number of features and L is a number of labels. Hence, this can be represented as maximization problem as shown in Eq. (3).

$$\underset{\mathbf{u}, \mathbf{v}}{\operatorname{argmax}} \frac{\mathbf{u}^T \mathbf{X}^T \mathbf{Y} \mathbf{v}}{\sqrt{(\mathbf{u}^T \mathbf{X}^T \mathbf{X} \mathbf{u})(\mathbf{v}^T \mathbf{Y}^T \mathbf{Y} \mathbf{v})}} \tag{3}$$

Since the normalization part in Eq. (3) will not change the objective function, two constraints can be added:

$$\mathbf{u}^T \mathbf{X}^T \mathbf{X} \mathbf{u} = 1 \tag{4}$$

$$\mathbf{v}^T \mathbf{Y}^T \mathbf{Y} \mathbf{v} = 1 \tag{5}$$

After solving this problem using *Lagrangian* method and eigenvectors decomposition technique, k pairs of projection vectors $((\mathbf{u}', \mathbf{v}') \in \mathbb{R}^K)$ are obtained, where $K \ll min(M, L)$. The projection vector (e.g., $\mathbf{u}'$) has been used to transform high-dimensional feature matrix $(\mathbf{X}_{N \times M})$ to lower-dimensional feature matrix $(\mathbf{X}'_{N \times K})$.

2.4 Multi-label Dimensionality Reduction via Dependence Maximization (MDDM)

In this subsection, the dimensionality reduction technique in MDDM is reviewed. The MDDM was proposed to find a projection matrix which maximizing the dependency between features and labels. To do such that, the MDDM employed the Hilbert-Schmidt Independence Criterion (HSIC) [3] that was introduced to measure dependence between two sets of variables. An empirical estimate of HSIC is given by

$$\mathrm{HSIC}(\mathbf{X}, \mathbf{Y}, \mathbf{P_{xy}}) = (N-1)^{-2} \mathrm{tr}(\mathbf{HKHL}), \tag{6}$$

where $\mathbf{P_{xy}}$ is joint distribution and $\mathrm{tr}(\cdot)$ represents trace of matrix. The $\mathbf{K}$ is a kernel matrix which $\mathbf{K} = \langle \phi(\mathbf{X}), \phi(\mathbf{X}) \rangle = \mathbf{X}^T \mathbf{u} \mathbf{u}^T \mathbf{X}$, where $\mathbf{u}$ is a projection vector. Hence, the matrix $\mathbf{K}$ can be substituted with $\mathbf{X}^T \mathbf{u} \mathbf{u}^T \mathbf{X}$. The $\mathbf{L}$ is the inner product of objects that are computed from the label matrix $(\mathbf{Y})$. The $\mathbf{H} \in \mathbb{R}^{N \times N}$, where $H_{ij} = \delta_{ij} - 1/N$, δ_{ij} is 1 when $i = j$ and 0 otherwise.

To search for an optimal linear projection, the Eq. 6 can be rewritten to the optimization problem

$$\mathbf{u}^* = \underset{\mathbf{u}}{\operatorname{argmax}} \ \mathrm{tr}(\mathbf{HX^T uu^T XHL}). \tag{7}$$

The normalization part is removed since it does not affect the optimization problem. It is noted that $\mathrm{tr}(\mathbf{HX^T uu^T XHL}) = \mathbf{u^T}(\mathbf{XHLHX^T})\mathbf{u}$. By using eigen decomposition, it can obtain the projection vectors $(\mathbf{u}')$. These projection vectors are selected from the eigenvectors which corresponding to the largest K eigenvalues, where $K \ll M$ and M is a number of features.

2.5   Boolean Matrix Decomposition (BMD)

This subsection explains the BMD that was proposed by Miettinen. The BMD aims to decompose a binary matrix into two binary factor matrices. Since label matrix ($\mathbf{Y}$) contains binary values, it is possible to employ BMD for constructing two smaller boolean matrices as shown in Eq. (8).

$$\mathbf{Y}_{N \times L} = \mathbf{Y'}_{N \times K} \times \mathbf{V'}_{K \times L}, \tag{8}$$

where N is a number of objects, L is a number of labels and K is a number of reduced dimensions. The $\mathbf{Y'}$ represents a lower-dimensional label matrix and $\mathbf{V'}$ is a factor matrix that can reconstruct the high-dimensional label matrix ($\mathbf{Y}$). As more details, each row in the $\mathbf{Y'}$ is selected from association matrix which computed from the label matrix ($\mathbf{Y}$). After each row is selected and inserted into the $\mathbf{Y'}$, the binary values in factor matrix $\mathbf{V'}$ are rearranged to minimize the label matrix reconstruction error. To improve the multi-label classification, the BMD was applied as described in [12].

3   Two-Stage Dual Space Reduction Framework (2SDSR)

As mentioned earlier, the Dependent Dual Space Reduction presented better performance comparing to traditional methods. In this work, we present an alternative dual space reduction framework, namely Two-Stage Dual Space Reduction (2SDSR), to transform both feature space and label space into the lower-dimensional spaces. The entire pseudo-code of 2SDSR framework is presented in Algorithm 1.

The 2SDSR framework is divided into three phases: *pre-processing* phase (line 1-2), *model training* phase (line 3-5) and *classification* phase (line 6-8). The first step in *pre-processing* phase is to transform the high-dimensional label matrix $\mathbf{Y}_{N \times L}$ into a lower-dimensional label matrix $\mathbf{Y'}_{N \times K}$, where $K < L$. To do such that, it is possible to apply various label space reduction methods such as SVD or BMD, into this framework. For more detail, the function $labelsSpaceReduction(\mathbf{Y}, K)$ (line 1) transforms a high-dimensional label matrix to K dimensional label matrix. When the SVD is exploited in that function, the lower-dimensional label matrix ($\mathbf{Y'}$) is computed from $\mathbf{Y'}_{N \times K} = \mathbf{Y}_{N \times L} \times \mathbf{V'}_{L \times K}$, where $\mathbf{V'}$ is a projection matrix. Likewise, the lower-dimensional label matrix ($\mathbf{Y'}$) can derive from Eq. (8) when the BMD is applied. This function returns two matrices which are the reduced label matrix ($\mathbf{Y'}$) and projection matrix ($\mathbf{V'}$) e.g., the projection matrix from SVD or BMD. This projection matrix is used to reconstruct the high-dimensional label matrix in the *Classification* phase.

The next step is to find the reduced feature space which maximizing the dependency between features and that reduced labels. The feature reduction method is embedded in function $featureSpaceReduction(\mathbf{X}, \mathbf{Y'}, D)$ (line 2). Similar to the label space reduction, various feature space reduction techniques can be exploited to the function. In this work, two feature space reduction methods i.e., MDDM

Algorithm 1. Two-Stage Dual Space Reduction (2SDSR)

Input: (1) a training set composed of
        (1.1) a feature matrix $\mathbf{X}_{N \times M}$
        (1.2) a label matrix $\mathbf{Y}_{N \times L}$
     (2) a test object $\hat{\mathbf{X}}_{1 \times M}$
     (3) a number of reduced features (D) and a number of reduced labels (K)
Output: the predicted label matrix $\hat{\mathbf{Y}}_{1 \times L}$ for the test object $\hat{\mathbf{X}}_{1 \times M}$

    [Pre-processing phase]
1: $(\mathbf{Y}'_{N \times K}, \mathbf{V}'_{K \times L}) \leftarrow labelsSpaceReduction(\mathbf{Y}_{N \times L}, K)$
2: $(\mathbf{X}'_{N \times D}, \mathbf{U}'_{M \times D}) \leftarrow featuresSpaceReduction(\mathbf{X}_{N \times M}, \mathbf{Y}'_{N \times K}, D)$

    [Model training phase]
3: **for** $k = 1$ **to** K **do**
4:    $h_k(\mathbf{X}') \leftarrow modelConstruction(\mathbf{X}'_{N \times D}, \mathbf{Y}'_{N \times 1}[k])$.
5: **end for**

    [Classification phase]
6: $\hat{\mathbf{X}}'_{1 \times D} \leftarrow \hat{\mathbf{X}}_{1 \times M} \times \mathbf{U}'_{M \times D}$
7: $\hat{\mathbf{Y}}'_{1 \times K} \leftarrow [h_1(\hat{\mathbf{X}}'), h_2(\hat{\mathbf{X}}'), ..., h_K(\hat{\mathbf{X}}')]$.
8: $\hat{\mathbf{Y}}_{1 \times L} \leftarrow labelsReconstruction(\hat{\mathbf{Y}}'_{1 \times K}, \mathbf{V}'_{K \times L})$.

---

and CCA are applied. These methods are well-known supervised dimensionality reduction techniques. In *featureSpaceReduction(*$\mathbf{X}, \mathbf{Y}', D$*)*, the matrices $\mathbf{X}$ is a high-dimensional feature matrix, $\mathbf{Y}'$ is a lower-dimensional label matrix and D is a number of reduced features. These two matrices ($\mathbf{X}$ and $\mathbf{Y}'$) are applied to Eq. (7) when the MDDM is used. Likewise, these matrices are substituted to Eq. (3) when the CCA is employed. After that, this function returns a reduced feature matrix ($\mathbf{X}'$) and projection matrix ($\mathbf{U}'$) that will be used in further steps.

In the *model training* phase, a classification model is built from these two lower-dimensional matrices, $\mathbf{X}'$ and $\mathbf{Y}'$. Among existing methods on multi-label classification, Binary Relevance (BR) is a simple approach and widely used. BR reduces the multi-label classification task to a set of binary classifications and then builds a classification model for each class. In this framework, the projected label matrix $\mathbf{Y}'$ contains numeric values when SVD is applied or it contains binary values when BMD is used. By this situation, a regression as well as a classification method can be applied to estimate these values. While the projected label matrix $\mathbf{Y}'$ has K dimensions, it is possible to build a regression or classification model for each dimension. That is K regression or classification models are constructed for K lower-dimensions. Moreover, each model, denoted by $h_k(\mathbf{X}')$ is a regression or classification model built for predicting each column $\mathbf{Y}'[k]$ using the matrix $\mathbf{X}'$ as shown in line 3-5 in the Algorithm 1. For regression model, the predicted values are continuous, therefore, we need a method to find the optimal threshold for mapping a continuous value to binary decision (0 or 1) as described in [1].

In the *classification* phase of Algorithm 1, an unseen feature vector $\hat{\mathbf{X}}$ is transformed to the lower-dimensional feature vector $\hat{\mathbf{X}}'$ using $\hat{\mathbf{X}}'_{1 \times D} = \hat{\mathbf{X}}_{1 \times M} \times \mathbf{U}'_{M \times D}$ (line 6). Then this vector is fed to a series of regression or classification models $h(\hat{\mathbf{X}}')$ to estimate the value in each dimension of the predicted lower-dimensional label vector $\hat{\mathbf{Y}}'_{1 \times K}$ as shown in line 7. After that, the projection matrix $\mathbf{V}'$ from SVD or BMD is multiplied to reconstruct the higher-dimensional label vector $\hat{\mathbf{Y}}_{1 \times L}$ using the *labelsReconstruction* function (line 8). If the predicted values are continuous values, the label vector $\hat{\mathbf{Y}}_{1 \times L}$ will be rounded to the value in $\{0,1\}$ by a threshold. Finally, the set of predicted multiple labels is the union of the dimensions which have the value of 1.

4   Datasets and Experimental Settings

To evaluate the performance of our proposed framework, the benchmark multi-label datasets are downloaded from MULAN[1]. Table 1 shows the characteristics of five multi-label datasets. For each dataset, N, M and L denote the total number of objects, the number of features and the number of labels, respectively. L_C represents the *label cardinality*, the average number of labels per example and L_D stands for *label density*, the normalized value of *label cardinality* as introduced by [11].

Table 1. Characteristics of the datasets used in our experiments

Dataset	Domain	N	M		L	L_C	L_D
			Nominal	Numeric			
corel5k	images	5,000	499	-	374	3.522	0.009
enron	text	1,702	1,001	-	53	3.378	0.064
emotions	music	593	-	72	6	1.869	0.311
scene	image	2,407	-	294	6	1.074	0.179
yeast	biology	2,417	-	103	14	4.237	0.303

Since each object in the dataset can be associated with multiple labels simultaneously, the traditional evaluation metric of single-label classification could not be applied. In this work, we apply two types of well-known multi-label evaluation metrics [8]. As the label-based metric, *hamming loss* and *macro F-measure*, are used to evaluate each label separately. As the label-set-based metric, *accuracy* and *0/1 loss* are applied to assess all labels as a set. Using ten-fold cross validation method, the results of the four evaluation metrics are recorded and shown in Table 2. All multi-label classification methods used in this work is implemented in R environment version 2.11.1[2] and linear regression is used for the regression model in the *model training* phase.

---

[1] http://mulan.sourceforge.net/datasets.html
[2] http://www.R-project.org/

Table 2. Performance comparison (mean) between BR, MDDM, CCA, PLST, MLC-BMaD, DDSR, 2SDSR-MS, 2SDSR-MB, 2SDSR-CS and 2SDSR-CB in terms of *Hamming loss (HL)*, *macro F-measure (F1)*, *accuracy* and *0/1 loss* on the five datasets. ($\downarrow$ indicates the smaller the better; $\uparrow$ indicates the larger the better; the superscript $<x>$ shows the percentage of dimensions reduced from the original feature space, the superscript $[x]$ shows the percentage of dimensions reduced from the original label space, and the superscript (x,y) shows the percentage of dimensions reduced from the original ones for the feature space and that for the label space.)

Dataset	Metrics	BR	MDDM	CCA	PLST	MLC-BMaD	DDSR	2SDSR-MS	2SDSR-MB	2SDSR-CS	2SDSR-CB
corel5k	HL $\downarrow$	0.0094	$0.0094^{<20>}$	$\mathbf{0.0093}^{<20>}$	$0.0094^{[20]}$	$0.0094^{[20]}$	$0.0145^{(30,40)}$	$0.0131^{(40,100)}$	$0.0133^{(20,20)}$	$0.0142^{(74.95,100)}$	$0.0771^{(14.99,20)}$
	F1 $\uparrow$	0.0284	$0.0284^{<100>}$	$0.0247^{<20>}$	$0.0286^{[40]}$	$0.0299^{[20]}$	$0.1215^{(15,20)}$	$0.1065^{(40,100)}$	$\mathbf{0.1282}^{(20,40)}$	$0.0948^{(74.95,100)}$	$0.1277^{(14.99,20)}$
	Accuracy $\uparrow$	0.0528	$0.0528^{<100>}$	$0.0440^{<20>}$	$0.0533^{[20]}$	$0.0537^{[20]}$	$0.1543^{(30,40)}$	$0.1352^{(20,100)}$	$\mathbf{0.1716}^{(20,40)}$	$0.1279^{(74.95,100)}$	$0.1117^{(74.95,100)}$
	0/1 Loss $\downarrow$	0.9948	$0.9948^{<100>}$	$0.9952^{<20>}$	$0.9944^{[45,60]}$	$0.9962^{[20]}$	$0.9944^{(45,60)}$	$\mathbf{0.8960}^{(40,100)}$	$0.9952^{(20,20)}$	$0.8974^{(74.95,100)}$	$0.9000^{(74.95,100)}$
enron	HL $\downarrow$	0.1019	$0.1019^{<20>}$	$0.1019^{<20>}$	$0.0721^{[20]}$	$0.0746^{[20]}$	$\mathbf{0.0529}^{(3.18,40)}$	$0.0576^{(20,80)}$	$0.0647^{(20,100)}$	$0.1234^{(8.33,100)}$	$0.1775^{(8.33,100)}$
	F1 $\uparrow$	0.1957	$0.2559^{<40>}$	$0.1957^{<20>}$	$0.2170^{[40]}$	$0.2628^{[40]}$	$\mathbf{0.3118}^{(5.29,100)}$	$0.2925^{(20,100)}$	$0.2855^{(20,60)}$	$0.1902^{(8.33,100)}$	$0.2836^{(3.33,40)}$
	Accuracy $\uparrow$	0.3328	$0.4132^{<40>}$	$0.3328^{<20>}$	$0.3475^{[20]}$	$0.4369^{[40]}$	$\mathbf{0.4723}^{(5.29,100)}$	$0.4406^{(20,100)}$	$0.3672^{(20,100)}$	$0.3111^{(8.33,100)}$	$0.4377^{(3.33,40)}$
	0/1 Loss $\downarrow$	0.9089	$0.8790^{<20>}$	$0.9089^{<20>}$	$0.9077^{[60]}$	$0.9206^{[60]}$	$\mathbf{0.8713}^{(5.29,100)}$	$0.8831^{(20,100)}$	$0.9084^{(20,100)}$	$0.9166^{(8.33,100)}$	$0.8930^{(8.33,100)}$
emotions	HL $\downarrow$	0.2068	$0.2048^{<80>}$	$0.2068^{<20>}$	$\mathbf{0.2037}^{[60]}$	$0.2068^{[100]}$	$0.2728^{(8.33,100)}$	$0.2130^{(100,80)}$	$0.2178^{(60,100)}$	$0.2130^{(4.24,80)}$	$0.3269^{(2.12,40)}$
	F1 $\uparrow$	0.6317	$0.6317^{<100>}$	$0.6317^{<20>}$	$0.6339^{[60]}$	$0.6317^{[100]}$	$0.6455^{(8.33,100)}$	$0.6757^{(100,80)}$	$\mathbf{0.6813}^{(60,100)}$	$0.6757^{(4.24,80)}$	$0.5915^{(5.29,100)}$
	Accuracy $\uparrow$	0.5091	$0.5091^{<100>}$	$0.5091^{<20>}$	$0.5091^{[100]}$	$0.5091^{[100]}$	$0.5090^{(8.33,100)}$	$\mathbf{0.5516}^{(100,80)}$	$0.5509^{(60,100)}$	$\mathbf{0.5516}^{(4.24,80)}$	$0.4160^{(5.29,100)}$
	0/1 Loss $\downarrow$	0.7467	$0.7435^{<80>}$	$0.7467^{<20>}$	$\mathbf{0.7300}^{[60]}$	$0.7467^{[100]}$	$0.8293^{(8.33,100)}$	$0.7316^{(100,60)}$	$0.7552^{(60,100)}$	$0.7316^{(3.18,60)}$	$0.9360^{(2.12,40)}$
scene	HL $\downarrow$	0.1105	$\mathbf{0.1051}^{<40>}$	$0.1105^{<20>}$	$0.1105^{[100]}$	$0.1105^{[100]}$	$0.1190^{(1.63,80)}$	$0.1140^{(20,100)}$	$0.1119^{(20,100)}$	$0.1213^{(2.04,100)}$	$0.3103^{(0.82,40)}$
	F1 $\uparrow$	0.6480	$0.6513^{<40>}$	$0.6480^{<20>}$	$0.6480^{[100]}$	$0.6480^{[100]}$	$0.7046^{(2,100)}$	$0.7156^{(20,100)}$	$\mathbf{0.7162}^{(20,100)}$	$0.6859^{(2.04,100)}$	$0.4574^{(2.04,100)}$
	Accuracy $\uparrow$	0.5302	$0.5302^{<100>}$	$0.5302^{<20>}$	$0.5302^{[100]}$	$0.5302^{[100]}$	$0.6109^{(1.63,80)}$	$0.6370^{(20,100)}$	$\mathbf{0.6371}^{(20,100)}$	$0.6048^{(2.04,100)}$	$0.2962^{(2.04,100)}$
	0/1 Loss $\downarrow$	0.5186	$0.5156^{<80>}$	$0.5186^{<20>}$	$0.5186^{[100]}$	$0.5186^{[100]}$	$0.5106^{(1.63,80)}$	$0.4886^{(20,100)}$	$\mathbf{0.4753}^{(20,100)}$	$0.5056^{(2.04,100)}$	$0.9273^{(0.82,40)}$
yeast	HL $\downarrow$	0.2008	$\mathbf{0.2000}^{<80>}$	$0.2008^{<20>}$	$0.2008^{[100]}$	$0.2010^{[80]}$	$0.2807^{(13.59,100)}$	$0.2686^{(80,80)}$	$0.2158^{(100,40)}$	$0.2711^{(13.59,100)}$	$0.2517^{(2.72,20)}$
	F1 $\uparrow$	0.4455	$0.4489^{<80>}$	$0.4455^{<20>}$	$0.4455^{[80]}$	$0.4451^{[80]}$	$0.4926^{(2.72,20)}$	$0.4913^{(40,40)}$	$\mathbf{0.5133}^{(40,60)}$	$0.4822^{(2.72,20)}$	$0.5092^{(8.16,60)}$
	Accuracy $\uparrow$	0.5019	$0.5030^{<80>}$	$0.5019^{<20>}$	$0.5019^{[80]}$	$0.5009^{[80]}$	$0.4884^{(8.16,60)}$	$0.4930^{(60,60)}$	$\mathbf{0.5154}^{(40,40)}$	$0.4877^{(13.59,100)}$	$0.4366^{(5.44,40)}$
	0/1 Loss $\downarrow$	0.851	$0.8465^{<60>}$	$0.8510^{<20>}$	$\mathbf{0.8506}^{[80]}$	$0.8510^{[60]}$	$0.9259^{(13.59,100)}$	$0.9143^{(40,100)}$	$0.8701^{(80,60)}$	$0.9143^{(10.87,80)}$	$0.9520^{(2.72,20)}$

Table 3. Performance comparison with a two-tailed paired t-test with 5% significance among nine methods. In total, 140 pairs are tested for each method. Three numbers (W/T/L) represent win, tie and loss. The scores of a win, a tie and a loss are set to 3, 1 and 0, respectively.

Methods	Metrics	MDDM	CCA	PLST	MLC-BMaD	DDSR	2SDSR-MS	2SDSR-MB	2SDSR-CS	2SDSR-CB	Total (W/T/L)	Rank
MDDM	HL	–	2/2/1	3/2/0	2/3/0	5/0/0	4/1/0	4/1/0	4/1/0	5/0/0	29/10/1	
	F1	–	2/3/0	1/4/0	0/5/0	0/1/4	0/0/5	0/0/5	1/0/4	2/0/3	6/13/21	
	Accuracy	–	2/3/0	1/3/1	0/3/2	1/1/3	1/0/4	1/0/4	2/0/3	3/0/2	11/10/19	4
	0/1 Loss	–	1/4/0	2/3/0	1/4/0	2/0/3	1/4/0	1/3/1	2/3/0	3/2/0	13/23/4	
	Overall	–	7/12/1	7/12/1	3/15/2	8/2/10	6/5/9	6/4/10	9/4/7	13/2/5	59/56/25	
CCA	HL	1/2/2	–	2/2/1	1/3/1	4/0/1	2/2/1	2/2/1	5/0/0	5/0/0	21/12/7	
	F1	0/3/2	–	0/3/2	1/2/2	0/1/4	0/0/5	0/0/5	0/1/4	2/0/3	3/10/27	
	Accuracy	0/3/2	–	0/3/2	1/2/2	1/1/3	0/0/5	0/0/5	2/0/3	3/0/2	8/9/23	8
	0/1 Loss	0/4/1	–	1/4/0	0/4/1	2/2/1	1/2/2	1/3/1	2/3/0	3/2/0	11/24/5	
	Overall	1/12/7	–	3/12/5	5/11/4	7/4/9	4/4/12	3/5/12	8/5/7	13/2/5	43/55/62	
PLST	HL	0/2/3	1/2/2	–	2/2/1	4/0/1	2/1/2	2/2/1	4/0/1	5/0/0	20/9/11	
	F1	0/4/1	2/3/0	–	1/3/1	0/1/4	0/0/5	0/0/5	1/0/4	2/0/3	6/11/23	
	Accuracy	1/3/1	2/3/0	–	1/3/1	1/1/3	1/0/4	0/1/4	2/0/3	3/0/2	11/11/18	7
	0/1 Loss	0/3/2	1/4/0	–	1/3/1	1/3/1	1/1/3	1/3/0	2/2/1	3/2/0	9/21/10	
	Overall	1/12/7	5/12/3	–	4/11/5	6/5/9	4/2/14	3/6/11	9/2/9	13/2/5	46/52/62	
MLC-BMaD	HL	0/3/2	1/3/1	1/2/2	–	4/1/0	4/1/0	4/1/0	4/1/0	4/1/0	22/13/5	
	F1	0/5/0	2/2/1	1/3/1	–	0/0/5	0/0/5	0/0/5	1/0/4	2/0/3	6/10/24	
	Accuracy	2/3/0	2/2/1	1/3/1	–	0/2/3	1/2/2	0/2/3	1/2/2	1/2/2	8/18/14	6
	0/1 Loss	0/4/1	0/4/1	1/3/1	–	2/3/0	1/3/1	2/3/0	1/3/1	2/3/0	9/26/5	
	Overall	2/15/3	5/11/4	4/11/5	–	6/6/8	6/6/8	6/6/8	7/6/7	9/6/5	45/67/48	
DDSR	HL	0/0/5	1/0/4	1/0/4	0/1/4	–	4/0/1	4/0/1	3/2/0	5/0/0	18/3/19	
	F1	4/1/0	4/1/0	4/1/0	5/0/0	–	1/2/2	1/0/4	4/0/1	3/0/2	26/5/9	
	Accuracy	3/1/1	3/1/1	3/1/1	3/2/0	–	1/2/2	1/0/4	1/3/1	5/0/0	20/10/10	3
	0/1 Loss	3/0/2	1/2/2	1/3/1	0/3/2	–	0/2/3	0/2/3	0/2/3	0/2/3	5/16/19	
	Overall	10/2/8	9/4/7	9/5/6	8/6/6	–	6/6/8	6/2/12	8/7/5	13/2/5	69/34/57	
2SDSR-MS	HL	0/1/4	1/2/2	2/1/2	0/1/4	1/0/4	–	1/3/1	3/1/1	4/1/0	12/10/18	
	F1	5/0/0	5/0/0	5/0/0	5/0/0	2/2/1	–	0/4/1	3/2/0	3/2/0	28/10/2	
	Accuracy	4/0/1	4/0/1	4/0/1	2/2/1	2/2/1	–	1/3/1	4/0/1	4/1/0	25/10/5	2
	0/1 Loss	0/4/1	2/2/1	3/1/1	1/3/1	3/2/0	–	0/3/2	1/3/1	4/1/0	14/20/6	
	Overall	9/5/6	12/4/4	14/2/4	8/6/6	8/6/6	–	5/13/2	9/9/2	14/5/1	79/50/31	
2SDSR-MB	HL	0/1/4	1/2/2	1/2/2	0/1/4	1/0/4	1/3/1	–	3/2/0	5/0/0	12/11/17	
	F1	5/0/0	5/0/0	5/0/0	5/0/0	4/0/1	1/4/0	–	3/2/0	2/3/0	30/9/1	
	Accuracy	4/0/1	5/0/0	4/1/0	3/2/0	4/0/1	1/3/1	–	4/1/0	4/0/1	28/7/5	1
	0/1 Loss	1/3/1	1/3/1	0/3/1	0/3/2	3/2/0	2/3/0	–	2/3/0	3/2/0	13/22/5	
	Overall	10/4/6	12/5/3	11/6/3	8/6/6	12/2/6	5/13/2	–	12/8/0	14/5/1	83/49/28	
2SDSR-CS	HL	0/1/4	0/1/4	2/0/3	0/1/4	0/2/3	1/1/3	0/2/3	–	1/0/4	5/9/26	
	F1	1/0/4	4/1/0	4/0/1	1/0/4	1/0/4	3/2/0	3/2/0	–	2/0/3	19/5/16	
	Accuracy	3/0/2	1/1/3	3/1/1	1/2/2	1/3/1	1/0/4	0/1/4	–	4/0/1	15/8/17	5
	0/1 Loss	0/3/2	0/3/2	1/2/2	1/3/1	3/2/0	1/2/2	0/3/2	–	3/2/0	9/21/10	
	Overall	7/4/9	7/5/8	9/2/9	7/6/7	5/7/8	5/6/9	0/8/12	–	12/3/5	48/43/69	
2SDSR-CB	HL	0/0/5	0/0/5	0/0/5	0/1/4	0/0/5	1/0/4	0/0/5	1/0/4	–	2/1/37	
	F1	3/0/2	3/0/2	3/0/2	3/0/2	2/0/3	0/2/3	0/3/2	2/0/3	–	17/5/18	
	Accuracy	2/0/3	2/0/3	2/0/3	2/2/1	0/0/5	0/2/3	1/0/4	1/0/4	–	10/5/25	9
	0/1 Loss	2/0/3	0/3/2	0/2/3	0/3/2	0/2/3	0/1/4	0/2/3	1/3/1	–	3/16/21	
	Overall	5/2/13	5/2/13	5/2/13	5/6/9	5/2/13	1/5/14	1/5/14	5/3/12	–	32/27/101	

5   Experimental Results

In this work, 2SDSR is compared with six multi-label classification techniques; BR, MDDM, CCA, PLST, MLC-BMaD [12] and DDSR. BR is a simple and widely used multi-label classification method but it does not employ dimensionality reduction techniques to both feature and label spaces. MDDM and CCA are feature space reduction methods, PLST and MLC-BMaD are label space reduction methods. In our proposed 2SDSR framework, MDDM and CCA were applied to reduce feature space and SVD and BMD were employed to reduce label space. The variation of our proposed frameworks are represented as 2SDSR-MS, 2SDSR-MB, 2SDSR-CS and 2SDSR-CB, where M, C, S and B stand for MDDM, CCA, SVD and BMD, respectively. Table 2 reports only the best value for each evaluation metric computed from each dataset and the comparison of nine multi-label classification methods are shown in Table 3.

The experimental results shown that the classification performance tends to be improved when the feature and label spaces are transformed to the lower-dimensional spaces. For instance, when the 2SDSR-MB is applied to *corel5k*, *scene* and *yeast*, it presented best performance in terms of the *macro F-measure* and *accuracy* as shown in Table 2. In the Table 3, we noticed that the proposed 2SDSR-MB achieved the best performance when MDDM and BMD were exploited in feature reduction and label reduction, respectively. In addition, the proposed 2SDSR framework that applied MDDM in feature reduction step i.e., 2SDSR-MS and 2SDSR-MB, shown better performance comparing to the other variation of 2SDSR frameworks. However, the 2SDSR framework that exploited the CCA i.e., 2SDSR-CS and 2SDSR-CB can reduced a large number of features as presented in the 11th and 12th columns of Table 2. Moreover, the dual space reduction methods e.g., 2SDSR-MS, 2SDSR-MB and DDSR show better performance, compared to the multi-label classification that applied only feature space reduction or label space reduction.

6   Conclusion

This paper presents an alternative framework to handle high dimensionality problem in the feature space as well as the sparseness problem in the label space. Our proposed framework, namely Two-Stage Dual Space Reduction (2SDSR), transforms a high-dimensional label space into the reduced label space after that a supervised dimensionality reduction technique is applied to project high-dimensional feature space to the lower-dimensional label space. Later, these reduced feature and label matrices are used to build a set of classification models. By this framework, four widely used dimensionality reduction methods i.e., MDDM, CCA, SVD and BMD can be applied to our proposed framework. Experiments with a broad range of multi-label datasets shown that our proposed framework achieved a better performance, compared to traditional method which reduce only the feature space or the label space.

Acknowledgement. This work has been supported by the TRF Royal Golden Jubilee Ph.D. Program [PHD/0304/2551]; and the Government Research Fund via Thammasat University, Thailand, and the National Research University Project of Thailand Office of Higher Education Commission.

References

1. Fan, R.E., Lin, C.J.: A Study on Threshold Selection for Multi-label Classification. National Taiwan University (2007)
2. Golub, G., Reinsch, C.: Singular value decomposition and least squares solutions. Numerische Mathematik 14, 403–420 (1970)
3. Gretton, A., Bousquet, O., Smola, A.J., Schölkopf, B.: Measuring statistical dependence with hilbert-schmidt norms. In: Jain, S., Simon, H.U., Tomita, E. (eds.) ALT 2005. LNCS (LNAI), vol. 3734, pp. 63–77. Springer, Heidelberg (2005)
4. Hotelling, H.: The most predictable criterion. Journal of Educational Psychology 26, 139–142 (1935)
5. Hsu, D., Kakade, S., Langford, J., Zhang, T.: Multi-label prediction via compressed sensing. Proceedings of the Advances in Neural Information Processing Systems 22, 772–780 (2009)
6. Miettinen, P.: The boolean column and column-row matrix decompositions. Data Mining and Knowledge Discovery 17(1), 39–56 (2008)
7. Pacharawongsakda, E., Theeramunkong, T.: Towards more efficient multi-label classification using dependent and independent dual space reduction. In: Tan, P.-N., Chawla, S., Ho, C.K., Bailey, J. (eds.) PAKDD 2012, Part II. LNCS, vol. 7302, pp. 383–394. Springer, Heidelberg (2012)
8. Read, J., Pfahringer, B., Holmes, G., Frank, E.: Classifier chains for multi-label classification. Machine Learning, 1–27 (2011)
9. Schapire, R., Singer, Y.: Boostexter: A boosting-based system for text categorization. Machine Learning 39(2/3), 135–168 (2000)
10. Tai, F., Lin, H.T.: Multi-label classification with principle label space transformation. In: Proceedings of the 2nd International Workshop on Learning from Multi-Label Data (MLD 2010), pp. 45–52 (2010)
11. Tsoumakas, G., Katakis, I., Vlahavas, I.: Mining Multi-label Data, 2nd edn. Data Mining and Knowledge Discovery Handbook. Springer (2010)
12. Wicker, J., Pfahringer, B., Kramer, S.: Multi-label classification using boolean matrix decomposition. In: Proceedings of the 27th Annual ACM Symposium on Applied Computing, pp. 179–186. Springer, Heidelberg (2012)
13. Yu, K., Yu, S., Tresp, V.: Multi-label informed latent semantic indexing. In: Proceedings of the 28th Annual International ACM SIGIR Conference on Research and Development in Information Retrieval, pp. 258–265 (2005)
14. Zhang, Y., Zhou, Z.H.: Multilabel dimensionality reduction via dependence maximization. ACM Transactions on Knowledge Discovery from Data (TKDD) 4(3), 1–21 (2010)

Effective Evaluation Measures
for Subspace Clustering of Data Streams

Marwan Hassani[1], Yunsu Kim[1], Seungjin Choi[2], and Thomas Seidl[1]

[1] Data Management and Data Exploration Group
RWTH Aachen University, Germany
{hassani,kim,seidl}@cs.rwth-aachen.de
[2] Department of Computer Science and Engineering
Pohang University of Science and Technology, Korea
seungjin@postech.ac.kr

Abstract. Nowadays, most streaming data sources are becoming high-dimensional. Accordingly, subspace stream clustering, which aims at finding evolving clusters within subgroups of dimensions, has gained a significant importance. However, existing subspace clustering evaluation measures are mainly designed for static data, and cannot reflect the quality of the evolving nature of data streams. On the other hand, available stream clustering evaluation measures care only about the errors of the *full-space* clustering but not the quality of subspace clustering.

In this paper we propose, to the first of our knowledge, the first subspace clustering measure that is designed for streaming data, called *Sub-CMM*: **Sub**space **C**luster **M**apping **M**easure. *SubCMM* is an effective evaluation measure for stream subspace clustering that is able to handle errors caused by emerging, moving, or splitting subspace clusters. Additionally, we propose a novel method for using available *offline* subspace clustering measures for data streams within the *Subspace MOA* framework.

1 Introduction

Data sources are increasingly generating more and more amounts of data. Additionally, the huge advances of data sensing systems resulted in cheap means for satisfying the eagerness for collecting data with a high number of attributes. The big size of the data together with its high dimensionality motivated the research in the area of high dimensional data mining and exploration. Data stream is a form of data that continuously and endlessly evolves reflecting the current status of collected values. Clustering is a well known data mining technique that aims at grouping similar objects in the dataset together into same clusters, and dissimilar ones into different clusters, where the similarity is decided based on some distance function. Thus, objects separated by far distances are dissimilar and thus belong to different clusters.

Stream clustering algorithms search for clusters that are formed out of the streaming objects when considering all dimensions of these objects. We call them

J. Li et al. (Eds.): PAKDD 2013 Workshops, LNAI 7867, pp. 342–353, 2013.

in this context: *full-space* stream clustering algorithms to differentiate them from other types of stream clustering algorithms which consider all subgroups of dimensions while searching for clusters.

Evaluating full-space stream clustering algorithms, can done mainly by assessing: (a) the **efficiency** represented by the runtime, the memory usage or the number of microclusters processed by the algorithm when mining the stream with different speeds, and (b) the **effectiveness** represented by the quality of the resulted clusters which mainly compares the found evolving clusters to the ground truth ones. Most of these were inherited from the offline clustering world, only one was mainly designed for streaming algorithm (cf. CMM [21]).

In many applications of streaming data, objects are described by using multiple dimensions (e.g. the Network Intrusion Dataset [1] has 42 dimensions). For such kinds of data with higher dimensions, distances grow more and more alike due to an effect termed *curse of dimensionality* [7] (cf. the toy example in Figure 1). Applying traditional clustering algorithms (called in this context: *full-space* clustering algorithms) over such data objects will lead to useless clustering results. In Figure 1, the majority of the black objects will be grouped in a single-object cluster (outliers) when using a full-space clustering algorithm, since they are all dissimilar, but apparently they are not as dissimilar as the gray objects. The latter fact motivated the research in the domain of *subspace* and *projected clustering* in the last decade which resulted in an established research area for static data.

In parallel to developing these static data subspace clustering algorithms, a group of measures for evaluating the clustering quality of offline subspace clustering algorithms were established. Additionally, other measures were inherited from traditional full-space clustering world (e.g. RNIA, CE [29], Entropy [30], Accuracy [9] and F1).

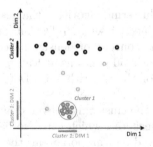

Fig. 1. An example of subspace clustering

For streaming data on the other hand, although a considerable research has tackled the full-space clustering, relatively limited work has dealt with subspace clustering. HPStream [3], PreDeConStream [17], HDDStream [27] and SiblingList [28] are the only works that have been done on projected/subspace stream clustering.

Almost all of the above mentioned algorithms have used the clustering purity [31] as the only measure for assessing the clustering quality. The purity was not mainly designed for subspace stream clustering, and does not reflect the cases when clusters hidden in some subspaces are completely not discovered.

In this paper we propose, to the first of our knowledge, the first subspace clustering measure that is designed for streaming data, called *SubCMM*: **Subspace Cluster Mapping Measure.** *SubCMM* is an effective evaluation measure for stream subspace clustering that is able to handle errors caused by emerging, moving, or splitting subspace clusters. Additionally, we propose a novel method for using available *offline* subspace clustering measures for data streams within the *Subspace MOA* framework [14].

The remainder of this paper is organized as follows: Section 2 gives a short overview of the related work from different neighboring areas to full-space and subspace stream clustering algorithms as well as the measured used there. Section 3 introduces the *Subspace MOA* framework [14] and the novel method that we use for adapting the offline subspace measures as well as our *SubCMM* measure for using it under streaming environments. Our SubCMM measure is introduced in Section 4. The suggested measures are then thoroughly evaluated using the Subspace MOA framework in Section 5. Then we conclude the paper with a short outlook in Section 6.

2   Related Work

In this section, we list the related work from three areas: subspace clustering measures for static data, full-space stream clustering measures, and available subspace stream clustering and measures. Finally we will detail CMM [21].

2.1   Subspace Clustering Measures for Static Data

SubClu [23] is a subspace clustering algorithm that uses the DBSCAN [12] clustering model of density connected sets. PreDeCon [8] is a projected clustering algorithm which adapts the concept of density based clustering [12]. and the preference weighted neighborhood contains at least μ points. IncPreDeCon [22] is an incremental version of the algorithm PreDeCon [8] designed to handle accumulating data.

Evaluating the quality of the clustering delivered by the above algorithms was performed using a set of measures, which can also be categorized according to [26] depending on the required information about the ground truth clusters into two categories:

1. **Object-Based Measures:** where only information on which objects should be grouped together to form a cluster are used. Examples are: **entropy** [30] which measures the homogeneity of the found clusters with respect to the ground truth clusters, **f1** [6] which evaluates how well the ground truth clusters are represented and **accuracy** [9].

2. **Object- and Subspace-Based Measures:** where information on objects as well as their relevant dimensions (i.e. the subspaces where they belong

to) are used. Examples are: (a)**RNIA** [29] (Relative Non Intersecting Area) which measures to which extent the ground truth subobjects are covered by the found subobjects and (b) **CE** [29] (Clustering Error) which is an advanced version of RNIA and differs that it maps each found cluster to at most one ground truth cluster and also each ground truth cluster to at most one found cluster.

2.2   Full-Space Clustering Measures for Streaming Data

There is a rich body of literature on stream clustering. Convex stream clustering approaches are based on a k-center clustering [2,16]. Detecting clusters of arbitrary shapes in streaming data has been proposed using kernels [18], fractal dimensions [24] and density based clustering [10,11]. Another line of research considers the anytime clustering with the existence of outliers [15].

To reflect the quality of the *full-space* clustering algorithm, many evaluation measures are used. Some of those are inherited from the offline clustering world (cf. for instance: **SSQ** [13], **Silhouette Coefficients** [19] and **purity** [31]). Other measures were mainly developed specifically for assessing the quality of full space stream clustering algorithms like **CMM** [21] (cf. Section 2.4).

2.3   Subspace Clustering Measures for Streaming Data

Sibling Tree [28] is a grid-based *subspace* clustering algorithm where the streaming distribution statistics is monitored by a list of grid-cells. Once a grid-cell is dense, the tree grows in that cell in order to trace any possible higher dimensional cluster. HPStream [3] is a k-means-based *projected* clustering algorithm for high dimensional data stream. PreDeConStream [17] and HDDStream [27] are recent density-based projected stream clustering algorithms that were developed developed upon PreDeCon [8] in the offline phase.

Almost all of the above mentioned subspace stream clustering algorithms have used the clustering **purity** [31] as the only measure for assessing the clustering quality. Although the purity has proved to be popular and good when used with full-space stream clustering, it was not mainly designed for subspace stream clustering, and does not reflect the cases when clusters hidden in some subspaces are completely not discovered. Additionally, because of its property of neglecting the shaped of the ground truth, errors occurring on the borders of detected microclusters are not correctly punished due to the fast change of the shape or the position of the cluster.

2.4   Review: CMM [21]

We will review CMM separately here, since it is the only stream clustering measure that was designed for streaming applications, and because it is the full-space version of our proposed measure: SubCMM. CMM (Cluster Mapping Measure) consists of three phases.

First, each found cluster is assigned to one of the ground truth clusters based on class distribution in each cluster. In Figure 2(a), a plain circle represents a ground cluster, and a dashed circle means a predicted cluster. Each dot is a data point having its class label expressed by colors. Class frequencies are counted for each cluster, and each prediction cluster is mapped to a ground truth cluster that has the most similar class distribution. For Figure 2(a), the found cluster is mapped to the gray circle ground truth cluster.

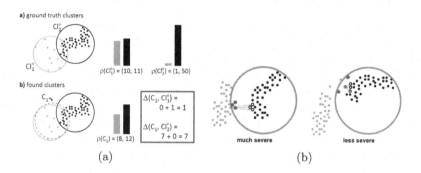

Fig. 2. CMM: (a) The mapping phase of the found cluster to a ground truth cluster, (b) Different penalties for two clusterings having the same accuracy

Second, the penalty for every incorrectly predicted point is calculated. In Figure 2(a), it can be seen that a lot of black points are included in the found cluster, which are incorrectly clustered, and some of the gray points are excluded in the cluster even if they are not noises. These points are "fault objects" and give they are penalized like this: $pen(o, C_i) = con(o, Cl(o)).(1 - con(o, map(C_i)))$ where C_i is a prediction cluster to which the object o belongs to, $Cl(o)$ is a ground truth cluster (hidden cluster) representing the original class label of o, and $map(C_i)$ is the hidden cluster on which C_i is mapped through the cluster mapping phase. The two clusters in Figure 2(b) have same accuracy, but it looks obvious that the left clustering has a bigger problem. If a fault object is closely connected to its hidden cluster, then the error becomes much severe since it was meant to be easily clustered. On the other hand, if the object has high connectivity to the found cluster, CMM allows a low penalty since it was hard to be clustered correctly. The connectivity $con(o, C)$ from an object to a cluster is exploiting the average k-neighborhood distance.

Third, derive a final CMM value by summing up all the penalties weighted over its own lifespan: $CMM(R, H) = 1 - \frac{\sum_{o \in F} w(o).pen(o,R)}{\sum_{o \in O} w(o).con(o,Cl(o))}$ Where R: represents the found clusters, H: represents the ground truth (hidden) clusters, O: is the set of objects o, F: is fault set, and $w(o)$: is the weight of o.

In the next section, we will explain our Subspace MOA tool, which we used to adapt the offline subspace clustering measures for the streaming scenario.

3   The *Subspace MOA* Framework [14]

OpenSubspace framework [25] was proposed to evaluate and explore subspace clustering algorithms in WEKA with a rich body of most state of the art subspace/projected clustering algorithms and measures. In *Subspace MOA* [14], we have used this framework within the MOA framework [20] to bring the powerful subspace evaluation measures from the offline to the streaming world. Additionally, we built all the required additional units:

3.1   Subspace Stream Generator

Subspace MOA offers a synthetic random RBF subspace generator with the possibility of varying multiple parameters of the generated stream and its subspace events. One can vary: the number of dimensions, the number of relevant dimensions (i.e. the number of dimensions of the subspaces that contain the ground truth clusters), the number of the generated clusters, the radius of the generated clusters, the speed of the movement of the generated clusters, the percentage of the allowed overlapping between clusters, and the percentage of noise. Please note that some dimensions of a point could represent a noise within some subspace, while other dimensions could be a part of a ground truth cluster in other subspace. The generated noise percentage in this case represents a guaranteed noise in all subspaces. Subspace MOA gives also the possibility of reading external ARFF files.

3.2   Subspace Stream Clustering Algorithms

In order to have a rich number of variants, Subspace MOA offers the possibility of making your own flavor of subspace stream clustering algorithm. It follows for this reason the online-offline model used in most stream clustering algorithms (cf. [2], [10], [17]). In the **online phase**, a summarization of the data stream points is performed and the resulting microclusters is given by sets of cluster features $CF_i = (N, LS_i, SS_i)$ which represent the number of points within that microcluster, their linear sum and their squared sum, respectively. Subspace MOA offers three algorithms to form these microclusters and continuously maintain them. These are: CluStream, DenStream, and the cluster generator. In the **offline phase**, the clustering features are used to reconstruct an approximation to the original N points using Gaussian functions to reconstruct spherical microclusters centered at $c_i = \frac{LS_i}{N}$ with a radius: $r = \sqrt{\frac{SS}{N} - (\frac{LS}{N})^2}$ ($SS = \frac{1}{d}\sum_{i=1}^{d} SS_i$ and $LS = \frac{1}{d}\sum_{i=1}^{d} LS_i$). The generated N points are forwarded to one of the five subspace clustering algorithms. These are SubClu [23], ProClus [4], Clique [5], P3C, and FIRES. This results with 15 different combinations of algorithms that can be tested.

3.3   Subspace Stream Evaluation Measures

Then we have adapted the most famous offline subspace clustering measures
(CE [29], Entropy [30], F1 [6], RNIA [29]) measures to the streaming scenario.
Additionally, we have implemented our novel **SubCMM** measure (cf. Section
4). The user has the possibility to select the evaluation frequency, the window
size is then set accordingly, and the evaluation measure is applied over the found
clusters when compared against the ground truth clusters within that window.
The output of these evaluation measures is delivered to the user according to the
MOA conventions in three ways: (a) in a **textual form**, where summarization
values are printed gradually in the output panel under the "Setup" tab as the
stream evolves, (b) in a **numerical form**, where recent values are of all measures
are printed instantly under the "Visualization" tab, and (c) in a **plotted** form of
a selected measure from the recent values. The evolving of the final clustering of
the selected subspace clustering algorithms as well as the evolving of the ground
truth stream is visualized in a two dimensional representation. Users can select
any pair of dimensions to visualize the evolving ground truth as well as the
resulted clustering. Different to MOA, Subspace MOA is able to visualize and
get the quality measures of arbitrarily shaped clusters.

4   *SubCMM*: Subspace Cluster Mapping Measure

We adopted important concepts of CMM (cf. Section 2.4) and revised its internal
structure to develop a novel evaluation measure for subspace clusterings. The
motivation for having a special subspace version of CMM becomes clear when
using CMM directly for subspace clustering scenarios. Consider the matrix representation of data in Figure 3, where columns represent the objects and rows
represent the attributes. Thus, each object is represented by a column, where its
lines represent the attributes of this object. Assume that neighboring columns
represent neighboring objects. Each circle is an attribute value of an object and
the color denotes its class label (gray means noise). Blue, red, purple and orange
subspace colors represent ground truth classes and the green dashed rectan-
gle represents the found cluster of some stream clustering algorithm. In Figure
3(a), the found cluster is delivered by a full-space stream clustering algorithm,
and thus it contains only complete columns in the matrix representation. CMM
would not be able to map the found cluster C to the class blue since no obvious
single class lable for each object can be found. Additionally, a subspace stream
clustering algorithm would deliver clusters that look like C in Figure 3(b). Here,
clusters could contain an arbitrary number of rows. Again, data objects in different clusters are defined in different spaces so we cannot simply count objects
to compute class distributions as in CMM. We propose checking the class label
of each attribute value (represented here by circle), instead of objects, we call
it: Subobjects e_{ij}. Thus, in the matrix representations in Figure 3(b), it seems
reasonable to assign the found cluster to class blue, since it contains 13 blue
circles, one red circle and one noise circle. A similar discussion was mentioned
in [29], to define the distance between subspace clusters.

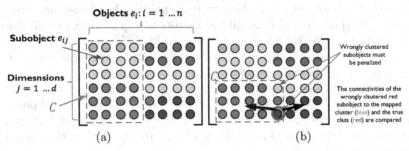

Fig. 3. (a) Full-space clustering and CMM over the matrix representation of subobjects, (b) Subspace clustering idea using SubCMM and penalizing fault subobjects

Thus, the penalty calculations in current CMM should be changed according to the revised clustering mapping phase. As we construct class distributions in a cluster in the matrix-element-wise way, the fault set consists of fault *matrix elements*, and a fault object o in $pen(o, C_i)$ is to be replaced with a fault matrix element e_{ij}, which is the $j - th$ subobject of $i - th$ object (cf. Figure 3(b)). Thus the penalty for each wrongly clustered subobject e_{ij} can be calculated as: $pen(e_{ij}, C) = con(e_{ij}, Cl(e_{ij})).(1 - con(e_{ij}, map(C_i)))$. To calculate the penalty in this fashion, we have to define the connectivity between a subobject e_{ij} and a subspace cluster C. In CMM, the connectivity is based on average k-neighborhood distance, which computes Euclidean distance between two data objects and only the difference between attribute values of a same dimension is needed. In the SubCMM, we consider additionally the distance between different dimensions: $con(e_{ij}, C) = subcon(e_{ij}, C).objcon(e_{ij}, C)$ where $subcon(e_{ij}, C)$, the subspace connectivity, represents how much e_{ij} is connected to the subspace of C, and $objcon(e_{ij}, C)$, the object connectivity, means how much e_{ij} is connected to the (sub)objects of C. We define the object connectivity as:

$$objcon(e_{ij}, C) = \begin{cases} 1 & \text{if } [e_{ij} \in C] \text{ or if } [e_{ij} \notin C] \text{ AND} \\ & [knhObjDist^S(e_{ij}, C) < knhObjDist^S(C)] \\ 0 & \text{if } C = null \\ \frac{knhObjDist^S(C)}{knhObjDist^S(e_{ij}, C)} & \text{else} \end{cases}$$

where $knhObjDist^S(e_{ij}, C)$ is the average k-neighborhood distance from e_{ij} to the subobjects in C within the subspace S, and $knhDist^S(C)$ is the average k-neighborhood distance between objects in C within S. The subspace connectivity $subcon(e_{ij}, C)$ is similarly defined as:

$$subcon(e_{ij}, C) = \begin{cases} 1 & \text{if } [j \in S] \text{ or if } [j \notin S] \text{ AND} \\ & [knhDimDist^{e_{ij}}(j, C) < knhDimDist^{e_{ij}}(C)] \\ 0 & \text{if } C = null \\ \frac{knhDimDist^{e_{ij}}(C)}{knhDimDist^{e_{ij}}(j, C)} & \text{else} \end{cases}$$

where: $knhDimDist^{e_{ij}}(j, C)$ is the average k-neighborhood distance from the vector $v_j = [e_{aj}]$ where $a \in C$ to all the vectors $v_l = [e_{al}]$ where $a \in C$ and all $l \in S$ constructed from the objects of C defined in S.

And $knhDimDist^{e_{ij}}(C)$ is the average k-neighborhood distance between vectors v_l constructed from C as above. One can regard this as performing the same procedure of calculating object connectivity on a transposed data matrix. Finally, we have to compute the final SubCMM value with the revised penalties. In this phase, we can just follow the CMM, but the fault object o must be a fault matrix element e_{ij}, and the weights of $e_{ij}s$ are equal when they belong to a same object.

$$SubCMM(R, H) = 1 - \frac{\sum_{e_{ij} \in F} w(i) \cdot pen(e_{ij}, R)}{\sum_{i \in DB} w(i) \sum_{j \in D} con(e_{ij}, Cl(e_{ij}))}$$

5 Experimental Evaluation

To test the performance of the suggested subspace stream clustering measures, we have used Subspace MOA [14] as the testing framework. We have used: CluStream+PROCLUS as the tested subspace stream clustering algorithm, and the RBF subspace stream generator as the ground truth stream. We compared the performance of SubCMM, RNIA, CE, Entropy and F1 as representatives of subspace stream clustering measures against the performance of CMM and Rand statistic as representatives of full-space stream clustering measures. In all of the following experiments, the stream and algorithm parameter settings, unless otherwise mentioned, are: number of stream attributes= 12, number of attributes of generated clusters= 4, number of generated clusters=5, noise level=10%, apeed of movement of clusters=0.01 per 200 points (which reflects the evolving speed of the concept drift of the stream), the evaluation frequency= 1000, and the decaying threshold= 0.1. Figure 4 compares the performance of subspace stream clustering measures (left) against full-space clustering algorithms when varying the pure noise percentage around the generated ground truth clusters. Apparently, most subspace measures are sensitive to the increasing of noise, different to the full-space ones. The stable high value that full-space measures give is due to the clusters which are accidentally created out the combination of clusters generated in the lower dimensions. Even for those clusters, when using the full-space measures, the quality does not decrease as in the subspace measures. Figure 5 shows the performance of both subspace and full-space measures when varying the number of generated ground truth clusters. Here the expected effect is a decreasing of the quality as the number of clusters increases. Again, full-space measures are relatively stable, while most subspace measures are sensitive.

Figure 6 depicts the quality of subspace and full-space measures when varying the radius of the generated clusters. Again the expected change here is a quality decrease as the radius increases. This is clear to see with most subspace measures, while only a slightly decrease can be seen on the full-space measures. The latter decrease, is due to the higher density of the noisy points around the accidentally

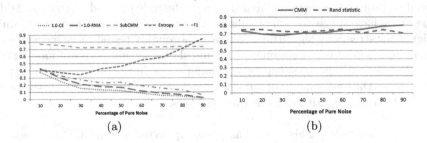

Fig. 4. Clustering quality of a subspace stream clustering algorithm when varying the noise level using: (a) Subspace measures, (b) Full-space measures

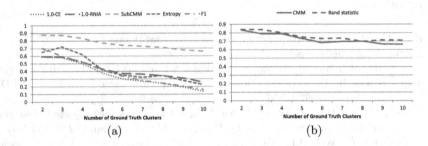

Fig. 5. Clustering quality of a subspace stream clustering algorithm when varying the number of clusters using: (a) Subspace measures, (b) Full-space measures

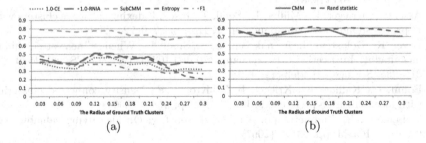

Fig. 6. Clustering quality of a subspace stream clustering algorithm when varying the radius of clusters using: (a) Subspace measures, (b) Full-space measures

generated clusters in the full space. This noise might wrongly be added to the clusters in the full-space, and only this noise is punished by full-space measures and not the noise in lower dimensions.

6 Conclusion and Future Work

In this paper we have suggested a new way for evaluating stream subspace clustering algorithms by making use of available offline subspace clustering algorithms as well as using the streaming environment to be able to handle streams. Additionally, we have suggested a first subspace clustering measure which was mainly designed for streaming algorithms. We have thoroughly tested these measures by comparing them to full-space ones. We could show the superiority of most of the suggested measures in the subspace streaming cases. In the future we plan to further improve the performance of SubCMM, and we want to test available subspace stream clustering algorithms using our measures.

Acknowledgments. This work has been supported by the UMIC Research Centre, RWTH Aachen University, Germany.

References

1. KDD Cup 1999 Data, http://kdd.ics.uci.edu/databases/kddcup99/kddcup99.html
2. Aggarwal, C.C., Han, J., Wang, J., Yu, P.S.: A framework for clustering evolving data streams. In: Proc. of the 29th Int. Conf. on Very Large Data Bases, VLDB 2003, vol. 29, pp. 81–92 (2003)
3. Aggarwal, C.C., Han, J., Wang, J., Yu, P.S.: A framework for projected clustering of high dimensional data streams. In: Proc. of VLDB 2004, pp. 852–863 (2004)
4. Aggarwal, C.C., Wolf, J.L., Yu, P.S., Procopiuc, C., Park, J.S.: Fast algorithms for projected clustering. SIGMOD Rec. 28(2), 61–72 (1999)
5. Agrawal, R., Gehrke, J., Gunopulos, D., Raghavan, P.: Automatic subspace clustering of high dimensional data for data mining applications. In: Proc. of SIGMOD 1998, pp. 94–105 (1998)
6. Assent, I., Krieger, R., Müller, E., Seidl, T.: Inscy: Indexing subspace clusters with in-process-removal of redundancy. In: ICDM, pp. 719–724 (2008)
7. Beyer, K., Goldstein, J., Ramakrishnan, R., Shaft, U.: When is "nearest neighbor" meaningful? In: Beeri, C., Bruneman, P. (eds.) ICDT 1999. LNCS, vol. 1540, pp. 217–235. Springer, Heidelberg (1998)
8. Bohm, C., Kailing, K., Kriegel, H.-P., Kroger, P.: Density connected clustering with local subspace preferences. In: ICDM, pp. 27–34 (2004)
9. Bringmann, B., Zimmermann, A.: The chosen few: On identifying valuable patterns. In: ICDM, pp. 63–72 (2007)
10. Cao, F., Ester, M., Qian, W., Zhou, A.: Density-based clustering over an evolving data stream with noise. In: 2006 SIAM Conference on Data Mining, pp. 328–339 (2006)
11. Chen, Y., Tu, L.: Density-based clustering for real-time stream data. In: Proc. of KDD 2007, pp. 133–142 (2007)
12. Ester, M., Kriegel, H.-P., Sander, J., Xu, X.: A density-based algorithm for discovering clusters in large spatial databases with noise. In: Proc. of KDD 1996, pp. 226–231 (1996)
13. Han, J., Kamber, M.: Data Mining: Concepts and Techniques. Elsevier Science & Tech. (2006)
14. Hassani, M., Kim, Y., Seidl, T.: Subspace moa: Subspace stream clustering evaluation using the moa framework. In: Meng, W., Feng, L., Bressan, S., Winiwarter, W., Song, W. (eds.) DASFAA 2013, Part II. LNCS, vol. 7826, pp. 446–449. Springer, Heidelberg (2013)

15. Hassani, M., Kranen, P., Seidl, T.: Precise anytime clustering of noisy sensor data with logarithmic complexity. In: Proc. 5th International Workshop on Knowledge Discovery from Sensor Data (SensorKDD 2011) in Conjunction with KDD 2011, pp. 52–60 (2011)

16. Hassani, M., Müller, E., Seidl, T.: EDISKCO: energy efficient distributed in-sensor-network k-center clustering with outliers. In: Proc. SensorKDD 2010 Workshop in Conj. with KDD 2009, pp. 39–48 (2009)

17. Hassani, M., Spaus, P., Gaber, M.M., Seidl, T.: Density-based projected clustering of data streams. In: Hüllermeier, E., Link, S., Fober, T., Seeger, B. (eds.) SUM 2012. LNCS, vol. 7520, pp. 311–324. Springer, Heidelberg (2012)

18. Jain, A., Zhang, Z., Chang, E.Y.: Adaptive non-linear clustering in data streams. In: Proc. of CIKM 2006, pp. 122–131 (2006)

19. Kaufman, L., Rousseeuw, P.J.: Finding groups in data: an introduction to cluster analysis. Wiley series in probability and mathematical statistics: Applied probability and statistics. Wiley (1990)

20. Kranen, P., Kremer, H., Jansen, T., Seidl, T., Bifet, A., Holmes, G., Pfahringer, B., Read, J.: Stream data mining using the MOA framework. In: Lee, S.-g., Peng, Z., Zhou, X., Moon, Y.-S., Unland, R., Yoo, J. (eds.) DASFAA 2012, Part II. LNCS, vol. 7239, pp. 309–313. Springer, Heidelberg (2012)

21. Kremer, H., Kranen, P., Jansen, T., Seidl, T., Bifet, A., Holmes, G., Pfahringer, B.: An effective evaluation measure for clustering on evolving data streams. In: Proc. of KDD 2011 (2011)

22. Kriegel, H.-P., Kröger, P., Ntoutsi, I., Zimek, A.: Towards subspace clustering on dynamic data: an incremental version of predecon. In: Proceedings of the First International Workshop on Novel Data Stream Pattern Mining Techniques, StreamKDD 2010, pp. 31–38 (2010)

23. Kröger, P., Kriegel, H.-P., Kailing, K.: Density-connected subspace clustering for high-dimensional data. In: SDM, pp. 246–257 (2004)

24. Lin, G., Chen, L.: A grid and fractal dimension-based data stream clustering algorithm. In: ISISE 2008, pp. 66–70 (2008)

25. Müller, E., Assent, I., Günnemann, S., Jansen, T., Seidl, T.: Opensubspace: An open source framework for evaluation and exploration of subspace clustering algorithms in weka. In: In Open Source in Data Mining Workshop at PAKDD, pp. 2–13 (2009)

26. Müller, E., Günnemann, S., Assent, I., Seidl, T.: Evaluating clustering in subspace projections of high dimensional data. PVLDB 2(1), 1270–1281 (2009)

27. Ntoutsi, I., Zimek, A., Palpanas, T., Kröger, P., Kriegel, H.-P.: Density-based projected clustering over high dimensional data streams. In: Proc. of SDM 2012, pp. 987–998 (2012)

28. Park, N.H., Lee, W.S.: Grid-based subspace clustering over data streams. In: Proc. of CIKM 2007, pp. 801–810 (2007)

29. Patrikainen, A., Meila, M.: Comparing subspace clusterings. IEEE Transactions on Knowledge and Data Engineering 18(7), 902–916 (2006)

30. Sequeira, K., Zaki, M.: Schism: A new approach to interesting subspace mining, vol. 1, pp. 137–160 (2005)

31. Zhao, Y., Karypis, G.: Criterion functions for document clustering: Experiments and analysis. Technical report (2002)

Objectively Evaluating Interestingness Measures for Frequent Itemset Mining

Albrecht Zimmermann

KU Leuven, Celestijnenlaan 200A, B-3001 Leuven, Belgium
albrecht.zimmermann@cs.kuleuven.be

Abstract. Itemset mining approaches, while having been studied for more than 15 years, have been evaluated only on a handful of data sets. In particular, they have never been evaluated on data sets for which the ground truth was known. Thus, it is currently unknown whether itemset mining techniques actually recover underlying patterns. Since the weakness of the algorithmically attractive support/confidence framework became apparent early on, a number of interestingness measures have been proposed. Their utility, however, has not been evaluated, except for attempts to establish congruence with expert opinions. Using an extension of the Quest generator proposed in the original itemset mining paper, we propose to evaluate these measures objectively for the first time, showing how many non-relevant patterns slip through the cracks.

1 Introduction

Frequent itemset mining (FIM) was introduced almost twenty years ago [1] and the framework has proven to be very successful. It not only spawned related approaches to mining patterns in sequentially, tree, and graph-structured data, but due to its relative simplicity it has been extended beyond the mining of supermarket baskets towards general correlation discovery between attribute value pairs, discovery of co-expressed genes, and classification rules, etc.

The original framework used frequency of itemsets in the data (support) as a significance criterion – often occurring itemsets are assumed not to be chance occurrences – and conditional probability of the right-hand side of association rules (confidence) as a correlation criterion. This framework has clear weaknesses and other interestingness measures have been proposed in the years since the seminal paper was published [18], as well as several condensed representations [13,5,10] that attempt to remove redundant information from the result set.

While each of these measures and condensed representations is well-motivated, there is as of yet no consensus about how effectively existing correlations are in fact discovered. A prime reason for this can be seen in the difficulty of evaluating the quality of data mining results. In classification or regression tasks, there is a clearly defined target value, often objectively measured or derived from expert labeling *a priori* to the mining/modeling process, that results can be compared to to assess the goodness of fit. In clustering research, the problem is somewhat more

J. Li et al. (Eds.): PAKDD 2013 Workshops, LNAI 7867, pp. 354–366, 2013.

pronounced but clusters can be evaluated w.r.t. intra-cluster similarity and inter-clusters dissimilarity, knowledge about predefined groups might be available, e.g. by equating them with underlying classes, and last but not least there exist generators for artificial data [15]. In FIM, in contrast, while the seminal paper introduced a data generator as well, that data generator has been used only for efficiency estimations and fell furthermore into some disregard after Zheng *et al.* showed that the data it generated had characteristics that were not in line with real-life data sets [22]. The current, rather small collection of benchmark sets, hosted at the FIMI repository [2], consists of data sets whose underlying patterns are unknown. As an alternative, patterns mined using different measures have been shown to human "domain experts" who were asked to assess their interestingness [8]. Given humans' tendency to see patterns where none occur, insights gained from this approach might be limited.

Interestingly enough, however, the Quest generator proposed by Agrawal *et al.* already includes everything needed to perform such assessments: it generates data by embedding source itemsets, making it possible to check mining results against a gold standard of predefined patterns. Other data generation methods proposed since [16,9,17,3] do not use clearly defined patterns and can therefore not be used for this kind of analysis.

The contribution of this work is that we repurpose the Quest generator accordingly and address this open questions for the first time:

– How effective are different interestingness measures in recovering embedded source itemsets?

In the next section, we introduce the basics of the FIM setting, and discuss different interestingness measures. In Section 3, we describe the parameters of the Quest generator and its data generation process. Equipped with this information, we can discuss related work in Section 4, placing our contribution into context and motivating it further. Following this, we report on an experimental evaluation of pattern recovery in Section 5, before we conclude in Section 6.

2 The FIM Setting

We employ the usual notations in that we assume a collection of *items* $\mathcal{I} = \{i_1, \ldots, i_N\}$, and call a set of items $I \subseteq \mathcal{I}$ an itemset, of size $|I|$. In the same manner, we refer to a transaction $t \subseteq \mathcal{I}$ of size $|t|$, and a data set $\mathcal{T} \subseteq 2^{\mathcal{I}}$, of size $|\mathcal{T}|$. An itemset I matches (or is supported by) a transaction t iff $I \subseteq t$, the support of I is $sup(I, \mathcal{T}) = |\{t \in \mathcal{T} \mid I \subseteq t\}|$, and its relative support or frequency $freq(I, \mathcal{T}) = \frac{sup(I, \mathcal{T})}{|\mathcal{T}|}$. The *confidence* of an association rule formed of two itemsets $X, Y \subset \mathcal{I}, X \cap T = \emptyset$ is calculated as $conf(X \Rightarrow Y, \mathcal{T}) = \frac{sup(X \cup Y, \mathcal{T})}{sup(X, \mathcal{T})}$. When the context makes it clear which data set is referred to, we drop $\mathcal{T}$ from the notation.

2.1 Interestingness Measures

The support/confidence framework has at least one major drawback in that it ignores prior probabilities. Assume, for instance, two items i_1, i_2 with $freq(i_1) = 0.6$, $freq(i_2) = 0.8$. While $freq(i_1, i_2) = 0.48$ would often denote the itemset as a high-frequency itemset, it is in fact exactly what would be expected given independence of the two items. Similarly, $conf(i_1 \Rightarrow i_2) = 0.8$, while clearly a high confidence value, would also indicate independence when compared to the prior frequency of i_2. Therefore, numerous other measures have been proposed to address these shortcoming [18].

Most of them have been proposed for assessing the quality of association rules, meaning that they relate two binary variables. Generally speaking, it is possible to use such measures more generally to assess the quality of itemsets in the following way. Given an interestingness measure $m : \mathcal{I} \times \mathcal{I} \mapsto \mathbb{R}$, itemset I, we can take the minimal value over all possible association rules with a single item in the right-hand side (RHS): $\min_{i \in I} \{m(I \setminus i \Rightarrow i)\}$. This is the approach taken in the FIM implementations of Christian Borgelt[1] and since we employ those in our experiments, we evaluated the included additional measures as well.

Our primary aim, however, is to test the recovery of itemsets, the precursors to association rules, and we therefore focus on measures that have been proposed to mine interesting *itemsets*. To make it easier to discuss those more sophisticated measures, we associate each itemset with a function $I : \mathcal{T} \mapsto \{0, 1\}$, with $I(t) = 1$ iff $I \subseteq t$ and $I(t) = 0$ otherwise, which allows us to define an equivalence relation based on a collection of itemsets $\{I_1, \dots, I_k\}$:

$$\sim_{\{I_1,\dots,I_k\}} = \{(t_1, t_2) \in \mathcal{T} \times \mathcal{T} \mid \forall I_i, I_j : I_i(t_1) = I_j(t_2)\}$$

Using this equivalence relation, the *partition* or quotient set of $\mathcal{T}$ over $\{I_1, \dots, I_k\}$ is defined as:

$$\mathcal{T} / \sim_{\{I_1,\dots,I_k\}} = \bigcup_{t \in \mathcal{T}} \{a \in \mathcal{T} \mid a \sim_{\{I_1,\dots,I_k\}} t\}$$

We label each block $b \in \mathcal{T} / \sim_{\{I_1,\dots,I_k\}}$ with a subscript denoting what the different itemsets evaluate to, e.g. b_{1010}. The first three measures are available as options for itemset evaluation in Christian Borgelt's implementations.

Lift. The lift measure was introduced in [7] and compares the conditional probability of an association rule's RHS to its unconditional probability: $lift(X \Rightarrow Y) = \frac{conf(X \Rightarrow Y)}{freq(X)}$. A lift value larger than one denotes evidence of a positive correlation, a value smaller than one negative correlation.

Information Gain. Information gain is best known for choosing the splitting test in inner nodes of decision trees. For a given RHS Y, it measures the reduction of its entropy:

$$H(Y, \mathcal{T}) = - \sum_{b \in \mathcal{T}/\sim_{\{Y\}}} \frac{|b|}{|\mathcal{T}|} \log_2 \frac{|b|}{|\mathcal{T}|}$$

---

[1] Downloadable at `http://www.borgelt.net/fpm.html`

by the presence of the LHS X:

$$IG(X \Rightarrow Y) = H(Y, \mathcal{T}) - \sum_{b \in \mathcal{T}/\sim_{\{X\}}} \frac{|b|}{|\mathcal{T}|} H(Y, b)$$

Normalized χ^2. The χ^2 test is a test for statistical independence of categorical variables. For the two-variable case given by RHS Y and LHS X, occurrence counts can be arranged in a contingency table:

	$Y = 1$	$Y = 0$	
$X = 1$	$|b_{11}|$	$|b_{10}|$	$sup(X)$
$X = 0$	$|b_{01}|$	$|b_{00}|$	$|\mathcal{T}| - sup(X)$
	$sup(Y)$	$|\mathcal{T}| - sup(Y)$	$|\mathcal{T}|$

To derive the χ^2 value, the observed values O_{xy} are compared to the expected value (the normalized product of the margins, e.g. $E_{11} = \frac{sup(X)}{|\mathcal{T}|} \cdot \frac{sup(Y)}{|\mathcal{T}|} \cdot |\mathcal{T}|$):

$$\chi^2(X \Rightarrow Y) = \sum_{i=0}^{1} \sum_{j=0}^{1} \frac{(|b_{ij}| - E_{ij})^2}{E_{ij}}$$

The χ^2 value scales with the number of cases the LHS occurs in. To normalize it, Borgelt's FIM implementations normalize this value by the support of the LHS.

Multi-way χ^2. Brin *et al.* proposed to use the χ^2 test to evaluate itemsets directly [6]. Each item $i \in I$ is considered its own itemset and instead of a 2×2 contingency table, a multiway table with $2^{|I|}$ cells is populated by the cardinalities of the blocks derived from $\mathcal{T}/ \sim_{\{i|i \in I\}}$. The χ^2-value is calculated as in the two-dimensional case. The degrees of freedom for such a table are $df(I) = 2^{|I|} - 1 - |I|$, and if the χ^2 value exceeds a given p-value for that many df, the itemset is considered significant. Brin *et al.* also propose an *interest* measure for individuals cells: $interest(b_v) = |1 - \frac{O_v}{E_v}|$, and propose to consider the combination of item presences and absences of the cell with the highest interest value the most relevant contribution of the found itemset.

Entropy. The entropy definition used for a binary variable above can be extended to partitions with more than two blocks and therefore used on the partition induced by the items of an itemset, similar to the preceding treatment of χ^2:

$$H(\{i \mid i \in I\}) = - \sum_{b \in \mathcal{T}/\sim_{\{i|i \in I\}}} \frac{|b|}{|\mathcal{T}|} \log_2 \left(\frac{|b|}{|\mathcal{T}|}\right)$$

The entropy is highest, equal to $|I|$, if all blocks are equally likely, and 0 if there is only one block. Heikinheimo *et al.* proposed mining low-entropy itemsets [12].

Maximum Entropy Evaluation. Not a measure *per se*, De Bie has proposed to use maximum entropy models to sample data sets conforming to certain constraints derived from $\mathcal{T}$, e.g. row and column margins, i.e. support of individual items and sizes of transactions, in the expectation [3]. Found patterns can be reevaluated on these databases and rejected if they occur in more than a certain proportion.

3   The Quest Generator

The Quest generator was introduced in the paper that jump-started the area of frequent itemset mining (FIM), and arguably the entire pattern mining field [1]. The generative process is governed by a number of parameters:

- L – the number of potentially large itemsets (source itemsets) in the data.
- N – the number of items from which source itemsets can be assembled.
- $|I|$ – the average size of source itemsets.
- $|t|$ – the average size of transactions in the data.
- $|\mathcal{T}|$ – the cardinality of the data set.
- c – the "correlation level" between successive itemsets.

The generator proceeds in two phases: it *first* generates all source itemsets, and in a *second* step assembles the transactions that make up the full data set from them. The authors, working in the shopping basket setting, aimed to model the phenomenon that certain items are typically bought together and several such groups of items would make up a transaction. This also means that the output of FIM operations can be compared to the source itemsets to get an impression of how well such mining operations recover the underlying patterns.

3.1   Source Itemset Generation

For each of the L source itemsets, the size is sampled from a *Poisson* distribution with mean I. A fraction of the items used in the source itemset formed in iteration i are taken randomly from the itemset formed in iteration $i - 1$. This fraction is sampled from an exponential distribution with mean c. The rest of the items are sampled uniformly from N. Each source itemset is assigned a weight, i.e. its probability of occurring in the data, sampled from an exponential distribution with unit mean, and a corruption level, i.e. a probability value for only the partial source itemset embedded into a transaction, sampled from a normal distribution with mean 0.5 and variance 0.1. Source itemsets' weights are normalized so that they sum to 1.0.

3.2   Transaction Generation

For each of the D transactions, the size is sampled from a Poisson distribution with mean T. Source itemsets to be embedded into the transaction are chosen according to their weight, and their items embedded according to their corruption level. Importantly, this means that source itemsets are selected independently from each other. If the number of items to be embedded exceeds the remaining size of the transaction, half the time the items are embedded anyway, and the transaction made larger, in the other half the transaction is made smaller, and the items transferred for embedding into the succeeding transaction.

4   Related Work

The seminal paper on FIM, which also introduced the Quest generator, was published almost twenty years ago [1]. The authors used the generator to systematically explore the effects of data characteristics on their proposed algorithm, using several different transaction and source itemset sizes, evaluating a number of values for $|\mathcal{T}|$ (9 values), N (5 values), and $|t|$ (6 values) while keeping the other parameters fixed, respectively, specifically the number of source itemsets L. It is unclear whether more than one data set was mined for each setting, an important question given the probabilistic nature of the correlation, corruption, and source itemset weight effects.

A similar kind of systematic evaluation can still be found in [20], although the authors did not evaluate different values for N (and also continue to keep L fixed throughout). The evaluation found in [11], however, already limits itself to only two Quest-generated data sets. In line with this trend, the authors of [19] used four Quest-generated data sets which they augmented by three UCI data sets [4], and PUSMB data sets that act as stand-ins for "dense" data, i.e. sets with few items coupled with large transaction sizes. The evaluation reported in [14] uses one artificial data set, one UCI data set, and the PUSMB data.

The systematic use of the Quest generator came to a virtual halt after Zheng *et al.* reported that one of the Quest-generated data sets shows different characteristics from real-life data and that algorithmic improvements reported in the literature did not transfer to real-life data [22]. Notably, the authors pointed out that CLOSET [14] scales worse than CHARM [19], a result that Zaki *et al.* verified in revisiting their work and comparing against CLOSET as well [21], and that runs contrary to the experimental evidence presented in [14] by the authors of CLOSET, probably due to the difference in used data sets.

The typical evaluation of FIM related approaches afterwards consisted of using two Quest-generated data sets, a number of UCI data sets, and the real-life data sets made available to the community, e.g. in the Frequent Itemset Mining Implementation competitions [2]. This has lead to the paradoxical situation that while techniques for FIM have proliferated, the amount of data sets on which they have been evaluated has shrunk, in addition to a lack of control over these data sets' characteristics. Also, all evaluations limited themselves to evaluating efficiency questions.

In the same period, data sets begun to be characterized by the distribution of the patterns mined from them, see e.g. [16]. These analyses have given rise to techniques for "'inverse itemset mining" that, starting from FIM results, generate data leading to the same distribution of mined itemsets. While these data sets could be used for efficiency evaluations, they are dependent on the data from which patterns are mined in the first place, and the lack of clearly defined patterns prevents quality evaluations. In a similar vein falls the generator proposed in [17] which uses the MDL principle to generate data sets that will lead to similar itemsets mined, even though it serves a different purpose, namely to protect the anonymity of original data sources.

Finally, FIM research has spawned a large number of interestingness measures and literature discussing what desirable characteristics of such measures are [18]. It is at present unknown, however, whether any of these measures manages to recover the patterns underlying the data, and the closest research has come to such evaluations are attempts to establish how well interestingness measures for association rules align with domain experts' interest [8].

5   Pattern Recovery

The fact that the Quest generator assembles transactions in terms of source itemsets gives us the unique opportunity to compare the output of a frequent itemset mining operation to the original patterns. Note that this is different from the approach taken in [16,17] – in those works databases were generated that would *result* in the itemsets (or at least of the same number of itemsets of certain sizes) being mined that informed the generating process. Contrary to this, we cannot be sure that the output of the frequent itemset mining operation has any relation to the source patterns from which the data is generated, although we of course expect that that would be the case. To the best of our knowledge, this is the first time that such an objective comparison of mined to source itemsets has been performed. Please note that we are not concerned with *ranking* patterns by interestingness in this study but only with removing spurious ones.

5.1   Experimental Setup

For reasons of computational efficiency, we use only few (10, 100) source itemsets in our experiments. This allows us to mine with high support thresholds without having to expect missing (too many) source itemsets. We generate data with $N = 2000, |t| = 10, |I| = 4$, with corruption turned off. We generate 100 data sets for each setting and average the results over them. We used Apriori in Christian Borgelt's implementation with support threshold $100/L\%$, a generous threshold given that we can expect each transaction to consist on average of $10/4 = 2.5$ itemsets. This corresponds to a relatively easy setting since the source itemsets have high support and apart from the correlation-induced overlap, items are unlikely to appear in several itemsets.

We mine three types of patterns: frequent, closed, and maximal itemsets. While frequent itemsets will be guaranteed to include all source itemsets recoverable at the minimum support threshold, they will also include all of their

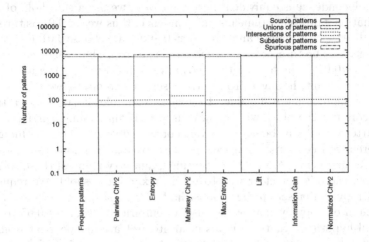

Fig. 1. Results for mining frequent itemsets for $L = 100$, no corruption

subsets, and possibly additional combinations of items. Closed itemsets might miss some source itemsets if the probabilistic process of the Quest generator often groups two itemsets together while generating transactions, an effect that should not be very pronounced over 100 data sets, however. On the other hand can closed itemsets be expected to avoid finding subsets of frequent sets unless those are intersections of source itemsets, and to restrict supersets of source itemsets to unions of them. Maximal itemsets, finally, can be expected to consist of unions of source itemsets. For each pattern type, we filter according to the different measures afterwards:

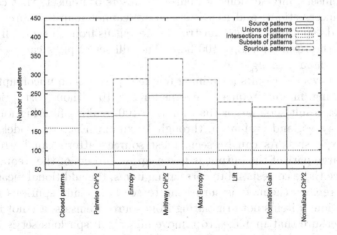

Fig. 2. Results for mining closed itemsets for $L = 100$, no corruption

a) Lift: independence is equivalent to a value of 1, we use a threshold of 1.01.
b) Information gain: $IG = 0$ means independence, thus we set 0.01 as threshold.
c) Normalized χ^2: the value can lie between 0 and 1, we choose 0.01 as threshold.
d) Multi-way χ^2: no threshold is needed for this measure but a significance level, we choose 0.05. A high score does not always indicate that the itemset as a whole is relevant, however. To interpret selected itemsets, we use the block with the highest interest value. To give an example, if $\{i_1, i_2, i_3\}$ attains a high score but the block with highest interest is b_{101}, we interpret $\{i_1, i_3\}$ as the pattern, and i_2 as being negatively correlated with it, hence coming from a different source itemset. For this measure, we can therefore also assess how many negative correlations were identified, and how many of those correctly.
e) Entropy: there is not clear way to set a maximal threshold. We require for the entropy of itemsets to be at most half of their size.
f) Maximum entropy evaluation: we use an empirical p-value of 0.05 to reject the null hypothesis that the items in an itemset are independent from each other, i.e. an itemset must not be frequent on more than 5% of the sampled data sets. We sample 100 times from the maximum entropy model of each data set. We will therefore risk false negatives but evaluating patterns on 10000 data sets already taxes our computational resources.
g) Pairwise χ^2: we also added an additional measure, calculating the χ^2 value for any pair of items in the set, normalizing and requiring a minimum of 0.01.

5.2   Data Sets Created without Corruption of Source Itemsets

Pattern counts are shown cumulatively so that the top of the bar corresponds to the total amount of itemsets mined, and vertical show the proportion taken up by different categories of itemsets. We show the actual itemsets recovered, unions of itemsets, intersections of itemsets, subsets of itemsets that cannot be mapped to intersections, and itemsets that we cannot map to source itemsets at all, labeled "spurious". Page constraints prevent us from showing all plots, so we focus on the results for $L = 100$ here. The full set of plots can be found at scientific-data-mining.org.

Figure 1 shows the results for mining frequent patterns on uncorrupted data. The first setting, mining frequent patterns for $L = 10$ without corruption, leads to the largest result sets, larger than for $L = 100$, making filtering for entropy and multi-way χ^2, and evaluation through Maximum Entropy models computationally expensive. As can be seen, most source pattern can be recovered, however a large part of the output is taken up by subsets of the frequent itemsets and since those correspond to correlating items, the additional measures are not able to remove them. It is surprising to see how many spurious itemsets, i.e. combination of items not originating from source itemsets, are not removed. The only measure that manages to remove almost all spurious set is the pairwise χ^2 measure, with the "association rule measures" (lift, information gain, normalized χ^2) coming next. In a sense, multiway χ^2 performs as well as the association rule measure, but not by removing spurious patterns but instead identifying relevant subsets via the most interesting cell.

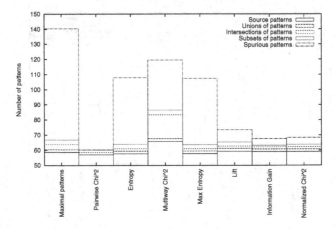

Fig. 3. Results for mining maximal itemsets for $L = 100$, no corruption

Mining closed patterns removes most of the subsets from the result set and leaves the output much more manageable (Figure 2), while keeping the correlation-factor induced intersection of itemsets. We see that pairwise χ^2 stays a very aggressive criterion, reducing not only the amount of spurious itemsets but also rejecting source itemsets, as does the Maximum Entropy evaluation due to the false negative effects. On the other hand are quite a few spurious sets not filtered out by the MaxEnt evaluation. The association rule measures are effective in filtering itemsets, as is multiway χ^2, which has the added advantage that it separates out negative correlations, recovering more intersections of itemsets.

Mining maximal itemsets, finally, reduces the result set to approximately L or even below, removing subsets and intersections. On the other hand, only half of those are related to source itemsets, as Figure 3 shows. Still, in particular in combination with additional interestingness measures, this figure seems to indicate that maximal itemsets should be the pattern semantic of choice.

When we take a closer look at Figure 4, however, we see that there are more unions of itemsets in the result set than source itemsets, even after interestingness measures are applied. The reason that this phenomenon does not appear for $L = 100$ can be explained by the fact that there are $\sum_{1 \leq i \leq 100} = 5050$ possible pairs of patterns, making it unlikely than any exceed the 1% threshold. For $L = 10$, however, that number is 55, increasing the likelihood. Whether maximal itemsets recover source itemsets or unions is therefore a result of the number of patterns occurring in the data, making them less reliable than closed patterns.

Interestingly, the association rule measures that have not been designed to evaluate itemsets as such are more effective in reducing the result sets than the itemset measures. In the case of multiway χ^2, this seems to be the price for recovering additional patterns by identifying negative correlations. All measures were used with rather lenient thresholds and stricter thresholds might improve

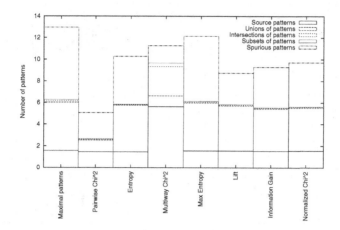

Fig. 4. Results for mining maximal itemsets for $L = 10$, no corruption

their performance. Deciding which threshold to use is not straight-forward when working with real life data.

Given that this uncorrupted embedding of source itemsets is the best-case scenario, an obvious next question is what effect pattern corruption has on the output. The authors of [1] motivated such corruption by shoppers that might not need all ingredients of a shopping basket, for instance, but in other settings, e.g. sensorial data, corruption might result from weak signals or malfunctioning equipment.

5.3   Data Sets Created with Corruption of Source Itemsets

The settings used in the preceding section are relatively easy: source itemsets are embedded without corruption so that they should be well recoverable. In real-life data, however, it is possible that patterns are being corrupted while they are being acquired, making the task of identifying them harder. Since the decision which items are not embedded is independently made for each item, corruption should occur uniformly and still enable itemset recovery.

As we see in Figures 5, however, the deterioration is significant. Only few itemsets in the result set correspond to source itemsets. Instead, the result set consists mainly of fragments of the source itemsets and while the interesting-ness measures are effective in filtering out spurious sets, reducing the rest of the result set would be up to the user. As our experiments have shown, FIM results should definitely be taken with a grain of salt. Even by using additional interestingness measures, it is not assured that the mining process recovers the patterns underlying the data.

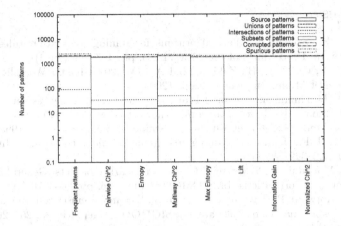

Fig. 5. Results for mining frequent itemsets for $L = 100$, with corruption

6   Summary and Conclusions

In this work, we have for the first time evaluated interestingness measures for frequent itemset mining objectively. Due to a lack of data whose underlying patterns are unknown and whose characteristics cannot be easily controlled, it had been unknown whether FIM approaches recover underlying patterns.

We have revisited the Almaden Quest data generator, and exploited the fact that it constructs data from explicit patterns. By generating data sets and performing frequent itemset mining on them, we could compare the mined patterns against the source itemsets used to construct the data. We found not only that mining frequent, closed, or maximal patterns leads to result sets that include many non-relevant patterns in addition to source itemsets but also that several interestingness measures that have been proposed in the literature are only partially effective in reducing the result set to the relevant patterns.

The ramifications of our results could be far-reaching: our experiments call the usefulness of itemset mining results into question since underlying patterns cannot be reliably recovered. Clear-cut evidence for such usefulness could take the form of implementing gained knowledge in the domains in which the data originate but such evaluations do not exist to the best of our knowledge. Using domain experts to evaluate itemset mining results, while easier and cheaper, has its pitfalls and current interestingness measures might not be up to the task of identifying the relevant itemsets. This is a challenge the community needs to take on to increase the utilization of itemset mining in non-academic contexts.

Acknowledgements. We are grateful to Christian Borgelt and Tijl De Bie for their support w.r.t. the Apriori implementation and the MaxEnt Database Generator, respectively, and to our colleagues Matthijs van Leeuwen and Tias Guns for helpful discussions. The author is supported by a post-doctoral grant by the Fonds Wetenschappelijk Onderzoek Vlanderen (FWO).

References

1. Agrawal, R., Srikant, R.: Fast algorithms for mining association rules in large databases. In: Proceedings of the 20th VLDB, pp. 487–499 (1994)
2. Bayardo, R., Goethals, B., Zaki, M. (eds.): FIMI 2004, ICDM Workshop on Frequent Itemset Mining Implementations (2004)
3. Bie, T.D.: Maximum entropy models and subjective interestingness: an application to tiles in binary databases. Data Min. Knowl. Discov. 23(3), 407–446 (2011)
4. Blake, C., Merz, C.: UCI repository of machine learning databases (1998)
5. Boulicaut, J.-F., Jeudy, B.: Mining free itemsets under constraints. In: IDEAS 2001, pp. 322–329 (2001)
6. Brin, S., Motwani, R., Silverstein, C.: Beyond market baskets: Generalizing association rules to correlations. In: SIGMOD Conference, pp. 265–276 (1997)
7. Brin, S., Motwani, R., Ullman, J.D., Tsur, S.: Dynamic itemset counting and implication rules for market basket data. In: SIGMOD Conference, pp. 255–264 (1997)
8. Carvalho, D.R., Freitas, A.A., Ebecken, N.F.F.: Evaluating the correlation between objective rule interestingness measures and real human interest. In: Jorge, A., Torgo, L., Brazdil, P., et al. (eds.) PKDD 2005. LNCS (LNAI), vol. 3721, pp. 453–461. Springer, Heidelberg (2005)
9. Cooper, C., Zito, M.: Realistic synthetic data for testing association rule mining algorithms for market basket databases. In: Kok, J., Koronacki, J., Lopez de Mantaras, R., et al. (eds.) PKDD 2007. LNCS (LNAI), vol. 4702, pp. 398–405. Springer, Heidelberg (2007)
10. Gouda, K., Zaki, M.J.: Genmax: An efficient algorithm for mining maximal frequent itemsets. Data Min. Knowl. Discov. 11(3), 223–242 (2005)
11. Han, J., Pei, J., Yin, Y.: Mining frequent patterns without candidate generation. In: SIGMOD Conference, pp. 1–12 (2000)
12. Heikinheimo, H., Seppänen, J.K., Hinkkanen, E., Mannila, H., Mielikäinen, T.: Finding low-entropy sets and trees from binary data. In: KDD, pp. 350–359 (2007)
13. Pasquier, N., Bastide, Y., Taouil, R., Lakhal, L.: Discovering frequent closed itemsets for association rules. In: Beeri, C., Bruneman, P. (eds.) ICDT 1999. LNCS, vol. 1540, pp. 398–416. Springer, Heidelberg (1998)
14. Pei, J., Han, J., Mao, R.: Closet: An efficient algorithm for mining frequent closed itemsets. In: DMKD, pp. 21–30 (2000)
15. Pei, Y., Zaïane, O.: A synthetic data generator for clustering and outlier analysis. Tech. rep (2006)
16. Ramesh, G., Zaki, M.J., Maniatty, W.: Distribution-based synthetic database generation techniques for itemset mining. In: IDEAS, pp. 307–316 (2005)
17. Vreeken, J., Leeuwen, M.v., Siebes, A.: Preserving privacy through data generation. In: ICDM, pp. 685–690 (2007)
18. Wu, T., Chen, Y., Han, J.: Re-examination of interestingness measures in pattern mining: a unified framework. Data Min. Knowl. Discov. 21(3), 371–397 (2010)
19. Zaki, M.J., Hsiao, C.J.: ChArm: An efficient algorithm for closed association rule mining. Tech. rep., CS Dept., Rensselaer Polytechnic Institute (Oct 1999)
20. Zaki, M.J.: Scalable algorithms for association mining. IEEE Trans. Knowl. Data Eng. 12(3), 372–390 (2000)
21. Zaki, M.J., Hsiao, C.J.: Charm: An efficient algorithm for closed itemset mining. In: SDM (2002)
22. Zheng, Z., Kohavi, R., Mason, L.: Real world performance of association rule algorithms. In: KDD, pp. 401–406 (2001)

A New Feature Selection and Feature Contrasting Approach Based on Quality Metric: Application to Efficient Classification of Complex Textual Data

Jean-Charles Lamirel[1], Pascal Cuxac[2], Aneesh Sreevallabh Chivukula[3], and Kafil Hajlaoui[2]

[1] SYNALP Team - LORIA, INRIA Nancy-Grand Est, Vandoeuvre-les-Nancy, France
`jean-charles.lamirel@loria.fr`
`http://www.loria.fr/`
[2] INIST-CNRS,Vandoeuvre-les-Nancy, France
`pascal.cuxac@inist.fr`
`http://www.inist.fr/`
[3] Center for Data Engineering,
International Institute of Information Technology, Gachibowli Hyderabad,
Andhra Pradesh, India
`aneesh.chivukula@gmail.com`
`http://www.iiit.ac.in/`

Abstract. Feature maximization is a cluster quality metric which favors clusters with maximum feature representation as regard to their associated data. In this paper we go one step further showing that a straightforward adaptation of such metric can provide a highly efficient feature selection and feature contrasting model in the context of supervised classification. We more especially show that this technique can enhance the performance of classification methods whilst very significantly outperforming (+80%) the state-of-the art feature selection techniques in the case of the classification of unbalanced, highly multidimensional and noisy textual data, with a high degree of similarity between the classes.

Keywords: feature maximization, clustering quality index, feature selection, supervised learning, unbalanced data, text.

1 Introduction

Since the 1990s, advances in computing and storage capacity allow the manipulation of very large data. Whether in bioinformatics or in text mining, it is not uncommon to have description space of several thousand or even tens of thousands of features. One might think that classification algorithms are more efficient if there are a large number of features. However, the situation is not as simple as this. The first problem that arises is the increase in computation time. Moreover, the fact that a significant number of features are redundant or irrelevant to the task of classification significantly perturbs the operation of the classifiers. In addition, as soon as most learning algorithms exploit probabilities, probability distributions

J. Li et al. (Eds.): PAKDD 2013 Workshops, LNAI 7867, pp. 367–378, 2013.

can be difficult to estimate in the case of the presence of a very high number of features. The integration of a feature selection process in the framework of the classification of high dimensional data becomes thus a central challenge.

In the literature, three types of approaches for feature selection are mainly proposed: the integrated (embedded) approaches, the wrapper methods and the filter approaches. An exhaustive overview of the state-of-the-art techniques in this domain has been achieved by many authors, like Ladha et al. [15], Bolón-Canedo et al. [4], Guyon et al. [10] or Daviet [7]. We thus only provide hereafter a rapid overview of existing approaches and related methods.

The integrated approaches incorporate the selection of the features in the learning process [5]. The most popular methods of this category are the SVM-based methods and the neural based methods. SVM-EFR (Recursive Feature Elimination for Support Vector Machines) [9] is an integrated process that performs the selection of features an iterative basis using a SVM classifier. The process starts with the complete feature set and remove the features given as the least important by the SVM. In an alternative way, the basic idea of the approaches of the FS-P (Feature Selection-Perceptron) family is to perform a supervised learning based on a perceptron neural model and to exploit the resulting interconnection weights between neurons as indicators of the features that may be relevant to provide a ranking [22]. On their own side, wrapper methods explicitly use a performance criterion for searching a subset of relevant predictors [13]. More often it's error rate (but this can be a prediction cost or the area under the ROC curve). As an example, the WrapperSubsetEval method evaluates the feature sets using a learning approach. Cross-validation is used to estimate the accuracy of the learning for a given set of features. The algorithm starts with an empty set of features and continues until adding features does not improve performance [30]. Forman presents a remarkable work of methods' comparison in [8]. As other similar works, this comparison clearly highlights that, disregarding of their efficiency, one of the main drawbacks of embedded and wrapper methods is that they are very computationally intensive. This prohibits their use in the case of highly multidimensional data description space. A potential alternative is thus to exploit filter methods in such context.

Filter approaches are selection procedures that are used prior and independently to the learning algorithm. They are based on statistical tests. They are thus lighter in terms of computation time than the other approaches and the obtained features can generally be ranked regarding to the testing phase results.

The Chi-square method exploits a usual statistical test that measures the discrepancy to an expected distribution assuming that a feature is independent of a class label [15].

The information gain is also one of the most common methods of evaluation of the features. This univariate filter provides an ordered classification of all features. In this approach, selected features are those that obtain a positive value of information gain [11].

In the MIFS (Mutual Information Feature Selection) method, a feature f is added to the subset M of already selected features if its link with the target Y

surpasses its average connection with already selected predictors. The method takes into account both relevance and redundancy. In a similar way, the CFS method (Correlation-based Feature Selection) uses a global measure of "merit" of a subset M of m features. Then, a relevant subset consists of features highly correlated with the class, and lowly correlated one to another [11].

The CBF (Consistency-based Filter) method evaluates the relevance of a subset of features by the resulting level of consistency of the classes when learning samples are projected onto that subset [6].

The MODTREE method is a correlation-based filtering method that relies on the principle of pairwise correlation. The method operates in the space of pairs of individuals described by co-labeling indicators attached to each original feature. For that, a pairwise correlation coefficient that represents the linear correlation between two features is used. Once the pairwise correlations are tabulated, the calculation of partial correlation coefficients allows performing a stepwise feature selection [16].

The basic assumption of the Relief feature ordering method is to consider a feature as relevant if it discriminates well an object from its nearest neighbor in the same class. Conversely, a feature will be irrelevant if it cannot distinguish between an object and its class nearest neighbor. ReliefF, an extension of Relief, adds the ability to address multiclass problems. It is also more robust and capable of handling of incomplete and noisy data [14]. This latter method is considered as one of the most efficient filter-based feature selection technique.

Like any statistical test, filter approaches are known to have erratic behavior for very low features' frequencies (which is common case in text classification) [15]. Moreover, we show in this paper that, despite their diversity, all the existing filter approaches also fail to successfully solve the feature selection task in case they are faced with highly unbalanced, highly multidimensional and noisy data, with a high degree of similarity between the classes. We thus propose a new filter approach which relies on the exploitation of a class quality measure based on a specific feature maximization metric. Such metric already demonstrated high potential in the framework of unsupervised learning.

The paper is structured as follows. Section 2 presents the feature maximization principle along with the new proposed technique. Section 3 describes our dataset and our experiment which is performed experimental is a dataset of 7000 publications related to patents classes issued from a classification in the domain of pharmacology. Section 4 draws our conclusion and perspectives.

2 Feature Maximization for Feature Selection

Feature maximization is an unbiased cluster quality metrics that exploits the features of the data associated to each cluster without prior consideration of clusters profiles. This metrics has been initially proposed in [17]. Its main advantage is to be independent altogether of the clustering method and of its operating mode. When it is used during the clustering process, it can substitute to usual distances during that process [20]. In a complementary way, whenever it is used after learning, it can be exploited to set up overall clustering quality indexes [19] or for cluster labeling [18].

Let us consider a set of clusters C resulting from a clustering method applied on a set of data D represented with a set of descriptive features F, feature maximization is a metric which favors clusters with maximum *Feature F-measure*. The *Feature F-measure* $FF_c(f)$ of a feature f associated to a cluster c is defined as the harmonic mean of *Feature Recall* $FR_c(f)$ and *Feature Precision* $FP_c(f)$ indexes which in turn are defined as:

$$FR_c(f) = \frac{\Sigma_{d \in c'} W_d^f}{\Sigma_{c' \in C} \Sigma_{d \in c'} W_d^f} \quad FP_c(f) = \frac{\Sigma_{d \in c} W_d^f}{\Sigma_{f' \in F_c, d \in c} W_d^{f'}} \tag{1}$$

$$FF_c(f) = 2 \left(\frac{FR_c(f) \times FP_c(f)}{FR_c(f) + FP_c(f)} \right) \tag{2}$$

where W_d^f represents the weight of the feature f for data d and F_c represent the set of features occurring in the data associated to the cluster C.

An important application of feature maximization metric is related to clusters labeling whose role is to highlight the prevalent features of the clusters associated to a clustering model at a given time. Labeling can thus be used altogether for visualizing or synthesizing clustering results and for optimizing the learning process of a clustering method [2]. It can rely on endogenous data features or on exogenous ones. Endogenous data features represent the ones being used during the clustering process. Exogenous data features represent either complementary features or specific validation features. Exploiting feature maximization metric for cluster labeling results is a parameter-free labeling technique [18]. As regards to this approach, a feature is then said to be maximal or prevalent for a given cluster iff its Feature F-measure is higher for that cluster than for any other cluster. Thus the set L_c of prevalent features of a cluster c can be defined as:

$$L_c = f \in F_c \mid FF_c(f) = \max_{c' \in C} (FF_{c'}(f)) \tag{3}$$

Whenever it has been exploited in combination with hypertree representation, this technique has highlighted promising results, as compared to the state-of-the-art labeling techniques, like Chi-square labeling, for synthetizing complex clustering output issued from the management of highly multidimensional data [18]. Additionally, the combination of this technique with unsupervised Bayesian reasoning resulted in the proposal of the first parameter-free fully unsupervised approach for analyzing the textual information evolving over time. Exhaustive experiments on large reference datasets of bibliographic records have shown that the approach is reliable and likely to produce accurate and meaningful results for diachronic scientometrics studies [21].

Taking into consideration the basic definition of feature maximization metric presented above, its exploitation for the task of feature selection in the context of supervised learning becomes a straightforward process, as soon as this generic metric can apply on data associated to a class as well as to those associated to a cluster. The feature maximization-based selection process can thus be defined as a parameter-free class-based process in which a class feature is characterized using both its capacity to discriminate a given class from the others ($FP_c(f)$ index) and its capacity to accurately represent the class data ($FR_c(f)$ index). The set S_c of features that are characteristic of a given class c belonging to an overall class set C results in:

$$S_c = \left\{ f \in F_c \mid FF_c(f) > \overline{FF}(f) \text{ and } FF_c(f) > \overline{FF}_D \right\} \text{ where} \qquad (4)$$

$$\overline{FF}(f) = \Sigma_{c' \in C} \frac{FF_{c'}(f)}{|C_{/f}|} \text{ and } \overline{FF}_D = \Sigma_{f \in F} \frac{\overline{FF}(f)}{|F|} \qquad (5)$$

and $C_{/f}$ represents the restriction of the set C to the classes in which the feature f is represented. Finally, the set of all the selected features S_C is the subset of F defined as $S_C = \cup_{c \in C} S_C$.

Features that are judged relevant for a given class are the features whose representation is altogether better than their average representation in all the classes including those features and better than the average representation of all the features, as regard to the feature F-measure metric. In the specific framework of the feature maximization process, a contrast enhancement step can be exploited complementary to the former feature selection step. The role of this step is to fit the description of each data to the specific characteristics of its associated class which have been formerly highlighted by the feature selection step. In the case of our metric, it consists in modifying the weighting scheme of the data specifically to each class by taking into consideration the "information gain" provided by the Feature F-measures of the features, locally to that class.

Thanks to the former strategy, the "information gain" provided by a feature in a given class is proportional to the ratio between the value of the Feature F-measure of this feature in the class $FF_c(f)$ and the average value of the Feature F-measure of the said feature on all the partition $\overline{FF}(f)$. For a given data and a given feature describing this data, the resulting gain acts as a contrast weight factorizing with any existing feature weight that can be issued from data preprocessing. Moreover, each data description can be optionally reduced to the features which are characteristic of its associated class. If it is present, normalization of the data descriptions is discarded by those operations. Optional renormalization can thus be performed in the curse of the process.

3   Experimental Data and Results

The data is a collection of patent documents related to pharmacology domain. The bibliographic citations in the patents are extracted from the Medline database[1]. The source data contains 6387 patents in XML format, grouped into 15 subclasses of the A61K class (medical preparation). 25887 citations have been extracted from 6387 patents [12]. Then the Medline database is queried with extracted citations

---

[1] http://www.ncbi.nlm.nih.gov/pubmed/

for related scientific articles. The querying gives 7501 articles. Each article is then labeled by the first class code of the citing patent. The set of labeled articles represents the final document set on which the training is performed. The final document set is highly unbalanced, with smallest class containing 22 articles (A61K41 class) and largest class containing 2500 articles (A61K31 class). Inter-class similarity computed using cosine correlation indicates that more than 70% of classes' couples have a similarity between 0.5 and 0.9. Thus the ability of any classification model to precisely detect the right class is curtailed. A common solution to deal with unbalance in dataset is undersampling majority classes and oversampling minority classes. However, sampling that introduces redundancy in dataset does not improve the performance in this dataset, as it has been shown in [12]. We thus propose hereafter to prune irrelevant features and to contrast the relevant ones as an alternative solution.

The abstract of each article is processed and converted into a bag of words model [26] using the TreeTagger tool [28] developed by the Institute for Computational Linguistics of the University of Stuttgart. This tool is both a lemmatizer and a tagger. As a result, each article is represented as a term vector filled with keyword frequencies. The description space generated by the tagger has dimensionality 31214. To reduce noise generated by the TreeTager tool, a frequency threshold of 45 (i.e. an average threshold of 3/class) is applied on the extracted descriptors. It resulted in a thresholded description space of dimensionality 1804. A final step of Term Frequency-Inverse Document Frequency (TF-IDF) weighting [27] is applied on resulting articles' descriptions.

To perform our experiments we firstly take into consideration different classification algorithms which are implemented in the Weka toolkit[2]: J48 Decision Tree algorithm [25], Random Forest algorithm [3], KNN algorithm [1], DMNBtext Bayesian Network algorithm [29], SMO-SVM algorithm [24].

Most of these algorithms are general purpose classification algorithms, except from DMNBtext which is a Discriminative Multinomial Naive Bayes classifier especially developed for text classification. As compared to classical Multinomial Naive Bayes classifier this algorithm cumulates the computational efficiency of Naive Bayes approaches and the accuracy of Discriminating approaches by taking into account both the likelihood and the classification objectives during the frequency counting. Other general purpose algorithms whose accuracy has especially been reported for text classification are SMO and KNN [32]. Default parameters are used when executing these algorithms, except for KNN for which the number of neighbors is optimized based on resulting accuracy.

We then more especially focus on the efficiency testing of the feature selection approaches including our new proposal. We include in our test a panel of filter approaches which are computationally tractable with high dimensional data, making again use of their Weka toolkit implementation. The panel of tested methods includes: Chi-square selector [15], Information gain selector [11], CBF subset selector [6], Symmetrical Uncertainty selector [31], ReliefF selector [14], Principal Component Analysis selector [23]. Defaults parameters are also used

---

[2] http://www.cs.waikato.ac.nz/ml/weka/

for most this methods, except for PCA for which the percentage of explained variance is tuned based on resulting accuracy. We first experiment the methods separately. In a second phase we combine the feature selection provided by the methods with the feature contrasting technique we have proposed. 10-fold cross validation is used on all our experiments.

3.1   Results

The different results are reported in Tables 1 to 5 and in Figure 1. Tables and figure present standard performance measures (True Positive Rate, False Positive Rate, Precision, Recall, F-measure and ROC) weighted by class sizes and averaged over all classes. For each table, and each combination of selection and classification methods, a performance increase indicator is computed using the DMNBtext True Positive results on the original data as the reference. Finally, as soon as the results are identical for Chi-square, Information Gain and Symmetrical Uncertainty, they are thus reported only once in the tables as Chi-square results (and noted Chi-square+).

Table 1 highlights that performance of all classification methods are low on the considered dataset if no feature selection process is performed. They also confirm the superiority of the DMNBtext, SMO and KNN methods on the two other tree-based methods in that context. Additionally, DMNBtext provides the best overall performance in terms of discrimination as it is illustrated by its highest ROC value.

Whenever a usual feature selection process is performed in combination with the best method, that is DMNBtext method, the exploitation of the usual feature selection strategies slightly alters the quality of the results, instead of bringing up an added value, as it is shown in Table 2. Alternatively, same table highlights that even if the feature reduction effect is less with the F-max selection method, its combination with F-max data description contrasting boosts the performance of the classification method (+81%), leading to excellent classification results (Accuracy of 0.96) in a very complex classification context.

Even if the benefit of the former use of F-max selection and contrasting approach is very high with the DMNBtext method, Table 3 shows that the added value provided by this preprocessing approach also concerns, to a lesser extent, all the other classifiers, leading to an average increase of their performance of 45% as compared to the reference DMNBtext result. Another interesting phenomenon that can be observed is that, with such help, tree-based classification methods significantly, and unusually, outperform the KNN method on text.

The results presented in Table 4 more specifically illustrates the efficiency of the F-max contrasting procedure that acts on the data descriptions. In the experiments related to that table, Fmax contrasting is performed individually on the features extracted by each selection method and, in a second step, DMNBtext classifier is applied on the resulting contrasted data. The results show that, whatever is the kind of feature selection technique that is used, resulting classification performance is enhanced whenever is a former step of F-max data description contrasting is performed. The average performance increase is 44%.

Table 1. Classification results on initial data

	TP Rate	FP Rate	Precision	Recall	F-measure	ROC	TP Incr. /Ref
J48	0.42	0.16	0.40	0.42	0.40	0.63	-23%
RandomForest	0.45	0.23	0.46	0.45	0.38	0.72	-17%
SMO	0.54	0.14	0.53	0.54	0.52	0.80	0%
DMNBtext	**0.54**	**0.15**	**0.53**	**0.54**	**0.50**	**0.82**	**0% (Ref)**
KNN (k=3)	0.53	0.16	0.53	0.53	0.51	0.77	-2%

Table 2. Classification results after feature selection (DMNBtext classification)

	TP Rate	FP Rate	Precision	Recall	F-measure	ROC	Nb of selected features	TP Incr./Ref
ChiSquare+	0.52	0.17	0.51	0.52	0.47	0.80	282	-4%
CBF	0.47	0.21	0.44	0.47	0.41	0.75	37	-13%
PCA (50% vr.)	0.47	0.18	0.47	0.47	0.44	0.77	483	-13%
Relief	0.52	0.16	0.53	0.52	0.48	0.81	937	-4%
F-max + C.	**0.96**	**0.01**	**0.96**	**0.96**	**0.96**	**0.999**	**1419**	**+81%**

Table 3. Classification results after F-max + Contrast feature selection (all classification methods)

	TP Rate	FP Rate	Precision	Recall	F-measure	ROC	TP Incr. /Ref
J48	0.80	0.05	0.79	0.80	0.79	0.92	+48%
RandomForest	0.76	0.09	0.79	0.76	0.73	0.96	+40%
SMO	0.92	0.03	0.92	0.92	0.91	0.98	+70%
DMNBtext	**0.96**	**0.01**	**0.96**	**0.96**	**0.96**	**0.999**	**+81%**
KNN (k=3)	0.66	0.14	0.71	0.66	0.63	0.85	+22%

Table 4. Classification results after feature selection by all methods + F-max contrasting (DMNBtext classification)

	TP Rate	FP Rate	Precision	Recall	F-measure	ROC	Number of selected features	TP Incr./Ref
ChiSquare+	0.79	0.08	0.82	0.79	0.78	0.98	282	+46%
CBF	0.63	0.15	0.69	0.63	0.59	0.90	37	+16%
PCA (50% vr.)	0.71	0.11	0.73	0.71	0.67	0.53	483	+31%
Relief	0.79	0.08	0.81	0.79	0.78	0.98	937	+46%
F-max + C.	**0.96**	**0.01**	**0.96**	**0.96**	**0.96**	**0.999**	**1419**	**+81%**

Table 5 and Figure 1 illustrate the capabilities of the F-max approach to efficiently cope with the class imbalance problem. Hence, examination of both TP rate changes (especially in small classes) in table 5 and confusion matrices of figure 1 shows that the data attraction effect of the majority class that

Table 5. Class data and number of F-max selected features/class

Class label	Class size	Selected features	TP Rate (F-max)	TP Rate (before)
a61k31	2533	223	**0.999**	0.79
a61k33	60	276	**0.77**	0.02
a61k35	459	262	**0.97**	0.31
a61k36	212	278	**0.89**	0.23
a61k38	1110	237	**0.99**	0.44
a61k39	1141	240	**0.99**	0.65
a61k41	22	225	**0.14**	0
a61k45	304	275	**0.83**	0.09
a61k47	304	278	**0.91**	0.21
a61k48	140	265	**0.76**	0.12
a61k49	90	302	**0.76**	0.26
a61k51	78	251	**0.90**	0.26
a61k6	47	270	**0.55**	0.04
a61k8	87	292	**0.74**	0.02
a61k9	759	250	**0.97**	0.45
Distinct features		1419		

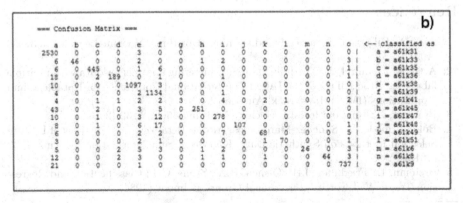

Fig. 1. Comparison of the confusion matrices of the optimal results before (1a) and after (1b) feature selection (Classification: DMNBtext, Feature selection: F-max + Contrast)

occurs at a high level in the case of the exploitation of the original data (figure 1(a)) is quite completely overcome whenever the F-max approach is exploited (figure 1(b)). The capability of the approach to correct class imbalance is also clearly highlighted by the homogeneous distribution of the selected features in the classes it provides, despite of their very different sizes (Table 5).

4   Conclusion

Feature maximization is a cluster quality metric which favors clusters with maximum feature representation as regard to their associated data. In this paper, we have proposed a straightforward adaptation of such metric, which has already demonstrated several generic advantages in the framework of unsupervised learning, to the context of supervised classification. Our main goal was to build up an efficient feature selection and feature contrasting model that could overcome the usual problems arising in the supervised classification of large volume of data, and more especially in that of large full text data. These problems relate to classes imbalance, high dimensionality, noise, and high degree of similarity between classes. Through our experiments on a large dataset constituted of bibliographical records extracted from a patents classification, we more especially showed that our approach can naturally cope with the said handicaps. Hence, in such context, whereas the state-of-the-art feature selection techniques remain inoperative, feature maximization-based feature selection and contrasting can very significantly enhance the performance of classification methods (+80%). Another important advantage of this technique is that it is a parameter-free approach and it can thus be used in a larger scope, like in the one of semisupervised learning.

Acknowledgment. This work was done under the program QUAERO[3] supported by OSEO[4] French national agency of research development.

References

1. Aha, D., Kibler, D.: Instance-based learning algorithms. Machine Learning 6, 37–66 (1991)
2. Attik, M., Lamirel, J.-C., Al Shehabi, S.: Clustering analysis for data with multiple labels. In: Proceedings of the IASTED International Conference on Databases and Applications (DBA), Innsbruck, Austria (2006)
3. Breiman, L.: Random forests. Machine Learning 45(1), 5–32 (2001)
4. Bolón-Canedo, V., Sánchez-Maroño, N., Alonso-Betanzos, A.: A Review of Feature Selection Methods on Synthetic Data. Knowledge and Information Systems, 1–37 (2012)
5. Breiman, L., Friedman, J.H., Olshen, R.A., Stone, C.J.: Classification and Regression Trees. Wadsworth International Group, Belmont (1984)

---

[3] http://www.quaero.org
[4] http://www.oseo.fr/

6. Dash, M., Liu, H.: Consistency-based search in feature selection. Artificial Intelligence 151(1), 155–176 (2003)
7. Daviet, H.: Class-Add, une procédure de sélection de variables basée sur une troncature k-additive de l' information mutuelle et sur une classification ascendante hiérarchique en pré-traitement. PhD, Université de Nantes, France (2009)
8. Forman, G.: An extensive empirical study of feature selection metrics for text classification. The Journal of Machine Learning Research 3, 1289–1305 (2003)
9. Guyon, I., Weston, J., Barnhill, S., Vapnik, V.: Gene selection for cancer classification using support vector machines. Machine Learning 46(1), 389–422 (2002)
10. Guyon, I., Elisseeff, A.: An introduction to variable and feature selection. The Journal of Machine Learning Research 3, 1157–1182 (2003)
11. Hall, M.A., Smith, L.A.: Feature Selection for Machine Learning: Comparing a Correlation-Based Filter Approach to the Wrapper. In: Proceedings of the Twelfth International Florida Artificial Intelligence Research Society Conference, pp. 235–239. AAAI Press (1999)
12. Hajlaoui, K., Cuxac, P., Lamirel, J.-C., François, C.: Enhancing patent expertise through automatic matching with scientific papers. In: Ganascia, J.-G., Lenca, P., Petit, J.-M. (eds.) DS 2012. LNCS, vol. 7569, pp. 299–312. Springer, Heidelberg (2012)
13. Kohavi, R., John, G.H.: Wrappers for feature subset selection. Artificial Intelligence 97(1-2), 273–324 (1997)
14. Kononenko, I.: Estimating Attributes: Analysis and Extensions of RELIEF. In: Bergadano, F., De Raedt, L. (eds.) ECML 1994. LNCS, vol. 784, pp. 171–182. Springer, Heidelberg (1994)
15. Ladha, L., Deepa, T.: Feature selection methods and algorithms. International Journal on Computer Science and Engineering 3(5), 1787–1797 (2011)
16. Lallich, S., Rakotomalala, R.: Fast Feature Selection Using Partial Correlation for Multi-valued Attributes. In: Zighed, D.A., Komorowski, J., Żytkow, J.M. (eds.) PKDD 2000. LNCS (LNAI), vol. 1910, pp. 221–231. Springer, Heidelberg (2000)
17. Lamirel, J.-C., Al Shehabi, S., Francois, C., Hoffmann, M.: New classification quality estimators for analysis of documentary information: application to patent analysis and web mapping. Scientometrics 60(3) (2004)
18. Lamirel, J.-C., Ta, A.P.: Combination of hyperbolic visualization and graph-based approach for organizing data analysis results: an application to social network analysis. In: Proceedings of the 4th International Conference on Webometrics, Informetrics and Scientometrics and 9th COLLNET Meeting, Berlin, Germany (2008)
19. Lamirel, J.-C., Ghribi, M., Cuxac, P.: Unsupervised recall and precision measures: a step towards new efficient clustering quality indexes. In: Proceedings of the 19th International Conference on Computational Statistics (COMPSTAT 2010), Paris, France (2010)
20. Lamirel, J.-C., Mall, R., Cuxac, P., Safi, G.: Variations to incremental growing neural gas algorithm based on label maximization. In: Proceedings of IJCNN 2011, San Jose, CA, USA (2011)
21. Lamirel, J.-C.: A new approach for automatizing the analysis of research topics dynamics: application to optoelectronics research. Scientometrics 93, 151–166 (2012)
22. Mejía-Lavalle, M., Sucar, E., Arroyo, G.: Feature selection with a perceptron neural net. Feature Selection for Data Mining: Interfacing Machine Learning and Statistics (2006)
23. Pearson, K.: On Lines and Planes of Closest Fit to Systems of Points in Space. Philosophical Magazine 2(11), 559–572 (1901)

24. Platt, J.: Fast Training of Support Vector Machines using Sequential Minimal Optimization. In: Schoelkopf, B., Burges, C., Smola, A. (eds.) Advances in Kernel Methods - Support Vector Learning. MIT Press (1998)

25. Quinlan, R.: C4.5: Programs for Machine Learning. Morgan Kaufmann, San Mateo (1993)

26. Salton, G.: Automatic processing of foreign language documents. Prentice-Hill, Englewood Cliffs (1971)

27. Salton, G., Buckley, C.: Term weighting approaches in automatic text retrieval. Information Processing and Management 24(5), 513–523 (1988)

28. Schmid, H.: Probabilistic part-of-speech tagging using decision trees. In: Proceedings of International Conference on New Methods in Language Processing (1994)

29. Su, J., Zhang, H., Ling, C., Matwin, S.: Discriminative parameter learning for bayesian networks. In: ICML (2008)

30. Witten, I.H., Frank, E.: Data Mining: Practical machine learning tools and techniques. Morgan Kaufmann (2005)

31. Yu, L., Liu, H.: Feature Selection for High-Dimensional Data: A Fast Correlation-Based Filter Solution. In: ICML 2003, Washington DC, USA, pp. 856–863 (2003)

32. Zhang, T., Oles, F.J.: Text categorization based on regularized linear classification methods. Inf. Retr. 4(1), 5–31 (2001)

Evaluation of Position-Constrained Association-Rule-Based Classification for Tree-Structured Data

Dang Bach Bui, Fedja Hadzic, and Michael Hecker

Department of Computing, Curtin University
Perth, Australia
dbuibach@postgrad.curtin.edu.au, F.Hadzic@curtin.edu.au,
Michael.Hecker@cbs.curtin.edu.au

Abstract. Tree-structured data is popular in many domains making structural classification an important task. In this paper, a recently proposed structure preserving flat representation is used to generate association rules using itemset mining techniques. The main difference to traditional techniques is that subtrees are constrained by the position in the original tree, and initial associations prior to subtree reconstruction can be based on disconnected subtrees. Imposing the positional constraint on subtreee typically result in a reduces the number of rules generated, especially with greater structural variation among tree instances. This outcome would be desired in the current status of frequent pattern mining, where excessive patterns hinder the practical use of results. However, the question remains whether this reduction comes at a high cost in accuracy and coverage rate reduction. We explore this aspect and compare the approach with a structural classifier based on same subtree type, but not positional constrained in any way. The experiments using publicly available real-world data reveal important differences between the methods and implications when frequent candidate subtrees on which the association rules are based, are not only equivalent structure and node label wise, but also occur at the same position across the tree instances in the database.

Keywords: Tree Mining, Structural Classification, Database Structure Model, Association Rule Mining.

1 Introduction

XML documents are popular across many domains and are typically modeled by ordered labeled tree structures. The classification task for XML documents and tree-structured data in general is one of the highly active research areas in recent years. Following the success of association-rule-based classification in relational/transactional data, first proposed in [1], and further studied and extended in works such as [2–4, 16], the *XRules* structural classifier was proposed in [19] based on association rules generated from frequent ordered embedded subtrees. This method first enumerates all frequent subtrees that satisfy a minimum support value, then association rules between set of frequent subtrees and their class are formed if they reach a certain confidence

J. Li et al. (Eds.): PAKDD 2013 Workshops, LNAI 7867, pp. 379–391, 2013.

threshold. The experimental evaluation of *XRules* shows that it outperforms the *CBA* association rule-based method [1] applied on the itemset representation of the tree data, thus highlighting the importance of preserving the structural information.

In this paper, we study a classification technique for tree-structured data based on association rules generated from a structure-preserving flat representation of the data, proposed in [7]. This representation was proposed with the motivation to overcome some complexity issues caused by inherent complexities in tree-structured data, as well as to enable the direct application of a wider range of methods, of which decision tree learning was used as a case in point. The implication of the method is that in contrast to traditional tree mining methods, the subtree patterns need to occur at the same position within the individual tree instances. As discussed in [7] this may be a desired property in applications such as process logs analysis [20]. This method is not so different to traditional approach when the structural characteristics and order in which the information is presented across instances is consistent. However, when structural variation is great, typically many patterns or rules will not be extracted which traditional approaches such as *XRules* would. In this work, we use tree-structured data coming from web access which is structurally-varied due to many different ways in navigating a website. The results are compared in detail with the *XRules* classifier for varying support thresholds limiting to those association rules that convert to valid embedded subtrees as is the case in *XRules*. The rest of the paper is organized as follows.

In Section 2 an overview of existing approaches to XML/tree-structured data classification is given. The related tree mining concepts and illustrative examples are provided in Section 3. Section 4 illustrates the approach adopted in this paper and the experimental evaluation is given in Section 5. The paper concludes in Section 6, with an outline of future work to be conducted.

2   Related Works

There are two main approaches for classifying XML documents in literature [18], one is to analyze the structure of the documents including node labels [10], [12], [19] and the other is to look into both structure and content [9], [13], [14]. In the structural classification family, some methods can only deal with attribute tree such as [15] and [17]. In [15] the emerging patterns are identified and then used as binary features in a decision tree algorithm. The work in [17] uses closed frequent subtrees as the structural units for the Support Vector Machine (SVM) algorithm and the Structured Link Vector Model (SLVM). The second XML classification family includes methods that use both structural and content information. In [9], tree edit distance and k-nearest neighbour algorithm are used. The authors claim that the edit distance can take into account both the content and structure of XML trees. In [14], Bayesian network is used as a generative model and a probabilistic network is then built for each document class. This model can capture both hierarchical structure among nodes and different type of contents such as image, text, audio etc. A recent approach is proposed by [13] using rule-learning technique to induct interpretable classification models.

Aside from these two general categories, the approach presented in [11] transforms trees into sets of attribute-values so that classification or clustering methods can be applied on. For example, the set of attribute-values can be the set of parent-child relations, the set of "next-sibling" relations and the set of paths starting from the root and the arity of the nodes. The work in [21] transforms XML documents to plain text while adhering to a set of rules. The structural properties of the tree remains in the text which enable the application of different probabilistic methods.

3 Related Tree Mining and Association-Rule-Based Tree Classification Concepts

For data mining purposes, XML documents are commonly modelled as rooted ordered labeled trees. Each tree is denoted as $t = (r, N, L, E)$ where r is the top-most node defined as the root, N the set of nodes or vertices, L is the vocabulary or a set of labels over the nodes, and E the set of edges in the tree, with each edge being denoted as (n_1, n_2), where $n \in N$ and $parent(n_2) = n_1$. An example of tree database (T_{db}) is shown in Fig. 1a. Below each tree in T_{db} is its pre-order string encoding which is generated by traversing the tree in a pre-order or depth-first traversal, listing the encountered node labels and using a special symbol '-1' when we backtrack up the tree [8]. The first and most complex task for discovering association rules from tree-structured data is known as frequent subtree mining, which given a tree database T_{db} and minimum support threshold π, finds all subtrees that occur in T_{db} at least π times. The absolute support of subtree st in T_{db} $(\pi^A(st, T_{db}))$ is defined as the number of trees in T_{db} having st as its subtree. The relative support of subtree st in T_{db} $(\pi(st, T_{db}))$ is expressed as the percentage of trees in T_{db} that contain st. While there are different definitions of support, that count repetition of subtrees within independent tree instances, in this work we focus on the definition that only counts records that contain a candidate subtree. For a comprehensive overview of the tree mining field, including formal definitions and algorithm implementation issues, please refer to [5, 6].

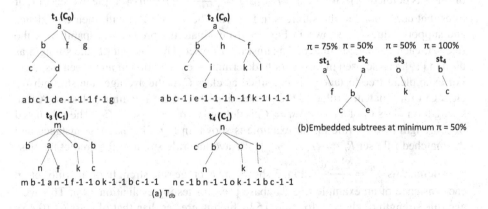

Fig. 1. The tree database T_{db} and example embedded subtrees

Several algorithms have been proposed in literature for mining different subtree types, among which the induced and embedded are most commonly considered. Induced subtrees restrict the relationships between the nodes in the paths to that of parent-child in the original tree, while a parent in an embedded subtrees can be separated from its child by several edges in the original tree. More formally, an embedded subtree $S = (r_S, N_S, L_S, E_S)$ of a tree $T = (r, N, L, E)$ has the following characteristics: (1) $N_S \subseteq N$; (2) $L_S \subseteq L$, and $L_S(n) = L(n)$; (3) if $(n_1, n_2) \in E_S$ then $parent(n_2) = n_1$ in S and n_1 is ancestor of n_2 in T_{db}, and (4) the left to right ordering of sibling nodes in the original tree is preserved. An example of some embedded subtrees of T_{db} at $\pi = 50\%$ is shown in Fig. 1b. Note that subtrees st_1, st_3 and st_4 are also induced subtrees, as all nodes are separated by a single edge in the original trees where they occur (i.e. st_1 is supported by t_1, t_2 and t_3, st_3 by t_3 and t_4 and st_4 by all trees). This is not the case for subtree st_2 because in the trees t_1 and t_2 where it occurs there are two edges separating nodes 'b' and 'e', (i.e. an embedded relationship between nodes 'b' and 'e').

Rule r_1: $st_1 \Rightarrow C_0$ with $\rho(r_1) = 66\%$ $\delta_{c_0}^{r_1} = 0.66$, $\delta_{c_1}^{r_1} = 0.34$
Rule r_2: $st_2 \Rightarrow C_0$ with $\rho(r_2) = 100\%$ $\delta_{c_0}^{r_2} = 1$, $\delta_{c_1}^{r_2} = 0$
Rule r_3: $st_3 \Rightarrow C_1$ with $\rho(r_3) = 100\%$ $\delta_{c_0}^{r_3} = 0$, $\delta_{c_1}^{r_3} = 1$
Rule r_4: $st_4 \Rightarrow C_1$ with $\rho(r_4) = 50\%$ $\delta_{c_0}^{r_4} = 0.5$, $\delta_{c_1}^{r_4} = 0.5$

(a) Confidence of rules   (b) Rule strengths

Fig. 2. Rules and rule strengths

In this paper, the focus is on the classification problem, where each individual tree instance is labelled with a class value. Thus, similar to the tree classification framework [19], a rule (r) corresponds to an implication of the form $st \Rightarrow C_i$ where st is an embedded subtree and C_i is the class value. The global support used in this work for a rule r is defined as $\frac{\pi^A(st, T_{db_i})}{|T_{db}|}$ where T_{db_i} is a set of trees in T_{db} labelled as C_i. The confidence of rule r is defined as $\rho(st \Rightarrow C_i) = P(C_i | st) = \frac{\pi^A(st, T_{db_i})}{\pi^A(st, T_{db})}$. As an example, we select four rules that correspond to the subtrees in Fig. 1b. The set of rules with their confidence and support values are shown in Fig. 2a. To evaluate the predictive capability of the rule set, each instance is matched against the rule set. The concept of rule strength as used in [19], is also used in this work to determine the prediction of an unseen instance. For example, a tree instance t is classified as class C_i if the average rule strength for class C_i of all matched rules of t is greater than that of the remaining classes. A rule strength for class C_i of a rule r_j: $st \Rightarrow C_i$ is defined as $\delta_{C_i}^{r_j} = \rho(st \Rightarrow C_i)$. The calculated rule strength of each rule in our example is shown in Fig. 2b. Given an instance and the matched rule set $R_m = \{r_1 \ldots r_{|R_m|}\}$, the average rule strength for predicting class C_i is defined as $\delta_{C_i}^{\mu} = \frac{\sum_{j=1}^{|R_m|} \delta_{C_i}^{r_j}}{|R_m|}$. Fig. 3 shows the average rule strength of the rule set on each instance of an example tree database used for testing/evaluation T_{eval}. The average rule strength of class C_0 for t_a is 0.54 which is greater than that of class C_1 (0.46). Thus, instance t_a is classified as C_0. Note that there is no average rule strength for t_c as it does not match with any rule. The coverage and accuracy rate for each class is then evaluated. Supposedly the number of instances in the evaluation data being labelled as class C_i is X. Among those, Y is the number of instances that matches with at least one rule. Z is the number of instances which are labelled as C_i and correctly classified. The coverage rate of class C_i is calculated as $CR(C_i) = \frac{Y}{X}$ and the accuracy rate is calculated as $AR(C_i) = \frac{Z}{Y}$. Applied this formula to the example in Fig. 3, we get the coverage and accuracy rate of class C_0 as follows, $CR(C_0) = \frac{2}{3} = 66\%$, $AR(C_0) = \frac{1}{2} = 50\%$ and $CR(C_1) = \frac{2}{2} = 100\%$, $AR(C_1) = \frac{1}{2} = 50\%$. The next section describes the approach studied in this work, and provides illustrative examples of embedded subtrees, associations based on disconnected subtrees as well as the difference caused by the positional constraint inherent in the approach.

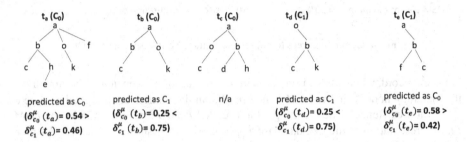

Fig. 3. Prediction on tree database T_{eval}

4   Illustration of the Position-Constrained Approach

In this section, we present a tree classification approach which combines features of the structure-preserving flat representation [7] and the association-rule-based tree classification [19]. This approach adopts the concepts introduced in the previous section. The main differences to the approach in [19] are how the trees are represented and how the rules are formed and interpreted.

Converting Trees to Flat Representation. The *DSM* is constructed from the pre-order string encodings of trees as described in [7]. The *DSM* captures the structural properties of all trees in the database, so that each node in the tree instance can be structurally matched to. Thus, the height of the *DSM* tree is equal to the maximum height among all tree instances, and each node in the *DSM*, has its fan-out equal to the maximum fan-out of the corresponding nodes among the tree instances. The *DSM* of the tree database T_{db} from Fig. 1a is shown in Fig. 4a. If we are only interested in examining the common characteristics of the majority of tree instances, the *DSM* can be simplified by eliminating the nodes where the number of tree instances having data at that position does not reach a certain threshold (minimum support). For example, the *DSM* extracted at the support of 50% (see Fig. 4b). Note that the two nodes at position X_7 and X_{10} of the original *DSM* were safely removed due to the lack of their frequency of occurrence. The pre-order string encoding of *DSM* will become the first row of the table with nodes X_i (i corresponds to the pre-order position of the node in the tree) used as the attribute names.

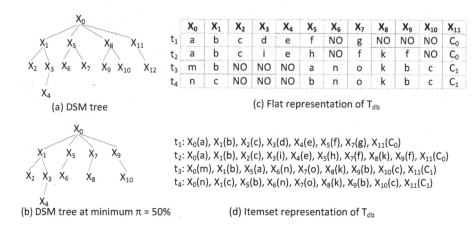

	X_0	X_1	X_2	X_3	X_4	X_5	X_6	X_7	X_8	X_9	X_{10}	X_{11}
t_1	a	b	c	d	e	f	NO	g	NO	NO	NO	C_0
t_2	a	b	c	i	e	h	NO	f	k	f	NO	C_0
t_3	m	b	NO	NO	NO	a	n	o	k	b	c	C_1
t_4	n	c	NO	NO	NO	b	n	o	k	b	c	C_1

(a) DSM tree

(c) Flat representation of T_{db}

t_1: $X_0(a)$, $X_1(b)$, $X_2(c)$, $X_3(d)$, $X_4(e)$, $X_5(f)$, $X_7(g)$, $X_{11}(C_0)$
t_2: $X_0(a)$, $X_1(b)$, $X_2(c)$, $X_3(i)$, $X_4(e)$, $X_5(h)$, $X_7(f)$, $X_8(k)$, $X_9(f)$, $X_{11}(C_0)$
t_3: $X_0(m)$, $X_1(b)$, $X_5(a)$, $X_6(n)$, $X_7(o)$, $X_8(k)$, $X_9(b)$, $X_{10}(c)$, $X_{11}(C_1)$
t_4: $X_0(n)$, $X_1(c)$, $X_5(b)$, $X_6(n)$, $X_7(o)$, $X_8(k)$, $X_9(b)$, $X_{10}(c)$, $X_{11}(C_1)$

(b) DSM tree at minimum π = 50%

(d) Itemset representation of T_{db}

Fig. 4. Converting trees to flat representation and itemset data format

For each record, when a label is encountered, it is placed in the matching column under the matching node X_i in the *DSM* structure. Remaining entries are assigned a value of 'NO' (non-existence). The resulting table is called *DSM-Flat*. For example, the *DSM-Flat* representation of the tree database T_{db} from Fig. 1a is shown in Fig. 4c. For more details on this conversion process, please refer to [7].

rule r_a: $X_1(b)$, $X_2(c)$ -> C_0 with $\rho(r_a)$ = 100% $\delta_{c_0}^{r_a}$ =1, $\delta_{c_1}^{r_a}$ =0
rule r_b: $X_9(b)$, $X_{10}(c)$ -> C_1 with $\rho(r_b)$ = 100% $\delta_{c_0}^{r_b}$ =0, $\delta_{c_1}^{r_b}$ = 1
rule r_c: $X_1(b)$, $X_2(c)$, $X_4(e)$ -> C_0 with $\rho(r_c)$ = 100% $\delta_{c_0}^{r_c}$ =1, $\delta_{c_1}^{r_c}$ =0
rule r_d: $X_6(n)$, $X_7(o)$, $X_8(k)$, $X_9(b)$, $X_{10}(c)$ -> C_1 with $\rho (r_d)$ = 100% $\delta_{c_0}^{r_d}$ = 0, $\delta_{c_1}^{r_d}$ = 1

(a) Rules with confidences

(b) Rule strengths

Fig. 5. *DSM*-based rules and strengths

Generating Association Rules. The *DSM-Flat* is converted to itemset format by attaching the position of each node to its value. Fig. 4d shows the itemset representation of T_{db}. An association rule mining algorithm is then used to extract rules that associate subtrees with a class. A subset of rules found by a association rule algorithm with confidence and support value set at 50% is shown in Fig. 5a. Using the same method described in Section 3, the rule strengths were calculated and displayed in Fig. 5b. The prediction performance of the *DSM*-based rule for each class when evaluated on the example database T_{eval} from Fig. 3, is $CR(C_0) = \frac{2}{3} = 66\%$, $AR(C_0) = \frac{2}{2} = 100\%$ and $CR(C_1) = \frac{1}{2} = 50\%$ and $AR(C_1) = \frac{0}{1} = 0\%$.

As mentioned in previous section, the antecedent part of the rule represents an induced/embedded or disconnected subtree. Thus, using the *DSM* as the reference model, one can reconstruct subtrees from their itemset representation. For example, in rule

$r_a : X_1b, X_2c - > C_0$, its antecedents can be re-mapped to subtree st_a. Fig. 6 and 1(b) shows the different results obtained by the *DSM* approach, namely position-constrained frequent subtrees and traditional ordered embedded subtree mining algorithm. Since the *DSM*-based subtrees are constrained by their position, this usually leads to the fewer number of embedded subtrees detected e.g. subtree st_1 is only detected by the traditional method for the 50% support threshold. However in some cases the former method produces more frequent subtrees, by further distinguishing a traditional subtree based on its occurrence. For example, the traditional subtree st_4 is distinguished into subtrees st_a and st_b where nodes occur at the indicated pre-order positions (displayed at the left of the node labels). Furthermore, since itemset mining techniques are used, and structural properties are ignored during the enumeration of itemsets, some itemsets after being matched to the *DSM* will result in disconnected subtrees. The disconnection occurs between two subtree nodes (sibling or cousin) for which no common ancestor. For example, the common ancestor connecting nodes X_6n, X_7o and X_9b from subtree st_d is not frequent. This characteristic could be desired in some applications, as frequent association existing in a tree database does not necessarily have to convert to a connected subtree, and may contain some useful information not captured by the connected subtrees.

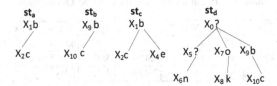

Fig. 6. Reconstructed subtrees from itemset representation

5 Evaluation Result

The purpose of this section is to compare the approach described in the previous section for association-rule-based structural classification and *XRules* which is a state-of-the-art XML document classification algorithm. The accuracy and coverage rate are the two main criteria for evaluating the result of the classification. There is a known trade-off between classification accuracy and coverage rate. The preference for higher accuracy or coverage rate is often application dependent. For example, in domains where any misclassifications are unacceptable (e.g. patient care), one may only be confident putting association rules to practice or for decision support purposes if they have high confidence and are specific enough not to misclassify any case. On the other hand, in business applications, one would allow for misclassifications given that sufficient number of cases are covered and overall profit is achieved. Furthermore, the number of rules is preferred to be kept to a minimum so that results are easier to analyse, understand and yield better generalisation power for unseen cases.

5.1 Experimental Setup

The CSLOG dataset used in [19] is selected for our experiment. It contains web access trees of an academic institute during three weeks. The log file for the first week is named as CSLOG1, the second week is CSLOG2 and the last week is CSLOG3. It contains user sessions which is labelled as "edu" or "other" depending on from where the web site is accessed from. The instances of "edu" class are in minority, and the exact class distribution is as follows: CSLOG1: edu = 24.3% other = 75.7%; CSLOG2: edu = 22.8% other = 77.2% and CSLOG3: edu = 23.6% other = 76.4%. In this experiment, the accuracy and coverage rate achieved when applying the *DSM* association-rule-based classifier is compared with the frequent-subtree based classifier of *XRules*. We select CSLOG data in one week for training and one other week for testing, as was performed in *XRules*. CSLOGx-y denotes that CSLOGx is the training set and CSLOGy is the test set. The structural properties of the CSLOG datasets are shown in Table 1 using the following notation: |Tr|= number of transactions, Avg(|L|) = average length of pre-order string encoding, Max(|T|) = maximum size of trees, Avg(|D|) = average height of trees, Avg(|F|) = average fan-out of trees, Avg(|T|) = average size of trees; Max(|D|) = maximum height of trees, Max(|F|) = maximum fan-out of trees.

Table 1. Structural characteristics of CSLOG datasets

Dataset	|Tr|	Avg|L|	Max|T|	Avg|D|	Avg|F|	Avg|T|	Max |D|	Max|F|
CSLOG1	8074	625	313	3.398	1.893	8.033	123	130
CSLOG2	7409	341	171	3.458	1.902	8.045	171	137
CSLOG3	7628	383	192	3.419	1.871	7.984	120	130

Using the *DSM*-based subtree generation, the initial set of rules may contain both disconnected and embedded ordered subtrees. In these experiments, several disconnected subtrees were detected at lower supports. However, their inclusion had no effect on the accuracy and coverage rate, and therefore all disconnected subtrees are removed and only valid embedded subtrees are used in evaluation. Note that in all experiments we use the 50% confidence threshold (default in *XRules*). Different confidence thresholds were applied which would increase accuracy at the cost of coverage rate, but similar trend in the differences between the methods was observed. The minimum support threshold used for frequent subtree mining ranged from 0.2% to 10%. At support below 0.2% the execution time was too long due to huge number of candidate subtrees being enumerated. Since the CSLOG data is imbalanced by nature, the frequent subtrees (in both *DSM* and *XRules*) were generated from the instances of each class separately using the same relative support.

5.2 Results and Discussion

Table 2 shows the predictive accuracy and Table 3 the coverage rate of different techniques when applied on the three pairs of training and test set. For each method, the number in the first row represents the overall performance, while the second row shows performance individually for majority (left) and minority (right) class. Please note that cells are bolded in rows of methods exhibiting best performance for the corresponding test case. The rows labeled *XRulesS* correspond to the results when *XRules* is evaluated on only those instances that are covered by the *DSM* method. Since *DSM* has lower coverage rate than *XRules* (see Table 3), it is important to measure accuracy of *XRules* relative to only those instances that *DSM* covered. Note that *XRules* typically covered all instances that *DSM* covers except for a few instances at 0.2% support. Another factor in evaluating pattern-based classifiers is the number of patterns/rules discovered. The less rules discovered the better (for comprehensibility purposes) as long as it does not decrease the accuracy and coverage rate. As Table 4 shows, *XRules* enumerates significantly more rules at lower support thresholds in comparison with other techniques. This makes the *XRules* approach achieve the best coverage rate, as can be seen in Table 3. The reason *XRules* produces much larger rule sets is that it detects frequent subtrees that occur at different positions of the tree. In the *DSM*-based approach, the number of frequent (connected) subtrees generated is generally smaller due to the fact that the frequent subtrees have to be located at the same position, but this comes at a cost or reduction in coverage rate. Generally speaking, the accuracy performance of the methods is comparable, while there is a larger degradation in coverage rate when position-constraint is imposed as part of the *DSM* approach. We now proceed to discuss the differences in more detail.

Table 2. Accuracy for test data

	Method	Accuracy Rate(%) for Support(%)					
		0.2	0.5	1	2	5	10
CSLOG1-2	DSM	83.24	83.88	83.93	**84.21**	**87.07**	**92.39**
		88.06 |**70.06**	88.09 |**71.65**	88.42 |**71.14**	90.51 |59.30	**92.05** |**62.44**	**100** |0
	XRules	**83.97**	**83.92**	**84.10**	84.07	84.32	81.30
		91.15 |61.01	**90.99** |62.56	**90.70** |65.36	89.90 |**67.31**	91.27 |62.20	88.64 |**56.36**
	XRulesS	83.57	**84.40**	**84.28**	84.11	**87.07**	**92.39**
		90.30 |65.20	90.80 |65.83	**91.02** |65.11	**92.20** |52.11	**92.05** |**62.44**	**100** |0
CSLOG2-3	DSM	83.67	83.98	84.43	84.19	**87.97**	**92.57**
		88.86 |**69.77**	89.26 |**68.71**	90.76 |64.90	91.87 |56.05	**93.06** |**62.33**	**100** |0
	XRules	**84.59**	**84.86**	84.25	**84.25**	84.99	82.00
		91.82 |62.79	**91.14** |67.17	90.72 |**67.22**	90.17 |**68.70**	92.84 |59.60	89.81 |**55.58**
	XRulesS	84.15	**84.86**	**84.49**	84.23	**87.97**	**92.57**
		90.77 |66.42	**91.17** |65.03	**92.82** |58.78	**93.22** |51.27	**93.06** |**62.33**	**100** |0
CSLOG3-1	DSM	83.96	84.71	83.20	83.63	80.08	80.17
		90.09 |67.59	89.91 |**70.89**	86.57 |**73.06**	88.52 |64.35	82.25 |**70.74**	82.37 |**70.65**
	XRules	**84.33**	84.48	**84.33**	84.27	85.58	82.66
		91.22 |63.85	**90.86** |66.23	**90.22** |68.79	89.66 |**69.71**	**93.79** |56.86	**90.99** |52.53
	XRulesS	**84.38**	**84.98**	**84.82**	**85.50**	83.23	83.20
		90.29 |**68.59**	90.36 |70.72	**91.55** |64.54	**93.93** |52.31	92.84 |41.80	**93.05** |40.65

Referring back to Table 2, we can see that overall the *XRules* and *XRulesS* achieve slightly better accuracy than *DSM* in most of cases except for CSLOG1-2: supports 2%, 5% and 10% and CSLOG2-3: supports 5% and 10%. Note that at 10% there were only 3 rules discovered by *XRules* for all dataset variations, while 1 rule was discovered by *DSM* for CSLOG1-2 and CSLOG2-3 and 2 rules for CSLOG3-1 (Table 4). These rules mostly cover less than 20% of the instances (Table 3), and as such the results for 10% are excluded from further discussion. Looking at the performances of the methods for each class individually, one can observe that *XRules* predicts the instances of majority class better, while the *DSM* approach predicts the instances of minority class better in all cases except when support = 2% (note that at 2% for CSLOG1-2 *DSM* actually achieved best overall accuracy indicating unusual results for this test case).

Table 3. Coverage for test data

	Method	Coverage Rate(%) for Support(%)					
		0.2	0.5	1	2	5	10
CSLOG1-2	DSM	**64.26**	**54.23**	**45.69**	**38.14**	**17.75**	**14.71**
		60.91 |75.64	52.22 |61.06	43.78 |52.16	39.43 |33.79	19.12 |13.10	17.60 |4.92
	XRules	**82.10**	**73.61**	**64.95**	**54.39**	**42.08**	**23.82**
		80.99 |85.89	71.60 |80.44	62.20 |74.27	52.25 |61.65	41.45 |44.22	23.84 |23.77
CSLOG2-3	DSM	**64.05**	**54.02**	**46.41**	**38.40**	**17.66**	**14.81**
		60.99 |73.97	52.54 |58.84	45.87 |48.16	39.47 |34.93	19.28 |12.40	17.94 |4.67
	XRules	**82.8**	**72.6**	**63.37**	**55.37**	**41.94**	**23.68**
		81.37 |87.43	70.12 |80.65	60.10 |73.97	52.50 |64.68	41.92 |41.99	23.91 |22.91
CSLOG3-1	DSM	**64.09**	**53.94**	**46.67**	**37.07**	**20.46**	**20.42**
		61.60 |71.87	51.75 |60.75	46.29 |47.86	39.05 |30.89	21.94 |15.85	21.91 |15.80
	XRules	**81.03**	**73.12**	**63.87**	**54.19**	**39.76**	**22.64**
		80.10 |83.89	71.60 |77.88	61.21 |72.17	52.24 |60.24	40.84 |36.39	23.43 |20.18

Table 4. Number of rules

	Method	#Rules for Support(%)					
		0.2	0.5	1	2	5	10
CSLOG1-2	DSM	8944	327	79	26	3	1
	XRules	50000	1764	367	105	19	3
CSLOG2-3	DSM	12103	381	89	28	3	1
	XRules	50000	3285	371	102	21	3
CSLOG3-1	DSM	15721	375	105	25	4	2
	XRules	50000	2671	401	114	20	3

Similar observations can be made when the performance of the methods is evaluated only using the instances that they both cover (i.e *DSM* and *XRulesS*). In majority of cases the *XRulesS* has slightly better overall accuracy stemming from better predicting the majority class instances, except at support 2% for CSLOG1-2. On the other hand, *DSM* has still consistently better accuracy in predicting minority class instances, except for CSLOG3-1 at support 0.2%. Note that at 5% support for CSLOG1-2 and CSLOG2-3 the performance between *DSM* and *XRulesS* is identical. Table 5 adds more detail to this comparison by showing the instances that *DSM* approach predicted correctly but *XRules* misclassified (called *DSM+ XRules-*) and instances that *DSM* approach misclassified but *XRules* classified it correctly (called *DSM- XRules+*). The left number of each cell in the table presents the majority class and the right number shows the minority class. From the table we see that, despite the higher accuracy of *DSM* on minority class, for most cases the total number of instances which *DSM* misclassified is higher than that of *XRules* which confirms the slightly lower accuracy of the *DSM* method seen in Table 2.

Table 5. Instances correctly(+)/incorrectly(-) classified by *DSM* and *XRulesS*

	Number of instances for Support(%)					
	0.2	0.5	1	2	5	10
DSM+ XRulesS-	16 |72	7 |62	12 |63	21 |53	0 |0	0 |0
DSM- XRulesS+	93 |10	88 |2	77 |10	59 |12	0 |0	0 |0
DSM+ XRulesS-	20 |67	10 |57	6 |61	16 |42	0 |0	0 |0
DSM- XRulesS+	86 |23	85 |18	61 |8	47 |12	0 |0	0 |0
DSM+ XRulesS-	47 |47	16 |22	0 |80	0 |73	0 |90	0 |93
DSM- XRulesS+	49 |62	30 |20	141 |0	129 |0	142 |0	143 |0

Generally speaking, one can see a clear trade-off between accuracy, coverage rate and number of rules for the different support thresholds. The observed difference in *XRules* predicting majority class with higher accuracy and *DSM* predicting minority class with higher accuracy, indicates that both approaches have some useful distinct properties, and that they could complement each other. This would result in overall better performance w.r.t accuracy as well as coverage rate. However, these initial findings need to be studied further and confirmed on a wider range of experimental data. It is also necessary to identify applications and dataset characteristics where it would be more effective to or not to constrain the subtrees by position and/or combine the subtrees from both approaches while ensuring non-redundancy and no contradictions. Furthermore, while we have used standard support and confidence measures here (as the focus was not so much on interestingness as is on subtree type implications), a number of important contributions exist in the data mining field that supply more robust interestingness measures [22, 23] and avoidance of the use of support threshold for which optimal setting is often unknown [24, 25], and these need exploration in the tree mining field.

6 Conclusion and Future Works

The paper presented an evaluation of a classification technique for tree-structured data based on association rules generated from a structure-preserving flat representation of the data. The main implication of the method of constraining the rules/subtree patterns by occurrence in the tree database for exhibiting same characteristics was studied in comparison to traditional subtree based classifier. Overall the results show comparable accuracy performance between the approaches. However, constraining subtrees by exact occurrence results in smaller rule sets which have less coverage than traditional subtrees, due to the number of rules extracted being less for structurally varied data on which the comparisons were made. Further, in majority of cases the position constrained approach had better accuracy for minority class, but worse for majority class, and this was the case when evaluated on commonly covered instances. This indicates the potential of the methods being combined to complement each other and achieve more optimal overall results.

Future work will involve comparisons across a wider range of data and between tree mining approaches that mine different subtree types including unordered, distance constrained and attribute trees, as well as the incorporation of now well established interestingness measures and methods for dealing with the class imbalance problem.

Acknowledgements. We would like to thank Professor Mohammed J. Zaki for making available the *XRules* classifier and the CSLOG dataset. We would also like to acknowledge the constructive comments and advice from Professor George Karypis during the QIMIE workshop, which has improved the experimental evaluation and the depth of the study.

References

1. Liu, B., Hsu, W., Ma, Y.: Integrating Classification and Association Rule Mining. In: 4th Int'l Conf. on Knowledge Discovery and Data Mining, pp. 80–86 (1998)
2. Li, J., Shen, H., Topor, R.W.: Mining the optimal class association rule set. Knowledge-Based Systems 15(7), 399–405 (2002)
3. Li, W., Han, J., Pei, J.: CMAR:Accurate and efficient classification based on multiple class-association rules. In: IEEE International Conference on Data Mining (ICDM), pp. 369–376 (2001)
4. Veloso, A., Meira, W., Zaki, M.J.: Lazy Associative Classification. In: 6th IEEE Inetrantional Conference on Data Mining (ICDM), pp. 645–654 (2006)
5. Hadzic, F., Tan, H., Dillon, T.S.: Mining of Data with Complex Structures. SCI, vol. 333. Springer, Heidelberg (2011)
6. Chi, Y., Muntz, R.R., Nijssen, S., Kok, J.N.: Freequent Subtree Mining - An Overview. Fundamenta Informaticae - Advances in Mining Graphs, Trees and Sequences 66(1-2), 161–198 (2005)
7. Hadzic, F.: A Structure Preserving Flat Data Format Representation for Tree-Structured Data. In: Cao, L., Huang, J.Z., Bailey, J., Koh, Y.S., Luo, J. (eds.) PAKDD Workshops 2011. LNCS, vol. 7104, pp. 221–233. Springer, Heidelberg (2012)
8. Zaki, M.J.: Efficiently mining frequent trees in a forest: algorithms and applications. IEEE TKDE 17(8), 1021–1035 (2005)

9. Bouchachia, A., Hassler, M.: Classification of XML documents. In: Computational Intelligence and Data Mining, CIDM (2007)
10. Bringmann, B., Zimmermann, A.: Tree^2: decision trees for tree structured data. In: 9th European Conference on Principles and Practice of Knowledge Discovery in Databases, PKDD, Berlin, Heidelberg, pp. 46–58 (2005)
11. Candillier, L., Tellier, I., Torre, F.: Transforming xml trees for efficient classification and clustering. In: 4th International Conference on Initiative for the Evaluation of XML Retrieval, INEX, Berlin, Heidelberg, pp. 469–480 (2006)
12. Chehreghani, M.H., Chehreghani, M.H., Lucas, C., Rahgozar, M., Ghadimi, E.: Efficient rule based structural algorithms for classification of tree structured data. J. Intelligent Data Analysis 13(1), 165–188 (2009)
13. Costa, G., Ortale, R., Ritacco, E.: Effective XML classification using content and structural information via rule learning. In: 23rd International Conference on Tools with Artificial Intelligence, ICTAI, Washington DC, USA, pp. 102–109 (2011)
14. Denoyer, L., Gallinari, P.: Bayesian network model for semi-structured document classification. Journal of Information Processing Management 40(5), 807–827 (2004)
15. De Knijf, J.: FAT-CAT: Frequent attributes tree based classification. In: Fuhr, N., Lalmas, M., Trotman, A. (eds.) INEX 2006. LNCS, vol. 4518, pp. 485–496. Springer, Heidelberg (2007)
16. Wang, J., Karypis, G.: On mining instance-centric classification rules. IEEE Transaction on Knowledge and Data Engineering 18(11), 1497–1511 (2006)
17. Wang, S., Hong, Y., Yang, J.: XML document classification using closed frequent subtree. In: Bao, Z., Gao, Y., Gu, Y., Guo, L., Li, Y., Lu, J., Ren, Z., Wang, C., Zhang, X. (eds.) WAIM 2012 Workshops. LNCS, vol. 7419, pp. 350–359. Springer, Heidelberg (2012)
18. Wu, J.: A framework for learning comprehensible theories in XML document classification. IEEE Transaction on Knowledge and Data Engineering 24(1), 1–14 (2012)
19. Zaki, M.J., Aggarwal, C.C.: Xrules: An effective algorithm for structural classification of XML data. Machine Learning 62(1-2), 137–170 (2006)
20. Bui, D.B., Hadzic, F., Potdar, V.: A Framework for Application of Tree-Structured Data Mining to Process Log Analysis. In: Proc. Intelligent Data Engineering and Automated Learning, Brazil (2012)
21. Campos, L.M., Fernández-Luna, J.M., Huete, J.F., Romero, A.E.: Probabilistic Methods for Structured Document Classification at INEX. Focused Access to XML Documents (2008)
22. Geng, L., Hamilton, H.J.: Interestingness Measures for Data Mining: A Survey. ACM Computing Surveys 38(3) (2006)
23. Lenca, P., Meyer, P., Vaillant, B., Lallich, S.: On selecting interestingness measures for association rules: User oriented description and multiple criteria decision aid. European Journal of Operational Research 184(2), 610–626 (2008)
24. Wang, K., He, Y., Cheung, D.W.: Mining confident rules without support requirement. In: 10th International Conference on Information and Knowledge Management, pp. 89–96 (2001)
25. Bras, Y.L., Lenca, P., Lallich, S.: Mining Classification Rules without Support: an Antimonotone Property of Jaccard Measure. In: Elomaa, T., Hollmén, J., Mannila, H. (eds.) DS 2011. LNCS, vol. 6926, pp. 179–193. Springer, Heidelberg (2011)

Enhancing Textual Data Quality in Data Mining: Case Study and Experiences

Yi Feng[1] and Chunhua Ju[1,2]

[1] School of Computer Science & Information Engineering,
Zhejiang Gongshang University, Hangzhou 310018, P.R. China
[2] Contemporary Business and Trade Research Center of Zhejiang Gongshang University,
Hangzhou 310018, P.R. China
yfeng@mail.zjgsu.edu.cn, juchunhua@hotmail.com

Abstract. Dirty data is recognized as a top challenge for data mining. Textual data is one type of data that should be explored more on the topic of data quality, to ensure the discovered knowledge is of quality. In this paper, we focus on the topic of textual data quality (TDQ) in data mining. Based on our data mining experiences for years, three typical TDQ dimensions and related problems are highlighted, including representation granularity, representation consistency, and completeness. Then, to provide a real-world example on how to enhance TDQ in data mining, a case study is demonstrated in detail in this paper, under the background of data mining in traditional Chinese medicine and covers three typical TDQ problems and corresponding solutions. The case study provided in this paper is expected to help data analysts and miners to attach more importance to TDQ issue, and enhance TDQ for more reliable data mining.

Keywords: Data Mining, Data Quality, Textual Data Quality, Traditional Chinese Medicine.

1 Introduction

With the advancement of data mining models and algorithms in last decades, the topic of data mining quality and reliability has attracted increasing interests in the community, such as PAKDD QIMIE workshops (2009-2013) [1] and ICDM RIKD workshops (2006-2012) [2]. Most existing researches on this topic are focused on interestingness, evaluation methods, and quality-aware models in data mining. However, few work has been done on another important issue which will greatly affect the quality of data mining, that is, the data quality in data mining. To ensure the discovered knowledge is of quality, the issue of data quality must be well considered and addressed. Violation of data quality requirements will lead to bias and even error in data, which is consequently possible to result in biased or untrustworthy model and knowledge. More importantly, in real-world data mining, data analysts is highly prone to encounter low-quality and unsatisfactory data as the input for the following data mining. According to an annual data miner survey conducted by Rexer Analytics, dirty data is listed as the top one challenge for data mining every year (2007-2010) [3]. The classical CRISP-DM

J. Li et al. (Eds.): PAKDD 2013 Workshops, LNAI 7867, pp. 392–403, 2013.

methodology also highlights data understanding and preparation as two major steps before modeling, in which identification and treatment of data quality problems become key tasks [4]. It is thus very necessary to explore how to enhance data quality in data mining in order to ensure the discovered knowledge is of quality.

With regard to data quality, a large number of researches have been devoted to identifying the dimensions of data quality, and their interrelationships. As early as in 1980s, Ballou et al. identified some key dimensions of data quality: accuracy, timeliness, completeness, and consistency [5]. Wang et al. followed by proposing a hierarchy of data quality dimensions in 1995, and defines accessible, interpretable, useful and believable as four basic dimensions in the hierarchy [6]. A more comprehensive study was conducted by Wang and Strong [7] in 1996, and a recent review on data quality could be found in 2009 [8]. These studies contribute greatly to data quality research and provide useful references for both industry and academy.

There is one type of data that should be explored more on the topic of data quality, that is, the textual data. At this age of information explosion, data represented in the textual form could be found almost everywhere: news in web pages and forums, product descriptions and customer reviews, emails, search results... Besides, each published literature itself could also be seen as a collection of textual data: the title, abstract, heading, and main-body text are all in the textual form. The issue of textual data quality (TDQ) is different from the generic data quality and non-textual data quality. Some dimensions in generic data quality framework might not be applicable or unimportant for textual data. For instance, the accuracy dimension might be more applicable for numerical data than textual data. Moreover, textual data have some data quality problems which are more typical and serious than that for non-textual data, such as problems related with representation granularity and consistency. Although there is a substantial amount of work discussing data quality, there is few work focusing on TDQ. O'Donnell et al. explored the additional information which needs to be specified to produce reasonable text quality when generating from relational databases [9]. Sonntag discussed the quality of natural language text data, and stated text quality for NLP could traces back to questions of text representation [10]. However, up to now there has been very few research particularly focusing TDQ from the view of data mining. This paper is an attempt in this aspect. Based on our data mining experiences in the field of medicine and business for more than 15 years, three important TDQ dimensions that have more TDQ problems are discussed, including representation granularity, representation consistency, and completeness,.

To provide a real-world example on how to handle these TDQ dimensions and related problems for data mining, a case study is also presented in this paper. A part of this case is mentioned in our preliminary work [11], and we extend the case and provide more detail in this paper. This case is under the background of data mining in traditional Chinese medicine (TCM). In order to conduct an association rule mining in Database of Chinese Medical Formula (DCMF), three TDQ problems are identified to be handled. The first one is the representation granularity problem in attribute *ingredients* in DCMF. To tackle this problem, a rule-based splitting system is developed to structurize *ingredients* values into smaller segments. The second one is the representation consistency problem in attribute *ingredients* in DCMF. To tackle this problem, the UTCMLS system [12] is used as the standardized terminological database, and a three-step verification and correction preprocessing is carried out based on UTCMLS.

The third data quality problem is textual value missing of attribute *efficacy* in DCMF. To tackle this problem, a closest-fit-based approach is presented to impute missing values. To effectively capture the similarity of two medical texts, an order-semisensitive similarity M-similarity [13] is used in this method. In summary, this case incorporates three important TDQ dimensions and problems, and shows how to effectively handle dirty textual data in data mining situations. Based on the case study and the experience accumulated during the long-year process of fighting with TDQ in data mining, five suggestions on TDQ in data mining are also provided in this paper. These suggestions are expected to help data analysts and miners to attach more importance to TDQ issue, and enhance TDQ for more reliable analysis and data mining.

The rest of the paper is organized as follows. Three typical TDQ dimensions are highlighted and discussed in Section 2. The case study in handling three TDQ problems is then provided in detail in Section 3. Finally, the conclusion and five suggestions are given in Section 4.

2   Typical TDQ Dimensions and Problems

In this section, three typical TDQ dimensions are highlighted. Many textual attributes are semi- and un-structured, which means representation-related problems are more prone to occur than non-textual attributes. Besides, according to our data mining experiences for years, textual data also suffers from the problem of data incompleteness.

2.1   Representation Granularity

This dimension means whether the data attributes represent textual information in the right granularity. Data mining algorithms usually have some requirements on input data, in which right representation granularity is usually an important one. That is, many data mining algorithms could not be applied on dataset with too large or too small representation granularity. Actually this type of data quality problem could possibly be avoided when the database model or data warehouse model is perfectly designed. However, this condition is not easy to fulfill in real world. As a result, such TDQ problem could easily be found in data mining.

There are two types of textual representation granularity problems. The first one is the problem of too small representation granularity, which means a certain piece of textual information should be stored in one attribute, but is separately recorded in several smaller segments (attributes). This is because data mining on such datasets usually need some integrating preprocessing to tackle the small granularity, which could otherwise be avoided in case of right representation granularity. The second type of textual representation granularity problems, is the one of too large granularity, which means multiple segments of textual information should be stored in separate attributes, but are recorded as only one attribute in database. In such cases, multiple textual data elements are collectively represented in one attribute, which as a result increases preprocessing burden for data mining. Take the case illustrated in [14] as an example, a data field containing "Mr. Frank M." can be easily understood by a human operator. However, this value actually includes three fields: the salutation "Mr.", the first name "Frank" and the middle initial "M.". Thus, if you want to know the number of male customers, you might get incorrect result if this data field is not treated. Identifying such problems of representation granularity and treating them is indispensable for data analysis and decision support.

2.2   Representation Consistency

Representation consistency means that data are continuously presented in the same format, consistently represented, consistently formatted and compatible with previous data [6]. Representation consistency could be found in both textual attributes and non-textual attributes. The inconsistent weight units used in commercial system is an example of representation consistency of non-textual attributes. However, such representation consistency occurs more often in textual attributes.

In real-world data mining, it is easy to find one concept represented by different textual expressions within one database. The reason behind such phenomena usually lies in the missing of terminological standard for the given area. When a standard terminology is available for the given application, such problem of representation inconsistency could be greatly alleviated. However, in real-world data analysis, such standard terminology could not be easily found for data miners, sometimes even not existing. The situation becomes even worse when data mining is conducted on some complex applications, such as TCM. Due to historical reasons, TCM experts in thousands of years tended to use different notions and expressions to describe one concept. When the information in different dynasties is collected in databases, the problem of representation inconsistency is also introduced. The existence of so many expressions and aliases for one concept, could very possibly influence the data distributions across the dataset. Data mining based on such biased data might result in unreliable or even wrong knowledge. Thus, before data analysis and knowledge discovery could be carried out on these data, the representation consistency issues must be addressed to ensure effective data mining.

2.3   Completeness

One of the biggest problems hampering the effective usage of textual data is the incompleteness of data. That is, the textual attribute value is missing for a portion of records. The reasons behind data incompleteness could also be related with the entire process of data collection, storage and usage. In the data collection stage, the data collection might be applied on only a part of data objects due to cost considerations. Another reason is the resistance from some data collecting objects. This phenomenon could easily be found in medical situations. Some patients might be unwilling to provide detailed personal information, or resist some medical examinations / treatments, which could lead to the missing of some attribute values in HIS/EMR system. In the data storage stage, sometimes the data scalability is not good enough. For example, the maximal length of some textual attributes might be not large enough, which make some large-length texts could not be stored in database. Such attribute values missing could also happen when multiple datasets of different attribute sets are integrated into one large dataset. In the data usage stage, the cost and/or security considerations could also prevent data owners open full data access. Sometimes only a part of dataset is open to access, and sometimes the data provider might replace original attribute values with missing values or noise values to protect data privacy, especially in medical situations. Note that, the problems discussed above are related with attribute values, that is, the missing of textual attribute values. In real-world data mining cases, sometimes one or even more attributes are not available as data source during the data mining process. That is, such attributes are totally missing.

3   Case Study on TDQ in Data Mining

This case is under the background of data mining in TCM. During the long-year process of data mining explorations using the TCM-Online Database System [15] (the largest TCM data collections in the world), we accumulate considerable experience on how to identify and tackle TDQ problems. One distinguishing feature of TCM lies in its emphasis on the usage of combinatorial medicines, as the form of Chinese Medical Formula (CMF). The Database of Chinese Medical Formula (DCMF) is just a large data resource that contains more than 85,000 CMFs. The Main contents of DCMF include formal name, efficacy, usage, adverse reactions and its treatment, ingredients, dosage form and specifications, compatibility of medicines, chemical composition, etc.[15]. Most of these attributes are stored in DCMF as the form of unstructured or semi-structured text. To discover compatibility rules of medicines in CMF data, frequent itemset analysis and associational rule mining are conducted on DCMF. However, we encounter serious data quality problems, especially in textual attributes. Among these problems, three main TDQ problems are identified and discussed below, as well as the methods utilized to remedy these TDQ problems.

3.1   Fighting with Representation Granularity Problems

When conducting data mining in DCMF, the first TDQ problem we encounter is the representation granularity problem found in the attribute *ingredients*. The contents of *ingredients* are the herbs or other medicinal materials constituting the CMF, which is thus the key attributes for frequent itemset analysis and associational rule mining. Note that CMF is usually composed of multiple Chinese herbal medicines. This means *ingredients* of CMF should contain the information of multiple drugs. However, the *ingredients* is stored in DCMF as a free-text attribute. Actually, this single data attribute contains not only the names of Chinese herbal medicines, but also the corresponding dosages, weight units and even preparation methods. A typical example of *ingredients* can be listed below: "*Ginseng 1 liang, Largehead Atractylodes Rhizome 1 liang, Tuckahoe (peeling) 1 liang, Liquorice Root 8 qian*". Such situation could be easily identified as a TDQ problem of too-large representation granularity, which must be handled before effective data mining could be carried out in DCMF.

The solution of this problem could be traced back to the level of database logical model. Actually, the current database model of DCMF is basically ok for simple application like browsing. However, this model is not applicable for more complex applications like data mining, which requires each Chinese herbal medicine in each CMF easy to index and count. So, a thorough solution for the current representation granularity problem is to modify the database logical model and physical model. After such modification, each data element in CMF *ingredients*, including each herb name, corresponding dosage, weight unit and preparation method, could be stored into separate attributes in DCMF.

Although the solution above is more thorough, it could be directly applied only on future CMF data. For existing CMF data, a preprocessing procedure is still needed to structurize the *ingredients* information into multiple separated data attributes. To conduct such structurizing, a concept of herb information unit (HIU) is defined, which is the name of Chinese herbal medicine, followed by the preparation method, dosage and weight unit. Under this perspective, we could see that the attribute *ingredients* usually consists of multiple HIUs separated by commas. To effectively use all information in this field, we should firstly split *ingredients* into multiple HIUs. Secondly, for each CIU, we further divide it into four fields: the name of Chinese herbal medicine, preparation method, dosage and weight unit. To perform this two-step extraction, there are a lot of details and exceptions that should be noticed in practice. For instance, in many records the delimiter comma might be replaced by semicolon / period, or even missing; the preparation method / dosage / weight unit is also missing or misspelled in many records. To implement the two-step splitting, a splitting-rule-based system named *field splitter* is developed by us to handle this problem. Tens of specific preprocessing and splitting rules, such as "keep between A and B", "replace A with B", "insert A after B", etc., are defined. Users can form their own splitting setting by organizing these rules. By using this system, the representation granularity problem above is resolved satisfactorily, which removes a great obstacle to following data mining.

3.2   Fighting with Representation Inconsistency Problems

The second TDQ problem we are faced with is an unwanted yet very common situation in TCM data mining, that is, the representation inconsistency. Due to historical reasons, TCM experts in thousands of years tended to use different notions and expressions to describe one concept. When the information in different dynasties is collected in databases, the problem of representation inconsistency is also introduced. This phenomenon could be easily found across the whole TCM database. As for the target database DCMF used in this case study, almost all of the textual attributes have the TDQ problem of representation inconsistency. Still take the attribute *ingredients* as an example: even this attribute is treated by the *field splitter* mentioned in section 3.1, the separated information, including the name of Chinese herbal medicine, and the preparation method, still suffer from the representation inconsistency problem. For the name of Chinese herbal medicine, for instance, ginseng Panax, and Radix ginseng could all refer to the Chinese herbal medicine ginseng in English. This situation becomes more complex in Chinese: there are ten aliases for ginseng. Before frequent itemset analysis and associational rule mining could be carried out on DCMF, such representation inconsistency issues must be addressed.

To tackle the above TDQ problem of representation inconsistency, the basic idea is to refer to the standardized terminology. In TCM context, this task could be done with the help of UTCMLS [12], which is the largest ontology-based language system in TCM. The basic procedure we apply could be illustrated in Figure 1.

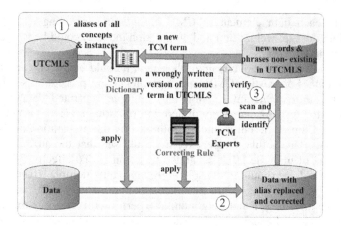

Fig. 1. Procedure to handle representation inconsistency

As Figure 1 shows, the procedure to handle textual representation inconsistency consists of three steps. In step one, the aliases of all concepts and instance are extracted from UTCMLS, forming a synonym dictionary. In step two, by scanning this dictionary from beginning to end, all of the aliases found in target data are replaced with their formal names. In step three, a manual check is conducted by the TCM experts to identify incorrect substitutions and new words / phrases that don't exist in UTCMLS. For each new word / phrase, a verification is conducted by experts to see whether it is a true new TCM term, or is just a wrongly written version of some term in UTCMLS. In the former case, this new term would be added into the synonym dictionary (or even UTCMLS after a period of time), so that the system could recognize this new term in the next round of scanning. In the latter case, the wrongly written version would be corrected to its right term, and such correcting operation with its context would be automatically recorded as a correction rule by the system. These newly-collected correction rules could be automatically applied or manually selected in following sessions. After the whole dataset is treated with these three steps, the synonym dictionary is updated, and some correction rules are collected. Then, we could go back to step two, performing scanning and substituting, and then to step three, checking and updating. After several rounds of processing like this, the problem of representation inconsistency in textual attributes could be relieved greatly. This procedure is applied by us in DCMF, which is found to greatly alleviate the TDQ problem of representation inconsistency.

3.3   Fighting with Incompleteness Problems

The third TDQ problem indentified in DCMF analysis is data incompleteness. This problem is found seriously in the attribute *Efficacy*, which is another textual attribute containing description of remedy principle in TCM background. Due to historical reason, among 85917 valid records wherein the attribute value of *ingredients* is not null, only 15671 records are stored with *efficacy* not null. That is, 81.76% of data in attribute *efficacy* is missing. Such data incompleteness becomes a great obstacle to the effective data mining on DCMF.

Typical methods to missing value problem include mean imputation, mode imputation and imputation by regression. However, these approaches are more applicable to structured data than unstructured text. To attack missing value problem in textual data, we propose closest fit approaches [13] to filling in textual missing values. In closest fit methods, we search the training set, compare each case with the one having missing value, calculate similarity between them, and select the case with largest similarity. Then, we substitute the attribute value of that case for the missing attribute value. Two versions of closest fit methods could be applied. The first is to search the best candidate in entire data set, which can be named *global closest fit*. The second is to restrict search space to all cases belonging to the same category, which can be named *concept closest fit*, or *category closest fit*.

A fundamental issue in this approach is how to evaluate the "closeness" of two given texts. In medical applications like TCM, a large portion of items in text has special meaning, while the order of item in text is not fully determinant for text comparison. To capture the similarity in this background more precisely and efficiently, a new order-semisensitive similarity M-similarity is proposed [13]. Given two texts S (with shorter length N) and L (with longer length M), and current position *curpos* within S, M-Similarity can be calculated as below:

$$\text{M-Similarity } (S, L) = \frac{\sum\limits_{curpos} \lambda_{lm}(S, L, curpos) + \lambda_{pm}(S, L)}{M \times W_s + (M-1) \times W_{ec}} \tag{1}$$

Where λ_{lm} is the sum of weights for maximum sequence matching, λ_{pm} is the value of potential matching, W_s represents weight of single item matching, and W_{ec} stands for extra weight of continuous matching [13].

The following is an experiment on handling missing textual values to show the performance of closest fit methods based on M-Similarity defined above. To evaluate the accuracy of closest fit method, another data set named DCMF-2 is used. DCMF-2 is a selected version of Database of Currently Application of Herbal Medicine Formula. It contains 4646 CMF derived from modern publications. Both the attribute *ingredients* and *efficacy* are not missing for each record. DCMF-2 has an attribute indicating the category of formula, enabling the category closest fit approach.

In theory of TCM, the closeness of formula ingredients reflects the resemblance of efficacy. The attribute *ingredients* in both DCMF and DCMF-2 are in the same textual form. As describe in section 3.1, the *field splitter* system is applied to extract components of formula from this attribute. Then, Jaccard coefficient is calculated to measure the degree of overlap between two sets of structured nominal ingredients derived from *field splitter*. Here, we define the similarity between two ingredients as the Jaccard coefficient multiplied by 100, that is, a value between 0 and 100. To fill in an assumed missing efficacy of certain formula, we search for the formula having the greatest similarity of ingredients with that case, and substitute its efficacy for missing one. M-similarity between the substitute and original efficacy is calculated subsequently to perform quantitative evaluation. The greatest similarity of ingredients mentioned above can be abbreviated as GSI for later reference. Both the global closest fit approach and category closest fit one are carried in our experiments. By analyzing the characteristic of TCM text and tuning parameter empirically, we set W_s, W_{ec} and P_{pm} to 0.8, 0.2 and 0.1 respectively. The experimental results are illustrated in Figure 2 and Figure 3.

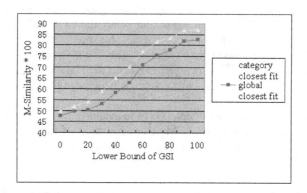

Fig. 2. Average M-Similarity (*100) for different scopes of data in DCMF-2

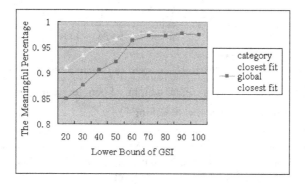

Fig. 3. The meaningful percentage of case processed by closest fit approach to DCMF-2

Figure 2 shows how the average M-similarity (*100) changes as a function of selection scope of records. Due to the diversity of expression for textual contents, our approach can't totally replace manual method. However, it can serve as a valuable reference to manual work. After carefully analyzing our result, experts of TCM point out, for missing value of efficacy, those cases with M-similarity no less than 0.2 are of great meaning for manual work. They also present that our method is reasonable only if GSI is no less than 20. Thus we calculate the following value as evaluation factor: *the meaningful percentage*, that is, the percentage of case with M-similarity no less than 0.2. Figure 3 shows how the meaningful percentage varies along with the lower bound of GSI. Among 3705 formulae (79.75% records of DCMF-2) with GSI no less than 20, nearly 85% of results derived from global closest fit approach are meaningful. This percentage reaches as high as 91.15% for category closest fit. That is, this method is effective for 67.79% records of DCMF-2 for global closest fit, and 72.69% for category closest fit. The experimental results above show that the closet fit methods based on M-similarity could serve as a valuable reference to manual work, to help data analysts determine missing textual values.

4   Conclusion

While the issue of data mining quality and reliability attracts increasing interest in the research community, the real-world data analysts might found data quality problems become great obstacle to overcome, in order to ensure the discovered knowledge is of quality. Textual data is one type of data that should be explored more on the topic of data quality, due to the ubiquity and diversity of textual information, as well as its distinguishing data quality dimensions and problems. In this paper, we focus on the topic of TDQ in data mining. Based on our data mining experiences for years, three important and typical TDQ dimensions are highlighted and discussed, including representation granularity, representation consistency and completeness. Then, a case study is also provided in this paper, which is under the background of data mining in TCM. In order to conduct an association rule mining in DCMF, three TDQ problems are identified to be handled. The first problem of representation granularity is tackled by a rule-based splitting system. The second problem of representation inconsistency is addressed by a three-step verification and correction preprocessing based on the standardized terminological database UTCMLS. The third problem of incompleteness is handled by closest fit methods based on a new text similarity measure M-similarity. In summary, this case incorporates three important TDQ dimensions and related problems, and shows how to handle dirty textual data in real-world data mining situations.

Based on the case study and the experience accumulated during the long-year process of fighting with TDQ in data mining, five suggestions on TDQ in data mining are also provided for data analysts in this paper, as the following:

1) **Never Neglect TDQ Problems.** Dirty data has already been listed as the top one challenge for data mining [3]. Because of the semi- and un-structured nature, textual data suffers more from the representation-related problems than non-textual data. Besides, some typical TDQ problems, such as data incompleteness, are also more difficult to solve for textual data than non-textual data. From this perspective, TDQ problems should never be neglected.

2) **Prepare Enough Time and Patience.** It was estimated that 50% to as much as 80% of the time and effort spent on knowledge discovery is utilized in preprocessing tasks [16]. The reason behind it is that today's real-world databases are highly susceptible to noise, missing, inconsistent, and other data quality problems. According to real-world experience, data quality problems in textual attributes are basically more complex and hard to handle than that in non-textual attributes, which means more time, effort and patience should be prepared for data miners to handle TDQ problems.

3) **Never Expect One Round of Preprocessing to Be a Total Solution.** In our data mining explorations in applications like medicine and business for years, it is seldom that TDQ problems could be perfectly addressed by a single round of preprocessing. That means multiple rounds of preprocessing are usually needed to handle TDQ problems. This is partly determined by the complexity and diversity of TDQ problems.

Another reason is that, multiple TDQ problems are usually interrelated. Thus, in order to address TDQ problems more effectively, multiple rounds of preprocessing should be needed to ensure a more satisfactory solution.

4) Construct Well-Designed and Standard-Terminology-Based Databases. Representation granularity and representation consistency are TDQ dimensions that always cause great troubles for data analysts. In fact, such kinds of problems could be largely avoided, or at least alleviated, by using well-designed data models and standard terminology during the building process of this database. However, in real-world situations data builders and data miners are typically not the same group of people, which means databases are usually constructed when the data analyzing requirements are not well-considered. A corresponding suggestion is that data builders should try their bests to design data models at a right granularity, and standard terminology should be encouraged to use as early as possible at the stage of database building.

5) Do Not Emphasize Too Much on Automatic Preprocessing Techniques. In our long-year process of data mining, almost every practical solution for TDQ problems would include the support from manual work. All of the three cases in this paper need manual work together with automatic preprocessing. Here is the corresponding suggestion: TDQ problems should be addressed based on the cooperation of automatic preprocessing techniques and manual efforts. Emphasizing too much on automatic preprocessing than manual work would mislead data miners to unwanted results.

The road towards satisfactory TDQ is never flat. By introducing key TDQ dimensions and presenting cases and suggestions to handle TDQ problems, this paper is expected to help data analysts and miners to attach more importance to TDQ issue, and acquire textual data with enhanced quality for more reliable analysis and decision making. Actually, the best way to handle data quality problems, whatever area it is, or whatever form of data it is, is to avoid them. However, total avoidance is a nearly impossible task in many cases. A realistic and workable strategy is to taking data quality into account throughout the process of data collection, storage and usage, which could help to diminish such problems to the minimum.

Acknowledgements. This work is supported by National Natural Science Fund of China (NO. 60905026, 71071141), Specialized Research Fund for the Doctoral Program of Higher Education of China (NO. 20093326120004), Natural Science Fund of Zhejiang Province (NO. Y1091164, Z1091224, LQ12G01007), Zhejiang Science and Technology Plan Project (NO. 2010C33016, 2012R10041-09), and the Key Technology Innovation Team Building Program of Zhejiang Province (No. 2010R50041).

References

1. PAKDD QIMIE'13 website,
   http://conferences.telecom-bretagne.eu/qimie2013/
2. ICDM RIKD'12 website, http://www.deakin.edu.au/~hdai/RIKD12/
3. Rexer, K.: 4th Annual Data Miner Survey - 2010 Survey Summary Report (2011),
   http://www.rexeranalytics.com

4. Chapman, P., Clinton, J., Kerber, R., Khabaza, T., Reinartz, T., Shearer, C., Wirth, R.: CRISP 1.0 Process and User Guide (2000), http://www.crisp-dm.org
5. Ballou, D.P., Pazer, H.L.: Cost/Quality Tradeoffs for Control Procedures in Information Systems. OMEGA: Int'l J. Management Science 15(6), 509–521 (1987)
6. Wang, R.Y., Reddy, M.P., Kon, H.B.: Toward Quality Data: an Attribute-based Approach. Decision Support Systems 13(3-4), 349–372 (1995)
7. Wang, R.Y., Strong, D.M.: Beyond Accuracy: What Data Quality Means to Data Consumers. Journal of Management Information Systems 4, 5–34 (1996)
8. Madnick, S.E., Wang, R.Y., Lee, Y.W., Zhu, H.W.: Overview and Framework for Data and Information Quality Research. ACM Journal of Data and Information Quality 1(1), 1–22 (2009)
9. O'Donnell, M., Knott, A.: Oberlander Jon., Mellish C.: Optimising Text Quality in Generation from Relational Databases. In: Proc. of 1st International Conference on Natural Language Generation, pp. 133–140 (2000)
10. Sonntag, D.: Assessing the Quality of Natural Language Text Data. Proc. of GI Jahrestagung 1, 259–263 (2004)
11. Feng, Y., Wu, Z.H., Chen, H.: j., Yu, T., Mao, Y.X., Jiang, X.H.: Data Quality in Traditional Chinese Medicine. In: Proc. of BMEI 2008, pp. 255–259 (2008)
12. Zhou, X.Z., Wu, Z.H., Yin, A.N., Wu, L.C., Fan, W.Y., Zhang, R.E.: Ontology Development for Unified Traditional Chinese Medical Language System. Artificial Intelligence in Medicine 32(1), 15–27 (2004)
13. Feng, Y., Wu, Z., Zhou, Z.: Combining an Order-Semisensitive Text Similarity and Closest Fit Approach to Textual Missing Values in Knowledge Discovery. In: Khosla, R., Howlett, R.J., Jain, L.C. (eds.) KES 2005. LNCS (LNAI), vol. 3682, pp. 943–949. Springer, Heidelberg (2005)
14. Schmid, J.: The Main Steps to Data Quality. In: Proc. of 4th Industrial Conf. on Data Mining, pp. 69–77 (2004)
15. Feng, Y., Wu, Z.H., Zhou, Z.M., Fan, W.Y.: Knowledge Discovery in Traditional Chinese Medicine: State of the Art and Perspectives. Artificial Intelligence in Medicine 38(3), 219–236 (2006)
16. Pipino, L., Kopcso, D.: Data Mining, Dirty Data, and Costs. In: Proc. of ICIQ 2004, pp. 164–169 (2004)

Cost-Based Quality Measures
in Subgroup Discovery

Rob M. Konijn, Wouter Duivesteijn, Marvin Meeng, and Arno Knobbe

LIACS, Leiden University, The Netherlands
{konijn,wouterd,meeng,knobbe}@liacs.nl

Abstract. In this paper we consider data where examples are not only
labeled in the classical sense (positive or negative), but also have costs associated with them. In this sense, each example has two target attributes,
and we aim to find clearly defined subsets of the data where the values
of these two targets have an unusual distribution. In other words, we
are focusing on a Subgroup Discovery task over somewhat unusual data,
and investigate possible quality measures that take into account both
the binary as well as the cost target. In defining such quality measures,
we aim to produce interpretable valuation of subgroups, such that data
analysts can directly value the findings, and relate these to monetary
gains or losses. Our work is particularly relevant in the domain of health
care fraud detection. In this data, the binary target identifies the patients
of a specific medical practitioner under investigation, whereas the cost
target specifies how much money is spent on each patient. When looking
for clear specifications of differences in claim behavior, we clearly need
to take into account both the 'positive' examples (patients of the practitioner) and 'negative' examples (other patients), as well as information
about costs of all patients. A typical subgroup will now list a number of
treatments, and how the patients of our practitioner differ in both the
prevalence of the treatments as well as the associated costs. An additional
angle considered in this paper is the recently proposed Local Subgroup
Discovery, where subgroups are judged according to the difference with
a local reference group, rather than the entire dataset. We show how the
cost-based analysis of data specifically fits this local focus.

1 Introduction

This paper is about data that involves a binary label for each example, as well as
a cost. The motivation comes from a real-life problem where we are interested in
benchmarking (comparing) the claim behavior of medical practitioners. When
a patient visits a medical practitioner, the practitioner charges an amount of
money, corresponding to the treatment the patient received, to a health insurance company. Several parties are involved in this treatment, each with its own
set of knowledge. The patient knows which treatments are performed, but he
is unaware of the communication between the practitioner and the insurance
company. The insurance company knows which treatments are claimed by the

J. Li et al. (Eds.): PAKDD 2013 Workshops, LNAI 7867, pp. 404–415, 2013.

practitioner, but it is unaware of what exactly happened when the patient visited the practitioner's office. The practitioner is the only party that has both sets of information: he knows what treatments he performed with this patient, and he knows what treatments he claimed at the insurance company. Because of this information advantage, a malevolent practitioner is in a unique position that gives leeway to inefficient claim behavior or even fraud.

Detecting fraud on this level is very interesting to the insurance company – much more so than fraud on the level of individual patients – since the commercial implications are substantial. Hence there is a market for a data mining solution to identify unusual claiming patterns that have a substantial economical impact. The problem of identifying interesting patterns in claim behavior is essentially an unsupervised learning problem. We have no claims that are labeled as interesting beforehand. The approach we take is to single out a practitioner and compare his claim behavior with the claim behavior of other practitioners. The data we consider describes patients and practitioners. A single record summarizes the care a patient received during a certain period. We are interested in finding patient groups (patterns), that describe the difference between a single medical practitioner and its peers. In other words, we would like to develop a data mining algorithm, of which the output would be: patients that are in subgroup S occur much more frequent for this medical practitioner, and indicate a difference with other practitioners. The task of identifying such interesting subgroups is known as Subgroup Discovery [5], and also as Emerging Pattern mining [2], and Contrast Set mining [1].

We are interested in patterns that distinguish one practitioner from the others. In order to find such patterns, we need quality measures to describe how 'interesting' a pattern is. We would like the quality measure to capture the distributional difference between one practitioner and the others: the higher the distributional difference, the more interesting a pattern is. Secondly, we are interested in including costs into the quality measure. The main motivation is that in our application, subgroups involving more money are more interesting. Also, a monetary-valued quality value for each subgroup greatly improves the interpretability of a subgroup, because the measure itself has a monetary value. In this paper we will describe how to take costs into account when calculating quality measures. Each patient is 'labeled' by a monetary value – in our application this is the total costs spent on treatments during a specific period – and the quality measures we develop use these monetary values. As a result, the subgroups we find should be easier to interpret by domain experts, since the groups have an associated value in a commodity the experts understand.

2   Preliminaries

Throughout this paper we assume this dataset D with N examples (typically patients). Each row can be seen as a $(h + 2)$-dimensional vector of the form $x = \{a_1, .., a_h, t, c\}$. Hence, we can view our dataset as an $N \times (h + 2)$ matrix, where each example is stored as a row $x^i \in D$. We call $a^i = \{a_1^i, .., a_h^i\}$ the *attributes* of the ith example x^i. The attributes are taken from an unspecified domain $\mathcal{A}$. The last two elements of each row are the targets. The first target, t, is binary. Its values are set by singling out a medical practitioner. This t-vector then indicates if a patient visited a medical practitioner (a positive example), or not (a negative one). The other target, c, indicates a monetary value. In our application this monetary value indicates the total costs spent on treatments, per year. For other applications c could indicate the profit or the per-customer value. Just like for the attributes, we will refer to the target values of a specific record by superscript: t^i and c^i are the targets of example x^i.

The goal of our approach is to find differences between the singled-out medical practitioner (positive examples) and the rest. Simultaneously, the difference should constitute a considerable amount of money; the more money involved, the better. For this purpose the second target vector c is used. These differences are described by subgroups. A subgroup can be seen as a bag of examples, it can be any subset S of the dataset $S \subseteq D$. We describe how interesting a subgroup is with the use of a quality measure. A quality measure $q : 2^D \rightarrow \mathbb{R}$ is a function assigning a numeric value to any subgroup. Generally, the larger the subgroup is, the better (very small subgroups are usually not preferred). Also, the bigger the distributional difference, the better. In our case, because we have two target vectors, this distributional difference can be measured in terms of the binary target vector t (the higher the frequency of $t = 1$ in the subgroup, the better), and the distributional difference can also be measured in the monetary-valued target vector c (the higher the values for c within the subgroup, the better). The quality measure combines these properties of interestingness in a single numeric value.

In traditional Subgroup Discovery, there is only one binary target attribute t. We denote the set of examples for which t is true (the *positives*) by T, and the set of examples for which t is false (the *negatives*) by F. When we consider a particular subgroup S, we denote its complement by $\neg S$. In this setting we denote the true/false positives/negatives in the traditional way: $TP = T \cap S$, $FP = F \cap S$, $FN = T \cap \neg S$, and $TN = F \cap \neg S$. For any subset of examples $X \subseteq D$, we let $\bar{c}_X$ denote the mean cost of the examples in X: $\bar{c}_X = \sum_{x^i \in X} c^i / |X|$, where $|X|$ is the cardinality of the set X.

2.1   The Local Subgroup Discovery Task

To deal with locality, in a previous publication we introduced the Local Subgroup Discovery (LSD) task [3]. The idea is to "zoom in" on a part of the data set, and detect interesting subgroups locally. In our application, we can think of the patient population as if they are distributed among different patient groups (for example one group could be patients having a type of cancer). Such a coherent group of patients on which we zoom in is called a *reference group*. LSD is a distance-based approach to find subgroups and reference groups, based on prototypes. A *prototype* can be any point in attribute space $x \in \mathcal{A}$. The *distance-based subgroup S_σ* based on x for parameter $\sigma \in \mathbb{N}$, consists of the σ nearest

Table 1. The *counts* cross table and the *costs* cross table

	T	F
S	TP	FP
$\neg S$	FN	TN

	T	F
S	$\bar{c}_{S \cap T}$	$\bar{c}_{S \cap F}$
$\neg S$	$\bar{c}_{\neg S \cap T}$	$\bar{c}_{\neg S \cap F}$

neighbors of x in D. The *reference group* R_ρ based on the same x for parameter $\rho \in \mathbb{N}$ s.t. $\rho \geq \sigma$, consists of the ρ nearest neighbors of x in D.

The goal of LSD is to find subgroups $S_\sigma \subseteq R_\rho$ for which the target distribution is different from the target distribution in the reference group. The reason for zooming in on a reference group is twofold. On the one hand, this allows us to provide information about the neighborhood of a found subgroup. On the other hand, it accounts for inhomogeneities in the dataset. The idea behind that is that R_ρ forms a region in input space where the target distribution is different from that distribution over the whole dataset. Subgroups that are interesting to report are not these reference groups: they are simply groups of patients sharing a disease that is relatively expensive to treat. The interesting subgroups from a fraud detection point of view, are those subgroups that represent a deviation in target distribution *relative to their peers*: we want to find subgroups $S_\sigma \subseteq R_\rho$ in which the target distribution is different from the distribution in the reference group.

We write $S(x, \sigma, \rho)$ for the subgroup S_σ in a reference group R_ρ, which we call a *reference-based subgroup*. The prototype can be seen as the center of this subgroup, and as the center of the reference group encompassing the subgroup. A quality measure calculated for a reference-based subgroup considers only examples inside the reference group.

3   Quality Measures

The quality measures we consider are defined in terms of two cross tables, both depicted in Table 1. The cross table on the left is common in traditional Subgroup Discovery. The cross table on the right is concerned with the mean costs for each of the categories. Our quality measures should satisfy the following criteria:

- in the first cross table, the higher the numbers on the diagonal ($TP + TN$) are, the more interesting the subgroup is;
- in the second cross table, the higher the mean cost value in the true positive cell $\bar{c}_{S \cap T}$ is, relative to those values in the other cells, the more interesting a subgroup is.

Furthermore, it would be desirable if the value of the quality measure has a direct interpretation in terms of money. In Sections 3.1-3.3 we introduce quality measures satisfying these criteria, but before that we will shortly discuss why a straightforward Subgroup Discovery approach does not suffice.

$$t = \{ \ + \ , \ - \ , \ - \ , \ - \ , \ + \ , \ - \ , \ + \ , \ + \ , \ + \ , \ - \ , \ - \ , \ - \ \}$$
$$c = \{ \ 1000, \ 2000, \ 2000, \ 1250, \ 2000, \ 3000, \ 200, \ 200, \ 200, \ 200, \ 200, \ 200 \ \}$$
$$c * t = \{ \ 1000, \quad 0 \ , \quad 0 \ , \quad 0 \ , \ 2000, \quad 0 \ , \ 200, \ 200, \ 200, \quad 0 \ , \quad 0 \ , \quad 0 \ \}$$
$$\uparrow$$
$$\sigma$$

Fig. 1. A dataset of twelve examples with a subgroup of six examples indicated

A naive way of dealing with the two targets in our dataset, is to multiply t by c for each observation, and use these new values as one numeric target variable of a traditional Subgroup Discovery run. By taking the difference in means between the subgroup and the mean of the data, the quality measure has a monetary value. Consider the dataset in Figure 1. The first 6 examples (up to σ) belong to the subgroup, and the other examples do not. Computing the difference in means for $c \cdot t$, the value of this naive quality measure would be $3000/6 - 3600/12 = 200$ (where we are comparing the subgroup mean with the mean of the total $c \cdot t$ column).

The disadvantage of this measure, is that the value of this monetary value of 200 does not have a direct meaningful interpretation: it does not directly relate to the amount of money that is present 'more' in the subgroup, or that could be recovered. But more importantly, the positive quality value for this subgroup is misleading. When we are looking for high average values for our target, this suggests that there is somehow more money involved than expected, but when we take a look at this subgroup, there is not more money involved for the positive examples than for the negative examples. In our application, suppose the reference group (12 examples) would indicate diabetes patients. The subgroup indicates patients receiving expensive diabetes treatments, and the rest of the reference group indicates patients receiving inexpensive diabetes treatments. A low number of true positives (lower than expected), would mean that there are less diabetes patients present at this practitioner than at other practitioners. Also the practitioner claims less money for diabetes patients than other practitioners do (the costs of the true positive patients is less than the false positives). Since overall the practitioner is claiming less money than expected, the quality measure should indicate this, but for this measure the positive quality value of 200 suggests more money than expected is claimed. The measure based on the average value of $c \cdot t$ is too much biased towards regions with high values for c only, and its quality value is not interpretable at all.

3.1 Measures Weighting Counts by Costs

When the emphasis of the measure should still be on the deviation in observed counts (rather than costs), the following measures can be used. The idea is to weight the deviation in counts in the true positive cell of the counts cross table. Such a positive deviation (so observing more true positives than expected), will be more interesting if more money is involved in those true positives. The measures we propose weight this deviation by costs.

$$CWTPD(S) = \left(TP - \frac{1}{N}(TP + FP)(TP + FN) \right) \cdot \bar{c}_{S \cap T} \tag{1}$$

This measure is called the Cost-Weighted True Positive Deviation (CWTPD). The first of the two factors in this equation is the deviation (in counts) within the subgroup from the expected value. This part is similar to the WRAcc measure [4] for binary targets. Only here the deviation is measured in number of observations instead of fraction of the whole dataset, as the WRAcc measure does. This deviation is then multiplied by the average costs of true positives. Hence the measure can be interpreted as: difference in counts × costs involved per count = total costs involved. The big advantage of this definition is that it has a direct interpretation in terms of money. The disadvantage of this measure, especially for the local subgroup discovery task, is that it does not take the costs outside the subgroup into account. It could be that the costs in the reference group outside the subgroup are also high.

The measure following equation 2 eschews this disadvantage, by compensating in the second factor with the costs outside the subgroup:

$$Relative\ CWTPD(S) = \left(TP - \frac{1}{N}(TP + FP)(TP + FN) \right) \cdot (\bar{c}_{S \cap T} - \bar{c}_{\neg S}) \tag{2}$$

This quality measure is called the Relative Cost-Weighted True Positive Deviation (Relative CWTPD). In our application, the measure can be interpreted as the amount of money that would be claimed less if the cross table of counts would be homogeneous. This can be viewed as moving examples from the TP cell into the FP cell until the expected costs cross table is obtained, where costs of non-subgroup examples are estimated by $\bar{c}_{\neg S}$.

The measure in Equation (2) is very suitable for local subgroup discovery because it searches for difference in counts and difference in costs between the subgroup and the examples outside the subgroup simultaneously.

3.2 Measures Based on Cost Difference

To find subgroups for which the mean costs of the target are different from the negative examples, the Total Mean Cost difference between Classes (TMCC) (3) can be used.

$$TMCC(S) = TP \cdot (\bar{c}_{S \cap T} - \bar{c}_{S \cap F}) \tag{3}$$

This measure compares the mean costs of the positive examples with those of the negative examples. Subgroups for which this difference is high are the most interesting. To obtain a total amount (as a monetary value), the difference in means is multiplied by the number of true positives.

$$t = \{ \ +\ , \ -\ , \ -\ , \ -\ , \ +\ , \ -\ , \dots \}$$
$$c = \{ \ 2000, \ 1000, \ 1000, \ 1000, \ 2000, \ 1000, \ \dots \}$$
$$\uparrow$$
$$\sigma$$

Fig. 2. A dataset with indicated subgroup of six examples. The mean value for c is higher for the positive examples than for the negative examples in the subgroup. This leads to quality $(2000 - 1000) \cdot 2 = 2000$, computed with Equation (3).

When the number of false positives is very small, the estimate of $\bar{c}_{S \cap F}$ can be based on too few examples. A more robust measure is obtained by using $\bar{c}_S$ instead:

$$TMC(S) = TP \cdot (\bar{c}_{S \cap T} - \bar{c}_S) \tag{4}$$

This measure is called the Total Mean Cost difference (TMC).

The advantage of the TMCC and TMC quality measures is the interpretability: the quality value corresponds directly to the amount of money that is involved. The disadvantage for local subgroup discovery is that these measures do not take the reference group into account at all. Figure 2 shows the calculation of the quality measure. This subgroup will not be found with quality measure (1) or (2) if the probability of the target being true is higher outside the subgroup than inside the subgroup.

3.3 Measures Based on the Proportion of Costs

The previous measures were detecting differences in one target vector, and weighing this distance with the other target vector. The following measure is based on another approach: it considers the difference in distribution of total costs. We can define a cross table of observed costs. This table can be obtained by simply multiplying cells of the two basic cross tables about counts and costs:

	T	F
S	$\sum_{x^i \in S \cap t} c^i$	$\sum_{x^i \in S \cap F} c^i$
$\neg S$	$\sum_{x^i \in \neg S \cap t} c^i$	$\sum_{x^i \in \neg S \cap F} c^i$

This quality measure operates on this cross table of observed total costs. It is based on the proportion of costs per cell relative to the total costs within the whole dataset. It does not take the size of the subgroup into account. We can calculate the $Costs - WRAcc$ measure (called WRAcc due to its similarity to the WRAcc measure for a single binary target vector t). When we denote $c_T = \sum_{i=1}^{N} c^i$ as the total costs in the dataset, the Proportional Costs Deviation (PCD) measure can be calculated as follows:

$$PDC(S) = \frac{1}{c_T} \sum_{x^i \in S \cap t} c^i \ - \ \frac{1}{c_T{}^2} \sum_{x^i \in S} c^i \sum_{x^i \in T} c^i \tag{5}$$

This measure can be interpreted as the fraction of costs that is observed beyond expectation in the true positive cell, relative to the total costs in the whole dataset.

In our application, suppose the subgroup indicates cancer patients. A value of 0.1 would mean that in the true positive cell, the fraction of costs compared to the whole data set is 10 % higher than expected. Because this interpretation as a fraction of the total costs in the data set is rather difficult, a much more intuitive measure is the one that has a monetary value. This can be obtained by multiplying equation (5) with the total costs:

$$MVPDC(S) = \sum_{x^i \in S \cap t} c^i - \frac{1}{c_T} \sum_{x^i \in S} c^i \sum_{x^i \in T} c^i \qquad (6)$$

This quality measure is called the Monetary Valued Proportional Costs Deviation (MVPCD). This monetary value can be interpreted as the amount of money that is observed beyond expectation in the true positive cell of the total costs cross table, if the total costs distribution would be the same for the positives and negatives. The higher the value of the measure, the more interesting a subgroup is. In our example of cancer patients, a value of $100,000$ would mean that the total amount spent on cancer patients by the target hospital is $100,000$ more than expected. The advantage of this measure is that this measure can detect both deviations in average costs in the subgroup as well as deviations in counts. A disadvantage can be that the calculation of the expected value depends on the total costs distribution of points in T. In our example of the subgroup of cancer patients, it can be that the cancer patients are not more present in this hospital, and also cancer patients are not more expensive than cancer patients at other hospitals, but due to the presence of 'cheap' patients (with a relative low value for c) outside the subgroup, the proportion of observed costs spent on cancer patients can still be higher than expected. The fact that the costs outside the subgroup also play a role in calculating the expected value can cause misinterpretation.

4   Experiments and Results

In this section we show how the quality measures are used to detect interesting local subgroups in a real-world application. Our health care application concerns fraud amongst dentists. Each patient is represented by a binary vector of treatments that the patient received during a year. The dataset contains 980,350 patients and 542 treatment codes. As a distance measure between patients we use the Hamming distance between the treatments they received. Note that because of the discrete nature of the data, there are many duplicate examples (many patients with an identical combination of treatments). Additionally, the distance of a point to different neighbors may be identical, which limits the number of subgroups that need to be tested.

Table 2. The *observed counts* cross table and the *observed costs* cross table, for the subgroup found with the weighted costs measure

	T	F
S	8	77
$\neg S$	0	101

	T	F
S	1,619	697
$\neg S$	0	686

We select a dentist with a markedly high claiming profile, and define the target vector t accordingly. The dentist is visited by 5,567 patients (0.57% of the total data set). The costs vector c is calculated by summing the costs spent on the treatments that the patient received during the year.

4.1   Results with the Relative Cost-Weighted True Positive Deviation

We start with results for quality measure (2). Because the Relative CWTPD measure in equation 2 is very suitable for local subgroup discovery, where the CWTPD measure from equation 1 is better suitable for normal subgroup discovery. Within local subgroup discovery we can alter the reference group size, and 'zoom in' to different resolutions. The following subgroup is found at reference group size 186, with a subgroup size of 85 patients. The prototype patient is using the treatments:

{221153, C11, C12, D22, D24, D32, D33, D42, M20, M50}

Treatment C11 and C12 are regular consults, treatment M20 and M50 are dental cleaning treatments, and treatment 22153, D22, D24, D33, and D42 are orthodontist treatments performed by a dentist. Table 2 (left) shows the counts within this part of the data set. When we observe the cross table with counts we see that there are 8 patients that visit the target dentist, and none in the reference group (outside the subgroup). Patients within the subgroup have treatments similar to the prototype, where patients outside the subgroup, but in the reference group, also use similar treatments, but use less, and use other treatments as well. The table on the right shows the corresponding mean costs. From the two tables we can see that the number of true positives is higher than expected, and the mean costs for observations in the true positive cell are also higher than the mean costs within the other cells. The expected value for the number of true positives is 3.66. This leads to a quality of $(8 - 3.66) \cdot (1,619 - 686) = 4,051$ euros.

To further investigate the observations within the subgroup, and compare them to the rest of the reference group, we observe Table 3, where the support and costs of all frequent treatments in the reference group are compared. Only treatments that have a support ≥ 0.1 are in the table, which means that the costs spent on the treatment are bigger than zero for more than 10 percent of the patients in the reference group.

The first line in Table 3 corresponds to these treatments. The next lines correspond to the supports in the set $S_1 \cap T$ (the true positives), the support

Table 3. Prototypes and their support in the subgroup, and their support in the reference group excluding the subgroup. The codes indicate treatments that were charged for a patient, the supports indicate the fraction of patients receiving those treatments respectively. The costs indicate the mean costs spent on each treatment.

Subgroup	Prototype, Supports, and Costs									
S_1 prototype	221153	C11	C12	D22	D24	D32	D33	D42	M20	M50
$S_1 \cap T$	1.00	1.00	0.63	0.18	0.75	0.25	0.50	0.63	0.88	0.25
S_1	0.78	1.00	0.44	0.05	0.31	0.22	0.31	0.85	0.72	0.26
$R_1 \setminus S_1$	0.75	1.00	0.57	0.38	0.20	0.13	0.13	0.88	0.56	0.26
$\overline{c}_{S_1 \cap T}$	169	37	17	175	197	90	131	233	46	5
$\overline{c}_{S_1}$	85	32	12	80	42	73	49	224	29	7
$\overline{c}_{R_1 \setminus S_1}$	73	34	16	22	18	41	19	233	24	5

in S_1 and the support in $R_1 \setminus S_1$ (the patients outside the subgroup, but in the reference group). For each treatment, we can also calculate the mean costs in these sets. These numbers are in the last three lines of Table 3. For this subgroup we can conclude that more orthodontist treatments are claimed (codes D22, D24, D32, D33) within the subgroup compared to the rest of the reference group. From the mean costs numbers, we can conclude that the D22 and D24 treatments are interesting for this subgroup, because of the high costs of those treatments for the true positives.

4.2 Detecting Outliers

When restricting the reference group to very small sizes it is possible to find very small groups of outliers, or even find individual outliers as a subgroup. For example, with a reference group size ρ of 13, the best subgroup found for this value of ρ has only one observation with costs of 3779 euros, compared to the mean costs of 1073 euros for its nearest neighbors. The quality value for this individual outlier (again using the Relative CWTPD measure in Equation 2) is $(1 - 1/13)(3779 - 1073) = 2,498$ euros.

4.3 Measure Based on Cost Difference

With the TMCC quality measure, using Equation (3), subgroup S_2 was found for the following prototype:

$$\{A10, C11, C12, C13, E01, E13, E40, H30, M50, M55, R25, R31, R74, V11,$$
$$V12, V13, V14, V20, V21, V40, V60, V80, X10, X21\},$$

which is a single patient using a combination of many treatments. Patients within the subgroup have a maximum distance of 7 treatments to this prototype. The mean costs of the true positives, $\overline{c}_{\{S_2 \cap T\}}$, is 983 euros, and the mean costs of patients for which the target is false is 773 euros. In the set $S \cap T$ there are 89

Table 4. The *observed count* cross table and the *observed costs* cross table, for the subgroup found with the costs wracc measure

	T	F
S	87	1236
$\neg S$	110	4390

	T	F
S	427	347
$\neg S$	411	307

Table 5. Prototypes and their support in the subgroup, and their support in the reference group excluding the subgroup. The codes indicate treatments that were charged for a patient, the supports indicate the fraction of patients receiving those treatments respectively. The costs indicate the mean costs spent on each treatment.

Subgroup	Prototype, Supports, and Costs										
S_3 prototype	C11	C12	M55	V12	V13	V14	V21	V40	V60	X10	X21
$S_3 \cap T$	1.00	0.93	0.97	0.85	0.31	0.49	0.99	0.47	0.84	0.89	0.74
S_3	1.00	0.90	0.99	0.85	0.21	0.54	0.99	0.49	0.56	0.91	0.29
$R_3 \setminus S_3$	1.00	0.86	0.96	0.82	0.21	0.35	0.97	0.28	0.29	0.87	0.17
$\bar{c}_{S_3 \cap T}$	37	29	58	51	19	44	69	4	24	21	36
$\bar{c}_{S_3}$	36	25	59	47	16	46	52	5	13	22	14
$\bar{c}_{R_3 \setminus S_3}$	35	24	55	45	16	28	46	3	7	21	9

patients, while in the set $S \cap F$ there are 592 patients. This leads to a quality value of 18, 665 euros. When we investigate the subgroup, the main difference in costs are due to the treatments R25 (a metal crown with porcelain on top), for which the difference between the target and non-target points is 66 euros, V21 (polishing a filling) with a difference of 31 euros, and V60 (a pulpa-coverage), and X21 (X-ray) each with a difference of 21 euros. With this measure we were also able to mine individual outliers: this comes down to a k-nearest neighbor outlier detection algorithm for which each target point is compared to the mean value of its k nearest neighbors.

4.4   Measure Based on the Proportion of Costs

We calculate the MVPCD measure (6). The best subgroup for a maximum reference group size ρ of 6,000, has a quality of 16, 476. The optimal quality value is found for a σ of 1,323 and a ρ of 5, 823. Table 5 shows the difference in treatments and treatment costs, to get an idea what is the difference between the subgroup and the rest of the reference group.

Patients in this reference group are using the following treatments: $C11$ and $C12$ are regular consults, $M55$ is a dental cleaning, $V12$, $V13$, and $V14$ stand for 2-hedral, 3-hedral, and 4-hedral fillings. $V40$ is for polishing amalgam fillings, $V60$ for a pulpa-covering, and $X10$ and $X21$ for an inexpensive and expensive X-ray respectively. From Table 5, we can see that the main difference between the subgroup and the reference group are the treatments V21 (costs for polishing a filling), and X21 (costs for an expensive X-ray picture). We can conclude that for patients using standard consults, a dental cleaning, and a few fillings, the treatments V21 and X21 are claimed much more often at this dentist. In total, for this patient group, an amount of $16,476$ euros is claimed more than expected.

5   Conclusion

In this paper, we have presented several suggestions for quality measures that involve both binary labels and costs. We demonstrated their effectiveness in producing interesting and actionable patterns in a fraud detection application. As is common in Subgroup Discovery, more than one definition of interestingness can be conceived, and it is up to the end user to determine which measure best fits the specific analysis. We have proposed several measures, and explained the specific benefits of each.

References

1. Bay, S.D., Pazzani, M.J.: Detecting group differences: Mining contrast sets. Data Mining and Knowledge Discovery 5(3), 213–246 (2001)
2. Dong, G., Li, J.: Efficient mining of emerging patterns: discovering trends and differences. In: Proceedings of KDD 1999, pp. 43–52 (1999)
3. Konijn, R.M., Duivesteijn, W., Kowalczyk, W., Knobbe, A.: Discovering local subgroups, with an application to fraud detection. In: Pei, J., Tseng, V.S., Cao, L., Motoda, H., Xu, G. (eds.) PAKDD 2013, Part I. LNCS(LNAI), vol. 7818, pp. 1–12. Springer, Heidelberg (2013)
4. Lavrač, N., Flach, P.A., Zupan, B.: Rule evaluation measures: A unifying view. In: Džeroski, S., Flach, P.A. (eds.) ILP 1999. LNCS(LNAI), vol. 1634, pp. 174–185. Springer, Heidelberg (1999)
5. Wrobel, S.: An algorithm for multi-relational discovery of subgroups. In: Komorowski, J., Żytkow, J.M. (eds.) PKDD 1997. LNCS, vol. 1263, pp. 78–87. Springer, Heidelberg (1997)

Applying Migrating Birds Optimization
to Credit Card Fraud Detection

Ekrem Duman[1,*] and Ilker Elikucuk[2]

[1] Özyeğin University, Faculty of Engineering, Industrial Engineering Department,
Istanbul, Turkey
ekrem.duman@ozyegin.edu.tr
[2] Intertech, Decision Support Systems Department, Istanbul Turkey
Ilker.elikucuk@intertech.com.tr

Abstract. We discuss how the Migrating Birds Optimization algorithm (MBO) is applied to statistical credit card fraud detection problem. MBO is a recently proposed metaheuristic algorithm which is inspired by the V flight formation of the migrating birds and it was shown to perform very well in solving a combinatorial optimization problem, namely the quadratic assignment problem. As analyzed in this study, it has a very good performance in the fraud detection problem also when compared to classical data mining and genetic algorithms. Its performance is further increased by the help of some modified neighborhood definitions and benefit mechanisms.

Keywords: migrating birds optimization algorithm, fraud, credit cards, genetic algorithms.

1   Introduction

Migrating birds optimization algorithm (MBO) is one of the newest nature inspired metaheuristic algorithms. In a recent study it has been applied successfully to the quadratic assignment problem [1]. Basically it gets use of the benefit mechanism between the migrating birds which fly in a V formation where birds at the back saves energy by the help of the air turbulence caused by birds flying in front. In this study, we apply the MBO to a different problem, namely the credit card fraud detection problem.

When a card is copied or stolen, the transactions made by them are labeled as fraudulent. These fraudulent transactions should be prevented or detected in a timely manner otherwise the resulting losses can be huge. Banks typically use two layers of fraud prevention/detection systems; rule based layer and statistical analysis layer. Here we are concerned with the statistical layer only where an incoming transaction is compared to card usage behavior of the card holder and if there is a considerable deviation, a high suspicion score is returned.

---

* Corresponding author.

J. Li et al. (Eds.): PAKDD 2013 Workshops, LNAI 7867, pp. 416–427, 2013.

Statistical fraud detection is not an easy problem at all due to several reasons. First, fraud data sets are extremely skewed; out of 100.000 transactions only a few turn out to be fraud. Secondly, the techniques used by fraudsters change in time gradually [2-4]. Thus, a model developed now may not be effective enough in future. In addition to these the idea exchanges between the banks are very limited because of the privacy issues; no one wants other banks know how many frauds they were faced with and no bank shares details of their solution if they think they have a good one. In this regard, our study differentiates from many in literature and although we will not be able to share all details, we will be talking about a fraud detection solution developed using real data and implemented in real life.

Due to its importance it is possible to find a lot of studies on fraud detection in literature. The most commonly used fraud detection methods are rule-induction techniques, decision trees, neural networks, Support Vector Machines (SVM), logistic regression, and meta-heuristics such as genetic algorithms [5-12]. These techniques can be used alone or in collaboration using ensemble or meta-learning techniques to build classifiers. Quah and Sriganesh [13], suggest a framework which can be applied real time where first an outlier analysis is made separately for each customer using self organizing maps and then a predictive algorithm is utilized to classify the abnormal looking transactions. Panigrahi et al. [14] suggest a four component fraud detection solution which is connected in a serial manner. The main idea is first to determine a set of suspicious transactions and then run a Bayesian learning algorithm on this list to predict the frauds. Sanchez et al. [15] presented a different approach and used association rule mining to define the patterns for normal card usage and indicating the ones not fitting to these patterns as suspicious. The study of Bolton and Hand [2] provides a very good summary of literature on fraud detection problems.

In most of the studies listed above the classical accuracy based model performance measures are used. Among these the accuracy ratio, the capture rate, the hit rate, the gini index and the lift are the most popular ones [16-17]. However, since the fraudsters use all available limit on the card they captured, an algorithm which is more successful in detecting the cards with higher available limits is more prominent. In this case the cost of making a false positive error and a false negative error will not be the same and actually false negative error (labeling a fraudulent transaction as legitimate) will be a variable. We will take this cost function here similar to few studies in literature [18-19]. A rather more detailed review of these two studies will be given in the next section.

The contributions of this study to the literature are three fold. First, we are talking on models built with real data and implemented in real life. Second, the new metaheuristic MBO is used to solve a credit card detection problem for the first time and this will be one of the very few studies where any member of the metaheuristic algorithms family is used. Third, the performance of MBO is improved further through the use of some modified neighborhood functions.

The rest of the paper is organized as follows. In the next section, the fraud detection problem we were faced is described in detail together with the explanation of closely related previous work. In the third section we describe the MBO algorithm as it is used to solve the quadratic assignment problem in [1]. Implementation of MBO on the credit card fraud detection problem and the modifications made on it to improve its performance are detailed in section four. The paper is finalized in section five by giving a summary of the study and the major conclusions.

2   Problem Definition and Previous Work

There has been a growing amount of financial losses due to credit card frauds as the usage of the credit cards become more and more common. As such, many papers reported huge amounts of losses in different countries [2, 20].

Credit card frauds can be made in many ways such as simple theft, application fraud, counterfeit cards, never received issue (NRI) and online fraud (where the card holder is not present). In online fraud, the transaction is made remotely and only the card's details are needed. A manual signature, a PIN or a card imprint are not required at the time of purchase. Though prevention mechanisms like CHIP&PIN decrease the fraudulent activities through simple theft, counterfeit cards and NRI; online frauds (internet and mail order frauds) are still increasing in both amount and number of transactions. According to Visa reports about European countries, approximately 50% of the whole credit card fraud losses in 2008 are due to online frauds [21].

When the fraudsters obtain a card, they usually use (spend) all of its available (unused) limit. According to the statistics, they do this in four - five transactions, on the average [18]. Thus, for the fraud detection problem, although the typical prediction modeling performance measures are quite relevant, as indicated by the bank authorities, a performance criterion, measuring the loss that can be saved on the cards whose transactions are identified as fraud is more prominent. In other words, detecting a fraud on a card having a larger available limit is more valuable than detecting a fraud on a card having a smaller available limit.

As a result, what we are faced with is a classification problem with variable misclassification costs. Each false negative has a different misclassification cost and the performance of the model should be evaluated over the total amount of saved available usable limits instead of the total number of frauds detected.

If we define;

TP = the number of correctly classified alerts
TN = the number of correctly classified legitimates
FP = the number of false alerts
FN = the number of transactions classified as legitimate but are in fact fraudulent
c = the cost of monitoring an alert
TFL = the total amount of losses due to fraudulent transactions
S = savings in TFL with the use of fraud detection system
ρ = savings ratio

Then,

TFL = sum of the available limits of the cards whose transactions are labeled as TP or FN c = cost of monitoring including staff wages, SMSs, phone calls. On the average, it is a small figure (less than a dollar)

S = (available limits of the cards of TP transactions) - c(FP+TP)

ρ = S/TFL

where the maximum value S can take is TFL and ρ can take is 1. A good predictor will be the one having a high ρ.

Duman and Ozcelik [18] tackled the same problem for another bank in Turkey. After putting the problem in the same way and pointing out the classical DM algorithms may not perform well for the objective of maximizing savings ratio they implemented a metaheuristic approach which is a hybrid of genetic algorithms and scatter search (the GASS algorithm). In GASS, the number of parent solutions was taken as 50 and child solutions were generated by the recombination operator. Each parent is recombined by every other parent so that the number of children was 1225 in each generation. One of the child solutions is selected randomly and one of its genes is mutated. As the fitness function the savings ratio is used. In the selection process, besides the fittest members which are determined by roulette selection, the most diverse solutions are also inherited to the next generation in [18]. GASS improved the savings ratio by more than 200% with a cost of 35% increase in the number of alerts. However, it had some limitations in that the authors were allowed to improve the score generated by some groups of variables only and the variables about MCCs (merchant categegory codes) and out of country expenditures were left out of the scope of the study. The problem was that a second score was being generated with these left out variables and the authors had no control on how these two scores were interfering.

The study of Duman and Sahin [19] gives a summary of previous results obtained in another bank where this study is carried out also. The results obtained by classical decision trees (C5.0, CART, CHAID), artificial neural networks, SVM, logistic regression and GASS are compared. The results obtained by a special cost sensitive decision tree where in splitting a node the savings ratios of the resulting leaf nodes are considered, is also given. It was shown that the GASS and the newly proposed cost sensitive decision trees were the two best performing methods.

The studies [22-24] are other studies that tackles with cost sensitive decision trees in literature.

3   The MBO Algorithm

Birds spend energy for two purposes while they are flying: to stay in the air (induced power) and to move forward (profile power). The induced power requirement can be less if more than one bird fly together. As such, while a bird moves through the air, air goes above and below the wings. The air flow over the upper surface has to move farther than the lower part of the wing (because upper part has a larger surface) and this causes the air on the upper part has a lower pressure than the air moving over the lower part (Figure 1). This pressure difference makes the lifting possible by the wing.

The regions of upwash may contribute to the lift of a following bird, thus reducing its requirement for induced power [25]. This explains why birds, especially the migrating birds which have to fly long distances fly together in specific formations.

The V formation is the most famous formation that the migrating birds use to fly long distances. As can be noticed easily, birds align themselves to upwash regions in this formation.

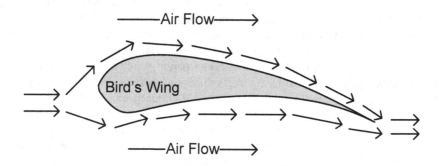

Fig. 1. Wing of a bird (taken from Duman et al. [1])

The pioneering study which brings a mathematical explanation to the energy saving in V formation is that of Lissaman and Schollenberger [25]. In that study, it was stated that as birds approach each other (a smaller WTS = wing tip spacing) and as the number of birds increase more energy will be saved. So that, a group of 25 birds for example would have approximately 71 per cent more flight range than a single bird. These results were obtained from aerodynamics theory where birds at the sizes of a plane were assumed. Also, for the WTS only positive values were assumed (i.e the case of overlapping were not considered).

Later it was shown that some overlap is useful [26]:

$$WTS_{opt} = -0.05b \tag{1}$$

Where, b is the wing span.

The solution algorithm MBO which is inspired by the V flight formation is explained below.

The MBO algorithm is a neighborhood search technique. It starts with a number of initial solutions corresponding to birds in a V formation. Starting with the first solution (corresponding to the leader bird), and progressing on the lines towards the tails, each solution is tried to be improved by its neighbor solutions (for the implementation of QAP (quadratic assignment problem), a neighbor solution is obtained by pairwise exchange of any two locations). If the best neighbor solution brings an improvement, the current solution is replaced by that one. There is also a benefit mechanism for the solutions (birds) from the solutions in front of them. Here we define this benefit mechanism as sharing the best unused neighbors with the solutions that follow (here "unused" means a neighbor solution which is not used to replace the existing solution). In other words, a solution evaluates a number of its own neighbors and a number of best neighbors of the previous solution and considered to be replaced by the best of them. Once all solutions are improved (or tried to be improved) by neighbor solutions, this procedure is repeated a number of times (tours) after which the first solution becomes the last, and one of the second solutions becomes first and another loop starts. The algorithm is stopped after a specified number of iterations.

Below, first the notation used and then the pseudocode of the MBO algorithm are given. Let,

n = the number of initial solutions (birds)
k = the number of neighbor solutions to be considered
x = the number of neighbor solutions to be shared with the next solution
m = number of tours
K = iteration limit

Pseudocode of MBO:

1. Generate n initial solutions in a random manner and place them on an hypothetical V formation arbitrarily.
2. $i=0$
3. while($i<K$)
4.   for ($j=0;j<m;j++$)
5.   Try to improve the leading solution by generating and evaluating k neighbors   of it.
6. $i=i+k$
7.   for each solution s_r in the flock (except leader)
8.   Try to improve s_r by evaluating $(k-x)$ neighbors of it and x unused best   neighbors from the solution in the front.
9. $i=i+(k-x)$
10.   endfor
11.   endfor
12. Move the leader solution to the end and forward one of the solutions following it to the leader position.
13. endwhile
14. return the best solution in the flock

As should already be noticed, the MBO algorithm has great similarities with the migrating birds' story. First it treats the solutions as birds aligned on a V formation. The number of neighbors generated (k) can be interpreted as the induced power required which is inversely proportional to the speed (recall the discussion above). With a larger k we would assume that birds are flying at a low speed where we can also make the analogy that while traveling at a low speed, one can explore the surrounding in more detail. The benefit mechanism between the birds is respected and by generating fewer neighbors for the solutions at the back, it was made possible that they get tired less and save energy by using the neighbors of the solutions in the front. The parameter x is seen as the WTS where an optimum value can be sought for. Its optimum value could be interpreted as the optimum overlap amount of the wingtips. In line 4, the parameter m can be regarded as the number of wing flaps or the profile power needed where we can assume that, as each bird travels the same distance, they all spend the same profiling energy. In line 12, similar to the real birds' story, the bird who spent the most energy and thus got tired moves back to get some rest and another bird fills its position.

For the MBO to perform better, it is necessary to determine the best values of some parameters. These are the number of birds to have in the flock (n), the speed of the flight (k), the WTS (x) and the number of wing flaps before a change in the order of the birds or the profiling energy spent (m). Similar to birds' story, one could expect some certain values of these parameters and their combinations might increase the performance of the algorithm. For the printed circuit board assembly originated quadratic assignment problem the best parameter values were obtained to be n = 51, m = 10, k = 11 and x = 1 in [1].

The philosophy of the MBO is that, by starting with a number of solutions, it is aimed to explore more areas of the feasible solution space. The exploration is made possible by looking at the neighbor solutions. Each time one of the solutions (the one in the front) is explored in more detail. When one of the solutions fails to improve itself by its own neighbors and if the solution in the front is more promising, it is replaced by one of the neighbors of the solution in the front. This way the neighborhood around the more promising solution will be explored in a greater detail (by the combined forces of two birds or solutions). Still after a few iterations these solutions may go to different directions as long as they find improvements along their ways. However, after some time we might expect most of the solutions converge to one or several neighborhoods where local optima or even the global optimum are contained. The convergence can be faster with larger values of x but in that case the termination could take place before the feasible region is thoroughly explored and thus the results obtained might not be good.

4   Results and Discussion

In the following subsections first the details of the experimental setting are given. Then, the results obtained by standard MBO and GASS are displayed together with their parameter fine tuning experiments. This is followed by some improvement attempts on MBO by employing different neighborhood functions.

4.1   Details of Experimental Setting

The original data of the time period used to form the training set have about 22 million transactions. The distribution of this data with respect to being normal or fraudulent is highly skewed so that only 978 transactions were fraudulent in this set. So, to enable the models to learn both types of profiles, some under sampling or oversampling techniques should be used. Instead of oversampling the fraudulent records by making multiple copies of them, we use stratified sampling to under sample the legitimate records to a meaningful number. Firstly, we identify the variables which show the most different distributions w.r.t. being fraudulent or normal. Then, we use these variables as the key variables in stratified sampling so that the characteristics of their distributions w.r.t. being fraudulent or not remains the same. For stratified sampling, we use those five variables which show the most different distributions to form a stratified sample with a ratio of nine legitimate transactions to one fraudulent transaction.

4.2   Results Obtained by MBO

The total number of variables in the data mart were 139 (all binary). Starting with the full set of variables, a variable reduction is made first. Each time the variables having coefficients close to zero (in the trained model) are eliminated and a new model is generated. This resulted in 15 variables where the coefficients of the variables were significantly different than zero. During these runs the MBO parameter values are used same as the best set obtained in [1].

Then a set of parameter fine tuning experiments are made on MBO where the findings are summarized in table 1 below. The number of runs made by each parameter set is 10. The average, minimum and maximum values obtained in these 10 runs are given in the appropriate columns.

According to this analysis the best set of parameters is determined to be:

Number of Birds:	15
Number of Neighbors :	7
Number of Flaps:	3
Number of Overlaps:	2

The parameter values of the GASS algorithm implemented here are determined in accordance with the study [18], namely:

Number of variables (genes): 15
Number of initial solutions: 15
Maximum number of tested solutions: 15000
Mutation procedure: One of the 15 genes is selected randomly and a uniform number between 0 and 1 ($U(0,1)$) is added to its value. If the result is greater than the upper bound (1.0), the final value is obtained by subtracting the upper bound from the new value.
Mutation rate: 8% of the intermediate solutions are selected for mutation.
Selection procedure: Roulette wheel

The results obtained by GASS and MBO are compared in Table 2 where we can see that MBO slightly outperforms GASS. In the Table TPR stands for true positives rate.

Table 1. MBO parameter fine tuning experiments

PARAMETER	SAVED LIMIT %				TRUE POSITIVES RATE		
NUMBER_OF_BIRDS	Average	Maximum	Minimum		Average	Maximum	Minimum
15	92.54	95.19	87.14		84.79	92.15	77.07
25	92.28	95.34	86.43		84.27	92.15	74.79
51	91.58	95.75	84.9		82.73	91.94	69.01
101	90.54	94.96	84.02		81.09	91.94	70.66
NUMBER_OF_NEIGHBOURS	Average	Maximum	Minimum		Average	Maximum	Minimum
3	91.69	95.19	84.9		83.09	92.15	70.66
7	92.11	95.19	84.63		83.96	92.15	72.73
11	91.73	95.34	84.93		82.96	92.15	74.79
15	91.4	95.75	84.02		82.81	92.15	69.01
NUMBER_OF_FLAPS	Average	Maximum	Minimum		Average	Maximum	Minimum
3	91.72	95.75	84.02		83.81	92.15	69.01
5	91.58	95.19	84.63		82.59	92.15	74.17
10	91.91	95.34	84.08		83.26	92.15	73.35
NUMBER_OF_OVERLAPS	Average	Maximum	Minimum		Average	Maximum	Minimum
0	91.09	95.19	84.02		81.87	92.15	69.01
1	91.82	95.19	84.63		83.5	92.15	74.17
2	92.11	95.75	85.66		83.77	92.15	75.83
3	92.11	95.34	85.83		84.09	92.15	75.21

Although we observe some slight improvements we cannot say it is statistically significant based on a t-test with alpha 5 per cent.

4.3   Modifications on MBO

The neighborhood function used in the standard MBO (above results) was making a mutation on a randomly selected variable coefficient. Specifically, one of the 15 coefficients is selected randomly and $U(0,1)$ is added to its value. If the result is greater than the upper bound (1.0), the final value is obtained by subtracting the upper bound from the new value.

Later, we implemented and compared five new neighborhood functions. Let,

A_i is a coefficient in solution A, and B_i is a coefficient of solution B.
A_i and B_i have values within [0,1] range.
r is a random number within (0, 1] range.
N_i is a coefficient of the neighbour solution N.

The following neighbourhood functions (NFx) have been tested on the value of a randomly determined coefficient.

NF1: $N_i = r * A_i + (1 - r) * B_i$
NF2: $N_i = A_i + (A_i - B_i) * (r - 0.5) * 2$
NF3: $N_i = r * (A_i - B_i) + (1 - r) * (A_i + B_i)$
NF4: $N_i = (1 - r) * (A_i - B_i) + r * (A_i + B_i)$
NF5: $N_i = A_i + 0.5$

Table 2. MBO versus GASS

INSTANCE	GASS			MBO	
	SAVED LIMIT %	TPR		SAVED LIMIT %	TPR
1	90,92	79,34		91,37	79,55
2	85,64	77,69		91,68	82,02
3	90,89	78,1		94,13	89,67
4	90,63	77,89		94,91	91,74
5	90,94	79,34		92,28	83,68
6	94,78	91,32		90,63	77,89
7	91,22	79,75		94,67	91,53
8	93,78	89,26		90,1	75,62
9	94,26	91,74		88,5	77,48
10	91,41	79,96		90,69	78,1
AVG	91,45	82,78		91,9	82,73

Table 3. Different neighborhood functions compared

	SAVED LIMIT %			TRUE POSITIVES RATE		
Function	Average	Maximum	Minimum	Average	Maximum	Minimum
NF1	86,13	89,07	83,91	75,35	82,23	72,93
NF2	89,16	91,3	85,62	80,47	91,32	74,59
NF3	**94,2**	95,19	91,46	89,82	92,15	79,96
NF4	91,9	95,22	90,13	82,34	92,36	77,48
NF5	88,9	91,41	86,95	77,85	89,46	72,52

For all functions, if the new value is greater than 1.0, 1.0 is subtracted from it; and if it is less than 0.0, 1.0 is added to it.

The results obtained in 10 runs are given in table 3 where we see that NF3 is significantly better than the others which also brings an improvement to standard MBO. NF3 is a type of neighborhood function used in the original artificial bee colony (ABC) algorithm [28] and its performance can be attributed to its search of a larger neighborhood as compared to other experiments.

5   Summary and Conclusions

In this study we solved the credit card fraud detection problem by the new metaheuristics migrating birds optimization algorithm. This study is one of the few studies where a metaheuristic algorithm is utilized in fraud detection and it performed better than a previous implementation of a combination of genetic algorithms and scatter search. The standard MBO is further improved by testing alternative neighborhood functions.

As future work, alternative benefit mechanisms on MBO could be developed.

References

1. Duman, E., Uysal, M., Alkaya, A.: Migrating Birds Optimization: A new metaheuristic approach and its performance on quadratic assignment problem. Information Sciences 217, 65–77 (2012)
2. Bolton, R.J., Hand, D.J.: Statistical fraud detection: A review. Statistical Science 28(3), 235–255 (2002)
3. Kou, Y., et al.: Survey of fraud detection techniques. In: Proceedings of the 2004 IEEE International Conference on Networking, Sensing and Control, Taipei, Taiwan, March 21-23 (2004)
4. Phua, C., et al.: A comprehensive survey of data mining-based fraud detection research. Artificial Intelligence Review (2005)
5. Sahin, Y., Duman, E.: An overview of business domains where fraud can take place, and a survey of various fraud detection techniques
6. Brause, R., Langsdorf, T., Hepp, M.: Neural data mining for credit card fraud detection. In: Proceedings of the 11th IEEE International Conference on Tools with Artificial Intelligence (1999)
7. Hanagandi, V., Dhar, A., Buescher, K.: Density-Based Clustering and Radial Basis Function Modeling to Generate Credit Card Fraud Scores. In: Proceedings of the IEEE/IAFE 1996 Conference (1996)
8. Juszczak, P., Adams, N.M., Hand, D.J., Whitrow, C., Weston, D.J.: Off-the-peg and bespoke classifiers for fraud detection. Computational Statistics & Data Analysis 52(9) (2008)
9. Quah, J.T., Sriganesh, M.: Real-time credit card fraud detection using computational intelligence. Expert Systems with Applications 35(4) (2008)
10. Shen, A., Tong, R., Deng, Y.: Application of classification models on credit card fraud detection. In: International Conference on Service Systems and Service Management, Chengdu, China (June 2007)
11. Wheeler, R., Aitken, S.: Multiple algorithms for fraud detection. Knowledge-Based Systems 13(2/3) (2000)
12. Chen, R.-C., Chiu, M.-L., Huang, Y.-L., Chen, L.-T.: Detecting credit card fraud by using questionnaire-responded transaction model based on SVMs. In: Yang, Z.R., Yin, H., Everson, R.M. (eds.) IDEAL 2004. LNCS, vol. 3177, pp. 800–806. Springer, Heidelberg (2004)
13. Han, J., Camber, M.: Data mining concepts and techniques. Morgan Kaufman, San Diego (2000)
14. Quah, J.T.S., Srinagesh, M.: Real-time credit fraud detection using computational intelligence. Expert Systems with Applications 35, 1721–1732 (2008)
15. Panigrahi, S., Kundu, A., Sural, S., Majumdar, A.: Credit Card Fraud Detection: A Fusion Approach Using Dempster-Shafer Theory and Bayesian Learning. Information Fusion, 354–363 (2009)
16. Sanchez, D., Vila, M.A., Cerda, L., Serrano, J.M.: Association rules applied to credit card fraud detection. Expert Systems with Applications 36, 3630–3640 (2009)

17. Kim, M., Han, I.: The Discovery of Experts' Decision Rules from Qualitative Bankrupcy Data Using Genetic Algorithms. Expert Systems with Applications 25, 637–646 (2003)
18. Gadi, M.F.A., Wang, X., do Lago, A.P.: Credit Card Fraud Detection with Artificial Immune System. In: Bentley, P.J., Lee, D., Jung, S. (eds.) ICARIS 2008. LNCS, vol. 5132, pp. 119–131. Springer, Heidelberg (2008)
19. Duman, E., Ozcelik, M.H.: Detecting credit card fraud by genetic algorithm and scatter search. Expert Systems with Applications 38, 13057–13063 (2011)
20. Duman, E., Sahin, Y.: A Comparison of Classification Models on Credit Card Fraud Detection with respect to Cost-Based Performance Metrics. In: Duman, E., Atiya, A. (eds.) Use of Risk Analysis in Computer-Aided Persuasion. NATO Science for Peace and Security Series E: Human and Societal Dynamics, vol. 88, pp. 88–99. IOS Press (2011)
21. Gartner Reports, May 10, 2010 from the World Wide Web, http://www.gartner.com
22. Mena, J.: Investigate Data Mining for Security and Criminal Detection. Butterworth-Heinemann, Amsterdam (2003)
23. Ling, C.X., Sheng, V.S., Yang, Q.: Test Strategies for Cost-Sensitive Decision Trees. IEEE Transactions on Knowledge and Data Engineering 18(8) (2006)
24. Liu, X.: A Benefit-Cost Based Method for Cost-Sensitive Decision Trees. In: 2009 WRI Global Congress on Intelligent Systems, pp. 463–467 (2009)
25. Cutts, C.J., Speakman, J.R.: Energy savings in formation flight of pink-footed geese. J. Exp. Biol. 189, 251–261 (1994)
26. Lissaman, P.B.S., Shollenberger, C.A.: Formation flight of birds. Science 168, 1003–1005 (1970)
27. Hummel, D., Beukenberg, M.: Aerodynamsiche Interferenseffekte beim formationsflug von vögeln. J. Orn. 130, 15–24 (1989)
28. Karaboga, D., Basturk, B.: A powerful and efficient algorithm for numerical function optimization: Artificial Bee Colony (ABC) Algorithm. Journal of Global Optimization 39(3), 459–471 (2007)

Clustering in Conjunction with Quantum Genetic Algorithm for Relevant Genes Selection for Cancer Microarray Data

Manju Sardana[1,*], R.K. Agrawal[1], and Baljeet Kaur[2]

[1] School of Computer and Systems Sciences, Jawaharlal Nehru University
New Delhi, India 110067
[2] Hansraj College, Delhi University, Delhi, India 110007
manjusardana12@yahoo.co.in, rkajnu@gmail.com,
baljeetkaur26@hotmail.com

Abstract. Quantum Genetic Algorithm, which utilizes the principle of quantum computing and genetic operators, allows efficient exploration and exploitation of large search space simultaneously. It has been used recently to determine a reduced set of features for cancer microarray data to improve the performance of the learning system. However, the length of the chromosome used is the original dimension of the feature vector. Hence, despite the use of the quantum variant of GA, it requires huge memory and computation time for high dimensional data like microarrays. In this paper, we propose a two phase approach, ClusterQGA, that determines a minimal set of relevant and non-redundant genes. Experimental results on publicly available cancer microarray datasets demonstrate the effectiveness of the proposed approach in comparison to existing methods in terms of classification accuracy and number of features. Also, the proposed approach takes less computation time in comparison to Genetic quantum algorithm proposed by Abderrahim et al.

Keywords: Quantum computation, Genetic algorithm, Microarrays, Feature selection, Clustering.

1 Introduction

Feature selection is important for many classification problems which are characterized with high dimension and small sample size, to avoid the curse of dimensionality and over-fitting. Examples of such applications are classification of web documents, images, microarray cancer data etc. Feature selection aims at finding a small set of relevant features by filtering out irrelevant, redundant and noisy features from the existing set. This improves the performance of the learning system in terms of classification accuracy, computation time and memory space requirement.

In literature, filter, wrapper and hybrid techniques have been suggested for selection of relevant features and applied to many classification problems [1,2]. Filter

---

* Corresponding author.

J. Li et al. (Eds.): PAKDD 2013 Workshops, LNAI 7867, pp. 428–439, 2013.

feature selection uses statistical properties of data at hand to identify a set of discriminative features for classification that is independent of a classifier. The selection is based on high relevance score value assigned to features. Univariate filter approaches such as Relief and its variants [3], cross entropy based feature elimination [4], and multivariate filter approaches namely mRMR [5], FCBF [6] have been proposed for efficient feature selection. Although these filter methods are scalable, the feature subset thus selected may not provide good accuracy with a particular classifier. Wrapper [1] select a set of discriminatory features by maximizing the classification accuracy of the learning algorithm. To mitigate the computational burden of wrapper approach, hybrid approaches [7,8] have been suggested. As the wrapper approach is computationally intensive, its applicability is limited to only low or middle dimensional data. To facilitate the use of wrapper approaches with high dimensional data, it is imperative to confine only to a relevant feature search space. For this, sequential and random search based variants of wrapper methods are suggested.

Sequential search may be forward, backward or bi-directional. Sequential forward search starts with an individual best feature and then works forward to add new features incrementally which improve the performance criteria. On the other hand, sequential backward search starts with whole set of features and repeatedly eliminates features. The bidirectional search is a combination of both. However the feature subset so obtained may not be optimal as a feature once added/eliminated incrementally is never revisited. To overcome this limitation, random search based methods such as Genetic algorithm (GA) have been extensively used. GA has been applied in conjunction with classifiers like K-nearest neighbor (KNN) and support vector machine (SVM) for selecting features [9,10]. GA not only requires huge time and memory to obtain an optimal solution, it may get trapped in local optima. To address these issues, the quantum approach is put in effect in conjunction with GA recently [11,12].

In literature, quantum computing has been suggested as a better alternative to classical computing both in terms of computational and storage requirements. Quantum computing uses Q-bits instead of bits and uses the principles of quantum mechanics such as interference, coherence and standing waves. Q-bit representation characterizes the property of exploration and exploitation simultaneously. Initially, it provides diversity in search space that disappears with convergence to a particular state. Q-bit representation of chromosomes is amalgamated with genetic operators of GA resulting in quantum genetic algorithm (QGA). QGA emulates parallel computation in classical sequential computer. Using Q-bit representation, QGA converges faster than classical GA.

QGA has been successfully employed for feature selection by researchers [12,13,14] in different domains as it allows compact feature space representation and exploration. Abderahhim et al [12] have effectively employed quantum genetic algorithm (GQA$_{SVM}$) on six binary class cancer microarray datasets. However, in their method, the length of chromosome is the dimension of the feature vector used to represent microarray data. Despite the use of the quantum variant of GA, their method requires huge memory and computation time. The fitness function used weighted average of classification accuracy and number of features in ratio of 3:1. This may at times compromise classification accuracy in lieu of reducing the number of features (genes). To handle these issues, this study extends the quantum GA paradigm to achieve better performance in terms of classification accuracy, number of features and computation time.

In this paper, we propose a simple two phase approach: ClusterQGA. In the first phase, clustering of genes is carried out to obtain a non-redundant and relevant set of genes. The second phase uses QGA to determine a minimal set of relevant genes from the genes obtained from the first phase. A fitness function is employed which gives more weight to classification accuracy and to fewer genes in case of comparable accuracy. To check the efficacy of the proposed method, experiments are carried out on both binary and multi-class publicly available cancer microarray datasets. Also, experiments have been conducted to compare the running time of GQA_{SVM} and ClusterQGA.

The outline of the paper is as follows. In section 2, a brief discussion of quantum genetic algorithm is included. Section 3 presents the proposed approach, ClusterQGA. Experimental setup and results are included in Section 4. Section 5 offers conclusions and future directions.

2   Quantum Genetic Algorithm

QGA is hybridization of genetic algorithm and quantum computation principle to get the benefit of both. Genetic algorithm uses bio-inspired computing concepts such as inheritance, mutation, selection, and crossover. The algorithm evaluates a population of chromosomes of candidate solutions using fitness function and evolves towards better solutions in subsequent generations. Genetic algorithm has the advantages of both random and parallel search. However, the success of GA depends on the choice of fitness function, mutation rate, population size etc. Moreover GA does not always provide global optimal solution. In addition GA requires more computation time and large memory space for the evaluation, evolution and storage of candidate solutions.

The quantum genetic algorithm is the quantum counterpart of classical genetic algorithm that uses the representations of quantum computing and operators from genetic algorithms with some adaptations. The basic unit of quantum computing representation, Q-bit is introduced below.

2.1   Q-Bit Representation

Quantum computers and algorithms use quantum bits (Q-bits) as basic unit of information. At a particular point in time, a Q-bit can be either in '0' state or '1' state or in a superposition of the two states. The state of a Q-bit is given by:

$$|\Psi\rangle = a|0\rangle + b|1\rangle \tag{1}$$

where $|0\rangle$ and $|1\rangle$ are used to represent '0' state and '1' state respectively; a and b are two complex numbers such that their respective squares represent the probability of finding a Q-bit in 0 state and 1 state.

The values of a and b are chosen in such a way that

$$|a|^2 + |b|^2 = 1 \tag{2}$$

A system of n Q-bits, Q(t) can simultaneously explore and exploit 2^n states, whose convergence will result in a single state, where each Q-bit will collapse to a binary value, w. The ith Q-bit with probability amplitudes $\begin{bmatrix} a_i \\ b_i \end{bmatrix}$ can be binarized using a simple procedure given below:

$$If\ |a_i|^2 < threshold\ then\ w_i \leftarrow 1\ else\ w_i \leftarrow 0 \tag{3}$$

The population of binary chromosomes B(t) so obtained from a population of Q-bit chromosomes Q(t) is evaluated for its fitness.

2.2   Quantum Genetic Operators

All evolutionary operators of GA namely selection, crossover and mutation are applicable in QGA[12] provided they do not violate the normalization condition given in equation (2). Update and Catastrophe operators are briefly introduced here.

The update operation is based on quantum computation theory. It drifts the population towards fitter states. Any quantum gate can be employed for population update, but the rotation gate is most frequently used. The rotation gate is given by

$$U(\theta) = \begin{bmatrix} \cos(\theta) & -\sin(\theta) \\ \sin(\theta) & \cos(\theta) \end{bmatrix} \tag{4}$$

and it is used to update the probability amplitude value of each Q-bit. For the ith Q-bit with probability amplitudes $\begin{bmatrix} a_i \\ b_i \end{bmatrix}$, it first determines rotation angle $\Delta\theta_i$ and the direction of rotation $s_i = s(a_i, b_i)$. The values for this computation are referred through the look-up table[12,13]. It then calculates the updated values $\begin{bmatrix} a_i' \\ b_i' \end{bmatrix}$ using

$$\begin{bmatrix} a_i' \\ b_i' \end{bmatrix} = U(\Delta\theta_i \times s_i) \times \begin{bmatrix} a_i \\ b_i \end{bmatrix} \tag{5}$$

The angle of rotation is critical to the convergence of the solution. A small value is generally preferred to avoid divergence and/or premature convergence [14].

When a certain number of successive generations do not show any improvement in the solution (stall generations), the catastrophe operation overcomes the problem of getting trapped in local optima thereby avoiding premature convergence [13]. This operation reserves a fraction of the current best population and reinitializes the rest of the population. This process propagates the search in different directions hence accelerating the efficiency of the search.

3   Clustering in Conjunction with QGA

QGA is a random search approach and exhibits compact representation based on superposition principle. However, memory and time requirements are huge while dealing with high dimensional data. To mitigate this limitation, one approach is to restrict the input feature space. As in high dimensional microarray data, features are highly redundant, the dimension of the input space should be reduced before exploration through QGA. Therefore instead of passing the whole set of available genes, a comparatively smaller set of non redundant and relevant genes can be selected and passed on to QGA for efficient selection of minimal set of informative features.

A two phase approach [15] is used to determine a reduced input relevant feature set. In the first phase, clustering is used to group similar genes and then a representative gene from each cluster is picked using t-statistics. This set of m representative genes is used in the second phase that involved the sequential forward feature selection framework to find a minimal set. To overcome the limitations of sequential search, we have used QGA in the second phase of our approach to determine the minimal set of features for better performance. In the first phase we have employed hierarchical agglomerative clustering. To simultaneously achieve maximum classification accuracy and minimal set of relevant features, the appropriate objective function needs to be defined. In [12] a fitness function that gives 0.75 weight to classification accuracy and 0.25 weight to number of features has been employed, thus sacrificing accuracy at times, to keep the number of features less, which may not be desirable. In the proposed work, the objective function is defined to give more weight to the classification accuracy, but it also attempts to minimize the number of features in case of comparable classification accuracy. The fitness of an individual binary chromosome z, is evaluated using the following fitness function:

$$f(z) = \text{Acc}(z) + 1 / (S * m * N(z)) \tag{6}$$

where Acc(z) denotes the classification accuracy of chromosome z, S is number of test samples, m is the number of input features and N(z) is the size of selected gene set (number of ones in z) used for classification. The term $1/(S * m * N(z))$ assures that the number of genes is not minimized at the cost of classification accuracy.

The initial quantum population is $Q(t) = \{q_1(t), q_2(t), \dots q_k(t)\}$ of size k, each $q_j(t), j = 1,2, \cdots, k$, consists of probability amplitudes $\begin{bmatrix} a_{ji} \\ b_{ji} \end{bmatrix}, i = 1,2, \cdots, m$, which are randomly generated. Binary population $B(t) = \{x_1(t), x_2(t), \dots, x_k(t)\}$ is extracted from the current quantum population Q(t) using equation (3). This binary population determines which genes among m supplied genes are selected. The fitness of an individual chromosome, $z = x_j(t)$, from the binary population so obtained is evaluated using the fitness function as given in equation (6). For the generation of subsequent populations, we have used roulette selection that probabilistically selects population according to its fitness. Single point crossover and one point Gaussian mutation are employed. The update operation is used to adjust quantum chromosomes towards fitter states. To update the population through rotation gate operation, we have used the lookup table [13]. The outline of the proposed approach is given below:

ClusterQGA Algorithm

Phase I
Set G=initial set of genes
F=∅ // set of selected genes
Cluster the genes using Hierarchical Agglomerative clustering into m clusters.
For each cluster
  Select gene g_i, the representative gene from each cluster using t-statistics.
  F=F ∪ {g_i}
end for
Phase II
t←0
Initialize Q(t) randomly
Consider B(t) based on Q(t) using equation (3)
Evaluate B(t) using fitness function from equation (6)
Store the best solution, y
Repeat
  i)   *t←t+1*
  ii)   *Generate next population using roulette selection, single point crossover and one point Gaussian mutation on current population Q(t).*
          Update population with quantum rotation gate using lookup table.
          Consider binary population B(t) based on Q(t) using equation (3).
  iii)   *Evaluate B(t) using fitness function (equation (6)) and store the best solution.*
  iv)   *If no_of_stall_ generations > threshold // apply catastrophe*
              Reserve a fraction of best population.
              Reinitialize the rest of the population.
Until (termination condition)

4   Experimental Section and Results

To evaluate the performance of the proposed approach, we have used six publicly available cancer microarray datasets which are considered challenging for cancer classification. Among these datasets, four are multiclass and two are binary class. The performance is evaluated in terms of classification accuracy and number of genes. Datasets used in our experiment are briefly described in Table 1. The datasets are preprocessed as in [15,16] and then normalized using z-score before carrying out the experiments. K-Nearest Neighbor (KNN) and Support Vector Machine (SVM) classifiers, which are commonly employed for classification in microarray domain, are used. SVM classifier is based on the LIBSVM library with linear kernel [17]. For CAR dataset, train and test data are separately available. Therefore classification accuracy is reported using test data. For other datasets Leave One Out Cross-Validation (LOOCV) is employed.

For this two stage algorithm, clustering of similar genes is performed in the first stage using Hierarchical Agglomerative Clustering (HAC) with Euclidean distance measure. Each dataset is clustered into a set of 60 clusters. Thereafter genes within each cluster are ranked using t-statistics and the top-most gene from each cluster is selected as a representative of that cluster. Thus a pool of sixty genes is formed, which is then passed on to the second stage of the algorithm.

Table 1. Datasets Used

S. no.	Dataset	Samples	Original genes	Preprocessed genes	Classes
1.	Glioma[18]	50	12625	4434	4
2.	NCI 60[19]	60	9706	2000	9
3.	CNS-v2[20]	40	7129	5548	5
4.	CAR[21]	174	12533	9182	11
5.	CNS-v1[20]	34	7129	2277	2
6.	Colon[22]	62	2000	2000	2

Table 2. Comparison of Cluster sequential forward selection approach and ClusterQGA approach in terms of classification accuracy(number of genes)

Dataset	Classifier	CSFS	ClusterQGA
Glioma	KNN	96(23)	**100(19)**
	SVM	98(5)	100(10)
Nci60	KNN	90(26)	94.82(29)
	SVM	91.67(15)	94.82(16)
CNS_v2	KNN	100(22)	**100(8)**
	SVM	100(7)	100(7)
CAR	KNN	98.65(48)	**100(45)**
	SVM	97.3(21)	100(24)
CNS_v1	KNN	100(14)	**100(4)**
	SVM	100(5)	100(5)
Colon	KNN	96.77(24)	**100(11)**
	SVM	96.77(20)	**100(16)**

In the second phase we use QGA for minimal feature selection. Length of each chromosome equals the size of the input feature set, which is 60 in our case. The population size is fixed to 100 with the elite count value set to 2. In the implementation of ClusterQGA, for the genetic selection operation, roulette selection is applied. Single point crossover, with probability 0.8 and random Gaussian mutation is carried out. For the update operation, rotation angle and sign is referred as per the lookup table The algorithm uses catastrophe in case the number of stall generations exceeds 8 which is the chosen threshold, wherein it reserves 20% of the fitter individuals and initializes rest of the population in random fashion. The best solution in terms of classification accuracy and number of genes over 10 runs is given in Table 2. This table also holds the observations for cluster sequential forward selection (CSFS) approach with hierarchical agglomerative clustering for comparison. Results that show improvements in classification accuracy and decrease in number of genes simultaneously are highlighted. Figure 1 depicts a graphical view of the comparison of classification accuracy and number of genes obtained by Cluster Sequential Forward Selection approach and the proposed ClusterQGA approach.

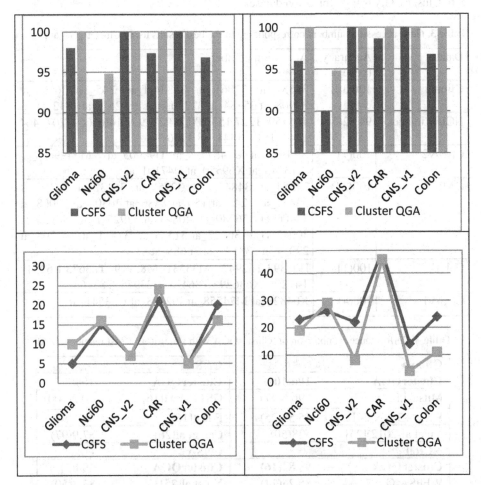

Fig. 1. Variation in terms of classification accuracy with (a) SVM and (b) KNN. Variation in number of genes with (c) SVM and (d) KNN.

Based on observations in Table 2 and Figure 1, it is clear that the proposed method, ClusterQGA shows improvement in classification accuracy of two class as well as multiclass datasets in comparison to CSFS. Both classifiers perform well, but KNN reduces the number of relevant genes in all datasets except in Nci60. Classification accuracy is same or more for all datasets for both KNN and SVM classifiers in comparison to CSFS.

Table 3 gives accession numbers of the genes selected corresponding to our best results. Table 4 makes a comparative assessment of our approach with respect to other well known approaches in literature. The comparison shows that our approach is better in terms of classification accuracy and the number of relevant genes selected. Comparing with the results of Abderrahim et al [12], the number of relevant genes with ClusterQGA is high for colon dataset.

Table 3. Gene accession numbers corresponding to the best results using ClusterQGA approach

Dataset	Accuracy (genes)	Accession numbers
Glioma	100(10)	34531_at 37061_at 32334_f_at 245_at 36996_at 39908_at 35784_at 32750_r_at 36924_r_at 1742_at
NCI60(indices)	94.82(16)	426 59 1227 153 2000 1927 997 1461 660 707 404 1244 1817 1441 88 1986
CNS-v2	100(7)	X14975_at U14577_s_at U90905_at M34996_s_at M13143_at X69550_at U47101_at
CAR	100(24)	33354_at 34845_at 33753_at 36132_at 39107_at 33449_at 245_at 150_at 1386_at 40303_at 38008_at 34406_at 36780_at 40898_at 37925_r_at 40735_at 40042_r_at 36627_at 31573_at 37511_at 41768_at 290_s_at 33179_at 36685_at
Colon	100(11)	H08393 T62947 M35531 M82919 T83673 R62549 T41204 X63629 T86473 H23975 T85165
CNS-v1	100(4)	X04828_at M74558_at J02783_at U63541_at

Table 4. Performance comparison of ClusterQGA with state-of-art (Best results in bold)

Glioma		CAR	
ClusterQGA	**100(10)**	**ClusterQGA**	**100(24)**
Mitsuaki et al[23]	96.6(67)	GS1+SVM[16]	90.2(100)
Relief+3-NN[24]	55.56(25)	F-test[16]	88.5(97)
Yu et al(2012)[25]	78(50)	Cho et al[26]	87.9(97)
NCI60		**CNS-v2**	
ClusterQGA	**94.82(16)**	**ClusterQGA**	**100(7)**
WFFSA-G [27]	85.25(14)	Yu et al[25]	87.8(50)
GA+SVM-RFE[28]	87.93(27)	OVR SVM[25]	85.6(50)
SVM-RFE+KNN[29]	94.89(150)	SVM-RFE+KNN[29]	100(150)
CNS-v1		**Colon**	
ClusterQGA	**100(5)**	**ClusterQGA**	100(11)
SVM-RFE+SVM [24]	75.49(100)	GQA$_{SVM}$ [12]	**100(1)**
TSP[30]	97.1(10)	WFFSA-G[27]	97.9(100)

To assess the computational efficiency in terms of time of our method in comparison to GQA_{SVM}, we have empirically determined average time of 10 runs over the Colon dataset which is shown in Table 5. The proposed method has clearly reduced the running time by one thirds.

Table 5. Comparison of computation time

GQA_{SVM}	ClusterQGA
31804.1 sec	10105.4 sec

5   Conclusion

We have proposed ClusterQGA as a two phase approach to determine minimal set of relevant genes of cancer microarray datasets. The first step determines a set of relevant representative genes using clustering that is further minimized using quantum GA. The fitness function is defined to reduce number of selected genes without compromising the classification accuracy. Experiments are performed on both binary class and multi-class cancer microarray datasets to check the efficacy of the proposed method, ClusterQGA. Experimental results demonstrate effectiveness of the proposed approach ClusterQGA on all the investigated cancer microarray datasets in terms of classification accuracy and number of genes. Also, the proposed approach takes less computation time in comparison to Genetic quantum algorithm proposed by Abderrahim et al [12]. Comparison with existing methods reaffirms the success of the proposed method. The improvement in classification accuracy along with a reduced set of relevant genes is attributed to optimal subset determination of genes by the proposed method in comparison to other feature selection approaches like sequential forward feature selection, sequential backward feature selection or combination of both.

We look forward to explore the proposed approach to determine minimal feature subset selection in other high dimensional datasets. A comparison with other feature selection approaches like sequential backward feature selection or combination of sequential forward and backward feature selection may be looked into to determine its suitability. Other evolutionary methods can be explored in conjunction with varied clustering techniques and classifiers.

References

1. Kohavi, R., John, G.: Wrapper for feature subset selection. Artificial Intelligence 97(1-2), 273–324 (1997)
2. Guyon, I., Elisseff, A.: An Introduction to variable and feature selection. Journal of Machine Learning Research 3, 1157–1182 (2003)
3. Kira, K.: Rendell,L.A.: The feature selection problem: traditional methods and a new algorithm. In: AAAI 1992 Proceedings, pp. 129–134 (1992)
4. Koller, D., Sahami, M.: Towards optimal feature selection. In: Proceedings of 13th International Conference on Machine Learning, Italy. Morgan Kaufmann, CA (1996)

5. Ding, C., Peng, H.C.: Minimum redundancy feature selection from microarray gene expression data. In: Second IEEE Computational Systems Bioinformatics Conf., pp. 523–528 (2003)
6. Yu, L., Liu, H.: Redundancy based feature selection for microarray data. In: International Conference on Knowledge Discovery and Data Mining, Seattle, Washington, pp. 22–25 (2004)
7. Xing, E., Jordan, M., Karp, R.: Feature selection for high-dimensional genomic microarray data. In: Proceedings of the Eighteenth International Conference on Machine Learning, pp. 601–608 (2001)
8. Guyon, I., Weston, J., Barnhill, S., Vapnik, V.: Gene selection for cancer classification using support vector machines. Machine Learning 46(1-3), 389–422 (2002)
9. Yang, J., Honavar, V.: Feature subset selection using a genetic algorithm. IEEE Intelligent Systems (1998)
10. Agrawal, R.K., Bala, R.: A hybrid approach for selection of relevant features for microarray datasets. International Journal of Computer and Information Engineering 1(2) (2007)
11. Han, K.H., Kim, J.H.: Genetic quantum algorithm and its application to combinatorial optimization problem. In: 2000 Congress on Evolutionary Computation, vol. 2, pp. 1354–1360. IEEE Press, Piscataway (2000)
12. Abderrahim, A., Talbi, G., Khaled, M.: Hybridization of genetic and quantum algorithm for gene selection and classification of microarray data. Journal of Foundations of Computer Science 23(2) (2012)
13. Zhang, G., Hu, L.-Z., Jin, W.-D.: Quantum computing based machine learning method and its application in radar emitter signal recognition. In: Torra, V., Narukawa, Y. (eds.) MDAI 2004. LNCS (LNAI), vol. 3131, pp. 92–103. Springer, Heidelberg (2004)
14. Zhang, G., Rong, H.: Parameter Setting of Quantum-Inspired Genetic Algorithm Based on Real Observation. In: Yao, J., Lingras, P., Wu, W.-Z., Szczuka, M.S., Cercone, N.J., Ślęzak, D. (eds.) RSKT 2007. LNCS (LNAI), vol. 4481, pp. 492–499. Springer, Heidelberg (2007)
15. Sardana, M., Agrawal, R.K.: A comparative study of clustering algorithms for relevant gene selection. Advances in Intelligent and Soft Computing 166, 789–797 (2012)
16. Yang, K., Cai, Z., Li, J., Lin, G.H.: A stable gene selection in microarray data analysis. BMC Bioinformatics 7(228) (2006)
17. Chang, C.C., Lin, C.J.: LIBSVM: A library for support vector machines (2002), http://www.csie.ntu.edu.tw/cjlin/libsvm
18. Nutt, C.L., Mani, D.R., Betensky, R.A., Tamayo, P., et al.: Gene expression based classification of malignant gliomas correlates better with survival than histological classification. Cancer Res. 63(7), 1602–1607 (2003)
19. Ross, D.T., Scherf, U., Eisen, M.B., Perou, C.M., Rees, C., Spellman, P., Iyer, V., et al.: Systematic variation in gene expression patterns in human cancer cell lines. Nature Genetics 24, 227–235 (2000)
20. Pomeroy, S.L., Tamayo, P., Gaasenbeek, M., Sturla, L.M., Angelo, M., McLaughlin, M.E., Kim, J.Y.H.: Prediction of central nervous system embryonal tumour outcome based on gene expression. Nature 415, 436–442 (2002)
21. Su, A.I., Welsh, J.B., Sapinoso, L.M., Kern, S.G., Dimitrov, P., Lapp, H., Schultz, P.G., Powell, S.M., Moskaluk, C.A., Frierson, H.F., Hampton, G.M.: Molecular classification of human carcinomas by use of gene expression signatures. Cancer Res. 61(20), 7388–7393 (2001)

22. Alon, U., Barkai, N., Notterman, D.A., Gish, K., Ybarra, S., Mack, D., Levine, A.J.: Broad patterns of gene expression revealed by clustering analysis of tumor and normal colon tissues probed by oligo-nucleotide array. Proc. Nat'l. Academy of Science 9612, 6745–6750 (1999)
23. Mitsuaki, S., Iwao, K.K., Sakai, S.: Gene expression based molecular diagnostic system for malignant gliomas is superior to histological diagnosis. Clinical Cancer Research 13, 7341–7356 (2007)
24. Alonso-Gonzalez, C.J., Moro-Sancho, Q.I., Simon-Hurtado, A.: Varela-Arrabal: Microarray gene expression classification with few genes: criteria to combine attribute selection and classification methods. Expert Systems with Applications 39, 7270–7280 (2012)
25. Yu, H.L., Gao, S., Qin, B., Zhao, J.: Multiclass microarray data classification based on confidence evaluation. Genetics and Molecular Research 11(2), 1357–1369 (2012)
26. Cho, J., Lee, D., Park, J.H., Lee, I.B.: New gene selection for classification of cancer subtype considering within-class variation. FEBS Letters 551, 3–7 (2003)
27. Zu, Z., Ong, Y.S., Dash, M.: Wrapper–Filter feature selection algorithm using a memetic framework. IEEE Transactions on Systems, Man and Cybernatics-Part B: Cybernatics 37(1) (2007)
28. Peng, S., Xu, Q.: Molecular classification of cancer types from microarray data using combination of genetic algorithm and Support Vector machine. Science Direct FEBS Letters 555(2), 358–362 (2003)
29. Li, X., Peng, S., Zhan, X., Zhang, J., Xu, Y.: Comparison of feature selection methods for multiclass cancer classification based on microarray data. In: 4th International Conference on Biomedical Engineering and Informatics (BMEI), vol. 3, pp. 1692–1696 (2011)
30. Tan, A.C., Naiman, D.Q., Xu, L., Winslow, R.L., Geman, D.: Simple decision rules for classifying human cancers from gene-expression profiles. Bioinformatics 21(20), 3896–3904 (2005)

On the Optimality of Subsets of Features Selected by Heuristic and Hyper-heuristic Approaches

Kourosh Neshatian* and Lucianne Varn

Department of Computer Science and Software Engineering
University of Canterbury, Private Bag 4800, Christchurch, New Zealand
kourosh.neshatian@canterbury.ac.nz

Abstract. The concepts of relevance and redundancy are central to feature selection algorithms that do not use a learning algorithm for subset evaluation. Redundancy is in fact a special form of relevance where there is a correlation (linear or nonlinear) between the input features of a problem. Therefore, having a good heuristic for measuring relevance can also help detect redundancy. In this paper, we show that there is a lack of generality in the solutions found by heuristic measures. Through some counter-examples we show that regardless of the type of heuristic measure and search strategy, filter methods cannot optimise the performance of all learning algorithms. We show how different measures may have different notions of relevance between features and how this could lead to not detecting important features in certain problems. We then propose a hyper-heuristic method that generates an appropriate relevance measure for each problem. The new approach can alleviate problems related to missing relevant features.

1 Introduction

Feature selection algorithms have, in abstract terms, two main components. The first component is a search mechanism that searches the space of power sets of features which grow exponentially ($O(2^n)$) with respect to the number of features in problems. The second component is an evaluation mechanism which measures the goodness of (candidate) subsets of features. There are two major approaches for evaluation: *wrapper* and *filter* (or non-wrapper) [9]. In the wrapper approach, the performance of a learning algorithm (e.g. a decision tree inducer) is used to guide the search. The wrapper approach is computationally intensive; every evaluation involves training and testing a model. In the filter approach, instead of using a learner's performance as a measure of the utility of a candidate subset of features, computationally-cheap heuristics are incorporated. The most common measure of utility in the filter approach is *relevance*. Relevance quantifies the degree of relatedness between a subset of features and another feature (that does not exist in the subset). Features with a significant degree of relevance to target

---

* Corresponding author.

J. Li et al. (Eds.): PAKDD 2013 Workshops, LNAI 7867, pp. 440–451, 2013.

concepts (such as class labels) are desired, while features with a considerable degree of relevance to each other are considered *redundant* and thus unwanted. Examples of commonly-used relevance measures are those based on information theory such as *Information Gain* (IG) and *Information Gain Ratio* (IGR) [11], and those based on statistical methods such as χ^2 (Chi-square) ranking [12] and *Logistic Regression* [6].

Filter-based feature selection methods are known to be computationally efficient in comparison with methods taking the wrapper approach. Since filter methods do not use any learning algorithms directly, they are usually described as being "independent of any learning algorithms" [9]. However, it is unclear whether the importance (utility) of features can be determined independently from any learning algorithms. Clearly, filter methods have improved the performance of some learning algorithms over some problems, but a question that remains to be answered is whether "independence from learning algorithms" implies that a highly relevant subset of features found by a filter method is expected to optimise the learning performance of any arbitrary learning algorithm. If the answer is 'no', then what can be done? This paper investigates these issues.

1.1 Problem Statement

Let $\mathcal{D}$ represent the set of all possible observations in a classification domain; for example $\mathcal{D}$ could be the population of patients receiving a medical diagnosis. A feature (attribute) is a mapping from $\mathcal{D}$ to a *co-domain*; for example, *height* and *gender* as features can be mappings of the form $height : \mathcal{D} \mapsto \mathbb{R}^+$ and $gender : \mathcal{D} \mapsto \{male, female\}$. If d is a member of the population (a data item), then $height(d)$ and $gender(d)$ represent the value of the two features for the given data item.

We use $\mathcal{F}$ to represent the set of all features that are available (defined or measurable) for all members of the population. In a supervised learning context $\mathcal{F}$ is partitioned into two sets $\mathcal{X} = \{X_1, X_2, \ldots, X_{|\mathcal{X}|}\}$ and $\mathcal{Y} = \{Y_1, Y_2, \ldots, Y_{|\mathcal{Y}|}\}$ such that $\mathcal{X} \cap \mathcal{Y} = \emptyset$, $\mathcal{X} \cup \mathcal{Y} = \mathcal{F}$ and thus $|\mathcal{X}| + |\mathcal{Y}| = |\mathcal{F}|$. $\mathcal{X}$ is known as the set of input features (*explanatory* variables), and $\mathcal{Y}$ is known as the set of concept or output features (*response* variables). For each data item $d \in \mathcal{D}$, $X_i(d)$ represent the value of the i-th feature. $|\mathcal{X}|$ shows the dimensionality of the problem (the number of features in the input space).

A subset of features $\mathcal{S} \subseteq \mathcal{X}$ is considered "good" if it is *relevant* to a response variable and has least *redundancy*. The first formal (mathematical) definition of relevance is almost a century old [8] and there has been several refinements to the definition since then [5,7]. Relevance is defined in terms of dependency using the concepts of *joint* and *conditional* probability distributions: a subset of features $\mathcal{S}$ is relevant to a response variable Y (on the basis of a prior evidence that is usually dropped for the sake of simplicity without loss of generality) if and only if

$$P\{Y(d) = y | \mathcal{S}(d)\} \neq P\{Y(d) = y\} \quad \forall d \in \mathcal{D} . \tag{1}$$

While this definition gives a good logical foundation for relevance, in practice, it cannot be *directly* used to find relevant features because:

1. We often need to measure (quantify) relevance on a scale such that we can compare subsets of features to each other and select ones that are more relevant. A logical definition (that takes values 'true' or 'false') is not adequate for this purpose.
2. In most problems (almost all real-world problems), it is infeasible to estimate the joint distribution of all variables as the training data required to do this is of exponential order. This problem is known as the curse of dimensionality.

In the remainder of this paper we first formalise the two current research directions in measuring relevance and discuss their advantages and disadvantages. We then use the developed formalism to prove that heuristic relevance measures (including many commonly-used measures) can misjudge the importance of features particularly by seeing relevant features as irrelevant. We then introduce a hyper-heuristic approach to measure relevance and illustrate how it can alleviate the current limitations.

2   Wrapping Learning Algorithms to Measure Relevance

The goal of learning is to find a model that predicts the value of features in $\mathcal{Y}$ based on the value of features in $\mathcal{X}$. Since in most regression and classification tasks there is only one response variable in $\mathcal{Y}$, without loss of generality we assume that $\mathcal{Y} = \{Y\}$. Using $\mathcal{C} = \{c_1, c_2, \dots c_{|\mathcal{C}|}\}$ as the set of target concepts (e.g. class labels) in the problem; Y represents the actual value of the target concept (e.g class label) for each observation: $Y : \mathcal{D} \mapsto \mathcal{C}$. Let $\mathcal{H}$ be a hypothesis space (e.g. the space of all possible decision trees for a classification problem). Then each hypothesis $h \in \mathcal{H}$ is a mapping from the population into the space of target classes (concepts), i.e. $h : \mathcal{D} \mapsto \mathcal{C}$.

A learning algorithm L (e.g. a decision tree inducer) is a function that takes three arguments and returns a hypothesis:

$$h = L(\mathcal{D}_{train}, \mathcal{S}, Y) , \qquad \mathcal{S} \subseteq \mathcal{X} , \ \mathcal{D}_{train} \subseteq \mathcal{D} . \qquad (2)$$

The arguments are a training data set $\mathcal{D}_{train}$ which is a sample from $\mathcal{D}$, a subset of features $\mathcal{S}$ which determines which input features are available to the learner, and the true (actual) output mapping Y. The algorithm induces and returns a hypothesis $h \in \mathcal{H}$ (e.g. a classifier). Deterministic learning algorithms—those that do not have any stochastic components—will always produce the same hypothesis, given the same three input arguments. On the other hand, learning algorithms with stochastic components such as Artificial Neural Networks (with random initial weights) and Genetic Programming (with random initial population and stochastic operators) may generate different hypotheses for even a fixed set of input arguments[1].

---

[1] These algorithms can become deterministic by introducing a fourth argument (known as random seed) that specifies the state (or an index to the state) of the random number generator used by the algorithm.

The quality (performance) of a hypothesis h is usually determined based on how closely it mimics Y and is quantified by a cost (error) function. The cost function is typically the approximation error in regression tasks and the misclassification cost in classification tasks. The cost function may also include a term for the length of the model (the model complexity or the number of bits required to encode the model) in order to penalise large and uninterpretable models. We use $e(h, \mathcal{D}', Y)$ to indicate the error (cost) of h for a given data set $\mathcal{D}'$ (a sample from $\mathcal{D}$). The expected error over $\mathcal{D}'$ is

$$E_{\mathcal{D}'}[e(h, \mathcal{D}', Y)|h] \ . \tag{3}$$

where h in equation (3) comes from equation (2).

From a wrapper point of view, the most relevant subset of features is the one that when passed to L yields the hypothesis with the lowest cost (in feature selection, we are, in addition to low costs, also interested in small subsets). In other words, the most relevant subset can be obtained by optimising the cost over the power set of features, denoted by $2^{\mathcal{X}}$.

Regardless of the search strategy (to navigate in the search space) that is used for optimisation , once a candidate solution has been selected, it must be evaluated. A candidate $\mathcal{S}$ can be directly evaluated by inserting it in equation (2) and then calculating the error of the resulting hypothesis:

$$Error_{(L,\mathcal{D}',\mathcal{S})} \ = \ E_{\mathcal{D}'}[e(L(\mathcal{D}', \mathcal{S}, Y), \mathcal{D}', Y)|\mathcal{S}] \ . \tag{4}$$

The error can then be used as a measure of the utility of $\mathcal{S}$. This is in fact a wrapper approach as L is directly used to find the worth of a candidate subset. The best subset of features is

$$\mathcal{S}^{\star} = \underset{\mathcal{S} \subseteq \mathcal{X}}{\arg\min}(Error_{(L,\mathcal{D}',\mathcal{S})}) \ . \tag{5}$$

The biggest issue in finding $\mathcal{S}^{\star}$ using the above equation is the computational cost associated with it. Using (4) to measure the utility of a candidate subset involves computing L; that is, inducing a new hypothesis and then estimating the cost of the resulting hypothesis which is computationally expensive. This is a motivation to use heuristic measures.

3   Heuristic Measures

Heuristic relevance measures are relatively simple and cheap-to-compute functions that do not depend on any learning algorithms. They allow for more thorough search strategies and bigger problems. Perhaps the most common heuristic measures are those based on *mutual information* [2,14].

Let $r(\mathcal{S}, Y, \mathcal{D}')$ denote the relevance between a subset of features $\mathcal{S}$ and a response variable Y over a data set $\mathcal{D}'$. Here, finding the most relevant subset reduces to maximising r:

$$\mathcal{S}_r^{\star} = \underset{\mathcal{S} \subseteq \mathcal{X}}{\arg\max}(r(\mathcal{S}, Y, \mathcal{D}')) \ . \tag{6}$$

In the context of feature selection, r may be combined with some other terms to penalise *redundancy*.

While heuristic measures enjoy computational efficiency, the fact that they quantify relevance independent of any learning algorithm raises a question concerning their generality: Given a relevance measure r, can $\mathcal{S}_r^\star$ maximise the performance of any arbitrarily chosen learning algorithm? The answer to this question can have important practical implications. In many data mining scenarios, selection of relevant features is considered a preprocessing step and is done without any particular learning algorithm in mind. If the answer to the question is 'no', then one needs to choose r based upon anticipated choices of learning algorithms. The next section answers this question.

4   The Lack of Generality in Wrapper and Heuristic Measures

This section shows, through some counter-examples, that for some classification problems, $\mathcal{S}_r^\star$ *cannot* optimise the learning performance of all algorithms. It also shows that for two arbitrary learning algorithms L and L', $\mathcal{S}_L^\star$ is not necessarily the same as $\mathcal{S}_{L'}^\star$.

Assume that there are enough computational resources available to find $\mathcal{S}_r^\star$ for a given classification/regression problem; this can be achieved by evaluating r on all subsets of features in $2^{\mathcal{X}}$; that is, performing an *exhaustive* search. Let $L_1, L_2,$ ... be learning algorithms applied to the same classification/regression problem. According to equation (5), the best subsets of features for these algorithms are $\mathcal{S}_{L_1}^\star$, $\mathcal{S}_{L_2}^\star$, and so forth. If $\mathcal{S}_r^\star$ could maximise the performance of all learning algorithms then we must have

$$\mathcal{S}_r^\star = \mathcal{S}_{L_1}^\star = \mathcal{S}_{L_2}^\star = \ldots . \tag{7}$$

To show that for some problems equation (7) does not hold, we show that for some problems at least one $\mathcal{S}_{L_i}^\star$, $i = 1, 2, \ldots$, differs from the others. In other words, we present examples where different learning algorithms have different optimal subsets and thus no unique solution can maximise their performance.

Two benchmark data sets from UCI machine learning repository [1] have been chosen for the examples. The two data sets are: **i)** Liver Disorders with 6 input (explanatory) features, 345 instances and 2 classes, and **ii)** Thyroid Disease with 5 input features, 215 instances and 3 classes. We have chosen relatively low-dimensional data sets so that we can use a brute-force search to find counter-examples. A number of classifiers—from different categories of learning algorithms—are applied to the data sets; they are enumerated in Table 1. All the algorithms are implemented in the Weka framework.

To find $\mathcal{S}^\star$ for each classifier and data set, an exhaustive (brute-force) search is conducted over $2^{\mathcal{X}}$—that is, the error of the classification is evaluated for all subsets of features. A common measure of error for classification is the misclassification ratio:

$$e(h, \mathcal{D}', Y) = \frac{\sum_{d \in \mathcal{D}'} \mathbf{1}_{\{h(d) \neq Y(d)\}}(d)}{|\mathcal{D}'|} . \tag{8}$$

Table 1. Learning (classification) algorithms used in the experiments

Category	Learning Algorithm (L)
Artificial Neural Networks	Multi-Layer Perceptrons (MLPs) with $\frac{\#features+\#classes}{2}$ sigmoid node in the middle (hidden) layer.
Support Vector Machines	LibSVM with Radial Basis kernels
Decision Trees	J48 implementation of C4.5 with pruning
Instance-based Learning	k-Nearest Neighbourhood with Euclidean distance measure
Probabilistic	Naive Bayes
Other	Logistic Regression

To estimate the expected value in equation (4), a sample data set D' is divided into 10 stratified folds $D'_1, D'_2, \ldots D'_{10}$ and then the average of equation (8) is calculated via 10-fold cross-validation:

$$\hat{Error}_{(L,\mathcal{D}',\mathcal{S})} =$$

$$\frac{1}{10} \sum_{i=1}^{10} e(L(\bigcup_{j\in\{1,2,\ldots 10\}:j\neq i} D'_j, \mathcal{S}, Y), D'_i, Y) .$$

The search results for the two data sets are presented in Tables 2 and 3. For each classification algorithm the best subset ($\mathcal{S}^\star$) and the second best subset ($\mathcal{S}''$)—the subset of features that yields the lowest error after the best subset—are reported. The corresponding estimated error for each subset of features is also reported. The tables show that in both problems, for most cases, the best subset of features for a given classifier differs from the best subset of features of the other classifiers.

Table 2. Liver Disorders Data set

Classifier	Best Subset			Second Best Subset		
	$\mathcal{S}^\star$	$|\mathcal{S}^\star|$	$Error$	$\mathcal{S}''$	$|\mathcal{S}''|$	$Error$
Decision Tree (J48)	$\{f_1, f_2, f_3, f_5, f_6\}$	5	0.307	$\{f_1, f_3, f_5, f_6\}$	4	0.316
Simple Logistic Regression	$\{f_1, f_3, f_4, f_5, f_6\}$	5	0.303	$\{f_1, f_3, f_4, f_5\}$	4	0.309
MLP	$\{f_1, f_3, f_4, f_5, f_6\}$	5	0.275	$\{f_3, f_4, f_5, f_6\}$	4	0.294
SVM	$\{f_3, f_4, f_5\}$	3	0.348	$\{f_2, f_3, f_4, f_5, f_6\}$	5	0.419
kNN	$\{f_1, f_3, f_4, f_5, f_6\}$	5	0.346	$\{f_2, f_3, f_4, f_5\}$	4	0.351
Naive Bayes	$\{f_3, f_5, f_6\}$	3	0.378	$\{f_1, f_3, f_6\}$	3	0.390

Based on Table 2 and Table 3, one can conclude that equation (7) does not hold for the two benchmark data sets and the presented classifiers. This conclusion is supported by the fact that in many cases the difference between classification errors is quite considerable and the best subset of features for a classifier is not even the second best for other classifiers. These observations serve as counter-examples and imply that no matter what relevance measure r is used,

Table 3. Thyroid Disease Data Set

Classifier	Best Subset			Second Best Subset		
	$\mathcal{S}^{\star}$	$|\mathcal{S}^{\star}|$	$Error$	$\mathcal{S}''$	$|\mathcal{S}''|$	$Error$
Decision Tree (J48)	$\{f_2, f_3\}$	2	0.061	$\{f_1, f_2\}$	2	0.072
Simple Logistic Regression	$\{f_2, f_3, f_5\}$	3	0.023	$\{f_2, f_5\}$	2	0.041
MLP	$\{f_2, f_3, f_5\}$	3	0.031	$\{f_2, f_3, f_4\}$	3	0.046
SVM	$\{f_1, f_2, f_3, f_4, f_5\}$	5	0.102	$\{f_1, f_2, f_3, f_5\}$	4	0.109
kNN	$\{f_1, f_2, f_3, f_5\}$	4	0.023	$\{f_1, f_2, f_5\}$	3	0.033
Naive Bayes	$\{f_1, f_2, f_5\}$	3	0.023	$\{f_2, f_5\}$	2	0.024

even the optimal solution $\mathcal{S}_r^{\star}$ cannot necessarily maximise the performance of all learning algorithms. This is in a way analogous to the no free lunch theorem [16]. While the original theorem is on the lack of difference over all permutations of a data scheme, the lack of generality observed in this section is over the set of all learning algorithms.

5   A Hyper-heuristic Relevance Measure

The lack of generality in heuristic measures is a two-fold problem: i) a subset of features that is highly relevant according to a relevance measure might not be useful to some classifiers; ii) a subset of features that is relevant to a classifier may not be detected as relevant by some relevance measures. The first issue is rather related to a poor choice of learning algorithm which can be solved by better design strategies; for example, by trying out a number of learning algorithms and choosing the best one. The second issue, however, is about failure in measuring relevance or more precisely a bad choice of heuristic measure. Similar to the first issue, one might think that a possible solution would be to try different heuristic measures, but the problem is that only a handful heuristic measures are available. This is where hyper-heuristics come into play.

Hyper-heuristics is a new direction in search and optimisation with very promising results [3,13]. In heuristic search, the space of solutions (for the problem in hand) is searched and the heuristic is used as a guide to move in the space in order to find better solutions. Heuristic search is subject to the no free lunch theorem; there is no single heuristic that would work for all problems. In Hyper-heuristic search, the space of possible heuristics is searched and the algorithm tries to find the right heuristic for the problem in hand. The promising news is that, there could be a free lunch in Hyper-heuristics [15]; that is, for a class of problems, a hyper-heuristic algorithm can be devised that can find the right heuristic for each instance of problem from that class.

We propose a hyper-heuristic algorithm that uses genetic programming (GP) to generate new heuristics on the fly. In terms of categorisation of hyper-heuristic algorithms, the proposed work is a heuristic generation algorithm [4].

For a binary classification problem with a (nominal) binary class variable $C \in \{c^+, c^-\}$, we define a new template relevance measure, r_φ, as

$$r_\varphi(\mathcal{S}, C) = \left(\frac{\mathrm{Cov}(\varphi(\mathcal{S}), \omega(C))}{\sigma(\varphi(\mathcal{S}))\, \sigma(\omega(C))} \right)^2 \tag{9}$$

where $\mathrm{Cov}(\cdot, \cdot)$ and $\sigma(\cdot)$ denote the covariance and the standard deviation, respectively. The function ω converts the binary class variable C into a numeric variable and is defined as

$$\omega(C) = \begin{cases} +\sqrt{\frac{n_N}{n_P}}, & C = c^+ \\ -\sqrt{\frac{n_P}{n_N}}, & C = c^- \end{cases} \tag{10}$$

where n_P and n_N are the numbers of instances belonging to class c^+ and class c^-, respectively, and $n_P + n_N = n$ is the total number of examples in the training set. The function φ is of the form $\varphi(X_1, X_2, \ldots, X_{|\mathcal{S}|})$ that takes the value of a subset of features for an object and returns a scalar value in $\mathbb{R}$. By the Cauchy-Schwarz inequality we have

$$|\mathrm{Cov}(\varphi(\mathcal{S}), \omega(C))| \leq \sqrt{\sigma^2(\varphi(\mathcal{S}))\, \sigma^2(\omega(C))}$$

Thus the r_φ function is bounded from below and above:

$$0 \leq r_\varphi(\mathcal{S}, C) \leq 1 \ .$$

If r_φ returns a high value (close to 1), then C depends on the image of input features under function φ. Therefore the subset $\mathcal{S}$ is relevant to the problem (the target concept C). We call r_φ a *template* relevance measure, because different relevance heuristics can be constructed by constructing different φs.

In order to find out whether $\mathcal{S}$ is relevant to C, one needs to find a function φ (of elements of $\mathcal{S}$) that maximises the value of r_φ. Note that not being able to find such a function does not necessarily mean $\mathcal{S}$ is irrelevant to the problem. We use GP to search a finite subset of the space of all functions constructable from a set of *primitive* functions. An evolved GP program defines a function over its variable terminals; the function maps a subset of features to the set of real numbers. The goal is to find a function that creates the largest output (close to 1) when it is inserted in the r_φ function. Therefore, in order to calculate the fitness in the GP search, for each candidate solution (program tree), a new r_φ (heuristic relevance measure) is generated such that φ in equation (9) is the candidate GP program. By using GP to discover the right heuristic, equation (9) can capture non-linear and complex relationships.

6   Case Studies

In this section, we demonstrate some preliminary results from the proposed hyper-heuristic measure on two families of classification problems that are deemed difficult to handle by two commonly-used heuristic measures in the literature:

- *Information-theory* family of relevance functions (such as IG [11]) measures the worth of features by first discretising them (via setting some split points) and then measuring the change in the entropy of the class variable.
- *Logistic regression*, as a uni-variate measure, that models the *logit* function for the probability of the positive class (log of odds). The value of $|\beta|$ returned by this measure is the coefficient of the feature in a linear expression. If it has a high magnitude the feature is considered relevant and when it is close to zero the feature is considered irrelevant [6].

For the proposed hyper-heuristic approach, we use the standard tree-based GP in all experiments [10]. In this model, each program produces a single floating-point number at its root as the result of its evaluation (output). There is one variable terminal for each feature in the problem. A number of randomly generated constants are also used as terminals. The four standard arithmetic operators were used to form the function set. The division operator, however, is *protected*— that is, it returns zero for division by zero. All the members of the function set are binary—they take two parameters. The population size is 1024 and the maximum number of generations is set to 50.

6.1   Multivariate Relationships

Consider a synthetic linear binary classification problem with two input features X_1 and X_2. The class boundary is set to $X_2 = -X_1 + 1$ and $X_1, X_2 \in [0, 1)$. According to (1), the two features are both useful for classification because a straight line (passing through the boundary of the two classes) can separate the classes. Indeed, a learning algorithm as simple as a single perceptron can learn the target concept completely.

Now, we look at two commonly-used heuristic relevance measures to see how they handle multivariate situations like this. We then compare the result to the new hyper-heuristic approach. We use a sample of 1000 observations from the described problem. The results have been summarised in the corresponding section of Table 4.

Information Entropy. The original entropy (without any input features) is 0.7. The best split points along X_1 and X_2 are at 0.5 which reduces the expected value of entropy to 0.55, which is a very small gain considering the high quality of these features—that is, to measures relying on changes in information entropy (such as mutual information), the two features are not very relevant.

Logistic Regression. The standard logistic regression method returns a $|\hat{\beta}|$ of less than 0.2 for each of these features, deeming them unimportant. A multivariate logistic regression, however, returns a high estimated coefficient for the two features, seeing them as important.

Hyper-heuristic. With this method, GP is used to find a φ for which the resulting heuristic relevance can detect the relationship between the explanatory variables (input features) and the response variable (the class label). One of the evolved solutions by GP is the s-expression (Sub (Add X1 X2) 1) which is actually the equation of the decision boundary. The relevance of $\{X_1, X_2\}$ measured by r_φ at late generations is above 0.9 indicating the two features are relevant.

Table 4. Three relevance measures on two case studies

Measure	Multi-Modal	Multivariate
Logistic Regression		
coefficient:	$|\hat{\beta}|_X \approx 0.03$	$|\hat{\beta}|_{X_1} \approx |\hat{\beta}|_{X_2} \approx 0.2$
Mutual Information		
entropy:	$H(C) \approx 0.61$	$H(C) \approx 0.7$
conditional entropy:	$H(C|X) \approx 0.43$	$H(C|X_1) \approx H(C|X_2) \approx 0.55$
gain:	$I(C; X) \approx 0.18$	$I(C; X_1) \approx I(C; X_2) \approx 0.15$
Hyper-heuristic		
relevance:	$r_{\varphi(X)} = 0.82$	$S = \{X_1, X_2\}$ and $r_{\varphi(S)} = 0.93$

6.2 Multi-modal Class Distribution

Now we examine a bimodal classification problem; that is, a problem where the probability density function of one of the classes has two peaks and between the two peaks, the density of the other class is higher. We look at a relatively simple case where probability densities are either normal or constructed from a number of normal distributions of the form $N(\mu, \sigma^2)$ where μ is the mean and σ is the standard deviation.

Consider a classification problem with one feature X where some of the positive objects are distributed by $N(2, 1)$ and some by $N(8, 1)$. The negative class is distributed by $N(5, 1)$. The feature X is observably a good feature because by setting up an interval around instances of the negative class (i.e. [3.5, 6.5]) the classification problem can be solved. This is equivalent to a simple decision tree with two nodes. Now we study the behaviour of some heuristic relevance measures and then the proposed hyper-heuristic measure on this problem. The results have been summarised in the corresponding section of Table 4.

Logistic Regression. Since the class probability does not change linearly with respect to X, the logistic regression method does not consider X to be a good feature, returning a $\hat{\beta}$ coefficient close to zero.

Information Entropy. Since measures based on information entropy need discretisation (in order to estimate probability densities) they try to find the best split point along X (using which, instances from different classes can be separated). However, since not all the instances can be separated around one split point, the feature is not considered relevant. While a more sophisticated discretisation may be able to handle low-dimensional problems like this, for a more complex problem, discretisation would fail.

Hyper-heuristic. One of the solutions GP evolved for φ is the s-expression (Add (Mul (Sub 5.1 X) (Sub 4.8 X)) -3.9) which is a second degree polynomial describing the decision boundary and thus enabling r_φ to detect the relevance of the feature to the target concept.

6.3   Discussion

In the multivariate case, although the two features were clearly useful (and sufficient) in separating the two classes, we observed that to some heuristic relevance measures, the features seemed irrelevant. No univariate relevance measure could judge X_1 or X_2 individually important. This is because very little separation can be obtained by using only one of the features. Multivariate measures can detect the importance of the two features. The features seem more useful to those measures that do not use discretisation.

If the distribution of one of the classes in the problem is multi-modal, then the features are likely to be dismissed as irrelevant by measures like logistic regression (due to non-linear relationships) and those depending on information entropy such as mutual information (due to poor discretisation).

Each heuristic relevance measure has its own notion of separability of data on the basis of which it assigns a relevance value to a subset of features (or just a single feature). If a group of features provides high separability between instances of different classes but not in a way that is recognisable to the relevance measure, then the features will receive low relevance score and be considered, consequently, irrelevant. Now if the measure was used in a feature selection algorithm (the filter approach), those good features would have been eliminated from the problem due to them being seen as irrelevant.

On the other hand, a hyper-heuristic approach like the one proposed searches for the right heuristic for the problem. In both cases, the proposed method detected the relevance of the features by finding a right heuristic by using GP to evolve a function φ that would lead to a right heuristic.

7   Conclusions

Heuristic relevance measures (filter-based feature selection algorithms) can *never guarantee* finding an optimal subset of features; that is, the best subset for any arbitrarily chosen learning algorithm (see the counter-examples). This is an intrinsic limitation of all filter methods. Being "independent from any learning algorithm" must not be interpreted as their results (selected subsets) being compatible with all learning algorithms.

Often feature selection is carried out as a preprocessing task, before it is known what type of learning algorithms will be used on data. It is therefore important to detect all relevant features in a problem regardless of whether a particular learning algorithm is able to use those features. A hyper-heuristic approach to measuring relevance seems to be a promising direction as it would be able to search for a right heuristic for the problem. The proposed hyper-heuristic approach uses GP to find (construct) a function that when inserted into a template, creates the right heuristic for the problem. Our results on two case studies show that the proposed approach can detect the relevance between input features and target concepts in difficult scenarios where commonly-used heuristic relevance measures are not able to detect the relationship between features.

While the paper focused on classification problems the conclusions can rationally be extended to a wider class of supervised learning algorithms including both classification and regression algorithms.

References

1. Asuncion, A., Newman, D.: UCI machine learning repository (2007), http://archive.ics.uci.edu/ml/index.html (last accessed 2010)
2. Bell, D.A., Wang, H.: A formalism for relevance and its application in feature subset selection. Machine Learning 41(2), 175–195 (2000), http://dx.doi.org/10.1023/A:1007612503587
3. Burke, E., Kendall, G., Newall, J., Hart, E., Ross, P., Schulenburg, S.: Hyperheuristics: An emerging direction in modern search technology. Handbook of Metaheuristics, 457–474 (2003)
4. Burker, E.K., Hyde, M., Kendall, G., Ochoa, G., Özcan, E., Woodward, J.R.: A classification of hyper-heuristic approaches. Handbook of Metaheuristics, 449–468 (2010)
5. Carnap, R.: Logical foundations of probability. University of Chicago Press (1967)
6. Cheng, Q., Varshney, P.K., Arora, M.K.: Logistic regression for feature selection and soft classification of remote sensing data. IEEE Geoscience and Remote Sensing Letters 3(4), 491–494 (2006)
7. Gärdenfors, P.: On the logic of relevance. Synthese 37(3), 351–367 (1978)
8. Keynes, J.: A treatise on probability. Macmillan & Co., Ltd. (1921)
9. Kohavi, R., John, G.: Wrappers for feature subset selection. Artificial Intelligence 97, 273–324 (1997)
10. Koza, J.R.: Genetic Programming: On the Programming of Computers by Means of Natural Selection. MIT Press, Cambridge (1992)
11. Last, M., Kandel, A., Maimon, O.: Information-theoretic algorithm for feature selection. Pattern Recognition Letters 22(6), 799–811 (2001), http://citeseerx.ist.psu.edu/viewdoc/summary?doi=10.1.1.22.5311
12. Liu, H., Setiono, R.: Chi2: Feature selection and discretization of numeric attributes. In: Proceedings of the Seventh International Conference on Tools with Artificial Intelligence, pp. 388–391. IEEE (1995)
13. Özcan, E., Bilgin, B., Korkmaz, E.E.: A comprehensive analysis of hyper-heuristics. Intelligent Data Analysis 12(1), 3–23 (2008)
14. Peng, H., Long, F., Ding, C.: Feature selection based on mutual information: criteria of max-dependency, max-relevance, and min-redundancy. IEEE Transactions on Pattern Analysis and Machine Intelligence, 1226–1238 (2005)
15. Poli, R., Graff, M.: There is a free lunch for hyper-heuristics, genetic programming and computer scientists. Genetic Programming, 195–207 (2009)
16. Wolpert, D., Macready, W.: No free lunch theorems for optimization. IEEE Transactions on Evolutionary Computation 1(1), 67–82 (1997)

A PSO-Based Cost-Sensitive Neural Network
for Imbalanced Data Classification

Peng Cao[1,2,*], Dazhe Zhao[1], and Osmar R. Zaïane[2]

[1] Key Laboratory of Medical Image Computing of Ministry of Education,
Northeastern University, China
[2] Department of Computing Science, University of Alberta, Canada
{Cao.p,zhaodz}@neusoft.com, zaiane@cs.ualberta.ca

Abstract. Learning from imbalanced data is an important and common problem. Many methods have been proposed to address and attempt to solve the problem, including sampling and cost-sensitive learning. This paper presents an effective wrapper approach incorporating the evaluation measure directly into the objective function of cost-sensitive neural network to improve the performance of classification, by simultaneously optimizing the best pair of feature subset, intrinsic structure parameters and misclassification costs. The optimization is based on Particle Swarm Optimization. Our designed method can be applied on the binary class and multi-class classification. Experimental results on various standard benchmark datasets show that the proposed method is effective in comparison with commonly used sampling techniques.

Keywords: classification with Class imbalance, Cost-sensitive learning, Neural network, Particle swarm intelligence.

1 Introduction

The classification of data with imbalanced data distributions has posed a significant drawback in the performance of the most traditional classification methods, which assume an even distribution of examples among classes [1]. This problem is growing in importance and has been identified as one of the 10 main challenges of Data Mining [2]. Much work has been done in addressing the class imbalance problem. These methods can be grouped in two categories: the data perspective and the algorithm perspective [3]. The significant shortcomings with the re-sampling approach are that the optimal class distribution is always unknown and the criterion in selecting instances is uncertain; furthermore, under-sampling may reduce information loss and over-sampling may lead to overfitting for model constructed. The cost-sensitive learning technique takes misclassification costs into account during the model construction, and does not modify the imbalanced data distribution directly. Assigning distinct costs to the training examples seems to be the most effective approach of class imbalanced data problems.

In the cost-sensitive learning, the misclassification costs play a crucial role in the construction of a cost-sensitive learning model for achieving expected classification

---

* Corresponding author.

J. Li et al. (Eds.): PAKDD 2013 Workshops, LNAI 7867, pp. 452–463, 2013.

results. However, in many contexts of imbalanced dataset, the appropriate misclassification costs are unknown. Besides the costs, the feature set and intrinsic parameter of some sophisticated classifiers also influence the classification performance, such as SVM and neural networks. Moreover, these factors influence each other. This is the first challenge. The other is that as we know, for evaluating the performance of cost-sensitive classifier on the skewed data set, the overall accuracy is not sufficient any more. An appropriate evaluation measure is critical in both assessing the classification performance and guiding the classifier in the imbalanced data distribution scenario, such as G-mean and AUC.

In order to solve the challenges above, we design a novel framework for training a cost-sensitive neural network driven by the imbalanced evaluation criteria. The training scheme can bridge the gap between the training and the evaluation of cost-sensitive learning, and it can learn the optimal factors associated with the cost-sensitive classifier automatically under the guidance of the performance metrics [4]. The search space is expanded exponentially as the class number increases. Moreover the factors to be searched are mixture including continuous and discrete variables. Therefore, we use Particle Swarm Optimization (PSO) [5] as the optimization strategy due to its fast and effective solution space exploration.

The contributions of this work can be listed as follows:

1) Optimizing the factors (misclassification cost, feature subset and intrinsic structure parameters) simultaneously for improving the performance of cost-sensitive neural network (CS-NN). We use G-mean [6] to guide the optimization of CS-NN.

2) Most existing imbalance data learning so far are still limited to the binary class imbalance problems. There are fewer effective solutions in multi-class imbalance problems, which exist in real world applications. Our method can be applied on the multi-class imbalance data.

2   Proposed Approaches

2.1   Cost-Sensitive Neural Network

The cost-sensitive learning technique takes misclassification costs into account during the model construction, and does not modify the imbalanced data distribution directly. The standard neural network is cost **in**sensitive. In standard neural network classifiers, the class returned is $C*$ by comparing the probability of each class directly for each instance x according to **Eq.**(1).

$$C* = \underset{C \in \{1,...,M\}}{argmax}(p_1(C_1 \mid x),...,p_M(C_M \mid x)) \tag{1}$$

where P_i denotes the probability value of each class from the neural network, $\sum_{i=1}^{M} P_i = 1$ and $0 \le P_i \le 1$. M is the number of the class.

The probabilities generated by a standard neural network are biased in the imbalanced data distribution, adjusting the decision threshold moves the output threshold toward inexpensive class such that instances with high costs become harder to be misclassified [7]. The idea is based on the classifier producing probability predictions rather than classification labels. Results suggest that threshold-moving, replacing the probability a sample belongs to a certain class with the altered probability, which takes into account the costs of misclassification, is found to be a relatively good choice in training CS-NN [8]. This method uses the training set to train a neural network, and the cost sensitivity strategy is introduced in the test phase. Given a certain cost matrix, the CS-NN with threshold-moving return the class $C*$, which is computed by injecting the cost according to **Eq.**(2).

$$
\begin{aligned}
C* &= \underset{C \in \{1,\dots,M\}}{argmax}(p_1^*(C_1 \mid x),\dots, p_M^*(C_M \mid x)) \\
&= \underset{C \in \{1,\dots,M\}}{argmax}(\eta_1 cost(C_1)p(C_1 \mid x),\dots, \eta_M cost(C_M) \times p(C_M \mid x))
\end{aligned}
\tag{2}
$$

where $Cost(C_i)$ denotes the cost of misclassifying instance of class $\underline{i}$. P_i^* denotes the class probabilities from the neural network combined with misclassification cost. η_i is a normalization term such that $\sum_{i=1}^{M} P_i^* = 1$ and $0 \le P_i^* \le 1$.

2.2   Particle Swarm Optimization

Swarm Intelligence (SI), an artificial intelligence technique for machine learning, is a research branch that models the population of interacting agents or swarms that are able to self-organize. SI has recently emerged as a practical research topic and has successfully been applied to a number of real world problems.

Particle swarm optimization (PSO) is a population-based global stochastic search method attributed to Kennedy and Eberhart to simulate social behavior [4]. Compared to Genetic Algorithms (GA), the advantages of PSO are that it is easy to implement and has fewer control parameters to adjust. Many studies have shown than PSO has the same effectiveness but is more efficient than GA [9]. PSO optimizes an objective function by a population-based search. The population consists of potential solutions, named particles. These particles are randomly initialized and move across the multi-dimensional search space to find the best position according to an optimization function. During optimization, each particle adjusts its trajectory through the problem space based on the information about its previous best performance (personal best, *pbest*) and the best previous performance of its neighbors (global best, *gbest*). Eventually, all particles will gather around the point with the highest objective value.

The position of individual particles is updated as follows:

$$
x_i^{t+1} = x_i^t + v_i^{t+1}
\tag{3}
$$

With v, the velocity calculated as follows:

$$
v_{id}^{t+1} = w \times v_{id}^t + c_1 \times r_1 \times (pbest_{id}^t - x_{id}^t) + c_2 \times r_2 \times (gbest^t - x_{id}^t)
\tag{4}
$$

where v_i^t indicates velocity of particle i at iteration t, w indicates the inertia factor, C_1 and C_2 indicate the cognition and social learning rates, which determine the relative influence of the social and cognition components. r_1 and r_2 are uniformly distributed random numbers between 0 and 1, x_i^t is current position of particle i at iteration t, $pbest_i^t$ indicates best of particle i at iteration t, $gbest^t$ indicates the best of the group.

2.3   PSO Based Cost-Sensitive Neural Network (PSOCS-NN)

In this section, we present a new measure oriented framework for optimizing the cost-sensitive neural network, which uses a particle swarm intelligence to carry out the meta-learning.

An important issue of applying the cost-sensitive learning algorithm to the imbalanced data is that the exact cost parameters are often unavailable for a problem domain. The misclassification cost, especially the ratio misclassification cost, plays a crucial role in the construction of the cost-sensitive approach. It is not correct to set the cost ratio to the inverse of the imbalance ratio (the amount of majority instances divided by the amount of minority instances).

Apart from the misclassification cost information, the intrinsic structure parameters and feature subset selection of the neural network have a significant bearing on the performance. Both factors are not only important for imbalanced data classification, but also for any other classification task. The proper intrinsic structure parameter setting of neural network (i.e. number of hidden layers and connection weights) can improve the classification performance. Feature selection is the technique of selecting a subset of discriminative features for building robust learning models by removing most irrelevant and redundant features from the data. The imbalanced data distribution are often accompanied by the high dimensional in real-world data sets such as text classification, or bioinformatics. Optimal feature selection can concurrently achieve good performance and dimensionality reduction [3]. Zheng et al[10] suggest that existing measures used for feature selection are not very appropriate for imbalanced data sets. Hulse et al. [11] investigate that the wrapper feature selection is a good approach for imbalanced data-sets, which can find potentially interesting feature information not captured by other filter techniques. Furthermore, the feature subset choice influences the appropriate intrinsic structure parameters as well as misclassification costs and vice versa, obtaining these optimal factors of CS-NN must occur simultaneously.

Based on the reason above, our specific goal is to devise a strategy to automatically determine the optimal factors during training of the cost-sensitive classifier oriented by the imbalanced evaluation criteria. In this paper, for the multivariable optimization, especially the hybrid multivariable, the best method is swarm intelligence technique [12]. We choose the particle swarm optimization (PSO) as our optimization method because it is very mature and easy to implement. In addition, many experiments claim that PSO has equal effectiveness but superior efficiency over GA [9]. The wrapper method is called PSOCS-NN, which empirically discovers the potential misclassification costs, the feature subset, and the intrinsic structure parameters for CS-NN.

Evaluation measures play a crucial role in both assessing the classification performance and guiding the classifier modeling. As we known, neural networks are driven by error based objective functions. We have known the overall accuracy is not an appropriate evaluation measure for imbalanced data classification. As a result, there is an inevitable gap between the evaluation measure by which the classifier is to be evaluated and the objective function according to the classifier trained [13]. The classifier for imbalanced data learning needs to be driven by the more appropriate measures. We inject the appropriate measures, G-mean into the objective function of the classifier in the training with PSO. The G-mean is the geometric mean of accuracies measured separately on each class, which is commonly utilized when performance of each class is concerned and expected to be high simultaneously [13-14]. The value of the evaluation metric is taken as the fitness function to adjust the position of a particle. Through training the CS-NN with G-mean, we can discover the best factors. The G-mean is defined as:

$$G-mean = (\prod_{i}^{M} R_i)^{1/M} \tag{5}$$

where R_i denotes the recall of class C_i, and M is the number of the classes.

In the binary class classification ($M=2$), given a certain cost matrix, the CS-NN will classify an instance x into positive (+) class if and only if:

$$P(+|x)Cost(+) > P(-|x)Cost(-) \tag{6}$$

Therefore the theoretical threshold for making a decision on classifying instances into positive is obtained as:

$$p(+|x) > \frac{Cost(-)}{Cost(+)+Cost(-)} = \frac{1}{1+C_{rf}} \tag{7}$$

where C_{rf} is ratio of two cost value, $C_{rf} = C(+)/C(-)$. The value of C_{rf} plays a crucial role in the construction of CS-NN for the classification of the binary class data .

Similarly, for the multiple class classification ($M>2$), we set the cost of the largest class to 1. The other $M-1$ ratio cost parameters need to be optimized.

PSO was originally developed for continuous valued spaces; however, the feature set is discrete, each feature is represented by a 1 or 0 for whether it is selected or not. We need to combine the discrete and continuous values in the solution representation since the costs and parameters we intend to optimize are continuous while the feature selection is discrete. The major difference between the discrete PSO [15] and the original version is that the velocities of the particles are rather defined in terms of probabilities that a bit will change to one. Using this definition a velocity must be restricted within the range [0, 1], to which all continuous values of velocity are mapped by a sigmoid function:

$$v''_i = sig(v'_i) = \frac{1}{1+e^{-v'_i}} \tag{8}$$

Equation 8 is used to update the velocity vector of the particle while the new position of the particle is obtained using Equation 9.

$$x_i^{t+1} = \begin{cases} 1 & if \quad r_i < v''_i \\ 0 & otherwise \end{cases} \tag{9}$$

where r_i is a uniform random number in the range [0, 1] .

In the training of the feed-forward neural network, it is often trained by adjusting connection weights with gradient descent. Another alternative is to use swarm intelligence to find the optimal set of weights [13]. Since the gradient descent is a local search method vulnerable to be trapped in local minima, we opted to substitute the gradient descent with PSO in our use of PSOCS-NN in order to alleviate the curse of local optima. We use a hybrid PSO algorithm similar to the PSO-PSO method presented in [16]. In the PSO-PSO Methodology, a PSO algorithm is used to search for architectures and a PSO with weight decay (PSO: WD) is used to search for weights. We also used two nested PSOs, where the outer PSO is used to search for architectures (including the feature subset which determines the input node amount as well as the number of the hidden nodes) and costs; the inner PSO is used to search for weights of the neural network defined by the outer PSO. In our work, we assume there is only one hidden layer. The solution of the outer PSO includes three parts: the cost, the number of the hidden nodes and the feature subset, and the solution of the inner PSO contains the vector of the connection weights. The amount of the variables to be optimized in the inner PSO is determined by the number of the hidden nodes in the   outer PSO. Figure 1 illustrates the mixed solution representation of the two PSOs. The detailed algorithm for PSOCS-NN is shown in Algorithm 1.

Algorithm 1. PSOCS-NN

Input: Training set D; Termination condition of two PSO T_{outer} and T_{inner}; Population size of two PSOs SN_{outer} and SN_{inner}

1. Randomly initialize outer-PSO population (including costs, number of the hidden nodes, and feature subset)

    repeat   *% outer PSO*
      foreach particle^i

2.   Construct D^i with the feature selected by the particle^i
3.   Separate D^i randomly into Trt^i (80%) for training *and* Trv^i (20%) for validation
4.   Randomly initialize inner-PSO population (connection weights) in each particle^i

      repeat   *% inner PSO*
        foreach particle^ij

5.   Obtain the number of the hidden nodes from the particle^i
6.   Construct a neural network with the weights optimized by the particle^ij
7.   Validate the neural network on the Trt^i and assign the fitness of particle^ij with the G-mean

      end foreach

8.   Inner-PSO particle population updates

    until T_{inner}

9.   Obtain the optimal connection weight vector in the $gbest^i_{inner}$ of the inner PSO
10.   Evaluate the neural network classifier with cost optimized by the particle^i as well as the connection weights optimized on the Trv^i, and obtain the value M^i based on G-mean
11.   Assign the fitness of particle^i with M^i

    end foreach

12. Outer-PSO particle population updates

    until T_{outer}

Output: the number of the hidden nodes, costs, feature subset and the connection weights of the $gbest_{inner}$ in the $gbest_{outer}$

Outer PSO	cost vector	number of the hidden nodes, N	F_1	F_2	...	F_{p-1}	F_p
Inner PSO	w_1	w_2		...		w_{N-1}	w_N

Fig. 1. Solution representations of outer and inner PSO

3   Experimental Study

We present two experiments separately, the binary class imbalanced data and multi-class imbalanced data. These datasets are from the public UCI benchmark [17]. In all our experiments, instead of the traditional 10-fold cross validation which can result in few instances of minority class, each dataset was randomly separated into training set (70%) for constructing classifiers and test sets (30%) for validating the classifiers. This procedure was repeated 20 times for obtaining unbiased results.

3.1   Binary Class Imbalanced Data

3.1.1   Dataset Description

To evaluate the classification performance of our proposed methods in different binary class classification tasks, and to compare with other methods specifically devised for imbalanced data, we tried several datasets from the UCI database. We used all available datasets from the combined sets used in [18]. This also ensures that we did not choose only the datasets on which our method performs better. There is no standard dataset for imbalanced classification, and most of these selected UCI datasets have multi-class labels. The minority class label (+) is indicated in Table 1.

Table 1. The data sets used for binary imbalanced data classification

The dataset name is appended with the label of the minority class (+)

Dataset (+)	Instances	Features	Class balance
Hepatitis (1)	155	19	1:4
Glass (7)	214	9	1:6
Segment (1)	2310	19	1:6
Anneal (5)	898	38	1:12
Soybean (12)	683	35	1:15
Sick (2)	3772	29	1:15
Car (3)	1728	6	1:24
Letter (26)	20000	16	1:26
Hypothyroid(3)	3772	29	1:39
Abalone (19)	4177	8	1:130

3.1.2   Experiment 1

In this experiment, we made the comparison between basic neural network (Basic NN) with and without the feature selection, cost-sensitive neural network (CS-NN), our method proposed using G-mean oriented training for CS-NN by PSO (PSO-CSNN) with and without the feature selection. For the Basic NN with feature selection, it is a common wrapper feature selection method with evaluating by classification performance. As for the CS-NN, the misclassification cost ratio is searched iteratively to maximize the measure score within a range of cost value. In the Basic NN and CS-NN, the number of neurons in the hidden layer was the average number between the input and output neurons. They are trained with gradient descent.

For the PSO setting of our method, PSOCS-NN, the initial parameter values in our proposed method were set according to the conclusion drawn in [19]. The parameters used were: C_1=2.8, C_2=1.3, w=0.5. For empirically providing good performance while at the same time keeping the time complexity feasible, the particle number was set dynamically according to the amount of the variables optimized (=1.5×|variables needed to be optimized|), and the termination condition could be a certain number of iterations (500 cycles) or other convergence condition (no changes any more within 2 × |variables needed to be optimized| cycles).

Along with these parameters in PSO, the other parameters are the upper and lower limits of CS-NN parameters to be optimized. For the intrinsic structure parameters of neural network, the upper and lower limits of the connection weights were set to 100 and -100 respectively in the inner PSO; the upper and lower limits of the number of hidden nodes were empirically set to 5 and 20 respectively in the outer PSO. The range of $Cost(C_i)$ of each class C_i was empirically chosen to [1, 100×$ImbaRatio_i$], where the $ImbaRatio_i$ is the size ratio between the largest class and each class C_i.

Table 2. Experimental results (average G-mean and size of the feature subset after feature selection)of the PSOCS-NN method with and without feature selection (FS), as well as Basic NN and CS-NN

Dataset	Basic NN		CS-NN	PSOCS-NN	
	without FS	FS	without FS	without FS	FS
Hepatitis	0.751	0.807 (11)	0.755	0.819	**0.848 (8)**
Glass	0.832	0.845 (5)	0.916	0.957	**0.970 (4)**
Segment	0.993	0.997 (10)	1	1	1 (11)
Anneal	0.736	0.798 (19)	0.818	0.909	**0.934 (12)**
Soybean	0.929	**1 (12)**	1	1	1 (12)
Sick	0.517	0.623 (10)	0.712	0.834	**0.907 (7)**
Car	0.783	0.796 (4)	0.928	0.960	**0.969 (4)**
Letter	0.955	0.962 (9)	0.972	**0.979**	0.971 (10)
Hypothyrid	0.651	0.763 (17)	0.813	0.928	**0.958 (14)**
Abalone	0.751	0.753 (6)	0.784	**0.891**	0.856 (5)

The average G-mean scores and the amount of feature subset are shown in Table 2. From the results in Table 2, we found that simultaneously optimizing the feature subset, intrinsic structure parameters and costs generally helps the CS-NN learn on the different data sets, regardless of whether there is feature selection or not. We also found the feature selection step for these classifiers when working on the imbalanced data classification for both the Basic NN and the PSOCS-NN. Therefore, we can draw the conclusion that simultaneously optimizing the intrinsic parameters, misclassification costs and feature subset with the imbalanced evaluation measure guiding, improves the classification performance of the cost-sensitive neural network on the different datasets.

3.1.3   Experiment 2

In this experiment, the comparisons are conducted between our method and the other state-of-the-art imbalanced data methods, such as the random under-sampling (RUS), SMOTE over-sampling [20], SMOTEBoost [21], and SMOTE combined with asymmetric cost neural network (SMOTE+CS-NN) [18]. For the re-sampling methods, the re-sampling rate is unknown. In our experiments, in order to compare equally, either under-sampling or over-sampling method, we also use the evaluation measure G-mean as the optimization objective of the re-sampling method to search the optimal re-sampling level. The increment step and the decrement step are set as 50% and 10% separately. This is a greedy search, that repeats, greedily, until no performance gains are observed. Thus, in each fold, the training set is separated into training subset and validating subset for searching the appropriate rate parameters. For the SMOTE+CS-NN, for each re-sampling rate searched, the optimal misclassification cost ratio is determined by grid search under the evaluation measure guiding under the current over-sampling level of SMOTE.

Table 3. Experimental comparison between PSOCS-NN and other imbalanced data classification methods on the binary imbalanced data

Dataset	Metric	RUS	SMOTE	SMB	SMOTE+CS-NN	PSOCS-NN
Hepatitis	G-mean	0.793	0.835	0.807	**0.851**	0.848
	AUC	0.611	0.74	0.815	0.827	**0.877**
Glass	G-mean	0.847	0.851	0.885	0.965	**0.970**
	AUC	0.919	0.964	0.988	0.953	**0.994**
Segment	G-mean	0.993	0.999	0.998	1	1
	AUC	0.999	1	1	1	1
Anneal	G-mean	0.702	0.799	0.848	0.914	**0.934**
	AUC	0.902	0.856	0.839	0.911	**0.932**
Soybean	G-mean	0.948	1	1	1	1
	AUC	1	1	1	1	1
Sick	G-mean	0.354	0.699	0.748	0.816	**0.907**
	AUC	0.721	0.817	0.856	0.885	**0.941**
Car	G-mean	0.786	0.944	0.939	**0.988**	0.969
	AUC	0.806	0.986	0.990	1	1
Letter	G-mean	0.957	0.959	0.966	0.963	**0.971**
	AUC	0.925	0.929	0.943	0.998	1
Hypothyrid	G-mean	0.673	0.841	0.853	0.917	**0.958**
	AUC	0.861	0.923	0.952	0.935	**0.972**
Abalone	G-mean	0.726	0.748	0.756	0.857	**0.856**
	AUC	0.751	0.793	0.771	0.828	**0.875**
Number of Wins / Ties	G-mean	0/0	0/1	0/1	2/2	**6/2**
	AUC	0/1	0/2	0/2	0/2	**7/3**

The experiment results of average G-mean and AUC are shown in Table 3. As shown in bold in Table 3, our PSOCS-NN outperforms all the other approaches on the great majority of datasets. From the results, we can see that the random under-sampling presents the worst performance. This is because it is possible to remove certain significant examples. Both the SMOTE and SMOTEBoost improve the classification for neural network. However, they have a potential disadvantage of distorting the class distribution. SMOTE combined with different costs is better than single only SMOTE over-sampling, and it is the method that share most of the second best results.

The feature selection is as important as the re-sampling in the imbalanced data classification, especially on the high dimensional datasets. However, the feature selection is always ignored. Our method conducts the feature selection in the wrapper paradigm, hence improves the classification performance on the data sets which have higher dimensionality, such as Anneal, Sick and Hypothyroid. Although all methods are optimized under the evaluation measure oriented, we can clearly see that PSOCS-NN is almost always equal to, or better than other methods. What is most important is that our method does not change the data distribution. The re-sampling based on the SMOTE may make the model overfitting, resulting in a weak generalization not as good as the training.

3.2   Multiclass Imbalanced Data

Most existing imbalance data learning so far are still limited to the binary class imbalance problems. There are fewer solutions in multi-class imbalance problems. They have been shown to be less effective or even cause a negative effect in dealing with multi-class tasks [8]. The experiments in [22] imply that the performance decreases as the number of imbalanced classes increases. We choose six multiclass datasets to evaluate our method. The data information is summarized in Table 4. The chosen datasets have diversity in the number of classes and imbalance ratio.

Table 4. The data sets used for multiclass imbalanced data classification

Dataset	Class	Instances	Features	Class distribution
Cmc	3	1473	9	629/333/511
Balance	3	625	4	49/288/288
Nursery	4	12958	8	4320/328/4266/4044
Page	5	5473	10	4913/329/28/88/115
Satimage	6	6435	36	1533/703/1358/626/707/1508
Yeast	10	1484	9	463/429/244/163/51/44/35/30/20/5

We compare our method with the other four methods on the datasets in Table 4. The average G-mean values are shown in the Table 5. Through the comparison, we found that our method is effective on the multiclass data.

Table 5. Experimental comparison between PSOCS-NN method and other imbalanced data classification methods on the multiclass imbalanced data

Dataset	RUS	SMOTE	SMB	SMOTE+CS-NN	PSO-CSNN
Cmc	0.719	0.741	0.749	0.755	**0.793 (4)**
Balance	0	0.507	**0.562**	0.525	0.542 (3)
Nursery	0.498	0.789	0.811	0.809	**0.853 (4)**
Page	0.684	0.707	0.739	0.758	**0.771 (6)**
Satimage	0.825	0.831	0.841	0.844	**0.872 (15)**
Yeast	0	0.311	0.327	0.335	**0.406 (6)**

4   Conclusion

Learning with class imbalance is a challenging task. Cost-sensitive learning is an important approach without changing the distribution because it takes into account different misclassification costs for false negatives and false positives. Since the costs, the intrinsic structure parameters and the feature subset are important factors for the cost sensitive neural network, and they influence each other, it is best to attempt to simultaneously optimize them using an object oriented wrapper approach. We propose a wrapper paradigm oriented by the evaluation measure of imbalanced dataset as objective function with respect to misclassification cost, feature subset and intrinsic parameter of classifier. The optimization processing is through an effective swarm intelligence technique, the Particle Swarm Optimization. Our measure oriented framework could wrap around an existing cost-sensitive classifier. The experimental results presented in this study have demonstrated that the proposed framework provided a very competitive solution to other existing state-of-the-arts methods, on the binary class and multiclass imbalanced data. These results confirm the advantages of our approach, showing the promising perspective and new understanding of cost-sensitive learning.

References

1. He, H., Garcia, E.: Learning from imbalanced data. IEEE Transactions on Knowledge and Data Engineering 21, 1263–1284 (2009)
2. Yang, Q., Wu, X.: 10 challenging problems in data mining research. Int. J. Inf. Technol. Decis. Mak. 5(4), 597–604 (2006)
3. Chawla, N.V., Japkowicz, N., Kolcz, A.: Editorial: special issue on learning from imbalanced data sets. SIGKDD Explorations Special Issue on Learning from Imbalanced Datasets 6(1), 1–6 (2004)
4. Li, N., Tsang, I., Zhou, Z.: Efficient Optimization of Performance Measures by Classifier Adaptation. IEEE Transactions on Pattern Analysis and Machine Intelligence (99), 1 (2012)
5. Kennedy, J., Eberhart, R.C.: Particle swarm optimization. In: IEEE Int. Conf. Neural Networks, pp. 1942–1948 (1995)
6. Kubat, M., Matwin, S., et al.: Addressing the curse of imbalanced training sets: one-sided selection. In: Proc. Int'l Conf. Machine Learning, pp. 179–186 (1997)

7. Ling, C.X., Sheng, V.S.: Cost-sensitive learning and the class imbalance problem. Encyclopedia of Machine Learning Springer (2008)
8. Zhou, Z.H., Liu, X.Y.: Training Cost-Sensitive Neural Networks with Methods Addressing the Class Imbalance Problem. IEEE Transactions on Knowledge and Data Engineering 18(1), 63–77 (2006)
9. Hassan, R., Cohanim, R., de Weck, O.: A comparison of particle swarm optimization and the genetic algorithm. In: Proceedings of the 46th AIAA/ASME/ASCE/AHS/ASC Structures, Structural Dynamics and Materials Conference (2005)
10. Zheng, Z., Wu, X., Srihari, R.: Feature selection for text categorization on imbalanced data. ACM SIGKDD Explorations 6, 80–89 (2004)
11. Van Hulse, J., Khoshgoftaar, T.M., Napolitano, A., Wald, R.: Feature selection with high dimensional imbalanced data. In: Proceedings of the 9th IEEE International Conference on Data Mining - Workshops (ICDM 2009), pp. 507–514. IEEE Computer Society (December 2009)
12. Martens, D., Baesens, B., Fawcett, T.: Editorial Survey: Swarm Intelligence for Data Mining. Machine Learning 82(1), 1–42 (2011)
13. Yuan, B., Liu, W.H.: A Measure Oriented Training Scheme for Imbalanced Classification Problems. In: Pacific-Asia Conference on Knowledge Discovery and Data Mining Workshop on Biologically Inspired Techniques for Data Mining, pp. 293–303 (2011)
14. Sun, Y., Kamel, M.S., Wang, Y.: Boosting for Learning Multiple Classes with Imbalanced Class Distribution. In: Proc. Int'l Conf. Data Mining, pp. 592–602 (2006)
15. Khanesar, M.A., Teshnehlab, M., Shoorehdeli, M.A.: A novel binary particle swarm optimization. In: Mediterranean Conference on Control & Automation, MED 2007, Athens, pp. 1–6 (2007)
16. Carvalho, M., Ludermir, T.B.: Particle swarm optimization of neural network architectures and weights. In: Proc. of the 7th Int. Conf. on Hybrid Intelligent Systems, pp. 336–339 (2007)
17. Blake, C., Merz, C.: UCI repository of machine learning databases (1998)
18. Akbani, R., Kwek, S.S., Japkowicz, N.: Applying support vector machines to imbalanced datasets. In: Boulicaut, J.-F., Esposito, F., Giannotti, F., Pedreschi, D. (eds.) ECML 2004. LNCS (LNAI), vol. 3201, pp. 39–50. Springer, Heidelberg (2004)
19. Carlisle, A., Dozier, G.: An Off-The-Shelf PSO. In: Particle Swarm Optimization Workshop, pp. 1–6 (2001)
20. Chawla, N.V., Bowyer, K.W., Hall, L.O., Kegelmeyer, W.P.: SMOTE: Synthetic minority over-sampling technique. J. Artif. Intell. Res. 16, 321–357 (2002)
21. Chawla, N.V., Lazarevic, A., Hall, L.O., Bowyer, K.W.: SMOTEBoost: Improving Prediction of the Minority Class in Boosting. In: Lavrač, N., Gamberger, D., Todorovski, L., Blockeel, H. (eds.) PKDD 2003. LNCS (LNAI), vol. 2838, pp. 107–119. Springer, Heidelberg (2003)
22. Wang, S., Yao, X.: Multiclass imbalance problems: Analysis and potential solutions. IEEE Transactions on Systems, Man, and Cybernetics, Part B: Cybernetics 42, 1119–1130 (2012)

Binary Classification Using Genetic Programming: Evolving Discriminant Functions with Dynamic Thresholds

Jill de Jong and Kourosh Neshatian

Department of Computer Science and Software Engineering
University of Canterbury, Private Bag 4800, Christchurch, New Zealand
kourosh.neshatian@canterbury.ac.nz

Abstract. Binary classification is the problem of predicting which of two classes an input vector belongs to. This problem can be solved by using genetic programming to evolve discriminant functions which have a threshold output value that distinguishes between the two classes. The standard approach is to have a static threshold value of zero that is fixed throughout the evolution process. Items with a positive function output value are identified as one class and items with a negative function output value as the other class. We investigate a different approach where an optimum threshold is dynamically determined for each candidate function during the fitness evaluation. The optimum threshold is the one that achieves the lowest misclassification cost. It has an associated class translation rule for output values either side of the threshold value. The two approaches have been compared experimentally using four different datasets. Results suggest the dynamic threshold approach consistently achieves higher performance levels than the standard approach after equal numbers of fitness calls.

1 Introduction

Binary classification is the problem of predicting which of two classes an input vector belongs to based on the values of a set of features or attributes. Classifiers model the relationship of all the variables in the input vector with the class. A classifier can be a decision tree, a set of rules, a discriminant function and various other things.

Genetic programming [1] is one option for formulating classifiers to carry out the task of Binary Classification. A random population of candidate classifiers is generated from a set of primitive functions, dataset attributes and constants. The performance of each candidate is then evaluated using a fitness function with one or more objectives. Candidates that perform well have a higher probability of being involved in the breeding of the next generation of candidate classifiers. Espejo et al. [2] look at decision trees, sets of rules and discriminant functions as classifiers, when applying genetic programming to the task of classification.

J. Li et al. (Eds.): PAKDD 2013 Workshops, LNAI 7867, pp. 464–474, 2013.

The standard approach (Static Model), when using genetic programming to evolve discriminant functions for use in binary classification, is to have a single classifier function. Each function is applied to the input vectors of a training dataset. The output value is compared to a static threshold set to zero. A positive output value indicates the vector belongs to one class and a negative output value points to the other class. Output values of zero are mapped to a predetermined class. Then the fitness of each candidate function is evaluated. A common fitness objective for binary classification is maximizing classification accuracy [3]. Classification is accurate when the function output value indicates the same class that appears in the class label of the input vector. A more generalised version of this is to minimize misclassification error cost with unequal costs for False Positive errors and False Negative errors. An explanation of cost sensitive classification is presented in [4].

An alternative approach is to dynamically determine the threshold(s) during the evolutionary process. Loveard and Ciesielski [5] use dynamic range selection to determine the class boundaries for each individual function with both binary and multi-class datasets. Outputs from a subset of the training data are rounded to the nearest integer between -250 and +250 and used to segment this range into regions corresponding to class boundaries. Zhang and Smart [6] look at two methods of changing the thresholds every five generations in multi-class object classification. One method determines the thresholds by calculating the centre of the function output for each class. The second method splits the output value of a function into slots and maps each slot to a class. Both methods are compared to the standard static threshold model.

The focus of this paper is a model that dynamically determines the optimum threshold for each generated function during the fitness evaluation (Dynamic Model). The whole training dataset is used for both threshold determination and evolution. The fitness evaluation has a single objective of minimizing misclassification cost, so the optimum threshold for each function is the one that achieves the lowest cost. An associated class rule specifies which class is below the threshold. The Static Model and Dynamic Model are compared on the basis of misclassification cost results after equal numbers of fitness function calls.

2   Dynamic Model Fitness Function Design

The Dynamic Model requires a number of steps in the fitness function to find the optimum threshold. These steps involve additional computation which increases with the number of rows in the training dataset.

The first step is to store the function output values in the dataset and sort it using these values as the key. This step has asymptotic computational complexity of $O(n \log_2 n)$ where n is the number of rows in the dataset.

The second step is to scan through the sorted dataset setting the threshold equal to the output value, incrementing the number of True Positives(TP) and False Positives(FP) as they occur. The class rule initially maps class P to be at or below the threshold. Therefore a TP occurs when the class label of an input vector is P and a FP occurs when the class label of an input vector is N. Each time the threshold changes the misclassification cost can be determined from:

$$Cost = (\#FP \times FPCost) + (\#FN \times FNCost) \tag{1}$$

This information is then used to update the best cost so far (Best Cost) and the worst cost so far (Worst Cost) over the dataset. We need to store the Worst Cost and the threshold where it occurs, so that we can quickly determine whether swapping each class to the opposite side of the threshold gives a better result. The scan has asymptotic computational complexity of $O(n)$ where n is the number of rows in the dataset.

It is possible to terminate the scan of the sorted dataset early if all rows with a class label equal to P or all rows with a class label equal to N have occurred. If the first situation occurs, then the best possible result from the dataset must have already eventuated. However it is still necessary to check whether the Cost at the end of the dataset needs to update the Worst Cost. This only involves a simple calculation and comparison as the total number of rows with each class label is known. If the second situation occurs, then the worst possible result from the dataset must have already happened, but it is still necessary to check whether the Cost at the end of the dataset needs to update the Best Cost.

Once the scan is complete, the misclassification cost ratio can be computed as follows:

$$MaximumCost = (\#P \times FNCost) + (\#N \times FPCost) \tag{2}$$

$$CostRatio = \min\{\frac{Best\ Cost}{Maximum\ Cost}, \frac{Maximum\ Cost - Worst\ Cost}{Maximum\ Cost}\} \tag{3}$$

The Cost Ratio has a minimum value of zero if all input vectors are correctly classified and a maximum of one if they are all incorrectly classified.

If the first calculation is smaller, the optimum threshold is where the Best Cost occurred and the class rule is set to P (Class P below the threshold). If the second calculation is smaller the optimum threshold is where the Worst Cost occurred and the class rule is set to N (Class N below the threshold).

An algorithmic view of the scan through the dataset is shown in Algorithm 1. There are three terminating conditions. The scan stops at a change in threshold value if all rows with a class label of P or all rows with a class label of N have occurred. Otherwise it stops when it reaches the end of the dataset.

Calculate Maximum Cost for dataset;
Initialize: Best Cost = Maximum Cost, Worst Cost = 0, Cost = 0, Best
Threshold = 0, Worst Threshold = 0, Current Threshold = Row 1 output
value, #TP = 0, #FP = 0, Class Rule = P;
for *each row in dataset* **do**
    read output value;
    if *output value > Current Threshold* **then**
        calculate Cost at Current Threshold;
        if *Cost < Best Cost* **then**
          | update Best Cost and Best Threshold
        end
        if *Cost > Worst Cost* **then**
          | update Worst Cost and Worst Threshold
        end
        if *all rows with class label = P have occurred* **then**
          calculate Cost at end of dataset;
          if *Cost > Worst Cost* **then**
            | update Worst Cost and Worst Threshold;
            | break
          end
        end
        if *all rows with class label = N have occurred* **then**
          calculate Cost at end of dataset;
          if *Cost < Best Cost* **then**
            | update Best Cost and Best Threshold;
            | break
           end
        end
        set Current Threshold to output value;
    end
    if *class label = P* **then**
      | increment #TP
    end
    if *class label = N* **then**
      | increment #FP
    end
    if *row is last row in dataset* **then**
        calculate Cost at end of dataset;
        if *Cost < Best Cost* **then**
          | update Best Cost and Best Threshold
        end
        if *Cost > Worst Cost* **then**
          | update Worst Cost and Worst Threshold
        end
    end
end
if *Best Cost ≤ (Maximum Cost - Worst Cost)* **then**
  | return Best Cost/Maximum Cost, Best Threshold, Class Rule = P
else
  | return (Maximum Cost-Worst Cost)/Maximum Cost, Worst
  | Threshold, Class Rule = N
end

Algorithm 1. Scan dataset to determine optimum threshold

3   Comparing the Models Using an Example

We examine both models using a simple dataset with four attributes, a class label of P or N and ten input vectors. This dataset is a subset of the Balance Scales dataset [7]. The fitness objective is to minimize misclassification cost. FP cost is 4.0 and FN cost is 1.0. The following function is used throughout the example.

Function: $Output\ Value = Var2 - (Var3 \times Var4)$

3.1   Static Model

In Table 1, three columns have been added to the basic dataset, one for output value, one for predicted class and one for the result. The Static Model uses a threshold of zero. An output value less than or equal to zero indicates class P.

The result column has five FP and two FN. The Maximum Cost if all items were misclassified is 25.0. So the misclassification Cost Ratio of this function is 22/25 or 0.88.

Table 1. Static Model Example

Var1	Var2	Var3	Var4	Class Label	Output Value	Predicted Class	Result
1	1	1	2	N	-1.0	P	FP
1	2	1	1	P	1.0	N	FN
1	4	5	3	N	-11.0	P	FP
3	2	3	1	P	-1.0	P	TP
2	3	2	4	N	-5.0	P	FP
2	4	2	3	P	-2.0	P	TP
5	2	5	4	N	-18.0	P	FP
5	2	4	5	N	-18.0	P	FP
5	3	1	2	P	1.0	N	FN
5	3	1	4	P	-1.0	P	TP

3.2   Dynamic Model

In Table 2 the dataset has been sorted in ascending order using the output value as the key. Six additional columns have been added to the basic dataset to show the output value, possible thresholds and the number of TP, FP, TN and FN at those thresholds. The final three columns show FP cost, FN cost and Cost .

In the Cost column the Best Cost with class P at or below the threshold is 13 at a threshold of -18.0. The Worst Cost is 22 at a threshold of -1.0. So using Equation 3:

$CostRatio = min\{13/25, (25 - 22)/25\} = 3/25$ or 0.12

The optimum threshold is -1.0 with a class rule of N(Class N below the threshold)

Table 2. Dynamic Model Example

Var1	Var2	Var3	Var4	Class Label	Output Value	Thres-hold	#TP	#FP	#TN	#FN	#FP * 4.0	#FN * 1.0	Cost
5	2	5	4	N	-18.0								
5	2	4	5	N	-18.0	-18.0	0	2	3	5	8	5	13
1	4	5	3	N	-11.0	-11.0	0	3	2	5	12	5	17
2	3	2	4	N	-5.0	-5.0	0	4	1	5	16	5	21
2	4	2	3	P	-2.0	-2.0	1	4	1	4	16	4	20
1	1	1	2	N	-1.0								
3	2	3	1	P	-1.0								
5	3	1	4	P	-1.0	-1.0	3	5	0	2	20	2	22
1	2	1	1	P	1.0								
5	3	1	2	P	1.0	1.0	5	5	0	0	20	0	20

3.3   Cost Comparison

The Static Model achieves a misclassification Cost Ratio of 0.88. The Dynamic Model looks at all the available threshold options for the function and chooses the option that achieves the lowest misclassification Cost. Using the Dynamic Model the example function appears to be a better candidate classifier with a misclassification Cost Ratio of 0.12.

4   Genetic Programming Implementation

All models were implemented in Python with the assistance of the DEAP (Distributed Evolutionary Algorithms in Python) framework [8]. The program was amended slightly to restrict growth during crossover and enable the required use of random seeds.

The genetic programming parameters used are displayed in Table 3.

Table 3. Genetic Programming Parameters

Function set	+ - * / (Safe Division)
Terminal set	Variables from dataset, 1 ephemeral constant
Fitness	Minimize misclassification costs
Selection	Tournament, size = 3
Population Size	200
Initial Max Tree Height	4
Overall Max Tree Height	12
Initial population	Ramped half-and-half
Probability crossover	0.9
Probability mutation	0.01
Termination	After 20 generations

5   Experiments

Table 4 shows the four datasets [7] used in this project, along with their size and number of attributes. The datasets were split 50 : 50 between training data and test data, with the same ratios of positive to negative classes.

Table 4. Dataset Details

Dataset	#P	#N	Total Rows	Attributes
Spambase	2788	1813	4601	57
Ionosphere	225	126	351	34
Sonar	97	111	208	60
Hill Valley With Noise	606	606	1212	100

Four different cost scenarios were used for the experiments as per Table 5. Unit costs were chosen arbitrarily in Scenario 1 and reversed in Scenario 2. Scenario 3 uses equal costs for both FP and FN, so is equivalent to minimizing error (maximizing accuracy). In Scenario 4, costs for misclassifying instances of particular classes are inversely proportional to the frequency of those classes in the dataset. The Hill Valley with Noise dataset is balanced so Scenario 4 is identical to Scenario 3.

Table 5. Misclassification Cost Scenarios

Scenario	Dataset	FP Cost	FN Cost
1	All	4.0	1.0
2	All	1.0	4.0
3	All	5.0	5.0
4	Spambase	6.1	3.9
	Ionosphere	6.4	3.6
	Sonar	4.7	5.3
	Hill Valley With Noise	5.0	5.0

Both models were run thirty times with each dataset for each cost scenario. A random seed was used to generate the same initial population for each model. This seed was generated independently for each run, to ensure diverse initial populations. The discriminant functions were evolved using the training datasets. The evolved functions were measured against the test datasets. The function achieving the lowest misclassification Cost Ratio to date was retained and updated as necessary. The lowest misclassification Cost Ratio achieved at each fitness call was output to a file for later analysis.

6   Results and Discussion

Figure 1 plots misclassification error Cost Ratio averaged over thirty runs on the test datasets against the number of fitness function calls, for cost Scenario 1. In all graphs the Dynamic Model is consistently achieving lower misclassification costs than the Static Model, after an equal number of fitness calls.

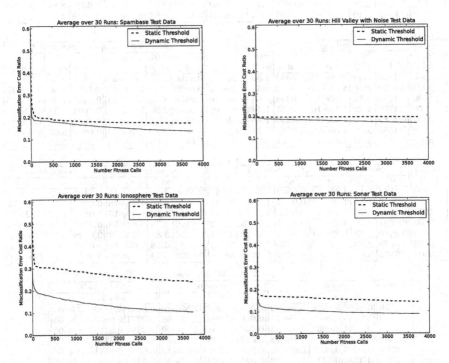

Fig. 1. Performance of Static vs Dynamic models on benchmark problems: Scenario 1

Statistical analysis has been carried out on the results from each dataset at every $500th$ fitness call. Table 6 shows the mean and standard deviation of the differences between the two models, calculated over thirty runs. The differences reflect the improved misclassification Cost Ratio achieved by the Dynamic Model. The p value has been calculated on the differences between the models using a Paired t test. All p values are less than 0.01 so we can say with 99 percent confidence that the differences in the results for these particular fitness calls are not from chance or sampling error.

The statistical results for the Spambase and Hill Valley with Noise datasets show the mean difference increasing as the fitness function call number increases, for all four cost scenarios. This suggests that even better results could have been achieved if the experiments had continued for additional generations.

Table 6. Statistical Analysis of Results

Spambase

Fitness	Scenario 1			Scenario 2			Scenario 3			Scenario 4		
Call	d	sd %	p	d	sd %	p	d	sd %	p	d	sd %	p
500	0.0121	1.70	2.58e-04	0.0020	0.44	9.66e-03	0.0188	1.93	4.96e-06	0.0142	1.64	2.49e-05
1000	0.0152	2.16	2.98e-04	0.0031	0.63	5.68e-03	0.0238	2.64	1.55e-05	0.0238	2.41	4.08e-06
1500	0.0202	2.65	1.29e-04	0.0057	0.93	1.04e-03	0.0272	2.98	1.27e-05	0.0259	2.69	6.02e-06
2000	0.0238	3.00	7.60e-05	0.0068	1.08	9.19e-04	0.0281	3.10	1.39e-05	0.0294	3.25	1.46e-05
2500	0.0282	2.98	7.63e-06	0.0068	1.08	9.20e-04	0.0300	3.47	2.63e-05	0.0305	3.27	9.26e-06
3000	0.0320	2.98	1.14e-06	0.0078	1.22	7.89e-04	0.0324	3.38	6.07e-06	0.0310	3.81	5.80e-05
3500	0.0341	3.10	7.38e-07	0.0087	1.24	3.28e-04	0.0334	3.64	1.20e-05	0.0316	4.01	8.45e-05

Ionosphere

Fitness	Scenario 1			Scenario 2			Scenario 3			Scenario 4		
Fitness Call	$\bar{d}$	Std sd %	p	$\bar{d}$	Std sd %	p	$\bar{d}$	Std sd %	p	$\bar{d}$	Std sd %	p
500	0.1295	1.54	5.68e-29	0.0403	1.56	7.25e-15	0.1160	2.35	2.14e-22	0.1588	4.46	1.63e-18
1000	0.1329	2.80	5.93e-22	0.0329	1.46	2.21e-13	0.0939	3.19	2.48e-16	0.1257	4.86	7.18e-15
1500	0.1390	4.18	9.97e-18	0.0284	1.65	1.25e-10	0.0850	3.55	5.28e-14	0.1130	4.30	4.97e-15
2000	0.1379	4.80	4.73e-16	0.0251	1.74	4.82e-09	0.0749	2.90	7.88e-15	0.1001	4.55	4.06e-13
2500	0.1383	5.26	4.72e-15	0.0230	1.88	1.24e-07	0.0688	3.17	5.65e-13	0.0924	4.81	1.03e-11
3000	0.1364	5.66	4.20e-14	0.0201	2.14	8.61e-06	0.0613	3.57	1.26e-10	0.0892	5.00	5.62e-11
3500	0.1362	5.99	1.83e-13	0.0167	2.30	2.10e-04	0.0570	3.60	7.80e-10	0.0844	5.05	2.41e-10

Sonar

Fitness	Scenario 1			Scenario 2			Scenario 3			Scenario 4		
Call	d	sd %	p	d	sd %	p	d	sd %	p	d	sd %	p
500	0.0547	1.17	9.80e-22	0.0502	1.55	1.94e-17	0.1146	3.44	1.01e-17	0.1150	3.49	1.33e-17
1000	0.0586	1.54	2.58e-19	0.0472	1.51	5.41e-17	0.0919	2.56	1.28e-18	0.0906	4.04	2.49e-13
1500	0.0576	1.74	1.08e-17	0.0463	1.87	2.33e-14	0.0832	3.19	6.00e-15	0.0834	4.07	2.32e-12
2000	0.0581	2.24	6.83e-15	0.0467	2.36	5.17e-12	0.0816	3.76	5.82e-13	0.0786	4.19	1.82e-11
2500	0.0580	2.33	1.92e-14	0.0472	2.54	2.11e-11	0.0757	3.89	7.40e-12	0.0743	4.32	1.26e-10
3000	0.0570	2.63	5.84e-13	0.0439	2.56	1.40e-10	0.0744	4.18	5.69e-11	0.0705	4.32	3.96e-10
3500	0.0555	3.01	2.58e-11	0.0414	2.83	3.78e-09	0.0702	4.49	9.61e-10	0.0678	4.29	7.56e-10

Hill Valley With Noise

Fitness	Scenario 1			Scenario 2			Scenario 3		
Call	d	sd %	p	d	sd %	p	d	sd %	p
500	0.0100	0.0050	4.36e-12	0.0066	0.0042	7.59e-10	0.0237	0.0303	9.34e-05
1000	0.0133	0.0070	1.35e-11	0.0092	0.0065	7.25e-09	0.0271	0.0304	1.73e-05
1500	0.0154	0.0069	3.50e-13	0.0135	0.0088	1.31e-09	0.0291	0.0313	9.86e-06
2000	0.0179	0.0080	2.44e-13	0.0171	0.0086	4.98e-12	0.0276	0.0348	7.93e-05
2500	0.0203	0.0097	1.42e-12	0.0186	0.0083	2.54e-13	0.0322	0.0433	1.65e-04
3000	0.0234	0.0118	4.39e-12	0.0215	0.0090	5.07e-14	0.0490	0.0405	1.46e-07
3500	0.0251	0.0124	2.92e-12	0.0240	0.0103	1.12e-13	0.0437	0.0444	4.37e-06

The Ionosphere and Sonar statistical results show the mean difference staying reasonably static for Scenario 1, but tending to decrease for the other three scenarios. A possible explanation is that once the Dynamic Model achieves something close to the best result, it struggles to improve any further and the Static Model starts to slowly catch up.

All experiments were run using a single set of genetic parameters. Further experiments could vary these parameters to identify their impact on the comparative results.

There are a couple of naive assumptions in the Dynamic Model algorithm that could be reviewed. The threshold is set to the output value. It is possible that additional efficiency gains could be achieved if the threshold was halfway between one output value and the next. Secondly, the best function so far only changes if there is an improvement in fitness. All equally fit functions are ignored.

Adding a secondary criteria to differentiate between equally fit functions may be worth investigating.

Table 7 compares the number of fitness calls required to achieve a certain misclassification Cost Ratio in two of the datasets in cost Scenario 1. The Spambase training dataset achieves a Cost Ratio of 0.17 with 2822 less fitness calls using the Dynamic Model. The Ionosphere training dataset achieves a Cost Ratio of 0.24 with 3688 less fitness calls using the Dynamic Model.

Table 7. Reduction in Fitness Calls

	Spambase Training Data		Ionosphere Training Data	
	Fitness Calls	Cost Ratio	Fitness Calls	Cost Ratio
Static Model	3,700	0.17	3,700	0.24
Dynamic Model	878	0.17	12	0.24
Reduction	2,822		3,688	

Table 8 attempts to quantify the level of computation required by the Dynamic Model to achieve these reductions in fitness calls. The sorting is treated as $n \log_2 n$ operations where n is the size of the dataset. The number of operations involved in sorting the Spam dataset is approximately 22 million, whereas for the Ionosphere dataset it is roughly 16 thousand. The size of the dataset has a large impact on the computational complexity of the Dynamic Model. Measuring the CPU time of both models during future experiments would give a useful indication of the additional time involved in sorting.

Table 8. Extra Operations for Sorting

	Spambase Training Data	Ionosphere Training Data
Training Data Size(n)	2,301	176
Operations($n \log_2 n$)	25,698	1,313
$\times$ Actual Fitness Calls	878	12
= Extra Operations	22,562,844	15,756

7   Conclusions and Future Directions

The Static and Dynamic models were compared experimentally using four cost scenarios with four different datasets. In all the experiments, the Dynamic model achieved statistically significantly better results than the Static model. Results suggest the dynamic threshold approach consistently achieves higher fitness levels than the standard approach after an equal number of fitness calls.

Sorting the dataset at each fitness call is the most computationally expensive part of the Dynamic Model algorithm and might be prohibitive for very large datasets. Further investigation is needed to find a more efficient method of determining the optimal threshold.

References

[1] Poli, R., Langdon, W., McPhee, N.: A Field Guide to Genetic Programming (2008), Published via http://lulu.com and freely available at, http://www.gp-field-guide.org.uk (With contributions by Koza, J.R.)

[2] Espejo, P.G., Ventura, S., Herrera, F.: A survey on the application of genetic programming to classification. IEEE Transactions on Systems, Man, and Cybernetics, Part C: Applications and Reviews 40(2), 121–144 (2010)

[3] Petrović, N.I., Crnojević, V.S.: Impulse noise detection based on robust statistics and genetic programming. In: Blanc-Talon, J., Philips, W., Popescu, D.C., Scheunders, P. (eds.) ACIVS 2005. LNCS, vol. 3708, pp. 643–649. Springer, Heidelberg (2005)

[4] Li, J., Li, X., Yao, X.: Cost-sensitive classification with genetic programming. In: Proceedings of the 2005 IEEE Congress on Evolutionary Computation, vol. 3, pp. 2114–2121 (2005)

[5] Loveard, T., Ciesielski, V.: Representing classification problems in genetic programming. In: Proceedings of the Congress on Evolutionary Computation, vol. 2, pp. 1070–1077 (2001)

[6] Zhang, M., Smart, W.: Multiclass object classification using genetic programming. In: Raidl, G.R., Cagnoni, S., Branke, J., Corne, D.W., Drechsler, R., Jin, Y., Johnson, C.G., Machado, P., Marchiori, E., Rothlauf, F., Smith, G.D., Squillero, G. (eds.) EvoWorkshops 2004. LNCS, vol. 3005, pp. 369–378. Springer, Heidelberg (2004)

[7] Frank, A., Asuncion, A.: UCI machine learning repository (2010), http://archive.ics.uci.edu/ml

[8] Fortin, F.-A., Rainville, F.-M.D., Gardner, M.-A., Parizeau, M., Gagné, C.: DEAP: Evolutionary algorithms made easy. Journal of Machine Learning Research 13, 2171–2175 (2012)

Incremental Constrained Clustering:
A Decision Theoretic Approach

Swapna Raj Prabakara Raj and Balaraman Ravindran

Department of Computer Science and Engineering,
Indian Institute of Technology Madras,
Chennai, 600 036, India
{pswapna,ravi}@cse.iitm.ac.in

Abstract. Typical constrained clustering algorithms incorporate a set of must-link and cannot-link constraints into the clustering process. These instance level constraints specify relationships between pairs of data items and are generally derived by a domain expert. Generating these constraints is considered as a cumbersome and expensive task.

In this paper we describe an incremental constrained clustering framework to discover clusters using a decision theoretic approach. Our framework is novel since we provide an overall evaluation of the clustering in terms of quality in decision making and use this evaluation to "generate" instance level constraints. We do not assume any domain knowledge to start with. We show empirical validation of this approach on several test domains and show that we achieve better performance than a feature selection based approach.

Keywords: Clustering, Constraints, Utility function, Decision theory.

1 Introduction

Cluster analysis is a useful tool for analyzing and understanding data. While typically the analysis is carried out in an unsupervised manner, in many occasions we have some background knowledge about the desired nature of the clusters. Constrained clustering methods typically consider background information or side information in the form of pairwise instance level constraints. Pairwise constraints specify the relationship between a pair of instances as *must-link* constraints that define pairs of data points which should belong to the same cluster, and *cannot-link* constraints that define pairs which should not be assigned to the same cluster [1], [2]. Constrained clustering algorithms attempt to find clusters such that these constraints are minimally violated.

While experts may have some knowledge about the intrinsic characteristics of the data it is difficult to predict the constraints that are relevant to the final use of the mined clusters. Consider the problem of grouping a set of commuters to a college. If the final goal is to allocate parking lots effectively, then it makes more sense to constrain people in the same department together. If the goal is to assign car pool partners, then putting people from the same locality in the

J. Li et al. (Eds.): PAKDD 2013 Workshops, LNAI 7867, pp. 475–486, 2013.

same cluster is more appropriate. But if two people are from the same family, it makes sense to group them even in the first case. While such information might be recoverable from repeated querying for expert input, automating the process of generating constraints to minimize the expert's involvement would be immensely beneficial.

Initial work on constrained clustering assumed that the constraints are specified in a batch style. However, in general not all the constraints are available apriori. We therefore use *Incremental constrained clustering* approach where, the constraints are added or removed incrementally so as to refine the clustering that are produced with existing set of constraints. The main approaches that incrementally add constraints are active learning, where experts are incrementally queried for more constraints [3]; similarity based approaches, where a small seed set of instances are used to generate further constraints [5]; and topology based approaches, which look at spatial distribution of points in order to generate constraints [4].

In our work we propose an architecture that incrementally generates constraints based on individuals preferences to be associated with a certain grouping. Each derived cluster is associated with a particular decision, say a parking lot or a car pool group [1]. Each individual comes with a preference to be associated with each decision. Once the clusters are decided the decisions are arrived at using an optimization procedure that depends on the elements clustered together. We model this process using a decision theoretic setting where the preferences are specified in terms of a utility function. A utility function assigns numerical values to decisions taken corresponding to given scenario. This numerical value represents payoff (either negative (expense/ cost) or positive (net revenue/ profit)). Different combinations of decisions and scenarios generate different payoffs and is represented in the form of table, which is also known as utility matrix.

We use the utility score of the derived decision on each element of the cluster to generate constraints for the clustering process. We attempt to identify pairs of data points which when constrained will result in a large improvement in the overall utility of the clustering. We empirically demonstrate that our approach finds clusters that yield higher utility decisions. Our approach is independent of the exact decision making process and only depends on having available the satisfaction (or utilities) of individuals with the decisions made. In this work we assume that the information is available for each data point, but our overall approach works even when only a subset of the data points express their preference in any given trial. The paper is organized as follows. In Section 2 we give a brief overview of existing work on constrained clustering. In Section 3 we present our incremental decision theoretic constrained clustering framework with an example and in Section 4 we present some empirical results.

---

[1] The motivation for our architecture comes from seminal work by George A. Miller, a cognitive psychologist. He argues that categorization is an important aspect of cognitive behavior and humans first categorize the inputs in order to simplify decision-making [6].

2   Related Work

In constraint clustering based approaches, the clustering algorithm itself is modified to respect the available constraints in order to obtain an appropriate clustering of the data. We observe from earlier work on constrained clustering that initial pairwise constraints are either initially assumed to exist and based on that either constraints can be incrementally added by querying from the user or can be propagated using neighborhood concept.

Cohn et al. [10] proposed a semi-supervised constrained clustering approach where unsupervised clustering method is used to obtain initial clustering of the data followed by presenting the data to the user so that they may critique it. User feedback is a set of constraints that the system tries to satisfy while generating new clustering. The clustering is refined repeatedly using the user feedback until the user is satisfied with the clusters. However, this process is time consuming when a large dataset is used as the clustering algorithm has to be re-run after each set of constraints is added.

Ian Davidson et al. proposed an efficient incremental constrained clustering [3], where the user is allowed to critique a clustering solution by providing positive and negative feedback via constraints. They address the problem of efficiently updating a clustering to satisfy the new and old constraints rather than re-clustering the entire data set.

Active learning scheme for selecting pairwise constraints has also been looked at in order to improve clustering in a semi supervised setting [4]. They acquire constraints or labels from domain experts apriori but use only informative pairwise constraints that are actively selected to improve the performance of clustering.

Eric Robert Eaton [5] focused on constraint propagation which assumes that the specified constraints are representative of their neighborhood. Essentially they perform adaptive constraint propagation based on data point similarity. They propose a method for propagating user-specified constraints to nearby instances using a Gaussian function, and provide an algorithm, GPK-Means, that uses these propagated constraints in clustering. The constraint clustering algorithms focus on finding clusters that merely follow either domain expert given constraints or random constraints.

3   Incremental Constrained Clustering Framework

We introduce an incremental constrained clustering approach where the constraints are generated using a decision theoretic approach. We then use the generated constraints to aid clustering. Our work on constrained clustering neither relies on batch style constraints as given by a domain expert nor randomly generated constraints. Our framework provides a mechanism to find better clusters by using the decision making process after the clustering algorithm. The details of the decision making process is not known to the clustering algorithm except the assumption that the same decision is applied to all data points in a cluster. Thus, the goal is to generate clustering such that the same decision when applied to the cluster is optimal for as many data points as possible.

In order to generate initial set of constraints, we partition the data using a traditional clustering process without considering any constraint information. Once we obtain the clustering an appropriate decision must be taken with respect to it and utility values must be associated with every data point in the cluster based on the utility function. The distribution of utility values are then used for generating a set of must-link and cannot-link constraints. We then perform clustering again based on these constraints until the stopping criterion is reached.

3.1   Decision Making

The usefulness of a pattern depends on the utility of the best decision that is supported by the pattern. Utility function quantifies the reward/penalty for taking different decisions in various contexts. Our focus is to use this utility in mining more useful patterns. The basic settings are as follows:

- We assume that there are fixed set of decisions.
- Decision making is at the level of the clusters i.e., we assign a single decision to each group.
- Same decision applies to all the points belonging to a cluster.
- We assume that the same decision can be applied to more than one cluster
- Goal : To find clustering such that the decisions taken with respect to clusters maximizes the overall utility of the clustering.

The generic form of the decision rule is as follows,

$$d(C_i) = max_j \sum_{k,s.t.,a_k \in C_i} v_{kj} \tag{1}$$

where, v_{kj} = Utility of applying decision j on data point a_k and $d(C_i)$ is the decision applied to cluster C_i. Specifying a v_{kj} for each decision and each data point is cumbersome.

It is more natural to specify the utility based on some intrinsic properties of data. In our work, we consider utility conditioned on class labels or category of data. The knowledge of the class labels is not essential for training purposes. We use class labels in order to define utility function for the purposes of simulation experiments alone. However, utility need not always be limited to class label, but can be conditioned on some other attribute of data. Now we can write the utility as: $v_{kj} = a_{kl}.u_{lj}$ where, a_{kl} = Label of a_k, u_{lj} = Utility of applying decision j to class l. We can now rewrite the generic form of the decision rule as,

$$d(C_i) = max_j \sum_l n_{il}.u_{lj} \tag{2}$$

where, n_{il} = Number of class l points in cluster C_i and u_{lj} = Utility of applying decision j to class l.

3.2   Generation of Constraints

Once a decision is taken with respect to the cluster, the best we can do is to try to separate the data points that have very different utilities. We generate cannot-link constraint between these data points since their utilities are an indicator that the same decision is not suitable for both the points as they reduce the overall utility of the cluster if they are assigned to same cluster. We present the algorithm to generate cannot-link in Algorithm 1.

Algorithm 1. Cannot-link constraint generation

1 **foreach** C_i *in clustering* **do**
2   An optimal decision j is taken in order to obtain a vector of utility values $U_{C_i} = \{v_{1j}, v_{2j}, v_{3j}, \cdots v_{kj}\}$ $\forall$ data points $a_k \in C_i$;
3   Sort the utility vector U_{C_i};
4   Compute the mean μ and standard deviation σ of U_{C_i} and consider data points $m\sigma$ above and below μ, where m is some positive constant;
5   Let $N1$ and $N2$ be the set of data points that fall above and below $\mu + m\sigma$ and $\mu - m\sigma$ of the utility distribution respectively. Consider the pairs from $N1 \times N2$ and form cannot-link constraints between them. These are instances which have larger standard deviation and hence should not belong to the same cluster;

Our intention is also to keep the data points close that have higher utilities. We generate must-link constraint between these data points since their utilities are an indicator that the same decision is suitable for both the points as they improve the overall utility of the cluster if they are assigned to same cluster. We present the algorithm to generate must-link in Algorithm 2.

Algorithm 2. Must-link constraint generation

1 **foreach** C_i *in clustering with utility* $U_{C_i} \geq median(U)$, *where* U *is the vector of all the cluster utilities in clustering* **do**
2   An optimal decision j is taken in order to obtain a vector of utility values $U_{C_i} = \{v_{1j}, v_{2j}, v_{3j}, \cdots v_{kj}\}$ $\forall$ data points $a_k \in C_i$;
3   Sort the utility vector U_{C_i};
4   Compute the mean μ and standard deviation σ of U_{C_i} and consider data points $m\sigma$ above μ, where m is some positive constant;
5   Consider all data points that fall above $\mu + m\sigma$ of the utility distribution and form must-link constraints between every pair of them;

Essentially all the instances that fall after $\mu + m\sigma$ correspond to instances with higher utility and we want such instances to fall in the same cluster, hence must-link relation must exist between all pairs of those instances. Now that we have a newly generated set of constraints, these are now used in the clustering process to yield better partitioning of the data by avoiding the violation of constraints. These sets of constraints acts as an aid for which a constrained clustering algorithm will attempt to find clusters in a data set which satisfy the specified must-link and cannot-link constraints. There exists constrained clustering algorithms that will abort if no such clustering exists which satisfies the specified constraints [1]. However, our approach will try to minimize the amount of constraint violation should it be impossible to find a clustering which satisfies the constraints by associating a weight to each constraint.

3.3 Handling Inconsistent Constraints

Constrained clustering algorithm returns a partition of the instances that satisfies all specified constraints. If a legal cluster cannot be found for the instance, an empty partition is usually returned [1]. This scenario of inconsistent constraint must be handled differently in our work since we must take a decision with respect to every data point. We handle this by assigning weights to the cannot-link constraints alone since the number of must-link constraints generated in our procedure is minimal.

The weight associated with a cannot-link constraint is computed as the difference in the utility values corresponding to the instances that must not belong to the same cluster i.e.,

$$weight(a_1, a_2) = v_{1j} - v_{2j} \qquad (3)$$

where, a_1, a_2 are a pair of data points with a cannot-link relation and v_{1j}, v_{2j} are utilities corresponding to data points a_1, a_2 when optimal decision j was taken with respect to them.

The weights suggests how far away are the utilities (farther away, stronger should the data points repel). The aim is now to generate clusterings with least weight on violated constraints. Obviously when a perfect clustering is possible, then no constraints are violated. The resulting clustering is then used to form a new set of constraints yet again as discussed above. Note that we do not delete constraints from the constraint list. This whole procedure of incrementally generating new constraints is repeated until stopping criterion is satisfied.

3.4 Stopping Criterion

Let the new number of constraints generated be A and the small percentage of total number of possible constraints be B. When A is greater than B we use the newly generated constraints as background information to perform clustering. The whole procedure is then repeated from clustering. If A lesser than equal to B we terminate. Since there are only a finite number of constraints that we can add our process will surely stop. In practice we observe that our process stops before the limit B is reached.

3.5 Example

Consider a scenario from the Vacation travel domain, where a travel agent wishes to segment his customer base so as to promote various vacation packages. Recent research on vacation traveling customers has identified three segments: *Demanders*, *Escapists* and *Educationalists*. Demander's are users who expect luxury service while escapists are users whose intention is to go on a vacation to relax and do not require costly service. Educationalists are users who want to gain more knowledge while traveling such as going out on safari trip, or visit culturally rich places.

Imagine that a travels agent designs two promotion packages say $P1$ and $P2$ for users. The package $P1$ provides facilities such as local tours at very cheap rates and hotel rates are quite moderate while package $P2$ offers great holiday experiences and corporate tours across international destinations. Trying to sell a package designed for a demander to an escapists would probably not succeed. Traditional clustering of the customers would yield compact clusters. But in this case trading compactness of the clusters for more homogeneity in the demographic of the users clustered together is a better approach.

Table 1. Utility function for vacation travel plan

	Demander	Escapist	Educationalist
$P1$	-2	-5	10
$P2$	8	-3	-8

Consider an example of utility function in Table 1 where, the decisions are the promotion packages $P1$ and $P2$. The preference of demander is assigned as a utility weight say 8 for package $P2$ since he is satisfied with the package and a weight of -2 for package $P1$ reflecting that he is least interested in it. Initially the data is partitioned using a traditional clustering process such as k-means clustering without considering any constraint information. Once we obtain the clustering as shown in Fig 1 an appropriate decision must be taken with respect to it.

According to our decision model we chose the decision among a set of finite decisions that provides maximum utility per cluster. In Fig 1 we also show the decisions taken with respect to each cluster. Consider cluster A, when decision $P1$ is applied to all data points in the cluster it results in utility of 12 ($4 \times -2 + 2 \times -5 + 3 \times 10 = 12$). Likewise when decision $P2$ is applied to cluster A it results in utility of 2. Hence $P1$ is the optimal decision that is taken with respect

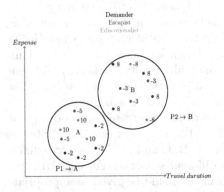

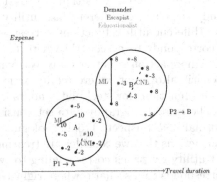

Fig. 1. Utility values assigned to Clustering

Fig. 2. Constraints generated on Travels Data

to cluster A. In the case of cluster B, the optimal decision would be $P2$ as it yields a utility of 7 ($4 \times 8 + 3 \times -3 + 2 \times -8 = 7$) while $P1$ would result in utility of -3.

We then generate the constraints once we have assigned utility values per instance in the cluster. We form *must-link* constraints between pairs of instances that have highest utility and create *cannot-link* between instances which have extreme utilities i.e., high and low utility as shown in Fig 2. We then incorporate these generated constraints into our clustering algorithm to produce new clustering configuration and the whole process is repeated i.e., decision making and generation of constraints with the new clustering till the maximum total utility for the clustering is obtained while respecting the constraints.

4   Experimental Results

In all the experiments we employ a slight variant of constrained k-means clustering algorithm - COP k-means [1] wherein we handle inconsistent data. Recall that the goal of clustering is to find groups such that we can assign a single decision to the clustering. We have to ensure that the value of the decision is optimized. For the purposes of validating our incremental constrained clustering (CC) approach we compared its performance to a feature selection (FS) approach proposed in [8] for utility based clustering. Feature selection chooses a subset of features by eliminating features with little or no predictive information. We compare CC and FS since both methods set up a mechanism for discovering clusters that support relevant decision making. Both CC and FS consider solving the problem as a two stage process with clustering stage followed by a decision making stage.

The data sets we have used in the experiments are the Steel plates faults data set and Cardiotocography data set adopted from UCI repository. The Steel plates faults data set consists of seven classes (158 Pastry, 190 Z-Scratch, 391 K-Scratch, 72 Stains, 55 Dirtiness, 402 Bumps, 673 Other faults) with 1941 instances and 27 attributes. The decisions that we consider are Ignore, Rectify and Recycle. We study the effect of different base utility functions on our architecture, by using two different utility functions corresponding to two different scenarios: Utility 1 corresponds to a scenario where for e.g., when we detect dirt as the fault the ignore action is better than rectifying the fault. Utility 2 reflects a different scenario altogether, where rectify action is suitable for fault such as dirt. The utility functions for steel plates faults is shown in Table 2 and Table 3.

The cardiotocography data set consists of three fetal state class codes (1655 Normal; 295 Suspect; 176 Pathologic) with 2126 instances and 23 attributes. The actions that we consider are treatments A, B, C and D. We used two different utility functions corresponding to two different scenarios. For e.g., Utility 1 corresponds to a scenario where right treatment should be given to appropriate fetal state code, i.e., we assume treatment A should be given to normal while treatment B should be given to suspect case, C to pathologic and D to either normal or pathologic. The utility functions are shown in Table 4.

Table 2. Utility function 1 - Steel Plates Fault dataset

	Pastry	Z scratch	K scratch	Stain	Dirtiness	Bumps	Other faults
				Utility 1			
Ignore	5	-8	-3	-6	10	-6	-2
Rectify	6	-5	-2	10	-9	-5	-3
Recycle	-9	-1	4	-7	-5	10	4

Table 3. Utility function 2 - Steel Plates Fault dataset

	Pastry	Z scratch	K scratch	Stain	Dirtiness	Bumps	Other faults
				Utility 2			
Ignore	-7	8	2	-3	-15	-10	15
Rectify	4	4	6	-7	10	6	-4
Recycle	7	-5	-5	10	-6	15	-10

Table 4. Utility function - Cardiotocography dataset

	Utility 1			Utility 2		
	Normal	Suspect	Pathologic	Normal	Suspect	Pathologic
Treatment A	10	-5	2	-2	-2	4
Treatment B	-3	8	-1	5	-2	-10
Treatment C	-2	-4	10	-2	5	-1
Treatment D	5	-4	5	-5	-5	10

Both CC and FS use the same decision making model where only that decision is selected among a set of decisions which maximizes the cluster utility. We ran both algorithms on these two data sets with different values of k : 5, 8 and 10. For the constrained clustering experiments, we used values of $m = 1$ and $m = 2$. The bound on the number of new constraints generated was set to 11000 for Steel faults dataset and 5000 for Cardiotocography dataset.

Table 5 tabulates the total number of constraints created and number of constraints violated when σ and 2σ were used in the experiments on Steel faults data set, utility 2, $k = 8$. We observe that with 2σ only few constraints are generated as compared to σ resulting in comparatively less constraint violation. Also the performance of the algorithm is much better with 2σ as can be seen from Table 5. Hence for further experiments we set $m = 2$. Table 6 shows the results for FS and CC that we conducted on steel plates data faults with different utility functions as specified in Tables 2 and 3. Likewise Table 7 tabulates the results for FS and CC experiments that we conducted on cardiotocography data set with utility functions specified in Table 4.

All the numbers are averages over ten learning trials. We compute the best utilities achieved before and after applying the two frameworks. The best before performance quantifies the best among ten random hyper-parameter settings in the case of FS and the best among the ten k-means performances without

Table 5. Experiment 2 with different values of $m : k = 8$, Steel faults dataset

Percentage Improvement	σ	2σ
Utility	35%	110%
Purity	8%	14%
Divergence	25%	30%
Total constraints	235687	44541
Violated constraints	8012	228

Table 6. Steel plates faults

	Utility 1						Utility 2					
	$k = 5$		$k = 8$		$k = 10$		$k = 5$		$k = 8$		$k = 10$	
	FS	CC	FS	CC	FS	CC	FS	CC	FS	CC	FS	CC
Best Before	1210	1209	1209	1209	1212	1211	3224	3449	3551	3495	3683	3665
Best After	2525	3029	1406	3399	1283	3033	3900	6251	3578	6487	4642	6126
% imp.	58%	97%	16%	110%	6%	120%	5%	51%	2%	63%	13%	56%

Table 7. Cardiotocography dataset

	Utility 1						Utility 2					
	$k = 5$		$k = 8$		$k = 10$		$k = 5$		$k = 8$		$k = 10$	
	FS	CC	FS	CC	FS	CC	FS	CC	FS	CC	FS	CC
Best Before	6162	5596	6425	5911	6692	6581	1379	1493	1210	1169	1414	1390
Best After	6822	6816	7106	6425	7071	7154	1532	1965	1801	2326	2070	2217
% imp.	6%	10%	5%	15%	4%	9%	23%	41%	79%	101%	30%	48%

constraint information in the case of CC. The best after quantifies the best obtained with the respective architectures, i.e., performance with respect to hyperparameters that are obtained during the local search in FS; performance with respect to new constraints that are generated in CC. We report the average performance improvement observed in the results as well.

We observe that the steel plates faults data set which has seven class labels performs well with $k = 8$ and 10. Also, the cardiotocography data set performs well with $k = 8$. The decision theoretic constrained clustering approach outperforms feature selection approach in all the cases since we are directly tuning the data instances in the case of constrained clustering. However, the feature selection method tries to tune the features and often there is no simple relation between the features and clustering. The quality of clusters are also evaluated using couple of intrinsic measures such as : Cluster purity and Cluster divergence (mean standard deviation). The Tables 8 and 9 shows the divergence and cluster purity values with constrained clustering approach on different data sets with various k values. Table 8 indicates that with $k = 5$ the average percentage increase in cluster divergence is high with 36 percent improvement with utility 1. Table 8 shows that divergence in most of the cases increases. On the other hand, there is not much change in purity values. This means that if we go just by divergence or purity, we may not get higher utility clusters.

Table 8. Constrained clustering, Steel plates fault

	Utility 1			Utility 2		
	$k = 5$	$k = 8$	$k = 10$	$k = 5$	$k = 8$	$k = 10$
Divergence Before	1162	850	905	1137	904	898
Divergence After	1586	1105	1054	1471	1114	1086
Purity Before	0.29	0.32	0.34	0.29	0.33	0.34
Purity After	0.36	0.41	0.39	0.36	0.40	0.40

Table 9. Constrained clustering, Cardiotocography dataset

	Utility 1			Utility 2		
	$k = 5$	$k = 8$	$k = 10$	$k = 5$	$k = 8$	$k = 10$
Divergence Before	11	10	10	11	10	9
Divergence After	17	13	12	13	12	13
Purity Before	0.70	0.71	0.72	0.69	0.70	0.73
Purity After	0.50	0.71	0.73	0.68	0.71	0.72

We initially compared the performance of CC to simple active learning based incremental constrained clustering baselines. The baseline queried a powerful oracle about constraints between selected pairs of data points. The oracle uses the true best-preference information of the data points, and returns a must-link constraint if the preferences are same and a cannot link constraint if they are different. At each round of the clustering, the baselines were allowed as many queries as the no. of constraints added by our method. The two variants that we used were to pick pairs at random from within a cluster; and to pick pairs that consisted of the centroids and the farthest points from them. To our dismay performing incremental clustering in this fashion caused a decrease in the overall utility score, as seen in Table 10. These experiments were conducted on the steel plates data sets with a utility function from Table 2. Therefore we decided to adopt baselines that looked at the utility information as well.

Table 10. Comparison of Incremental CC approaches

	$k = 3$			$k = 5$		
	CC	Random	Pairs	CC	Random	Pairs
Best Before	1209	1209	1209	1209	1209	1209
Best After	3693	980	1129	3213	747	742
% imp.	185%	-23%	-14%	149%	-53%	-56%

Note that utility functions are just one form of preferences that we can use in our framework. It is generic enough to accommodate other forms of feedback as-well. We can use a much weaker utility information like satisfaction estimate on a 1-10 scale. For e.g., if data points X and Y get clustered together and X is satisfied with the decision (say 10/10) and Y is not (say 2/10), then we can insert a cannot-link constraint between them.

5   Conclusion

In this paper we have presented an incremental constrained clustering approach where we add clustering constraints, based on the utility assigned to points in a cluster using decision theoretic framework. Clustering is then repeated to incorporate these constraints and improve utility of the cluster. Decision theoretic measure is a task-oriented evaluation where the patterns performance is tied to an application task. Our work on constrained clustering neither relies on batch style constraints as given by a domain experts nor randomly generated constraints. Our approach generates constraints based on the derived utility and not merely based on background knowledge.

We have compared our framework with a feature selection framework and observe that our approach performs better than the feature selection method. The proposed architecture consists of a clustering stage followed by a decision making stage where the goal of the clustering algorithm is to find clusters that maximize the utility. The clustering process is unaware of the details of the decision making stage. The utility of decisions made are then used to tune certain hyper-parameters of the clustering algorithm. The hyper-parameters of the constrained clustering we consider are the pair-wise constraints.

References

1. Wagstaff, K., Cardie, C., Rogers, S., Schroedl, S.: Constrained K-means Clustering with Background Knowledge. In: 18th International Conference on Machine Learning (ICML), pp. 577–584. Morgan Kaufmann, San Francisco (2001)
2. Wagstaff, K., Cardie, C.: Clustering with instance-level constraints. In: 17th International Conference on Machine Learning (ICML), pp. 1103–1110. Morgan Kaufmann, Stanford (2000)
3. Davidson, I., Ravi, S.S., Ester, M.: Efficient incremental constrained clustering. In: 13th ACM SIGKDD International Conference on Knowledge Discovery and Data Mining, pp. 240–249. ACM, San Jose (2007)
4. Basu, S., Banerjee, A., Mooney, R.J.: Active Semi-Supervision for Pairwise Constrained Clustering. In: SIAM International Conference on Data Mining (SDM). SIAM, Florida (2004)
5. Eaton, E.: Clustering with Propagated Constraints. University of Maryland Baltimore County (2005)
6. Miller, G.A.: The Magical Number Seven, Plus or Minus Two: Some Limits on Our Capacity for Processing Information. Psychological Review 63, 81–97 (1965)
7. Kleinberg, J., Papadimitriou, C., Raghavan, P.: A Microeconomic View of Data Mining. Data Mining Knowledge Discovery 2, 311–324 (1998)
8. Swapna Raj, P., Ravindran, B.: Utility Driven Clustering. In: 23rd International Florida Artificial Intelligence Research Society Conference (FLAIRS). AAAI Press, Florida (2011)
9. Tasi, C.-Y., Chiu, C.-C.: A purchase-based market segmentation methodology. Expert System Applications 27, 265–276 (2004)
10. Cohn, D., Caruana, R., Mccallum, A.: Semi-supervised clustering with user feedback. Technical report (2003)

Querying Compressed XML Data

Olfa Arfaoui and Minyar Sassi-Hidri

Université Tunis El Manar,
Ecole Nationale d'Ingénieurs de Tunis,
BP. 37. Le Belvédère 1002 Tunis, Tunisia
{olfa.arfaoui,minyar.sassi}@enit.rnu.tn

Abstract. The exploitation of large volume of XML (eXtensible Markup Language) data with a limited storage space implies the development of a special and reliable treatment to compress data and query them. This work studies and treats these processes in order to combine them via a mediator while facilitating querying compressed XML data without recourse to the decompression process. We propose a new technique to compress, re-index and query XML data while improving XMill and B+Tree algorithms. We show the reliability and the speed up of the proposed querying system towards response time and answers' exactitude.

Keywords: XML, Compression, Querying, B+Tree, XMill, eXist.

1 Introduction

XML [1] becomes one of the most reliable and important technologies which followed the appearance of the popular technology *HTML* (HyperText Markup Language) [2] and the *WWW* (World Wide Web).

The main use of this technology is to store data in a structured format in order to exploit them via a querying process.

Indeed, *XML* is often considered as self-describing data because it is designed so that the scheme is repeated for each record in the document. This feature provides its flexibility, but it also introduces the problem of what we called verbose *XML* documents which entails huge volumes of data.

Several studies have been proposed to develop and improve approaches and methods of compressing *XML* data [3–9].

The main objectif of these tools is essentially to establish reliable solutions to solve the problems resulting from the large *XML* data volume.

They present several advantages such as the decreasing of both transmission costs of *XML* data over the network (at the client-server communication) and disk space responsible for the document storage and the minimization of needs in main memory for the processing and the querying of *XML* documents.

Several works have been developed and proposed in order to improve *XML* querying process while using compression techniques [10, 11]. However, with the large volume of *XML* data, these solutions become insufficient to insure an efficient compression and decompression in terms of size and run time.

J. Li et al. (Eds.): PAKDD 2013 Workshops, LNAI 7867, pp. 487–498, 2013.
© Springer-Verlag Berlin Heidelberg 2013

The purpose of this paper is to try to find solutions to this problem by i) improving a compression *XML* data technique; ii) re-indexing compressed data; iii) querying *XML* data resulting from the compression process and finally iv) studying the performance of this approach on compressed data.

The rest of the paper is organized as follows: section 2 presents backgrounds on compressing and indexing *XML* data. Section 3 presents our approach for querying compressed *XML* data. Section 4 evaluates the proposed approach by giving some experimentations. Section 5 concludes the paper and highlights future work.

2   Backgrounds

2.1   About Indexing XML Data

As in many markup languages, an *XML* document relies heavily on three fundamental building blocks: elements, attributes, and values. An element is used to describe or contain a piece of information.

To handle and process such data, *XML* documents can be represented as trees whose leaves contain textual data. This tree has several types of nodes.

Recall that the essential purpose of indexing techniques is to find methods that ensure faster access to a given well-defined data and thus avoid a sequential scan of the entire document.

Two approaches are used for indexing *XML* documents: indexing based on the values and structural indexing [12]. To index data according to their values, the data structure commonly used in DB are the *B+Tree* [13].

The structural indexing is considered as the basis of research on *XML* indexing. It is based exclusively on the notion of vertex numbering plan. Several works were been done in order to perform and improve these numbers. We distinguish between the following methods [14] :

- Dietz numbering plan;
- Numbering based on the position of nodes;
- The XISS system;
- K-ary tree level Numbering;
- Dynamic level numbering;
- Virtual level numbering.

2.2   About Compressing XML Data

During recent years, a large number of *XML* compressors were been proposed in the literature. These compressors can be classified into three main characteristics which are: (1) The consideration of the *XML* documents structure, (2) the ability to support queries, (3) the operating speed of the compressor.

In the first characteristic, the compressors can be divided into two main groups. In the first group, text file compressors, *XML* data can be stored as text files, so the first logical approach to compress this data is to use traditional tools for compressing text documents.

This group of compressors is called *blind* since it traits *XML* documents exactly by the same way as text documents by applying traditional compression of text. We can give as an example *GZip* [15] and *BZip2* [16] compressors. The second group of compressor is designed so that to be specific to the *XML* format, by taking into account the structure of the *XML* document to achieve a compression ratio better than that achieved by text compressors.

These compressors can be further classified according to their dependence or not to the *XML* schema.

XML Schema dependent compressors need to have access to the *XML* schema of the document to start the compression process such as *XAUST* [17].

In *XML* Schema independent compressors, the existence of the *XML* diagram is not necessary to start the process of compression such as *SCMPPM* [18]. For the second feature, we distinguish those that allow the querying of those which do not allow.

The first compressors allow the execution of queries on compressed *XML* documents. However, the main objective of this type is to avoid decompressing of the document during query execution. By default, all queried *XML* compressors are not really perfect such as *XGrind* [19].

Others *XML* compressors do not allow the execution of queries on compressed *XML* data. The main objective of these compressors is to achieve the highest compression ratio. By default, the text file compressors belong to the group of non queried compressors such as *XAUST* [17] and *SCMPPM*[19] compressors.

The third feature indicates whether the operating speeds of the compressor is so online or off line.

Based on comparative study presented in [20], we deduced that *XMill* [7] is the most efficient algorithm thats why our intervention will start from an *XML* document compressed by *XMill*.

The aim of our work is to find an algorithm that solves the problem of adapting an indexing algorithm to compressed *XML* data while keeping the performance offered by the *XMill* compressor [7].

3   Querying Compressed XML Data

3.1   Overview of the Approach Steps

The aim of our work is to find a model that solves the problem of adapting an indexing algorithm to compressed *XML* data while keeping the performance offered by the *XMill* compressor [7].

For this, we will try to find a combination of an *XML* indexing method and compressed *XML* data [20] .

So, the structure of a compressed *XML* file given by *XMill* [7] is composed by several parts: the first contains the document structure and the other contains data. For this, our work consists in intervening in the separation of the structure step from the data during the compression process [20].

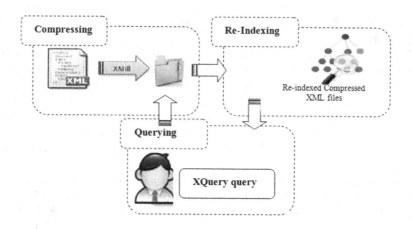

Fig. 1. Overview of the approach steps

As shown is Fig. 1, we have as input a set of compressed *XML* files given by *XMill* and the user *XQuery* query [11].

The purpose of our approach is to index the compressed data by *XMill* [7] so that the user can make a query for a research on these data.

3.2   Re-indexing Compressed XML Data

Based on Dietz numbering plan [21], our idea is to involve us in the construction step of the container structure. So, instead of linking each node of the *XML* tree symbols and numerical identifiers, we associate them to each node a quadruplet obtained by applying the Dietz numbering plan and the tag identifier (obtained by applying the *XMill* algorithm).

That is to say, in the traversal of the *XML* file and during the preparation of different containers, instead of associating symbol (defined by the algorithm *XMill*) to data dictionary, we allocate it the values of the quadruplet.

Let us take the following example of an *XML* file. It describes a *paper* presented through its *title*, the *publication date* and the *conference* in which it is presented.

```
<paper><entryyear="2003">
<journal> <title>Secret Sharing</title>
</journal></entry>
<entry year="2003"><conference><title>{\em XML} Water Mark
</title></conference></entry>
</paper >
```

To make understand easier, the following notations are used in the rest of the paper:

- *TB* : Traversal of the tree from Top to Bottom and from left to right;
- *BT* : Traversal of the tree from Bottom to Top and from left to right;

- *Lev* : The depth of the tree;
- *Idi* : The node identifier.

As a result, a node is identified by the quadruplet (TB, BT, Lev, Idi).

The new format of the *XML* document is illustrated in Fig. 2 which presents an explanatory diagram of our theoretical method applied to the previous example.

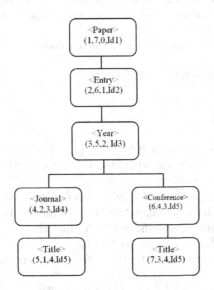

Fig. 2. Rewriting of the *XML* tree

We take for example the case of the tag *Title*, this tag has the quadrupled *(5,1,4,Id5)*. The first integer (5) shows the position of the *XML* tree traversal from top to down. The second integer (1) shows the position of the *XML* tree traversal from bottom to top. The third integer (4) defined the depth of this node (the level) in the *XML* file and the Id5 corresponds to the node identifier obtained through the application of the *XMill* algorithm.

The purpose of re-indexing and compression procedure is to improve the indexing step by the introduction of the Dietz numbering plan in the B+Tree indexing algorithm. Thus, this procedure can improve the compression process through the assignment of a quadruplet *(TB,BT,Lev,Idi)* at each node of the *XML* tree. These integers (the quadruplet) will be recorded later in the container structure.

We run the following algorithm for each node of the *XML* tree.

Algorithm 1. Re-indexing and compressing

Require: The tree corresponding to the input *XML* file

Ensure: The new *XML* tree where each node is identified by the quadruplet (TB, BT, Lev, Idi)

1: *XML* tree traversal by adopting the TB traversal
2: Determination of the integer obtained following the TB traversal
3: *XML* tree traversal by adopting the BT traversal
4: Determination of the integer obtained following the BT traversal
5: Determination of the integer Lev corresponding to the node depth in the *XML* tree

6: Application of the *XMill* compressor on the tree nodes to retrieve the node identifier Idi
7: Recording of the quadruplet (TB, BT, Lev, Idi)

3.3   Querying Process

In the indexing step, the structure container is decompressed. In which case, we can find the sought node by applying the B+Tree algorithm which requires that the nodes of the tree are ordered.

This property is verified by the application of the Dietz numbering plan.

To perform a search in a tree, we need to define relationships between navigation nodes by applying specific relations like that of *father-son, ancestor-descendant, next-brother* and *previous-brother*.

These relationships are shown by the following equations:

$$ancestor(n, n') = preceding(n, n') \wedge n.post > n'.post . \tag{1}$$

$$descendant(n, n') = ancestor(n', n) = n'.pre < n.pre \wedge n'.post > n.post . \tag{2}$$

$$parent(n, n') = ancestor(n, n') \wedge n.pre + 1 = n'.pre . \tag{3}$$

$$preceding - sibling(n, n') = preceding(n, n') \wedge \exists n''(parent(n'', n) \wedge parent(n'', n')) . \tag{4}$$

where n, n' and n'' are nodes belonging to the tree of the *XML* file.

The following algorithm, called *Q2XD* (Querying *XML* by *XMill* compressor and Dietz numbering plan), allows to find the sought node and display the data of each node of the *XML* tree.

4   Evaluation

4.1   Experimental Data

We experiment our approach on large *XML* data such as the DBLP.*XML*. We perform a comparison of the results given by our approach and the initial source file.

The size of this file is 127 MB in non-compressed form and 23MB in the compressed one. It contains 3,332,130 elements and 404,276 attributes.

Algorithm 2. Q2XD

Require: Compressed *XML* file, Indexed query
Ensure: A set of query answers
  1: Recovery of compressed *XML* file
  2: Reading of the query
  3: Extraction of searched key-words
  4: Decompression of the *XML* file
  5: Recovery of the structure container
  6: **repeat**
  7:   **for** Each E **do**
  8:     Recovery of the associated quadruplet" (PH, PB, Niv, Idi)
  9:     **if** E verifies the key-words of the query **then**
 10:       **if** E is a parent node **then**
 11:         Decompression of containers associated to father and child nodes
 12:         Application of the equation (4) in the child nodes of E
 13:         Display the attributes of each node
 14:       **else**
 15:         Display the attributes of each node
 16:       **end if**
 17:     **else** {E don't verifies the query}
 18:       Display *NO-DATA-FOUND*
 19:     **end if**
 20:   **end for**
 21: **until** End structure

4.2   About Response Exactitude

We mention that our goal is to seek information corresponding to each file node.
We try to test in two cases: simple and complex element.

- Simple Query: the purpose is to index a single element. We take the following
  query *Looking for the list of all authors*. Fig. 3 shows the result of running
  Q2XD for author attribute.
- Complex Query: if we want to look different books, the system displays the
  book title, the name of author, the year, the publication reference etc. Fig.
  4 shows the result of running *Q2XD* for book attribute.
  According to Fig. 4, a list of all books is displayed. To check this, we take
  for example the book *ElmasriN89*. Our algorithm displays the following in-
  formations:

  - ElmasriN89
  - RamezElmasri
  - Shamkant B. Navathe
  - Fundamentals of Database Systems
  - Benjamin/Cummings
  - 1989

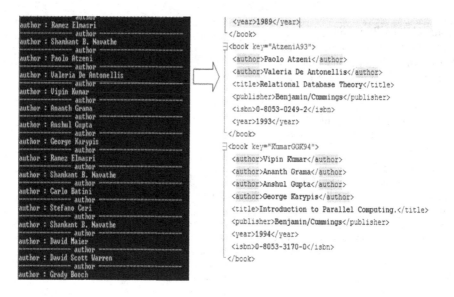

Fig. 3. Running Q2XD for author attribute

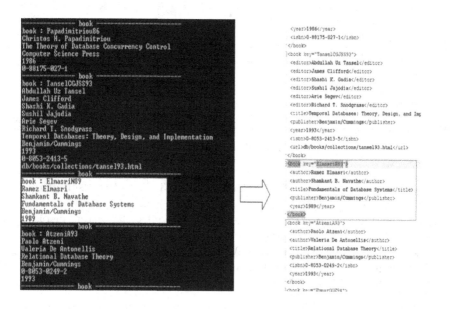

Fig. 4. Running Q2XD for book attribute

If we check the results obtained with the source *XML* file, we find that the displayed information is consistent.

Despite the reduction in the speed and efficiency of the system, the proposed system has proven its performance in querying compressed *XML*.

The contribution of our model has also very remarkable when we examined the execution time of this algorithm in the case of large data set. We note that the speed of execution time and the efficiency result we have get is very important, which leads us to say that the data volume does not have a large impact on execution time.

4.3   About Performance Evaluation

To investigate some indexing approaches, we performed a series of comparative experiments to study their performance.

We use the query processing time as a criterion for measuring performance.

The specification parameters we should take into consideration for a given *XML* source are: the document size, the number of nodes and their values, the path complexity (nesting level) and the average size (short chains or long chains).

In our *Q2XD* algorithm, we define three steps to evaluate a query. The first involves the decompression of the structure container of the compressed file.

The second selects the sought attribute and the container to which it belongs.

The third extracts, decompress and displays founded data.

To compare the performance of the querying process for a given query, we are using different documents on which we have execute some queries. We classify these queries according to the selected data positions in the *XML* tree (for each document) and the response size corresponding to this query (also for each document).

Table 1 gives an example of queries ranking according to these criteria.

Table 1. Queries' classification

Query	*XML* file	Characteristics
Q1	/DBLP.*XML*/book	Large query answer Lots of information
Q2	/DBLP.*XML*/incollection	Small query answer No lots of information
Q3	/Weblog.*XML*/statusCode	Small query answer No lots of information
Q4	/TPC.*XML*/referer	Large query answer Lots of information

Let us take the example of the first query Q_1. The purpose is to seek the element $< book >$ in the *DBLP*.XML document. According to Table 1, it concerns a query with a wide set of answers and so much information.

4.4   About Run Time

We evaluated the performance of *Q2XD* for a wide range of experiences. All experiments were performed on a *Ubunto* machine with a Pentium 4 processor, 2.13 GHz and 3 GB of main memory.

We compared the execution time of a search query from a file element belonging to the *DBLP XML* file to time needed to decompress the same file but using the *XMill* algorithm.

This is well illustrated in Fig. 5 which shows a comparison of execution times required for indexing the *Book, Author, Book title, Pages, Year* and *Publisher* nodes and the time required for decompression *Dec. Time* of the *XML* file.

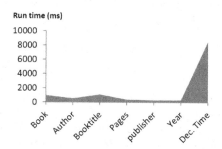

Fig. 5. Run time comparison

We conclude that *Q2XD* is a querying algorithm which includes a decompression process is most efficient in terms of execution time and response time compared to algorithms that developed only for decompression.

4.5   About Complexity

Q2XD algorithm requires that all elements must be ordered. This property is ensured by the numbering system and the different equations defined above.

The complexity of this algorithm is about $O(l \log(n))$ in the worst case, which explains the rapidity of its implementation.

Instead to decompress the entire document, we decompress only two containers, the first one is for the structure and the second one is for content.

Let be consider:

− *T*: the total decompression time;
− *n*: the containers number.

The decompression run time will be:

$$Td = 2 * \frac{T}{n} .$$

$$(5)$$

If the file is very large, the time required for decompression operation will be very negligible compared to the time required for the decompression of the total file.

Similarly the overall complexity of the system is equal to the sum of the complexity of the search and decompression algorithms.

5 Conclusion

The compression of *XML* data remains an inevitable solution to solve problems related to the coexistence of large data volumes. In this context, mining compressed *XML* documents begins to take its place in the data mining research community.

In this work, we have proposed a new querying model which ensures two major processes: the re-indexing and the querying compressed *XML* data.

This constitutes a combination of an adapted *XML* indexing plan such as Dietz numbering plan with an *XML* documents compressor such as *XMill* to facilitate querying compressed *XML* data. So, compressed data are re-indexed based on an adapted Dietz numbering plan to be suitable to our case. The querying process is also developed through the application of the B+Tree algorithm following the re-indexing process.

Hence, the work is done during the separation of the structure from the content in the compression process.

As future work, we propose to i) improve the compression ratio with improved existing methods and to take into account the flexibility in the querying process.

References

1. World Wide Web Consortium, eXtensible Markup Language (XML) 1.0, W3C Recommendation (2006), http://www.w3.org/TR/2006/REC-{XML}-20060816
2. World Wide Web Consortium, XHTML 1.0 The Extensible HyperText Markup Language (2000), http://www.w3.org/TR/xhtml1
3. Cheney, J.: Tradeoffs in XML Database Compression. In: Data Compression Conference, pp. 392–401 (2006)
4. Bača, R., Krátký, M.: TJDewey – on the efficient path labeling scheme holistic approach. In: Chen, L., Liu, C., Liu, Q., Deng, K. (eds.) DASFAA 2009. LNCS, vol. 5667, pp. 6–20. Springer, Heidelberg (2009)
5. Girardot, M.: Sundaresan. N.: Millau: An encoding format for efficient representation and exchange of XML over the Web. Computer Networks 33(1-6), 747–765 (2000)
6. League, C., Eng, K.: Schema Based Compression of XML data with Relax NG. Journal of Computers 2, 1–7 (2007)
7. Liefke, H., Suciu, D.: XMill: An efficient compressor for XML data. In: ACM SIGMOD International Conference on Management of Data, pp. 153–164 (2000)
8. Cheney, J.: Compressing XML with Multiplexed Hierarchical PPM Models. In: Data Compression Conference, pp. 163–172 (2001)
9. Liefke, H., Suciu, D.: An extensible compressor for XML Data. SIGMOD Record 29(1), 57–62 (2000)

10. Tagarelli, A.: XML Data Mining: Models, Methods, and Applications. University of Calabria, Italy (2011)
11. Chamberlin, D.: XQuery: An XML Query Language. IBM Systems Journal 41(4) (2002)
12. Wluk, R., Leong, H., Dillon, T.S., Shan, A.T., Croft, W.B., Allan, J.: A survey in indexing and searching XML documents. Journal of the American Society for Information Science and Technology 53(3), 415–435 (2002)
13. Bayer, R., McCreight, E.M.: Binary B-trees for virtual memory. In: ACM SIG-FIDET Workshop, pp. 219–235 (1971)
14. Nelson, M., Gaily, J.L.: The data compression Book. 2nd Edition M&T Books (1996)
15. Gailly, J.-L.: Gzip, version 1.2.4, `http://www.gzip.org`
16. Seward, J.: bzip2, version 0.9.5d, `http://sources.redhat.com/bzip2`
17. Subramanian, H., Shankar, P.: Compressing XML Documents Using Recursive Finite State Automata. In: Farré, J., Litovsky, I., Schmitz, S. (eds.) CIAA 2005. LNCS, vol. 3845, pp. 282–293. Springer, Heidelberg (2006)
18. Adiego, J., De la Fuente, P., Navarro, G.: Merging prediction by partial matching with structural contexts model. In: IEEE Data Compression Conference, p. 522 (2004)
19. Tolani, P.M., Haritsa, J.R.: XGRIND: A query-friendly XML compressor. In: 18th International Conference on Data Engineering, pp. 225–234 (2002)
20. Jedidi, A., Arfaoui, O., Sassi-Hidri, M.: Indexing Compressed XML Documents, Web-Age Information Management: XMLDM 2012, Harbin, China, pp. 319–328 (2012)
21. Dietz, P., Sleator, D.: Two Algorithms for Maintaining Order in a List. In: 19th Annual ACM Symposium on Theory of Computing, pp. 365–372. ACM Press (1987)

Mining Approximate Keys Based on Reasoning from XML Data

Liu Yijun, Ye Feiyue, and He Sheng

School of Computer Engineering, Jiangsu University of Technology, Changzhou,
Jiangsu, 213001, China
Key Laboratory of Cloud Computing & Intelligent Information Processing of Changzhou City,
Changzhou, Jiangsu, 213001, China
{lyj,yfy,hs}@jsut.edu.cn

Abstract. Keys are very important for data management. Due to the hierarchical and flexible structure of XML, mining keys from XML data is a more complex and difficult task than from relational databases. In this paper, we study mining approximate keys from XML data, and define the support and confidence of a key expression based on the number of null values on key paths. In the mining process, inference rules are used to derive new keys. Through the two-phase reasoning, a target set of approximate keys and its reduced set are obtained. Our research conducted experiments over ten benchmark XML datasets from XMark and four files in the UW XML Repository. The results show that the approach is feasible and efficient, with which effective keys in various XML data can be discovered.

Keywords: XML, keys, data mining, support and confidence, key implication.

1 Introduction

XML is a generic form of semi-structured documents and data on the World Wide Web, and XML databases usually store semi-structured data integrated from various types of data sources. The problem that how to efficiently manage and query XML data has attracted lots of research interests.

Much work has been done in applying traditional integrity constraints in relational databases to XML databases, such as keys, foreign keys, functional dependency and multi-valued dependency, etc.[1,2,3,4,5,6]. As the unique identifiers of a record, keys are significantly important for database design and data management[7]. Various forms of key constraints for XML data are to be found in [6,8,9,10,11]. In this paper we use the key definition proposed by Buneman et al. in [12,13]. They propose not only the concepts of absolute keys and relative keys independent of schema, which are in keeping with the hierarchically structured nature of XML, but also a sound and complete axiomatization for key implication. By using the inference rules, the keys can be reasoned about efficiently.

Though key definitions and their implication are suggested, there are still some issues needed to be considered in the practical mining of XML keys, as pointed out in

J. Li et al. (Eds.): PAKDD 2013 Workshops, LNAI 7867, pp. 499–510, 2013.

[14]. Firstly, there could be no clear keys in XML data which is semi-structured and usually integrated from multiple heterogeneous data sources. Secondly, an XML database may have a large number of keys and therefore we should consider how to store them appropriately. Thirdly, the most important problem is how to find out the keys holding in a given XML dataset in an efficient way. Currently there is not much work in the literature in practical mining of keys from XML data. G''osta Grahne et al. in [14] define the support and confidence of a key expression and a partial order on the set of all keys, and finally a reduced set of approximate keys are obtained. In this paper, we also study the issue of mining keys from XML data. Considering the characteristics of XML data, we propose another universal approach for mining keys.

2   Key Definitions and Related Concepts

The discussions in this section are mainly based on the definitions by Buneman et al.[12,13].

2.1   The Tree Model for XML

An XML document is typically modeled as a labeled tree. A node of the tree represents an element, attribute or text(value), and edges represent the nested relationships between nodes.

Node labels are divided into three pairwise disjoint sets: E the finite set of element tags, A the finite set of attribute names, and the singleton $\{S\}$, where S represents text (PCDATA). An XML tree is formally defined as follows.

Definition 1. An XML tree is a 6-tuple $T=(r, V, lab, ele, att, val)$, where

- r is the unique root node in the tree, i.e. the document node, and $r \in V$.
- V is a finite set containing all nodes in T.
- *lab* is a function from V to $E \cup A \cup \{S\}$. For each $v \in V$, v is an element if $lab(v) \in E$, an attribute if $lab(v) \in A$, and a text node if $lab(v)=S$.
- Both *ele* and *att* are partial functions from V to V^*. For each $v \in V$, if $lab(v) \in E$, $ele(v)$ is a sequence of elements and text nodes in V and $att(v)$ is a set of attributes in V; For each $v' \in ele(v)$ or $v' \in att(v)$, v' is the child of v and there exists an edge from v to v'.
- *val* is a partial function from V to string, mapping each attribute and text node to a string. For each $v \in V$, if $lab(v) \in A$ or $lab(v)=S$, $val(v)$ is a string of v.

2.2   Path Expressions

In the XML tree, a node is uniquely identified by a path of node sequence. Because the concatenation operation does not have a uniform representation in XPath used in XML-Schema, Buneman et al.[12] have proposed an alternative syntax. For identifying nodes in an XML tree, we use their path languages called PL_s, PL_w and PL, where ε represents the empty path, l is a node label in $E \cup A \cup \{S\}$, and "." is concatenation.

In PL_s, a valid path is the empty path or the sequence of labels of nodes. PL_w allows the symbol "_" which can match any node label. PL includes the symbol "_*" which represents any sequence of node labels. The notation $P \subseteq Q$ denotes that the language defined by P is a subset of the language defined by Q. For the path expression P and the node n, the notation $n[P]$ denotes the set of nodes in T that can be reached by following a path that conforms to P from n. The notation $[P]$ is the abbreviation for $r[P]$, where r is the root in T. The notation $|P|$ denotes the number of labels in the path. $|\varepsilon|$ is 0, and "_" and "_*" are both counted as labels with length 1. The paths which are merely sequences of labels are called simple paths.

2.3 Definitions on Keys

Definition 2. A key constraint φ for XML is an expression $(Q', (Q, \{P_1,..., P_k\}))$ where Q', Q and P_i are path expressions. Q' is called the context path, Q is called the target path, and P_i is called the key paths of φ. If $Q' = \varepsilon$, φ is called an absolute key, otherwise φ is called a relative key. The expression (Q, S) is the abbreviation of $(\varepsilon, (Q, S))$, where $S = \{P_1,..., P_k\}$.

Definition 3. Let $\varphi = (Q', (Q, \{P_1,..., P_k\}))$ be a key expression. An XML tree T satisfies φ, denoted as $T \models \varphi$, if and only if for every $n \in [Q']$, given any two nodes n_1, $n_2 \in n[Q]$, if for all i, $1 \leq i \leq k$, there exist $z_1 \in n_1[P_i]$ and $z_2 \in n_2[P_i]$ such that $z_1 =_v z_2$, then $n_1 = n_2$. That is,

$$\forall n_1, n_2 \in n[Q]$$

$$\left(\left(\bigwedge_{1 \leq i \leq k} \exists z_1 \in n_1[P_i] \exists z_2 \in n_2[P_i](z_1 =_v z_2) \right) \to n_1 = n_2 \right)$$

The definition 3 of keys is quite weak. The key expression could hold even though key paths are missing at some nodes. This definition is consistent with the semi-structured nature of XML, but does not mirror the requirements imposed by a key in relational databases, i.e. uniqueness of a key and equality of key values. The definition 4 which meets both two requirements is proposed in [12].

Definition 4. Let $\varphi = (Q', (Q, \{P_1,..., P_k\}))$ be a key expression. An XML tree T satisfies φ, if and only if for any $n \in [Q']$,

(1) For any n' in $n[Q]$ and for all $P_i (1 \leq i \leq k)$, P_i exists and is unique at n'.

. (2) For any two nodes n_1, $n_2 \in n[Q]$, if $n_1[P_i] =_v n_2[P_i]$ for all i, $1 \leq i \leq k$, then $n_1 = n_2$.

The definition 4 of keys is stronger than the definition 3, and the key paths are required to exist and be unique. Note that there probably are empty tags in XML documents. A consequence is that some nodes in $n'[P_i]$ are null-valued, which is allowed in the definition 4. However the attributes of the primary key in relational databases are not allowed null. Here we explore a strong key definition which captures this requirement.

Definition 5. Let $\varphi=(Q', (Q, \{P_1,..., P_k\}))$ be a key expression. An XML tree T satisfies φ, if and only if for any $n \in [Q']$,

(1) For any n' in $n[Q]$ and for all $P_i (1 \leq i \leq k)$, P_i exists and is unique at n', and all nodes in $n'[P_i]$ are not null valued.

(2) For any two nodes n_1, $n_2 \in n[Q]$, if $n_1[P_i] =_v n_2[P_i]$ for all i, $1 \leq i \leq k$, then $n_1 = n_2$.

In the definition 5 of strong keys, the key paths are required to exist, be unique and not have a null value. In relational databases, a tuple can be identified by more than one group of key attributes. Analogously, given a context path Q' and a target path Q in the XML tree T, there exist probably multiple sets S of key paths such that $T \models (Q', (Q, S))$.

Definition 6. Let $\varphi=(Q', (Q, S))$ be a key expression satisfied in the XML tree T. If for any key expression $\varphi'=(Q', (Q, S'))$ satisfied in T, $|S| \mathrel{<=} |S'|$, then φ is called the minimal key.

In other words, a minimal key has the least number of key paths with the determined Q' and Q. Note that there are probably multiple minimal keys with the fixed Q' and Q.

2.4   Node Equality and Value Equality

The key definition involves the issue of node equality and value equality, etc.

Value Equality. Value equality in XML-Schema is restricted to text nodes. Buneman et al.[12] propose a more general way of describing value equality by using tree equality. The example they provided is that when **name** is treated as a key for **person** nodes, **name** may have a complex structure consisting of **first-name** and **last-name** subelements. However, since S in $(Q', (Q, S))$ is the set consisting of multiple key paths, the key with a complex structure can be decomposed to several simple key paths. For **person** nodes, the union of name.first-name and name.last-name can substitute for **name**. Hence in this paper we use the equality of text nodes but not tree quality. $n_1 =_v n_2$ denotes that n_1 and n_2 are value equal.

Node Equality. In an XML tree, a path starting from the root uniquely identifies a node. The nodes n_1 and n_2 are equal, denoted as $n_1 = n_2$, indicating that n_1 and n_2 represent one node in the tree. In a relational database, the key uniquely identifies a record. In XML data, the key is analogously considered to uniquely identify a node, that is, the two distinct nodes n_1 and n_2 certainly cannot have identical values on key paths. However, XML data is flexibly organized, and different nodes may indicate the same entity in real-world. In the example in Figure 1, both the **teacher** nodes represent Li Wen. Node equality needs more consideration especially when discovering absolute keys in the large range of the entire document.

```
<root>
  <course>
    <cno> 009 </cno>
    <cname>Data Stucture</cname>
    <teacher>
      <name> Li Wen </name>
      <gender> Male </gender>
      <age> 35 </age>
    </teacher>
  </course>
  <course>
    <cno> 010 </cno>
    <cname>Operating System</cname>
    <teacher>
      <name> Li Wen </name>
      <gender> Male </gender>
    </teacher>
  </course>
</root>
```

Fig. 1. An example of XML document

We redefine the node equality. If one of the two nodes n_1 and n_2 contains all information of the other, the two nodes are considered to represent the same entity, and consequently they are equal. In XML trees, Let $T(n)$ be the subtree rooted at node n. n_1 and n_2 represent the same entity if and only if $T(n_1)$ is the subgraph of $T(n_2)$, or vice versa, where n_1 matches n_2.

3   Approximate Measures for Keys

Due to the hierarchical and flexible structure of XML, there could be no clear keys in XML data. An XML document possibly has enormous number of keys meeting weak key definitions, and it is time consuming to find out all of them. While among them many keys are uninteresting and even meaningless. G¨osta Grahne et al.[14] propose the concept of approximate keys for XML based on the support and confidence of a key expression, which are similar to those of association rules. The support and confidence is defined respectively according to the number of branches of key paths and the number of distinct values on key paths. We now give the measures in another way.

For simplicity, we consider every element node having a child of text node, and the text node is treated as null-valued if the element has no text.

3.1   The Support of Keys

Given a node n, let $size(n)$ be the number of child nodes of n, indicating the size of n. For a key expression $\varphi=(Q', (Q, S))$ in an XML tree, the size of φ in the tree T is

$$size(T, \varphi) = \max\{size(n) | n \in [Q'.Q]\}$$

The size of φ is the maximum size of nodes reached by $Q'.Q$ of φ from root. For those nodes in $[Q'.Q]$ with extremely small size, e.g. those leaf nodes without children whose size is zero, it becomes meaningless to find their key paths. Therefore *min_size* is set to be the minimum threshold of node size. The support of φ in the whole XML tree T is

$$support(T, \varphi) = \begin{cases} 0 & \text{if } size(T, \varphi) < \text{min\_size} \\ \sum_{n' \in [Q']} |n'[Q]| & \text{otherwise} \end{cases}$$

The support of φ is assigned to 0 when the size of φ is less than *min_size*. Consequently, the category of nodes with too small size is abandoned. When the size of φ is not less than *min_size*, the support of φ is the number of nodes in $[Q'.Q]$.

3.2 The Confidence of Keys

Section 2.3 gives several definitions on keys for XML, among which the definition 3 is the weakest, the definition 4 is stronger, and definition 5 is the strongest. The choice of key definitions, which will affect the final mining results, should be ultimately determined by practice. In the process of mining keys, when choosing the strong key definition, probably no keys are discovered in semi-structured XML documents. However, if the weak key definition is chosen, probably meaningless key paths appear. Therefore we define the confidence to achieve a compromise.

Given a key expression $\varphi=(Q', (Q, S))$ in an XML tree, $S=\{P_1, P_2, ...,P_k\}$. Define a two-valued function *vals(n, P)*, where n is a node and P a path expression. If there exists $z \in n[P]$ and z is not null valued, *vals(n, P)* is assigned to 1, and otherwise 0. The confidence of φ in the tree T is

$$confidence(T, \varphi) = \frac{\min\left\{ \sum_{n \in [Q']} \sum_{n \in n'[Q]} vals(n, P_i) | P_i \in S \right\}}{support(T, \varphi)}$$

In particular, we set *confidence(T, φ)=1* when *support(T, φ)=0*.

The support of φ is defined associated with target paths and the confidence associated with key paths. The key paths of φ are computed if φ satisfies the specified support threshold *min_sup*. Specify the confidence threshold *min_conf*, allowing the null values or missing paths but confine their number. In particular, with *min_conf=0*, the null values or missing paths have no impact on satisfaction of φ, and with *min_conf=1*, they are not allowed.

3.3 The Measures of Absolute Keys

An absolute key is a special case of a relative key. Given an absolute key expression $\varphi= (Q, S)$ in the XML tree T, where Q' is ε and omitted. The size, support and confidence of φ are

$$size(T,\varphi) = \max\{size(n)|n \in [Q]\}$$

$$support(T,\varphi) = \begin{cases} 0 & \text{if } size(T,\varphi) < \text{min\_size} \\ \|[Q]\| & \text{otherwise} \end{cases}$$

$$confidence(T,\varphi) = \frac{\min\left\{ \sum_{n \in [Q]} vals(n, P_i)|P_i \in S \right\}}{support(T,\varphi)}$$

4   Mining Approximate Keys Based on Reasoning

4.1   Target Keys to Be Mined

Philosophically, if a tuple is treated as representing some real world entity, the key provides an invariant connection between the tuple and entity. In relational databases, the key uniquely identifies a tuple, and is the link between the tuple and entity[12]. In XML databases, the node set of $n[Q](n \in [Q'])$ is analogous to a set of tuples in a relation and the key paths to the key attributes of the relation. Due to the irregular semi-structure of XML, the nodes associated with a special category of entities may appear at an arbitrary position in the XML tree. The keys that can accurately and globally identify those nodes are the absolute keys in form of $(\_*.l, S)$, where l is an element label.

Proposition 1. If $T\models(\_*.l, S)$, and for the pairwise context path Q' and target path Q in T, Q has the suffix of l, then $T\models(Q', (Q, S))$.

$[Q'.Q] \subseteq [\_*.l]$ since Q has the suffix of l. Obviously, S can certainly identify the l nodes in the scope within the subtree if it can identify them in the entire XML tree. The absolute keys of $(\_*.l, S)$ are of special significance.

This paper aims to find out the set K_G of key expressions holding in T. K_G contains all absolute keys of (Q, S) and relative keys of $(Q', (Q, S))$, where $S=\{P_1,...,P_k\}$, which meet the following requirements:

(1) The path expressions of Q', Q and $P_i(1 \leq i \leq k)$ are all in PL_s.
(2) Let l be the suffix node label of Q. If $T\models(Q', (Q, S)$ or $T\models(Q, S)$, then $T\models(\_*.l, S)$.

For the second requirement, we find the key paths for Q' and Q that can globally identify a special category of nodes.

Let K_I be the set of key expressions in form of $(\_*.l, S)$ satisfied in T, that is $K_I=\{(\_*.l, S)| T\models(\_*.l, S)\}$. K_G can be obtained by two-phase reasoning starting from K_I.

4.2   Reasoning about Keys

Logical Implication on Keys. Similar to functional dependency, XML keys also have the issue of logical implication. Here the definitions about logical implication on keys by G"osta Grahne et al. is adopted. Further details are provided in[14].

Inference Rules for Key Implication. Buneman et al.[12] propose the sound and complete axiomatization, solving the problem of key implication for XML. In this paper, to compute the K_G starting from K_I the initial set of absolute keys, only two inference rules are needed.

R_1: $(Q', (Q_1, S))$, $Q_2 \subseteq Q_1 \Rightarrow (Q', (Q_2, S))$

R_2: $(Q', (Q_1.Q_2, S)) \Rightarrow (Q'.Q_1, (Q_2, S))$

R_1 is the rule of target-path-containment and R_2 is the rule of context-target[14]. Let K be the set of absolute keys in K_G. We firstly compute K from K_I by applying rule R_1, and then K_G can be obtained from K by applying rule R_2.

The Inference Procedure. A two-phase inference process for keys is followed.

1. Phase I: Infer K from K_I

K can be inferred from K_I with R_1. The context path Q' in R_1 is ε since K_I and K contain only absolute keys.

The rule R_1 is complete for K. That is, for every key expression $\varphi \in K$, φ is inferable from K_I by applying R_1. For a key expression (Q, S) in K, Q is a simple path and has the suffix of node label l. Because $(\_^*.l, S) \in K_I$ and $Q \subseteq \_^*.l$, (Q, S) can be inferred from $(\_^*.l, S)$ by using R_1.

It should be noted that if we set interestingness thresholds, the keys inferred from K_I are probably fake keys which don't satisfy the specified thresholds.

2. Phase II: infer K_G from K

K_G can be inferred from K by using R_2. Here we prove that K is a minimal set of key expressions from which K_G can be inferred by R_2.

Proposition 2. By applying the rule R_2, $K^+ = K_G$ and K has no redundant keys.

We prove $K^+ = K_G$ and then that K is non-redundant.

(1) $K^+ = K_G$.

For an absolute key (Q, S), (Q, S) is in K_G if and only if (Q, S) is in K.

Consider relative keys of $\varphi_1 = (Q'.Q, S)$ and $\varphi_2 = (Q', (Q, S))$. By the definitions of support and confidence we have $support(T, \varphi_1) = support(T, \varphi_2)$ and $confidence(T, \varphi_1) = confidence(T, \varphi_2)$. Hence, no fake key is generated in reasoning by the rule R_2. That φ_1 is in K iff. φ_2 is in K_G can be achieved as follows. On the one hand, if $\varphi_1 = (Q'.Q, S)$, equivalent to $(\varepsilon, (Q'.Q, S))$, is in K, by the rule R_2 we obtain $\varphi_2 = (Q', (Q, S))$. $Q'.Q$ is in PL_s, and then Q' and Q are both in PL_s. Hence, φ_2 is in K_G by the requirements of keys in K_G. On the other hand, if φ_2 is in K_G, by the rule R_2, φ_2 can be inferred from φ_1, equivalent to $(\varepsilon, (Q'.Q, S))$. Q' and Q are both in PL_s, and then $Q'.Q$ is also in PL_s. Hence, φ_1 is in K.

(2) K is minimal. The set of K contains no relative keys. For any key expression φ in K, φ is an absolute key and is not inferable from $K \setminus \{\varphi\}$ by applying R_2. Therefore K is non-redundant.

4.3   A Sketch of Key Mining Process

A two-step key mining process is followed, consisting of discovery and inference. In practice, the measures of support and confidence can be used if needed.

The Discovery Step. We find out K_I, the set of key expressions in form of $(\_*.l, S)$ which hold in the XML tree T. This step is divided into two phases. In the first phase, the target paths of $\_*.l$ satisfying the support threshold are generated. In the second phase, for each target path, the set S of key paths, satisfying the confidence threshold, is generated. Note that here only minimal keys are discovered.

The Inference Step. There could be a large number of key expressions in K_G, while K is a compact representation for K_G by proposition 2, therefore this paper only discovers the set K, which is inferable from K_I with R_1. Apply the rule R_1 to every key expression $(\_*.l, S)$ in K_I. By traversing the XML tree, the target path set of $QS=\{Q_1, Q_2,...,Q_n\}$ is generated, where Q_i is in PL_s and $Q_i \subseteq \_*.l$, that is, Q_i is a simple path with the suffix of l. The key expressions of $(Q_i, S)(1 \leq i \leq n)$ are generated. Here we mine approximate keys with the support and confidence thresholds, and therefore need to examine whether the keys of (Q_i, S) $(1 \leq i \leq n)$ satisfy both the thresholds and remove those fake keys.

5   Experimental Study

In this section, we perform experiments on two categories of XML datasets to evaluate our approach. The first category of datasets is from XMark which is an XML benchmark project, and the second is from UW XML Repository. The algorithms are implemented in the C/C++ language and programs are executed on Microsoft Visual C++ 6.0. All experiments are conducted on computers with an INTEL Core 2DuoProcessorG630 and 3G memory, running Windows XP.

5.1   Experiments on the XMark Datasets

XML data generator **xmlgen** produces scaled documents according to the DTD specified in the project of XMark. Further details are provided on http://www.xml-benchmark.org. Ten XML documents D1-D10 with different size are generated as benchmark datasets for our experiments.

Here some experiments have been performed to monitor the time needed to discover the keys in the set K_I and infer new keys from K_I. Figure 2 shows the empirical results obtained on the ten documents, given the minimum support threshold *min_sup*=30 with *min_size*=2 and the minimum confidence threshold *min_conf*=80%. T0 is the time of discovering the keys in K_I, T1 corresponds to the inference time for deriving new keys from K_I, and T2 is the sum of T0 and T1. Obviously, T0, T1 and

T2 all increase as the document size increase. However, T1 increases much more slowly than T0. The process of finding K_I is expensive, compared with which the cost of inference is negligible.

Figure 3 shows the performance of the time T2 on the documents D1, D5 and D10 with various confidence thresholds, given *min_sup*=30. All the three time curves are downward generally. The curves seem smooth when *min_conf* is less than 85%. The reason is that almost all the keys with confidence greater than 50% have a confidence not less than 85%. But the time T2 decreases slightly when *min_conf* is greater than 85%, because the keys with confidence not satisfying the threshold are removed, saving a small amount of inference time.

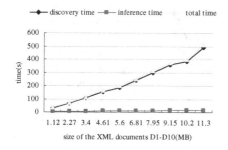

Fig. 2. Performance on D1-D10   **Fig. 3.** Performance on D1, D5 and D10

5.2   Experiments on the UW Datasets

In mining keys from UW datasets, we set a minimum length threshold for key paths. In other words, a depth bound is used to prevent the search process from running away toward nodes of unbounded depth from the node at the target path. We select four xml files of SIGMODRecord, reed, uwm and wsu with various node depth. Further details are provided on http://www.cs.washington.edu/research/xmldatasets/. The *min_sup* is set to 5 with *min_size*=2 for all, while the *min_conf* is set to 80% for SIGMODRecord, reed and wsu and 50% for uwm.

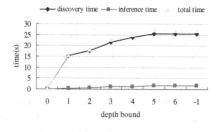

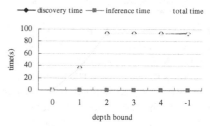

Fig. 4. Performance on SIGMODRecord.xml   **Fig. 5.** Performance on reed.xml

The time costs on the four test files are shown in figure 4-7, where "-1" represents a unbounded depth, and the keys discovered are listed in Table 1. Generally the curves rise and then flatten with the depth bound increasing. In the case of SIGMODRecord with max-depth 6 and avg-depth 5.14107, the key paths discovered with unbounded depth are all have length 1, and therefore the depth bound 1 is sufficient to find out all key paths. From figure 4, setting the depth bound to a smaller value help reduce the discovery time significantly. Intuitively, this is due to that the attribute or element nodes as keys are usually close to the target nodes in hierarchical XML data.

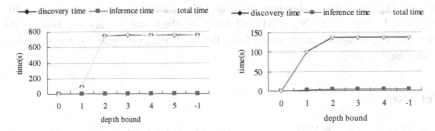

Fig. 6. Performance on uwm.xml   **Fig. 7.** Performance on wsu.xml

Table 1. Keys discovered in four UW XML files

filename	key	S	support	confidence
SIGMOD Record	(_*.issue, S)	{number, volume}	67	100%
	(_*.article, S)	{endPage, initPage, title}	1504	100%
reed	(_*.course, S)	{days, reg_num}	703	98%
	(_*.time, S)	{start_time, end_time}	703	98%
	(_*.place, S)	{Building, room}	703	93%
uwm	(_*.course_listing, S)	{course}	2112	100%
	(_*.hours, S)	{start, end}	4575	53%
	(_*.bldg_and_rm, S)	{bldg, rm}	4575	74%
wsu	(_*.course, S)	{sln}	3924	95%
	(_*.place, S)	{bldg, room}	3924	100%

6 Conclusions

In this paper, we discuss definitions on keys for XML without considering foreign keys and DTDs and have proposed an approach for mining keys from XML data. Due to that keys are usually not be satisfied at 100% in XML data which has a hierarchical and flexible structure and is usually integrated from heterogeneous sources, we use the support and confidence proposed in[14] for key expressions, but propose novel measure formulae. To find out all satisfiable absolute keys and relative keys with simple target and key paths in an XML tree, we firstly discover an initial set of keys and then two phases of reasoning are used. A reduced set of all target keys are obtained after the first phase of reasoning. Based on the results of our experiments on ten benchmark datasets of XMark and the four chosen files of UW repository, it can be concluded that our approach is effective. During the mining process new keys can be reasoned about efficiently but the discovery of initial keys is time consuming. In this discovery stage, very basic approaches are used. Alternative approaches and further tunings are possible for improving computational efficiency.

Acknowledgement. This work is supported by National Natural Science Foundation of China (61142007) and University Science Research Project of Jiangsu Province (12KJD520003) and Key Laboratory of Cloud Computing & Intelligent Information Processing of Changzhou City (CM20123004). Furthermore, we are indebted to the support and encouragements received from the staff and colleagues of the school of computer engineering.

References

1. Fan, W., Libkin, L.: On XML integrity constraints in the presence of DTDs. J. ACM 49(3), 368–406 (2002)
2. Fan, W.: XML constraints. In: DEXA Workshops (2005)
3. Fan, W., Siméon, J.: Integrity constraints for XML. J. Comput. Syst. Sci. 66(1), 254–291 (2003)
4. Hartmann, S., Link, S.: More Functional Dependencies for XML. In: Kalinichenko, L.A., Manthey, R., Thalheim, B., Wloka, U. (eds.) ADBIS 2003. LNCS, vol. 2798, pp. 355–369. Springer, Heidelberg (2003)
5. Hartmanna, S., Link, S.: Numerical constraints on XML data. Information and Computation 208, 521–544 (2010)
6. Hartmann, S., Köhler, H., Link, S., Trinh, T., Wang, J.: On the Notion of an XML Key. In: Schewe, K.-D., Thalheim, B. (eds.) SDKB 2008. LNCS, vol. 4925, pp. 103–112. Springer, Heidelberg (2008)
7. Kroenke, D.M.: Database Processing: Fundamentals. Design and Implementation. Prentice Hall (2010)
8. Bray, T., Paoli, J., Sperberg-McQueen, C.M.: Extensive Markup Language (XML) 1.0. World Wide Web Consortium(W3C) (February 1988), http://www.w3.org/TR/REC-xml
9. Layman, A., Jung, E., Maler, E., Thompson, H.S.: XML-Data. W3C Note (January 1998), http://www.w3.org/TR/1998/NOTE-XML-data
10. Thompson, H.S., Beech, D., Maloney, M., Mendelsohn, N.: XML Schema Part 1:Structures, W3C Working Draft (April 2000), http://www.w3.org/TR/xmlschema-1/
11. Sumon Shahriar, M., Liu, J.: On Defining Keys for XML. IEEE 8th International Conference on Computer and Information Technology Workshops, 86–91
12. Buneman, P., Davidson, S., Fan, W., Hara, C., Tan, W.-C.: Keys for XML. Comput. Networks 39(5), 473–487 (2002)
13. Buneman, P., Davidson, S., Fan, W., Hara, C., Tan, W.: Reasoning about Keys for XML. Inform. Syst. 28(8), 1037–1063 (2003)
14. Grahne, G., Zhu, J.: Discovering Approximate Keys in XML Data. In: CIKM, pp. 453–460 (2002)

A Semantic-Based Dual Caching System for Nomadic Web Service

Panpan Han, Liang Chen, and Jian Wu

Zhejiang University, Hangzhou, Zhejiang, China
ronson@zju.edu.cn

Abstract. As mobile devices become more widely used, they will emerge as a standard platform for hosting Web Service clients. Since mobile devices tend to be connected via a wireless network, they have to work with significantly less and fluctuating bandwidth as well as sudden and unexpected loss of connectivity. Moreover, mobile devices have other constraints, such as limited CPU, memory, or energy resources. To handle the above problems, we proposed a dual caching architecture and development method of web services for mobile devices. With the caching system between the client and server, we can cache the computing result and data downloaded from the server, which can reduce the latency and network load for workloads of web service. Meanwhile, the client side caching system can store the upload and download data.

Keywords: web service, caching, mobile devices.

1 Introduction

Currently, the Web services are spreading widely throughout the world. Web Services are an enabling technology for interoperability within a distributed, loosely coupled, and heterogeneous computing environment. The W3C defines a "Web Service" as "a software system designed to support interoperable machine-to-machine interaction over a network". It has an interface described in a machine-processable format (specifically Web Services Description Language, known by the acronym WSDL). Other systems interact with the Web service in a manner prescribed by its description using SOAP messages, typically conveyed using HTTP with an XML serialization in conjunction with other Web-related standards.

The "standard" Web Services scenario assumes service providers and consumers as static and connected entities. But as mobile devices become more resource-rich and pervasive this is bound to change. As mobile devices become widely used, they are emerging as a means for hosting applications that consume Web Services(shown in Fig.1). However, since mobile devices tend to be connected to the Internet via very different kinds of networks, such as wireless LAN(802.11b), cellphone network(WAP), broadband network(cable modem), or

J. Li et al. (Eds.): PAKDD 2013 Workshops, LNAI 7867, pp. 511–521, 2013.

local area network(Ethernet), they have to work with significantly less and fluctuating bandwidth as well as sudden and unexpected loss of connectivity. While fluctuations in the available bandwidth impact only the transmission speed of SOAP messages, the total loss of connectivity is more serious since it interrupts all SOAP traffic. Consequently, the use of mobile devices will introduce the novel notion of a nomadic Web Services participant that can suddenly disappear from the network and reappear at a later point in time.

The growth in the number of Web services has been phenomenal, hence, applying changes to existing Web services is impractical. For the same reason, the solution should be scalable and general enough to apply to all Web services. A good solution to improve availability of Web services should be transparently deployable and generally applicable[1]. Transparent deployment means that the solution must not require changes to the implementation of the Web services, either to the server and client side modules or to the communication protocol between them. Caching satisfies both the required characteristics of transparent deployment and general applicability. Caches are transparent to both the client and server components of the Web services.

This paper focuses on how to support nomadic Web Services clients by the use of dual caching system. With the combination of service characteristics and requirement of service, we can get cache semantic description(CSD). CSD is a XML which can show the type of the service operation(read or write), the service response characteristics and so on. Then the cache system can choose the corresponding caching strategy. The paper is structured as follows. Section three focuses on the novel dual SOAP caching system. An empirical evaluation of the dual caching system is presented in section four. A discussion of the results and a summary and future work section conclude the paper.

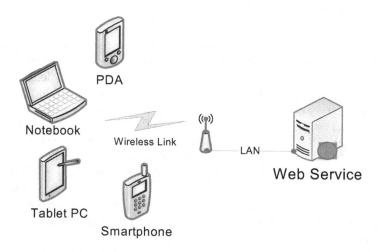

Fig. 1. Examples of mobile devices

2   Related Work

The concept of a cache [2] was first introduced for processor-memory communication; the concept then spread to file systems, computer networks, database systems and distributed object systems. Caches have been used to overcome disconnectivity, to decrease the latency of responses, and to increase throughput. A cache requires the identification of two cache semantics. These are cacheability and consistency maintenance.

There is much research on software caches in client-server architectures, with many objectives ranging from providing transactional guarantees, through providing consistency based on relaxed consistency models, to providing availability (e.g., [3], [4], [5] - just to name a few). It should be noted that although the hardware for mobile devices is improving at a tremendous rate, mobile devices still have limitations in terms of memory, processing power, communication bandwidth, and, in particular, power consumption. Consequently, caches targeted to mobile devices, in general, are smaller and simpler than caches targeted to servers or desktops.

A variety of systems have employed caching on mobile devices in support of disconnected access to files, databases, objects, and Web pages[6]. With the popularity of web service, several researches have been done on the caching of web services. [7] proposed a "HTTP-like" caching system. Upon receiving a response with a particular code in its content (for example, 304, as in HTTP), clients would know that their cached data were still up-to-date. This method reduces the wirelessly transmitted data to some extent. However, it would not eliminate the need of establishing a connection each time we need data.

To reduce the latency perceived by the user, [8] present a caching architecture for web services and an adaptive prefetching algorithm. The key characteristics of their approach are the compatibility with major mobile browsers and the independence of the caching proxy from the front-end application and the back-end services.

[9] introduces a dual caching approach to overcome problems arising from temporarily loss of connectivity and fluctuations in bandwidth. [10] present Differential Caches, with the accompanying Differential Updates method and the Mobile SOAP (MoSOAP) protocol, to avoid transfer of repeated data, sent by a web service to an application. The protocol is flexible in that other optimization techniques, such as encoding, can also be applied.

3   Dual Caching System

3.1   System Architecture

Fig.2 shows the architecture of the implemented semantic-based dual caching system. As mentioned in the previous sections, two transparent caches, one on the client side and one on the proxy side are required to overcome the loss of connectivity during SOAP traffic and to reduce the runtime overhead of mobile devices. The pair of caches is used to store the data sent by the web service to the invoking application and are managed by the respective client and server Cache Managers.

The Cache Managers controls all cache operations. The Cache Manager interfaces with the CSD preliminary to making cache decisions (e.g. read from cache, read from server side). The detailed description of caching strategy is described in the next chapter.

The proxy side cache(PSC) resides on a proxy server which has a reliable connection to the service provider. The proxy can alter the network traffic and can be a load balancing gateway, or a buffer to an intermittently available resource (e.g. WS).

The incoming requests from the client side cache(CSC) are sent directly to the proxy server. Responses from the service provider are first cached in the PSC and then sent to the CSC. In case the CSC can't be reached the PSC will wait for the CSC to issue a reconnect message upon which the PSC will resubmit all queued responses. To the client, the client side cache(CSC) appears as a local proxy residing on the mobile device.

When connected to network, the request sent by client side is intercepted by cache manager. Depends on the cache requirement and service semantic, we determine to return the client side cache data or to fetch response from server side. And when disconnected, for read operation, we also use CSD to determine whether to read data from cache or from server side. For write operation, we store the request data in the writer queue. If the client detect the network connected, we replay the request queue.

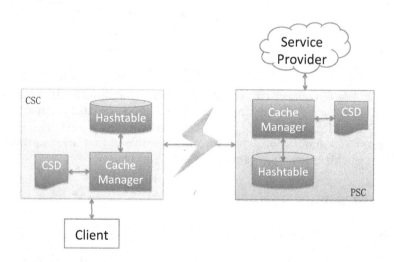

Fig. 2. The dual caching architecture

3.2   Caching Strategy

Cacheability of a request is the property stating that responses can be cached without the creation of an undesired program state [11]. Cacheability is always true for a request that is state-reading and non state-altering. The cached response, however, remains in cache until it is determined as invalid, or until the cache size is too large and the response was not recently used. A response is invalid if it has expired by an age value (e.g. HTTP time-to-live). An invalid response must be requested again from the live resource.

A cache is supported by strategies for maintaining equality between local responses and live responses. Consistency maintenance is the term used to describe these strategies. Hence, cached responses should closely resemble the responses of the live resource (e.g. WS). A strategy (e.g. implicit invalidation) removes or refreshes a cached response when a condition is true (e.g. response age is more than maximum age).

Requests which read the state of a resource are called READ requests (or READs). A READ request is synonymous with the terms query, state-reading, and state-dependent. Requests which alter (a.k.a. modify) the state of a resource are called WRITE requests. A WRITE request is synonymous with the terms update, and state-altering. A client receiving a local reply to a READ has performed a read-local operation. However, a client receiving a remote response to a READ has performed a read-through operation. A delayed state-alteration is known as a write back. However, an immediate state-alteration on the live resource is the result of a write-through operation.

Table 1 shows the attributes and corresponding values of CSD, and Fig 3 shows the key structure of CSD. In which the "type" attribute can be read, write and query, "response" attribute can be permanent, stable, predictable and random, "writeRequest" can be last-write-wins, context-free and other.

Server Side Caching Strategy. The server side caching strategy depends on the CSD, which is shown in table 2. And the write strategy for server side is No-Cache. No-Cache means all requests sent to proxy side, do not use cache.

Client Side Caching Strategy. The client side caching strategy is not only affected by service semantics but also has relation with service consistency requirement, which is shown in table 3 and 4. There are three consistency requirements: strong consistency means we must provide the newest response for each request, eventual consistency means after a period of time, we can return the newest response, and unconstrained consistency means there is no need to return the newest response for each request.

And the read strategy during connections is Automatic Update, the write strategy during connections is Write-through.

Table 1. CSD schema

Attribute Name	Attribute Value	Attribute Description
Name	Operation Name	the name of the operation
Type	Read	type of the operation: read operation, response is related to service state, operation doesn't change service state
Type	Write	type of the operation: write operation, response may be related to service state, operation changes service state
Type	Query	type of the operation: evaluate operation, response isn't related to service state but is related to parameters
Response	Permanent	feature of the response: permanent, response value is always the same for the same request value
Response	Stable	feature of the response: stable, response value is the same over a period of time for the same request value
Response	Random	feature of the response: random, response value is totally random
WriteRequest	last-write-wins	feature of the write request: latest write overwrites the previous ones
WriteRequest	context-free	feature of the write request: the order of write request has no effect to the response
WriteRequest	other	feature of the write request: different from the previous ones

Table 2. Server side cache read strategy

Service semantics	Permanent	Stable	Random
Server side caching strategy	Cache-Only	Passive Update	Automatic Update

Table 3. Client side cache read strategy during disconnections

	Strong consistency	Eventual consistency	unconstrained consistency
Permanent	Cache-Only	Cache-Only	Cache-Only
Stable	Failure	Cache-Only	Cache-Only
Random	Failure	Cache-Only	Cache-Only

Table 4. Client side cache write strategy during disconnections

	Strong consistency	Eventual consistency	unconstrained consistency
last-write-wins	Failure	LWW	LWW
context-free	Failure	Failure	Write-back
other	Failure	Failure	Failure

```
<complexType name="operationType">
    <sequence>
        <element name="resDepend" minOccurs="0"
                maxOccurs="unbounded">
            <complexType>
                <attribute name="resName" type="string"></attribute>
            </complexType>
        </element>
    </sequence>
    <attribute name="name" type="string"></attribute>
    <attribute name="type">
        <simpleType>
            <restriction base="string">
                <enumeration value="read"></enumeration>
                <enumeration value="write"></enumeration>
                <enumeration value="query"></enumeration>
            </restriction>
        </simpleType>
    </attribute>
    <attribute name="responce">
        <simpleType>
            <restriction base="string">
                <enumeration value="permanent"></enumeration>
                <enumeration value="stable"></enumeration>
                <enumeration value="predictable"></enumeration>
                <enumeration value="random"></enumeration>
            </restriction>
        </simpleType>
    </attribute>
    <attribute name="writeRequest">
        <simpleType>
            <restriction base="string">
                <enumeration value="last-write-wins"></enumeration>
                <enumeration value="context-free"></enumeration>
                <enumeration value="other"></enumeration>
            </restriction>
        </simpleType>
    </attribute>
</complexType>
```

Fig. 3. Structure of CSD

4   Performance Evaluation

In order to evaluate the dual caching system, several experiments were performed. In the experiments Axis 2 was used as the Web Services middleware.

4.1   Experimental Setup

Web Service. The experimental WS implements methods supporting a game recommendation application. Users can get a list of recommended games, view game details and score the game. The WS implements the following Three methods, in no particular order:

- Get the game list (READ)
- Get the description of a certain game (READ)
- Give a game score (WRITE)

Metrics

- Mean Latency: the total time spent between a method call and receiving the method return
- Cache Hit ratio: the ratio of locally found responses

The client is instrumented to collect the metrics while it is subjected to a set of scenarios (e.g. Workloads). The client executes dependently on a request/connectivity pattern, and the metrics are collected after every request.

Workloads. The experimental workloads are a set of synthetic request patterns. A synthetic workload is a set of WS requests following the Zipf distribution. The requests are characterized by the ratio X (READ operations) to Y (WRITE operations), such that a workload is composed of X% READs and (100- X)% WRITEs. For all workloads, optimistic concurrency is assumed and an experimental run assumes no write-write conflict.

- P1; 100% READs, 0% WRITEs
- P2: 70% READs, 30% WRITEs
- P3: 40% READs, 60% WRITEs

Execution Environment. The experiments are executed within Samsung Galaxy Note 10.1 N8010 with android 4.1 OS. The Galaxy Note are configured to contain 2G Ram, and a Samsung Exynos 4412 Quad-core 1.4 GHz processor.

4.2   Experiment Result

To measure the impact of the dual caching system each experiment is performed with and without cache. Firstly, we measure the mean latency as the response message size changes from 1k to 100k with workload P1.

Fig.4 shows that the mean latency as the response message size changes from 1k to 100k. This figure shows a linear increase of mean latency as a function of the request message size. And it's obvious that with dual caching system the

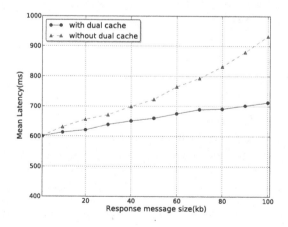

Fig. 4. Mean latency for workload P1 with cache and without cache

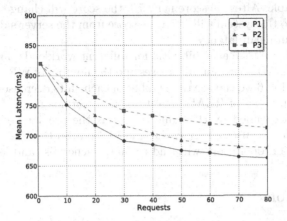

Fig. 5. Mean latency for different workloads

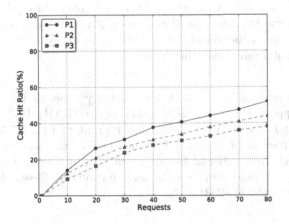

Fig. 6. Effect of Workload on Cache Hits

mean latency decreases notably. This is because the locally answered READ requests reduces the execution and network costs for the mobile device.

After evaluating the dual cache system with very basic workloads, we observe the effect of varying workloads on the latency of requests [Fig.5].

In the workloads P1-P3, the number of READ operations starts at 100% (in P1) and decreases by 30% for each workload (e.g. 40% in P3). The reduction in the number of READ operations is combined with a proportional increase of the number of WRITE operations. As a result, the mean latency decreases linearly with the decrease in number of READ operations in a workload.

This can be explained that many READ records are invalidated by WRITE operation. For example, before we score a game, the score is 87, which is cached in client hash table. After we score it by 70, the score will change and the cache is invalidated. So the system will fetch the score from the server side, which leads to the increase in mean latency.

Then we evaluate the cache hit ratio for different workloads. From P1 to P3, the number of READ operations decreases and the number of WRITE operations increases. From Fig.6 we can see the number of cache hits decreases linearly with the decrease in number of READ operations in a workload.

This can be explained by the same reason as the previous experiment, the WRITE operations caused many cache invalidation. So the the increase of the number of WRITE operations will lead to more cache miss and less cache hits.

5   Conclusions

This paper focuses on the challenges of enabling PDAs to host Web Services consumers and introduces a dual caching approach to overcome problems arising from temporarily loss of connectivity and fluctuations in bandwidth. Using a dual caching it becomes possible to handle loss of connectivity during the transmission of requests and the transmission of responses. An additional advantage of the dual caching is the reduction of latency and network load for workloads that contain significantly more read than writes.

Acknowledgement. This research was partially supported by the National Technology Support Program under grant of 2011BAH15B05, the National Natural Science Foundation of China under grant of 61173176, Science and Tech- nology Program of Zhejiang Province under grant of 2008C03007, National High- Tech Research and Development Plan of China under Grant No. 2009AA110302, National Key Science and Technology Research Program of China (2009ZX01043- 003-003).

References

1. Elbashir, K., Deters, R.: Transparent Caching for Nomadic WS Clients. Arch. Rat. Mech. Anal. 78, 315–333 (1982)
2. Barbara, D., Imielinski, T.: Sleepers and Workaholics: Caching Strategies in Mobile Environments (Extended Version). VLDB Journal 4(4), 567–602 (1994)
3. Garrod, C., et al.: Scalable query result caching for web applications. VLDB 1(1), 550–561 (2008)
4. Haas, L., Kossmann, D., Ursu, I.: Loading a cache with query results. In: VLDB 1999, pp. 351–362 (1999)
5. Oh, S., Fox, G.C.: HHFR: A new architecture for Mobile Web Services Principles and Implementations. Community Grids Technical Paper (2005)
6. Ramasubramanian, V., Terry, D.B.: Caching of XML Web Services for Disconnected Operation,www.cs.cornell.edu/People/ramasv/WebServiceCache/ WebServiceCache(techfest).pdf

7. Papageorgiou, A., Schatke, M., Schulte, S., Steinmetz, R.: Enhancing the Caching of Web Service Responses on Wireless Clients. In: ICWS 2011, July 4-9, pp. 9–16 (2011)
8. Schreiber, D., Aitenbichler, E., Göb, A., Mühlhäuser, M.: Reducing User Perceived Latency in Mobile Processes. In: ICWS 2010, pp. 235–242 (2010)
9. Liu, X., Deters, R.: An efficient dual caching strategy for web service-enabled PDAs. In: ACM Symposium on Applied Computing 2007, pp. 788–794 (2007)
10. Qaiser, M.S., Bodorik, P., Jutla, D.N.: Differential Caches for Web Services in Mobile Environments. In: ICWS 2011, July 4-9, pp. 644–651 (2011)
11. Friedman, R.: Caching Web Services in Mobile Ad-Hoc Networks: Opportunities and Challenges. In: Proceedings of the Second ACM International Workshop on Principles of Mobile Computing, pp. 90–96 (2002)

FTCRank: Ranking Components for Building Highly Reliable Cloud Applications

Hanze Xu, Yanan Xie, Dinglong Duan, Liang Chen, and Jian Wu

Zhejiang University, Hangzhou, China
{xhz1992,xyn,ddl,cliang,wujian2000}@zju.edu.cn

Abstract. With the increasing popularity of cloud computing[2], building highly reliable applications on cloud is very important. However, it's hard to give an optimal solution for large-scale cloud applications. In order to provide an effective solution on this research problem, we propose a component ranking approach named as FTCRank for applying fault-tolerant strategies to the significant components. FTCRank considers not only structure information but also component characteristics to obtain the result. Experiments show that FTCRank achieves better results than other existing algorithms in Top-K fault-tolerant cloud tasks.

Keywords: Cloud application, component ranking, fault tolerance, software reliability.

1 Introduction

Cloud computing is a kind of Internet-based computing, whereby shared resources, software, and information provided to computers and other devices on demand. In recent years, cloud computing is becoming increasingly popular under the promotion of many leading industrial companies (e.g., Amazon, Google, IBM, Microsoft, etc.). The cloud applications which mean the software systems in the cloud typically involve multiple cloud components communicating with each other[9]. Obviously, before trying to transfer the critical systems to the cloud environment, it should be affirmed that the reliability of the cloud applications is almost perfect[7]. But unfortunately, the reliability of the cloud applications is far from people's expectation. So how to build highly reliable cloud environment develops into an increasingly popular and challenging topic.

As the cloud applications tend to be more complex and larger in scale as well as structure, not all of the traditional main approaches (i.e., fault prevention, fault removal, fault tolerance and fault forecasting[6]) used for building reliable software systems are able to be applied conveniently. The most widely employed is fault tolerance. But usually it is only implemented on critical systems (e.g., payment system, traffic control system, etc.) due to the high cost of developing and maintaining redundant components.

In fact, it is a waste of resources to provide fault-tolerance mechanism for the noncritical components (e.g., advertise on web). On the basis of the well-known 80-20 rule[5], only a small number of critical components need fault-tolerance

J. Li et al. (Eds.): PAKDD 2013 Workshops, LNAI 7867, pp. 522–532, 2013.

strategy to make the application quite reliable. FTCRank identifies the most significant components to which we need apply fault-tolerance strategy to. Moreover, FTCRank is efficient and extensible, which means it can be implemented on various occasions flexibly.

The rest of this paper is organized as follows: Section 2 introduces related work, Section 3 proposes three ranking algorithms for discovering significant components, Section 4 shows experiments and Section 5 concludes this paper.

2   Related Work

2.1   Fault-Tolerance Strategies

The approaches to build reliable software systems have been studied for years. As an important one of those approaches, software fault tolerance is widely employed for building reliable distributed systems and cloud-computing environment. Three well-known fault-tolerance strategies are introduced in the following with formulas for calculating the failure probabilities of the fault-tolerant modules.

- **Recovery Block (RB).** Recovery block[8] is a well-known mechanism employed in software fault tolerance. With recovery block, a standby components will be started one by one when the primary component fails to pass through the structuring redundant program modules. The failure probability f of a recovery block can be calculated by:

$$f = \prod_{i=1}^{n} f_i \qquad (1)$$

  where n is the number of redundant components and f_i is the failure probability of the ith component.
- **N-Version Programming (NVP).** N-version programming, also known as multi-version programming, is a software fault-tolerance method where multiple functional equivalent programs (named as versions) are independently generated from the same initial specifications[1]. When we apply the NVP approach to the cloud applications, the independently implemented functionally equivalent cloud components are invoked in parallel and the final result is determined by majority voting. The failure probability f of an NVP module can be computed by:

$$f = \sum_{i=\frac{n+1}{2}}^{n} F(i) \qquad (2)$$

  where n is the number of functionally equivalent components which is usually an odd number and F_i is probability that i alternative components from all the n components fail.

- **Parallel.** Parallel strategy invokes all the n functional equivalent components and the first returned response will be the final result. A parallel module fails only if all the redundant components fail. The failure probability f of a parallel module can be computed by:

$$f = \prod_{i=1}^{n} f_i \tag{3}$$

where n is the number of redundant components and f_i is the failure probability of the ith component.

2.2 FTCloud

A lot of work has been done to solve research problems about fault-tolerant cloud applications. Z. Zheng et al. propose a component ranking framework named FTCloud for building fault-tolerant cloud applications. The procedure of FTCloud is as follows[12]:

1. The system designer provides the initial architecture of a cloud application to FTCloud. A component graph is built based on the component invocation relationships.
2. Significance values of the cloud components are calculated by component ranking algorithms according to the components can be ranked based on the significance values.
3. The Top-K most significant components in the cloud application are identified according to the ranking results.
4. The performance of various fault-tolerance strategy candidates is calculated and the most suitable fault-tolerance strategy is selected for each significant component.
5. The component ranking results and the selected fault-tolerance strategies for the significant components are returned to the system designer for building a reliable cloud application.

Differing from our approach, FTCloud considers only structure information while ignores the probability of different components during component ranking. However, FTCRank combines the probability of different components and structure information for component ranking so that it can get better performance.

2.3 PageRank

PageRank is a link analysis algorithm used by the Google web search engine, which assigns a numerical weight to each element of a hyperlinked set of documents, such as the World Wide Web, with the purpose of "measuring" its relative importance within the set[10]. In our algorithm, PageRank is applied on ranking components of the cloud application whose structure is similar to World Wide Web. In Section 3 we will show the detail of the usage of PageRank in our algorithm and in Section 5 we will show that it works efficiently.

3   Significant Component Ranking

The target of the significant component ranking algorithm is to find out Top-K percent significant components in a cloud application upon available information (e.g., component invocation link, component characteristics, etc.). Our algorithm includes three strategies (i.e., building component graph, component ranking based on the significance and selection of the significant component) which will be described in Section 3.1 to 3.3, respectively.

3.1   Component Graph Building

We can model a cloud application as a weighted directed graph G, where a node c_i represents a cloud component in the application and a directed edge e_{ij} from c_i to c_j represents a component invocation link (i.e., c_i invokes c_j). Assuming that each node c_i in the graph G has a nonnegative significant value $I(c_i)$ and a nonnegative relative visiting frequency $V(c_i)$ in the range of (0,1). Each edge e_{ij} in the graph has a nonnegative weight value $W(e_{ij})$ in the range of [0,1]. The weight value of an edge e_{ij} can be calculated by:

$$W(e_{ij}) = \frac{frq_{ij}}{\sum_{j=1}^{n} frq_{ij}} \tag{4}$$

where frq_{ij} is the invocation frequency of component c_j by component c_i, n is the number of components. If an edge e_{ij} has a larger weight value, c_i invokes c_j more frequently compared with other components invoking c_j. For a component graph with n components, an $n \times n$ transition probability matrix W can be generated by (4) to get the invocation weight values of the edges[12]. Each entry w_{ij} in the matrix is the value $W(e_{ij})$. For $\forall i$, the transition probability matrix W satisfies:

$$\forall i, \sum_{j=1}^{n} w_{ij} = 1 \tag{5}$$

3.2   Component Ranking

In view of the component graph and the failure probability of each component, three component ranking algorithms named as Baseline1, Baseline2 and FTCRank are proposed in this section. The first approach only employs the failure probability of each component in a cloud application for ranking components. The second approach only considers the component information of system structure. The third approach combines techniques proposed in Baseline1 and Baseline2 together through a certain basic function.

Baseline1: Failure-Probability-Based Component Ranking. In a cloud application, some components have higher failure probability. These components are considered to be more important than the components with lower failure probability because they are easier to make the application fail. So we can propose a ranking algorithm based on failure probability:

1.Get the failure probability $f(c_i)$ of each component c_i from the existent information.

2.Obtain the significance value for a component c_i by:

$$I(c_i) = f(c_i) \tag{6}$$

With the above approach, the significance values of the cloud components can be achieved. A component with larger significance value is more important.

Baseline2: Structure-Based Component Ranking. This approach is first introduced as FTCloud in [12]. In a cloud application, some components are frequently invoked by many more other components. These components are deemed to be more important because the failure of them impacts on the system more greatly. Intuitively, the significant value of a component is also affected by the visiting frequency, which is determined by the amount of relative invocation link from other components.

In order to rank the components as accurate as possible, we propose a ranking approach according to PageRank algorithm:

1. Randomly assign initial numerical scores between 0 and 1 to the components in the graph.

2. Compute the visiting frequency for a component c_i by:

$$I(c_i) = V(c_i) = \frac{1-a}{n} + a \sum_{k \in N(c_i)} V(c_k)W(e_{ki}) \tag{7}$$

where n is the number of components and $N(c_i)$ is a set of components that invoke component c_i. The parameter a in (7) is used to balance the frequency values derived from other components that invoked c_i and the basic value of itself. In vector form, (7) can be written as:

$$\begin{bmatrix} I(c_1) \\ \vdots \\ I(c_n) \end{bmatrix} = \begin{bmatrix} V(c_1) \\ \vdots \\ V(c_n) \end{bmatrix} = \begin{bmatrix} (1-a)/n \\ \vdots \\ (1-a)/n \end{bmatrix} + aW^t \begin{bmatrix} V(c_1) \\ \vdots \\ V(c_n) \end{bmatrix} \tag{8}$$

where W^t is the transposed matrix of the transition probability matrix W.

3. Solve (8) by computing the eigenvector with eigenvalue 1 or by repeating the computation until all significance values become stable[12]. With the above algorithm, the significance values of the cloud components can be obtained. Components with larger value will be more important.

FTCRank: Functional Combination of Baseline1 and Baseline2. According to Baseline1 and Baseline2, it is obvious that both structure information and component probability have an impact on component significance. In

FTCRank, we try to combine them together through a certain basic function to get more accurate $I(c_i)$. As mentioned, $V(C_I)$ reflects the visiting frequency of component c_i and $f(c_i)$ stands for the failure probability of component c_i. Once a component in a cloud application is visited, its failure probability is $f(c_i)$. So if it has been visited $n(c_i)$ times, its failure probability will be $f(c_i)^{n(c_i)}$. Furthermore, $n(c_i)$ is usually larger when $V(c_i)$ is larger, indicating that component c_i is invoked by a lot of other significant components frequently. Therefore we propose a power function to calculate the significant value of component c_i as follows:

$$I(c_i) = f(c_i)^{V(c_i)} \tag{9}$$

4 Experiments

4.1 Prototype Implementation

Our experiment includes several modules as follows:

- Component and Invocation extraction. The component and the invocation relationships of different components are both extracted from a cloud application.
- Component graph building. Each node stands for a component and each edge represents an invocation link, the weight of an edge is calculated by (4).
- Component ranking. The component ranking algorithms introduced in Section 3.2 are implemented in this step. The input is the component invocation probability matrix and output is a list of ranked components based on their significance values. We will show the results of different ranking algorithms after.
- FT strategy selection. In this step, we implement the suitable fault-tolerance strategy for every Top-k important component.

4.2 Experimental Setup

Our significant component ranking algorithms are implemented by C++ language. To study the performance of reliability improvement, we compare approaches as follows:

- NoFT. No fault-tolerance strategies are employed for the components in the cloud application.
- Baseline1. Fault-tolerance strategies are employed to mask faults of the Top-K percent significant components. The component ranking algorithm is Baseline1.
- Baseline2. Fault-tolerance strategies are employed to mask faults of the Top-K percent significant components. The component ranking algorithm is Baseline2.

- FTCRank. Fault-tolerance strategies are employed to mask faults of the Top-K percent significant components. The component ranking algorithm is FTCRank.
- AllFT. Fault-tolerance strategies are employed for all the cloud components.

The graph we implement in this experimental is scale-free graph whose degree distribution follows a power law. We use C++ to generate scale free directed component graphs. For a cloud component, we implement the fault-tolerance strategy determination algorithm[12] to select the optimal fault-tolerance strategy for tolerating faults. When a cloud application is executing, it is considered to be failed if an invoked component is failed and there is no fault-tolerance strategy applied for it. If a fault-tolerance strategy is applied, it is failed only if the fault-tolerance strategy also fails. In Baseline2 and FTCRank, the parameter a balances the significance value derived from the other components and the basic value of the component. In our experiments, we set a to be 0.85 to make component rank fairly stable[12].

4.3   Performance Comparison

We implement random walk to simulate the invocation behavior in cloud applications. To start a random walk, we randomly select a node in the invocation graph to be the start node. A very small stop rate can guarantee the invocation coverage of almost all nodes in graph. A cloud application finishes successfully only if none of the invoked components is failed. So the failure probability of a cloud application is:

$$f = 1 - \prod_{i=1}^{n}(1 - f_i) \tag{10}$$

where n is the number of component invoked during execution of a cloud application and f_i if the failure probability of the ith component. In our experiments, we assume that the failure probabilities of components in a cloud application obey uniform distribution. The uniform distribution is randomly generated on $(0, 2 \times E)$ where E is the expectation of component failure probability in a cloud application.

In our experiments, 10000 invocation sequences are randomly generated for each set of nodes (e.g., 100, 1000 and 10000 nodes). Five types of fault-tolerance mechanisms (i.e., NoFT, Baseline1, Baseline2, FTCRank and AllFT) are applied on these invocation sequences and the average results are reported in Fig.1. and Table 2.

In Fig. 1. and Table 2, *Component FP* represents the expectation of failure probabilities of the cloud components, *Top-K* (K=1, 5, 10 and 20 percent) indicates that fault-tolerance mechanisms are applied for the K percent most significance components. The experimental results in Fig.1. and Table 2 show that:

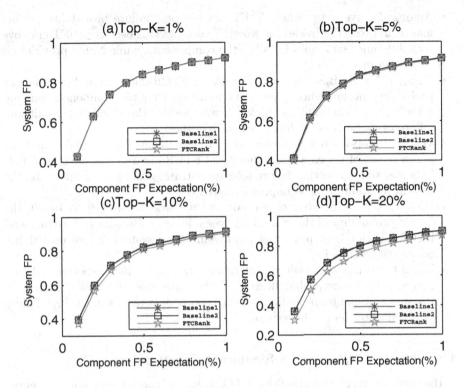

Fig. 1. Performance Comparison of Failure Probability

Table 1. Performance Comparison of Failure Probability

Nodes	Methods	Component FP=0.1%			Component FP=0.5%			Component FP=1.0%		
		Top1%	Top5%	Top10%	Top1%	Top5%	Top10%	Top1%	Top5%	Top10%
100	NoFT	0.0245	0.0245	0.0245	0.0903	0.0903	0.0903	0.2353	0.2353	0.2353
	Baseline1	0.0244	0.0229	0.0227	0.0901	0.0821	0.0741	0.2352	0.2136	0.1948
	Baseline2	0.0244	0.0225	0.0203	0.0901	0.0825	0.0818	0.2264	0.2140	0.2111
	FTCRank	0.0243	0.0227	0.0201	0.0900	0.0803	0.0719	0.2183	0.2070	0.1654
	AllFT	0.0000	0.0000	0.0000	0.0010	0.0010	0.0010	0.0034	0.0034	0.0034
1000	NoFT	0.4332	0.4332	0.4332	0.8438	0.8438	0.8438	0.9230	0.9230	0.9230
	Baseline1	0.4300	0.4177	0.4020	0.8422	0.8360	0.8268	0.9229	0.9190	0.9133
	Baseline2	0.4270	0.4140	0.3961	0.8402	0.8324	0.8222	0.9221	0.9175	0.9125
	FTCRank	0.4253	0.4021	0.3711	0.8398	0.8288	0.8080	0.9222	0.9145	0.9034
	AllFT	0.0013	0.0013	0.0013	0.0310	0.0310	0.0310	0.0870	0.0870	0.0870
10000	NoFT	0.8684	0.8684	0.8684	0.9862	0.9862	0.9862	0.9960	0.9960	0.9960
	Baseline1	0.8667	0.8581	0.8436	0.9859	0.9841	0.9810	0.9959	0.9955	0.9948
	Baseline2	0.8665	0.8601	0.8496	0.9859	0.9843	0.9815	0.9959	0.9956	0.9950
	FTCRank	0.8654	0.8510	0.8250	0.9856	0.9827	0.9773	0.9959	0.9955	0.9937
	AllFT	0.0083	0.0083	0.0083	0.0981	0.0981	0.0981	0.4724	0.4724	0.4724

- Among the five approaches, AllFT has the best failure probability performance and NoFT provides the worst. This is obvious because AllFT employs fault-tolerance strategies for all of the components, while NoFT provides no fault-tolerance strategy.
- Compared with Baseline1 and Baseline2, FTCRank obtains better failure probability performance. The result indicates that the component ranking achieves more accurate results when we consider the PageRank result and failure probability of each component together.
- When the Top-K value increases from 5 to 20 percent, the failure probabilities performance of Baseline1, Baseline2 and FTCRank decrease obviously. This indicates that by setting failure tolerance strategy on more components, the system reliability can be improved distinctly.
- When the node number of components increases from 100 to 10000, the failure probability of the system increases, however Baseline1, Baseline2 and FTCRank can keep providing improvement on system failure probability compared with NoFT.
- When the component failure probability expectation increases from 0.1 to 1 percent, the failure probabilities of all the approaches are greatly increased. Because high failure probability of each component results in the high failure probability of the whole system.

4.4   Impact of Component Significant Function

In the component ranking algorithm FTCRank, the function that is implemented to calculate the final component significance is of great importance. In this section, we try to demonstrate that

$$S(c_i) = f(c_i)^{V(c_i)} \tag{11}$$

is a better function than some other tested basic functions. We study the fault-tolerance performance of FTCRank under different component significance calculation functions. The experimental results in Table 2 show that:

Table 2. Impact of Signification Function on Application Failure Probability

Nodes	Methods	Component FP=0.1%			Component FP=0.5%			Component FP=1.0%		
		Top1%	Top5%	Top10%	Top1%	Top5%	Top10%	Top1%	Top5%	Top10%
100	$V(c_i) \times f(c_i)$	0.0249	0.0241	0.0206	0.0942	0.0857	0.0847	0.2345	0.2289	0.2161
	$V(c_i) \times f(c_i)^2$	0.0249	0.0240	0.0204	0.0934	0.0849	0.0825	0.2321	0.2266	0.2117
	$V(c_i)^{f(c_i)}$	0.0249	0.0239	0.0203	0.0934	0.0847	0.0819	0.2315	0.2265	0.2110
	$f(c_i)^{V(c_i)}$	0.0248	0.0211	0.0180	0.0933	0.0614	0.0748	0.2095	0.1965	0.1701
1000	$V(c_i) \times f(c_i)$	0.4198	0.3958	0.3668	0.8339	0.8206	0.8009	0.9226	0.9216	0.9067
	$V(c_i) \times f(c_i)^2$	0.4170	0.3808	0.3431	0.8317	0.8119	0.7802	0.9215	0.9116	0.8965
	$V(c_i)^{f(c_i)}$	0.4169	0.3800	0.3401	0.8316	0.8114	0.7774	0.9216	0.9138	0.8951
	$f(c_i)^{V(c_i)}$	0.4110	0.3636	0.3187	0.8293	0.8091	0.7698	0.9213	0.9103	0.8938
10000	$V(c_i) \times f(c_i)$	0.8638	0.8576	0.8480	0.9862	0.9852	0.9862	0.9960	0.9960	0.9838
	$V(c_i) \times f(c_i)^2$	0.8633	0.8544	0.8396	0.9860	0.9846	0.9810	0.9959	0.9955	0.9826
	$V(c_i)^{f(c_i)}$	0.8633	0.8534	0.8382	0.9860	0.9846	0.9815	0.9959	0.9956	0.9824
	$f(c_i)^{V(c_i)}$	0.8621	0.8446	0.8123	0.9859	0.9840	0.9773	0.9959	0.9955	0.9812

- When Top-K is small, there is no obvious difference between these four kinds of functions because fault-tolerance strategies are implemented on only a few components.
- When Top-K increases, the effect of the function we select becomes more and more obvious. So with gradually applying fault-tolerance strategies on more components, the quantity of the significant components selected by component ranking becomes more and more important.

5 Conclusion

This paper proposes a component ranking algorithm for building fault-tolerant cloud applications. Both component failure probability and component structure information are considered to rank components in our proposed algorithm. The structural significance value of a component which is determined by the number of components that invoke this component, is computed by employing a PageRank-like algorithm. Experiments show that our algorithm outperforms other available component ranking algorithms in various component graphs.

Our FTCRank algorithm considers only component failure probability and component graph. In the future, we will investigate more factors of component to extend the FTCRank algorithm.

The PageRank-like algorithm used in our FTCRank algorithm may not be the best approach to estimate the component structure characteristics for all kinds of component graph. In our future work, we will also study more algorithms to employ different types of component graphs, especially those generated in real-world cloud applications (e.g., employing the NASA NPB benchmark).

Acknowledgments. This research was partially supported by the National Technology Support Program under grant of 2011BAH15B05, the National Natural Science Foundation of China under grant of 61173176, 71171077, Science and Technology Program of Zhejiang Province under grant of 2008C03007, National High-Tech Research and Development Plan of China under Grant No. 2009AA110302, National Key Science and Technology Research Program of China (2009ZX01043- 003-003).

References

1. Avizienis, A.: The methodology of n-version programming. Software Fault Tolerance 3, 23–46 (1995)
2. Buyya, R.: Cloud computing: The next revolution in information technology. In: 2010 1st International Conference on Parallel Distributed and Grid Computing (PDGC), pp. 2–3. IEEE (2010)
3. Chen, L., Feng, Y., Wu, J., Zheng, Z.: An enhanced qos prediction approach for service selection. In: 2011 IEEE International Conference on Services Computing (SCC), pp. 727–728. IEEE (2011)

4. Chen, L., Kuang, L., Wu, J.: Mapreduce based skyline services selection for qos-aware composition. In: 2012 IEEE 26th International Parallel and Distributed Processing Symposium Workshops & PhD Forum (IPDPSW), pp. 2035–2042. IEEE (2012)
5. Lipovetsky, S.: Pareto 80/20 law: derivation via random partitioning. International Journal of Mathematical Education in Science and Technology 40(2), 271–277 (2009)
6. Lyu, M.R., et al.: Handbook of software reliability engineering, vol. 3. IEEE Computer Society Press, CA (1996)
7. Petruch, K., Stantchev, V., Tamm, G.: A survey on it-governance aspects of cloud computing. International Journal of Web and Grid Services 7(3), 268–303 (2011)
8. Randell, B., Xu, J.: The evolution of the recovery block concept (1995)
9. Wikipedia. Cloud-computing (2013), http://en.wikipedia.org/wiki/Cloud_Computing
10. Wikipedia. Pagerank (2013), http://en.wikipedia.org/wiki/PageRank
11. Wu, J., Chen, L., Xie, Y., Zheng, Z.: Titan: a system for effective web service discovery. In: Proceedings of the 21st International Conference Companion on World Wide Web, pp. 441–444. ACM (2012)
12. Zheng, Z., Zhou, T., Lyu, M., King, I.: Component ranking for fault-tolerant cloud applications (2011)

Research on SaaS Resource Management Method Oriented to Periodic User Behavior

Jun Guo, Hongle Wu, Hao Huang, Fang Liu, and Bin Zhang

College of Information Science and Engineering, Northeastern University, Shenyang, China
{guojun,zhangbin}@ise.neu.edu.cn,
{woshihongle,jxfchuanghao}@126.com

Abstract. With the development of Internet technology, SaaS is gaining popularity as a kind of innovative mode of software applications. In order to meet the
needs of the periodic user behavior better, allocate virtual resource more reasonable and achieve the targets of SaaS Service performance optimization and
energy conservation, this paper puts forward one SaaS resource management
method oriented to periodic user behavior. This method takes the periodic user
behavior as the research object, predicts future resource demand by predicting
and matching concurrent requests and resource occupancy, then allocates the
resource by demands. The results show that this strategy has good usability and
validity and it can predict the user future demand for resources accurately. This
method also lays a foundation for further performance optimization and energy
conservation.

Keywords: SaaS, periodic user behavior, VM resource, energy conservation.

1   Introduction

With the rapid development of service computing and cloud computing, software as a
service (SaaS) becomes a software development trend as a new kind of software
service operation mode, SaaS delivers in form of services, and provides customized
service through multi-tenancy to users with personalized service [1]. In this mode, SaaS
service providers need building network infrastructure, software and hardware platforms for enterprises. Besides, SaaS service providers are also responsible for the
deployment, upgrade and maintenance of SaaS service. Customers simply reserve
the services on demand and pay according to the time and the quality of service [2].
SaaS service could reduce the cost and risk of customers' software deployment and
implementation.

Normally multiple SaaS services are implemented on a cloud platform, however, the
user behavior of these SaaS services may show a certain periodicity and each
SaaS service's peak or trough is desynchronized, which causes the resource consumption among different SaaS services differ sharply, with a large uncertainty [3]. The
traditional resources allocation management methods are mainly based on load

J. Li et al. (Eds.): PAKDD 2013 Workshops, LNAI 7867, pp. 533–542, 2013.

characteristic and special load resource allocation. In these methods, we need to undertake certain capacity planning and load analysis, assessment demand of resource status of workloads to establish an appropriate resource allocation and management model. However, this static allocation model has certain limitations due to its fixed model and the allocation of resource can't change with the load [4]. According to the relevant features of periodic user behavior, how to allocate resource real-time, dynamically, and reasonably to achieve the goals of service performance and energy-saving, becoming a core research hotspot of Cloud computing.

In order to achieve the double goals of optimization performance and energy-saving, this paper presents a SaaS resource management mechanism oriented to periodic user behavior. Firstly, it predicts the number of periodic user behavior concurrent requests, and then calculates the resource occupation prediction value. Secondly adjusts resource supplement in SaaS environment, to ensure that the virtual machine cluster scale changes with the traffic load change, meanwhile ensure the user request QoS by optimizing system and resource allocation spontaneously. Finally this paper carries out some application experiments to verify the validity and availability; the experimental result shows that the dynamic adjustment of the allocation of resources reached the goals of the service performance optimization and energy-saving.

2   The Characteristic Analysis of Periodic User Behavior

Periodic user behavior is an important user behavior of SaaS application. During using SaaS services, these users' behavior is regular, which means, SaaS service users change regularly in every time intervals, and this situation repeat appearance regularly with time changing.

2.1   The Periodic User Behavior's Data Characteristics

The process data of periodic user behavior that real-time measured can be expressed as a three dimensional array: $U(I \times J \times K)$, and the physical meaning of each dimension is as follows: I represents the cycle of periodic user behavior ($i=1,2,3\ldots,I$), J represents the number of periodic user behavior's process variable($j=1,2,3\ldots,J$), in SaaS platform, the process variables include concurrent requests, CPU utilization, memory consumption, bandwidth, the failure rate and the system overhead; K represents the number of the virtual machine that using in different time used by periodic users in SaaS service ($k=1,2,3\ldots,K$).

The qualitative data of periodic user behavior can be expressed as a two dimensional matrix: $V(M \times N)$, and the physical meaning of each dimension is as follows: M represents different periodic user behavior types ($m=1,2,3\ldots,M$); N represents the corresponding QoS requirements of periodic user behavior ($n=1,2,3\ldots,N$), in this paper, QoS includes execution time, reliability, availability, price and throughout.

Therefore, the typical form of periodic user behavior data are a three dimensional process variable array $U(I \times J \times K)$ and a two dimensional quality variable matrix $V(M \times N)$.

2.2   The Periodic User Behavior Characteristics

In SaaS applications, periodic user behavior is a dynamic process, and a SaaS application generally includes a plurality of periodic user behavior. But the service cycle and business peak and valley of each individual behavior are different, which leads to the complexity of periodic user behavior's process. As shown in Figure 1, there are three periodic user behaviors S1, S2 and S3, each user behavior shows different periodicities according to the different number of concurrent requests.

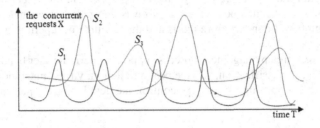

Fig. 1. Periodic user behavior

Generally speaking, the process of periodic user behavior has the following characteristics:

(1) The similarity of every periodic user behavior's cycle

Unlike the continuous processes in general, the SaaS application supporting periodic user behavior is a cyclical service process. And periodic user behavior shows cyclical with time due to the concurrent requests present different trend in different time. The Cloud platform includes many periodic user behaviors, but the cycle of user behavior service is relatively limited, and the cycle shows regular change with the number of concurrent requests, which causes these periodic user behaviors shows a certain similarity.

(2) The volatility of every periodic user's resources occupancy rate

The dynamic feature of periodic user behavior leads to the occupation of the system resources in each time is different,, and the resources occupancy show regular changes according to the concurrent requests.

(3) The independence of each periodic user's service cycle

Periodic user behavior has the certain repeatability, but these periodic user behaviors have no relationship and are independent with each other. Therefore, the resources occupancy shows a status of trading off and takes turns.

(4) The boundedness of each service's total resources occupancy

In the cloud platform, system resource is shared by multiple SaaS services supporting periodic user behavior. But the total amount of resources is limited, if one SaaS service occupies too many resources at one moment, it will affect other SaaS services at that moment, causing the lack of system resource of them.

3   The Process of SaaS Resource Management Oriented to Periodic User Behavior

The process is put forward by the periodicity of SaaS service user behavior and the flexibility of system resource management, and the process takes full consideration to the behavior characteristics of SaaS service and the scalability characteristics virtual machines clusters [5]. SaaS resource management methods make the corresponding adjustment based on resources occupancy, and resources occupancy are closely related with concurrent requests. Therefore, the method proposed in this paper is to reach the adjustment of virtual machines scale based on isomorphic virtual machines by predicting the number of concurrent requests and the resource occupation in future period of time.

The SaaS resource management process supporting periodic user behavior includes four steps: request classification, service peak prediction, virtual machine performance analysis and virtual machine start/stops control, the details of each part are introduced as following.

(1) Request classification

The request classifier focuses on user request description and classification. When the user requests arrive, the request classifier begins to analysis with a certain model, including learning users' intentions, extracting the user's request level and QoS demand, and getting the type result of periodic user behavior. Service quality attributes contain execution time, reliability, availability, cost and throughout. Different periodic user behaviors require different service quality, and also pay the corresponding expenses based on certain QoS. When the user requests are classified, the result will be transmitted to the service peak predictor and the concurrent request database.

(2) Service peak prediction

Service peak predictor is to forecast concurrent requests of each periodic user behavior. In order to realize the efficient management of resources, it needs to determine the virtual machines scale according to the number of concurrent requests. At the same time, in order to avoid scheduling lag, it also needs to predict the number of concurrent requests. Service peak predictor predicts the number concurrent requests by monitoring the time of each periodic behavior of user requests simultaneously and using the improved Gray - Markov prediction model [6].

(3) Virtual machine performance analysis

Virtual machine performance analyzer is to predict the resource occupancy of each VM. It regularly predicts resources demand in next time period according to the number of concurrent requests and resources occupancy in a certain period of time, and then use the prediction as the evident to Schedule virtual machine, so as to ensure that the resource is available when service is peak while the resource can be retrieved when service is low [7].

(4) Virtual machine start/stop control

In the SaaS environment, the number of users request often presents a fluctuating phenomenon erratically. The VM scale should change along with the load changes;

otherwise, the VM resource may be wasted or inadequate, so it needs to control the virtual machines scale [8].

As shown in figure 2, the PM start/stop controller manages a number of physical machines; every physical machine also controls a number of virtual machines. Once receiving scheduling information, the PM start/stop controller needs to update the virtual machine start/stop status, in order to reduce the unnecessary energy consumption. When a virtual machine is in zero load status, the virtual machine should be closed; only when all the virtual machines in one physical machine are dormant or closed, it needs to close the physical machine [9]. When the load peak comes and the opened virtual machines are not able to meet all user requests, the dormant or closed virtual machines have to be waked up. When it needs to wake up virtual machines, it is firstly to consider open the virtual machines controlled by a same physical machine. When the virtual machines can't meet the requirements, it is essential to open a new physical machine. In a word, the virtual machines should be scheduled on fewer physical machines to realize the management optimization [10].

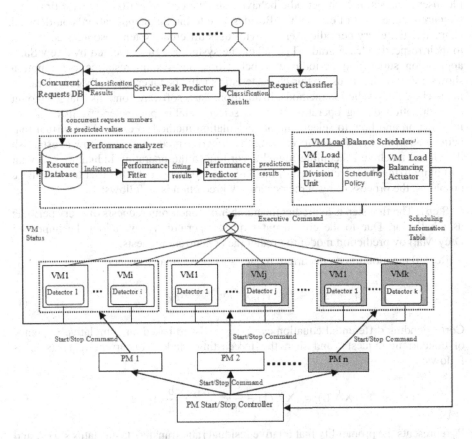

Fig. 2. Framework of SaaS resource management supported to periodic user behavior

4   SaaS Resource Prediction Method of Periodic User Behavior

The SaaS application supporting periodic user behavior is a dynamic process, and it generally has some periodic user behaviors running on it at the same time. The business peak and valley of periodic user behaviors are not identical, which cause the complexity of SaaS application process. Dynamic concurrent requests simultaneously will lead to the system resource demand dynamic change, which makes the software system face various random and unpredictable changes. However, when new user requests arrive, request scheduler adjust the scale of virtual machines according to the requests and the system resources occupancy, this process will delay the service time and have a significant impact on QoS. In order to deal with these problems, it needs to predict service performance, and to arrange system resources reasonably, so that it can meet the requirement for system working.

Compared with the general prediction problem, virtual machine resources prediction of SaaS application supporting periodic user behavior has its particularity. For example, user requests of each periodic behavior show a certain periodicity over time, but they are independent of each other. Besides, due to the SaaS application's on-demand characteristic, every periodic user behavior uses different system resources according to their respective lease grade [11]. When the system are implemented by a few SaaS application supporting periodic user behaviors, the system resource consumption shows a shift in the status, so this characteristic should be taken into fully consideration in the choice of prediction methods. In addition, SaaS software contains a large amount of information during operation, how to select suitable parameters from the above information and how to select suitable calculation method to express the virtual machine load is the foundation of realizing the effective prediction. And how to establish the virtual machine scheduling model according to the operating indicators is a vital part of realizing the effectiveness of SaaS resource management. In order to solve these problems, the process of resource occupancy prediction is as follows:

Step1: The first step is to predict the number of concurrent requests of every periodic user behavior. Due to the concurrent requests' periodicity, we adopt the improved Grey-Markov prediction model to predict the concurrent requests.

Regard the monitored concurrent requests as an original sequence:

$$X^{(0)} = \{X^{(0)}(1), X^{(0)}(2),..., X^{(0)}(n)\} \tag{1}$$

Corresponding differential equation can be established based on cumulative sequence of concurrent requests, and then the forecasting model concurrent requests is as follows:

$$X^{(0)'}(i) = [X^{(0)}(1) - \frac{b}{a}]e^{-a(i-1)} + \frac{b}{a}, i \geq 1 \tag{2}$$

P_{ij} represents the probability that relative residual ratio transfers from status s_i to s_j, and thus the transition probability matrix can be gained:

$$P = (P_{ij})_{n \times n} = \begin{pmatrix} p_{11} & \cdots & p_{1n} \\ \cdots & & \cdots \\ p_{n1} & \cdots & p_{nn} \end{pmatrix} \tag{3}$$

The future state of relative residual ratio sequence can be predicted by using improved Grey-Markov. Get the prediction interval by state transfer matrix, recover the prediction sequence, and finally the final prediction sequence can be obtained.

Step2: The second step is to use the RBF neural network model [12] to do curve fitting between concurrent requests and the resource consumption under the condition of multiple periodic user behaviors, and find out the function relationship between them.

Step3: The third step is to use the fitted relationship and predicted concurrent requests as the performance predictor's inputs, and to predict resource occupancy in the next period, then use the results to guide the scheduling of virtual machines resources.

The improved Grey-Markov model is to predict the number of concurrent requests. Compared with the traditional Grey-Markov model, the improved Grey-Markov is based on the normal distribution of sample mean-variance classification, and it defines n-dimensional status even division to provide a theoretical basis for different granularity of status division. Using resource occupancy volume prediction algorithm based on the radial basis neural network to determine the resource occupancy by the number of concurrent requests, then, predicting the resource and finding the fitting relationship between concurrent requests and resource occupancy of every periodic user behavior. When, the predicted value of concurrent requests is given, the resource occupancy also can be predicted. Finally the prediction of the resources occupancy of every periodic user behavior can be realized.

5   Experiment

5.1   Experimental Environment and Data Acquisition

Experimental environment is composed of a Web server and Web clients in a same LAN, including a Web server running on the Linux platform and a Windows client.

In order to finish data acquisition and prediction, we use LoadRunner to stimulate the behavior of users, and to obtain the number of concurrent requests and performance indicators. LoadRunner is a system performance prediction tool, which can obtain some system performance indicators (such as CPU utilization, memory utilization, concurrent requests and so on) real-timely by stimulating a large number of users with concurrent requests and monitoring performance data.

5.2   Concurrent Request Number and Resource Occupation Prediction

Monitoring the number of concurrent requests of three different grads of periodic user behavior through IE client respectively, and the monitoring interval is 10s. So in this paper, there are 450 sets monitored data, and we use the first 350 sets as sample data and the last 100 sets as comparison data.

Step1: Monitoring a certain periodic behavior's concurrent requests and then using Grey-Markov model to predict, finally restoring data, and selecting the maximum probability interval as the predictive value interval, and the mean of the maximum probability interval is the predictive value of concurrent requests (Figure 3).

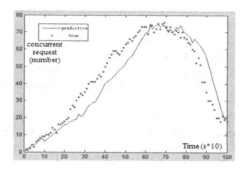

Fig. 3. The comparative result between predictive and true value based on Grey-Markov

Step2: In this experiment, some indicators are used including concurrent requests of three different periodic user behaviors in different grades, the CPU utilization and memory consumption. Then preprocessing the sample data, establishing the RBF nerve network model, finally predicting the resource occupation (Figure 4), and the final resource usage is the weighted summation method of various resources.

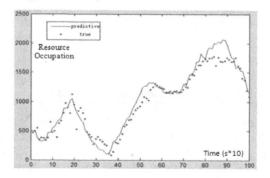

Fig. 4. The comparative result between predictive value based on RBF Neural Network and true value

Step3: By adjusting isomorphism virtual machines, SaaS resource management method can be realized. When the number of concurrent requests increases, the system resource demand also increases. If the current resources remain the same, it will decrease the user experience and can't meet the user's QoS, it is time to adjust the isomorphic virtual machined scale by increasing the number of virtual machine, in order to shorten the response time and meet the user's QoS; One the contrary, when system resource demand decreases, it needs to close some virtual machines in order to realize energy-saving as well as satisfy users' QoS. In this experiment, the virtual machine cluster scale is adjusted according to the predicted resource consumption. The effectiveness of resource management is verified by the users average response time.

As shown in the Figure 5, the horizontal axis represents time and the vertical axis represents the response time. When the virtual machine resource is deficient, user request response time will increase significantly, in that case, the virtual machine scale should be adjusted, the user response time will be maintained in a certain range. Therefore, it can verify the effectiveness of the SaaS resource management method based on isomorphism virtual machines.

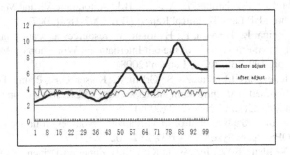

Fig. 5. Contrast of response time

6   Summary

In this paper, we proposed a mechanism of SaaS resource management oriented to periodic user behaviors based on the current SaaS service research and deep consideration of periodic user behavior characteristic. The resource management is reached by adjusting the isomorphic virtual machines, the experimental results show that user's resource demand can be predicted accurately and the method can achieve the goals of performance optimization and energy-saving to some extent.

Acknowledgment. This work was supported by the Key Technologies R&D Program of Shenyang City (F12-029-2-00), the Key Technologies R&D Program of Shenyang City (No. F11-034-2-00), the Special Fund for Fundamental Research of Central Universities of Northeastern University (No.100404003) and National Natural Science Foundation of China (No.60903008 and No. 61100028).

References

1. Ju, J., Wang, Y., Fu, J., Wu, J., Lin, Z.: Research on Key Technology in SaaS. In: 2010 International Conference on Intelligent Computing and Cognitive Informatics (ICICCI), Kuala Lumpur, pp. 384–387 (2010)
2. Kwok, T., Laredo, J., Maradugu, S.: A Web Services Intergration to Manage Invoice Identification, Metadata Extraction, Storage and Retrieval in a Multi-tenancy SaaS Application. In: IEEE International Conference on e-Business Engineering, Xi'an China, pp. 359–366 (2008)

3. Sun, W., Zhang, K., Chen, S.-K., Zhang, X., Liang, H.: Software as a Service: An Integration Perspective. In: Krämer, B.J., Lin, K.-J., Narasimhan, P. (eds.) ICSOC 2007. LNCS, vol. 4749, pp. 558–569. Springer, Heidelberg (2007)
4. Barham, P., Dragovi, B., Fraser, K., et al.: Xen and the art of virtualization. In: Proceedings of the 19th ACM SOSP, pp. 164–177. ACM Press, New York (2003)
5. Wang, X., et al.: Virtualization-based autonomic resource management for multi-tier Web applications in shared data center. J. Syst. Softw. 81(9), 1591–1608 (2008)
6. Saucedo, V.M.: On-line optimization of stochastic processes using Markov Decision Processes. Computer and Chemical Engineering 20(suppl. 1), 701–706 (2006)
7. Hyser, C., McKee, B., Gardner, R., Watson, B.J.: Autonomic Virtual Machine Placement in the Data Center. HP Labs Technical Report HPL-2007-189 (2007)
8. Silva, J.N., Veiga, L., Ferreira, P.: Heuristic for resources allocation on utility computing infrastructures. In: Proceedings of the 6th International Workshop on Middleware for Grid Computing, pp. 129–138. ACM, Leuven (2008)
9. Yixin, D., Hellerstein, J.L., Parekh, S., Grfith, R., Kaiser, G.E., Phung, D.: A control theory foundation for self-managing computing system. IEEE Journal on Selected Areas in Communications 23(12), 2213–2222 (2005)
10. Padala, P., et al.: Adaptive control of virtualized resources in utility computing environments. SIGOPS Open. Syst. Rev. 41(3), 289–302 (2007)
11. Gerald, T., Wliilam, E.W., Jeffrey, O.K.: Utility-Function-Driven Resource Allocation in Autonomic Systems. In: Proceeding of the Second International Conference on Automatic Computing. IEEE Computer Society (2005)
12. Rao, W.B., Li, Z.Q., Shang, G.: Dynamic damage identification by neural network. In: Proceedings of International Conference on Advanced Problems in Vibration Theory and Applications, Beijing (2000)

Weight Based Live Migration
of Virtual Machines

Baiyou Qiao, Kai Zhang, Yanpeng Guo, Yutong Li,
Yuhai Zhao, and Guoren Wang

College of Information Science & Engineering, Northeastern University, China
qiaobaiyou@ise.neu.edu.cn

Abstract. Due to having many advantages, virtualization has been widely used and become a key technology of cloud computing. Live migration of virtual machines is the core technique of virtualization fields, but the existing pre-copy live migration approaches have problems of low copy efficiency and long total migration time, so we propose a weight based live migration algorithm of virtual machines in this paper, which adds weights to the dirty page information collected, preferentially selects and transfers the dirty pages that are not modified frequently, the dirty pages that are modified frequently are transferred after virtual machine is suspended. The algorithm effectively reduces the amount of memory pages transferred and the total migration time. Experiment results show that when virtual machine is under heavy load, the proposed algorithm considerably reduces the number of transferred memory pages and shortens the total migration time without significantly increment of the virtual machine downtime.

Keywords: Xen, Virtual Machine, Live Migration, Cloud Computing.

1 Introduction

Virtualization technology first appeared in the 1960's, and plays an important role in the development of the computer; it is widely used in the fields of services and resources integration, system security and distributed computing. Since virtualization technology can enhance the resilience and flexibility of system architecture, implement resources partition and aggregation, package services transparently and so on, it can greatly enhance the efficiency of resource usage, reduce the computing cost. Virtualization has become one of the important supporting technologies of current mainstream cloud computing systems. As one of the key techniques of virtualization, live migration of virtual machines can seamlessly and completely migrate a running virtual machine from one physical machine to another. It is usually used along with the resource monitoring and load balancing algorithm to schedule resources automatically in the cloud computing systems, achieving load balancing among physical machines. This technique greatly increases automatic resource management capabilities of cloud computing center, reducing operating and maintenance costs and enhancing the system

J. Li et al. (Eds.): PAKDD 2013 Workshops, LNAI 7867, pp. 543–554, 2013.

availability and scalability, so live migration of virtual machines has attracted more and more people's attention.

Xen[1] is a very excellent open source virtualization hypervisor of x86 platform, which has high performance approximate of the original system, it is able to support full virtualization and has been widely used. However, virtualization platforms including Xen mainly use pre-copy migration algorithm to implement live migration of virtual machines. The main drawback of this algorithm is that its iterative pre-copy process needs to transfer many memory pages repeatedly when the migration memory pages are modified frequently. This leads to the repeated transmission of a large number of memory pages, not only adding the total migration time, but also taking up network bandwidth, and thus reducing system performance. To solve this problem, in this paper we present a weight based migration algorithm (WBMA) on the basis of deeply analyzing the original pre-copy memory migration algorithm. The algorithm weighs the dirty pages information collected, and gives priorities to send the pages which have low modification frequency and are not used in the period of time, for the pages which has high modification frequency will be transferred after the virtual machine is suspended. The experiment results show that the proposed algorithm can effectively reduce the number of memory pages transferred and the total migration time, and not significantly increase the virtual machine downtime.

2   Related Works

In recent years, virtual machine live migration techniques are given much attention by scholars at home and abroad, and a lot of relative researches have been done. Live migration algorithm of virtual machines is one of the main research directions, and many research results have been made. Several typical migration algorithms of virtual machines are presented such as stop-and-copy[2], pre-copy[3], post-copy[4] and etc.. The stop-and-copy migration algorithm is suitable for small memory system. Pre-copy algorithm is the mainstream live migration algorithm of virtual machines currently, which copies memory pages on the source machine to the target machine iteratively. However, this algorithm has a problem which is that the total migration time is too long. Hines proposed post-copy algorithm, which first transfers the state of the CPU and necessary memory information to the target host, at the same time starts the virtual machine and transfers necessary memory pages from the source host to the target host dynamically. Paper [5] proposed a new fast and transparent virtual machine migration mechanism which uses Re Virt framework and combines the checkpoint recovery idea with the track playback technology, but the method wastes some performance. Paper[6] proposed an adaptive data compression algorithm, which selects the appropriate compression algorithm to compress memory pages based on the characteristics of the memory page data. Paper[7] proposed an improved pre-copy scheme, which adds a data structure called *to_send_last* bitmap to mark memory pages that modified frequently. In the final round of the iterative process of copy, it transfers memory pages marked by the *to_send_last* bitmap. Paper[8] proposed a hierarchical copy algorithm based on Xen pre-copy algorithm, which layers memory pages according to its modification frequency, and adjusts the transferring strategy of memory pages in the first iterative copy. The first iterative copy does not send all memory pages, but sets writable working set testing in advance of the stage of pre-migration and resource reservation of original algorithm. Paper[9] proposed a slowdown scheduling algorithm, decreasing the CPU resources that have been assigned to migration domain, and reduces the dirtying page rate according to the decrease of CPU activity, but it increases response time. Paper[10] proposed a memory migration mechanism named Microwiper. Microwiper includes two policies, which are transferring according to memory page modification rate and transferring regulator. The former divides the memory of virtual machines into a series of regions, migrates according to the rate of modification of the region, while the latter adjusts the page transferring according to the network bandwidth.

3   Analysis of Xen Pre-copy Migration Algorithm

The virtual machine (VM) migration is mainly related to two important performance indicators, which are downtime and total migration time. According to the weight of two indicators, different algorithms are designed to meet different application requirements. Pre-copy method well balances the contradiction between downtime and total migration time, and it is used by the live migration of the VMware, Xen and other mainstream virtualization platform. Assume that the source host is A, the destination host is B, and then the whole Xen pre-copy algorithm consists of the following five steps:

Step1: Source Reservation. At this stage, the source host A sends a request to the destination host B, the first thing need to be done is to make sure whether there are enough resources to run the migration virtual machine. If so, it reserves the resources which have the same size as the VM migrated, or the VM is still running in A, and it may choose another host as the destination host.

Step2: Iterative Pre-Copy. At this stage, the memory of the VM will be copied to the destination host B by A in an iterative manner; the VM in A is still in the state of running and offer service. In first round of iteration copy, all the VM memory pages should be copied from A to B. In the latter iteration, only the memory pages modified on the last transmission process are copied.

Step3: Stop-and-Copy. The copy process of the iteration will be stopped once meeting the given conditions. Then suspend the migration VM in the host A, and redirect the network connection of VM to destination host B, transmit the state of the CPU and the left dirty pages from A to B. After this stage, A and B have the same copy of the suspended VM. If the migration fails, the VM in A could still restore to run.

Step4: Commitment. The target host B informs Host A that virtual machine image has been successfully received. Once the message is conformed, the source host A will destroy the original VM.

Step5: Activation. In this phase, host B activates the migrated VM, binds the device drivers to the destination host B, and broadcasts the new IP address.

In the above migration algorithm of Xen, memory iterative pre-copy is the important factor affecting migration performance. The VM memory migration of Xen is copy memory pages from the source host to the destination host iteratively. The first round of transmission includes all pages of memory of the VM. For later iterations, the n-th iteration of the transmission only includes the modified pages in the n-1th iteration process. But from the point of view of systems, the memory pages frequently modified are to be repeatedly transferred for many times. This increases the number of memory pages for each iteration transmission and total migration time, it has a negative impact on the migration performance. These pages changed frequently are called Writable Working Set (WWS). Precisely determining WWS can avoid repeat transmission of the pages and reduce the iteration times. In order to accurately determine WWS and migrate memory efficiently, Xen divides virtual machine memory pages into three categories[11], using three page bitmap variables, which are to_send, to_skip and to_fix. To_send denotes the pages that become dirty in the former round of the iterative process and those pages need to be transmitted in this iteration; To_skip is the bitmap that introduced by Xen in order to reduce the memory pages retransmission, it marks the pages that are modified more frequently and can be skipped in the current round of iteration. To_fix marks the pages that have not been mapped and will be transferred in the final round of stop and copy stage.

We can see from above analysis, Xen pre-copy algorithm mainly through two consecutive collection of dirty page information to two bitmaps to_send and to_skip, then compares this two bitmaps information to determine the WWS. Obviously, such a method of testing WWS is too simple, especially under the memory pages being modified frequently, the information collected is not sufficient to predict modification state of a page, and this leads the WWS measurement inaccurate, and makes many memory pages transmitted repeatedly more times, which increases the total migration time, and makes the performance of pre-copy migration algorithm not high.

4   Weight Based Live Migration Algorithm

We can draw from above analysis that under the heavy load environment, the performance of Xen pre-copy algorithm is low, the main reason is that its WWS measurement is inaccurate. To solve the problem, we presents a weight based live migration algorithm. We will describe the main idea, data structures, collection approach of dirty pages and other aspects of the proposed algorithm in detail.

4.1   Main Idea

In accordance with the principle of program locality, the more recently used instructions or data will be likely to be used later, so the greater the probability of recently modified pages are modified again. According to this principle we propose a weight based pre-copy algorithm, which is based on the Xen original pre-copy algorithm, and improve the WWS measuring method. the main ideas is that in each round of the iterative process, repeatedly collects dirty page information of VM and assign an appropriate weight, then compute the weight of each dirty page. A larger weight value of a dirty page shows its higher modification frequency and higher possibility to be used again in the next period of time. A smaller weight value of a dirty page shows the lower modification frequency and in the future over a period of time it is not likely to be used. After setting a threshold value, dirty pages whose weight values are less than the threshold are transferred in each iteration copy process. This can predict the virtual machine memory page modification trends and accurately measure the WWS, thereby reducing the pages to be transmitted and improving page transmission efficiency, hence reducing the migration time and optimizing the migration performance.

4.2   The Main Data Structures and Variables

To predict dirty page information accurately and implement efficient migration of virtual machines, we improve the original pre-copy migration algorithm based on the above design ideas. The important data structures and variables used by the algorithm are as follows:

$Dirtymaps[i][j]$: used to record the modification information of a memory page which is collected in a iterative copy process, i denotes the i-th iterative process and j denotes the j-th dirty page.

$Collect\_times$: used to specify the times of dirty pages to be collected in an iterative process, abbreviated as CT.

$Dirty\_maps\_tag$: bitmap label array, i.e. values of the $dirty\_maps$ elements, it is an important variable to process page transferring, if a page is modified (dirty), its $dirty\_maps$ corresponding to $dirty\_maps\_tag$ is set to 1; otherwise set to 0. The initial values of $dirty\_maps\_tag$ array are 0.

$Dirty\_weight_i$: the weight of a dirty page i, representing the modifying degree of dirty page i in one iteration, the parameter is used to determine WWS.

$Threshold$: transferring threshold of memory page, which is used to mark memory pages, if the $dirty\_weight$ of a memory page is greater than the threshold, the memory page will not be transferred in this iteration copy process. The threshold value is set according to the weights set.

$Time\_slot$: the time slot, i.e. time interval to collect dirty page bitmap information.

$Mem\_page\_send[]$: the array is used to record the information of memory pages which will be transferred. This array corresponds to the to_send bitmap of original Xen pre-copy algorithm, if $mem\_page\_send[i]$ equals to 1, the memory page i needs to be transferred in this iteration; otherwise it will not be transferred.

Max_iters: maximum time of iterative pre-copy. Original maximum time of iterations is 29 in Xen3.4.2, which does not include the downtime (the last round of iterative copy time).

In addition to the above data structures and variables, we also use data structures and variables of Xen original pre-copy algorithm as much as possible, and make the changes of Xen3.4.2 source code smallest. The function name and parameter lists are remained unchanged to ensure that the upper layer services calling interface of Xen3.4.2 platform unchanged.

4.3   Compute Weights of Memory Dirty Pages

The proposed algorithm first collects memory pages information, and then computes the weight for each dirty page to determine WWS. Collection of dirty pages directly use shadow page table operation XENDOMCTL_OP_CLEAN provided by Xen platform, memory dirty page bitmap information are copied to *dirty_maps* array, then empty the memory dirty page bitmap, after a given time slot (specified by *time_slot* parameter) executes the next dirty page information collection operation, and do such operations repeatedly, until it reaches a given collection times. The time slot is given by *Time_slot* variable which can be specified by user. In Xen3.4.2 *time_slot* initial value is set to 900 milliseconds, it decreased by 80 milliseconds after one round of iteration. Fig. 1 shows the procedure of collecting memory dirty page information.

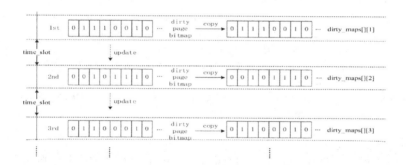

Fig. 1. The demonstration of collecting dirty Page information

We can see from Fig. 1 that the dirty page information of memory are collected many times. All of them are stored in the *dirty_maps* array, and then used to calculate the weight of each dirty page. If we use $Dirty\_Weight_i$ to express the weight of dirty page i, the calculation is as equation (1):

$$Dirty\_Weight_i = Dirty\_maps\,[i]\,[1] * Weight_1 + Dirty\_maps\,[i]\,[2] * \\ Weight_2 + \cdots + Dirty\_maps\,[i]\,[ct] * Weight_{ct} \tag{1}$$

In the equation above, $dirty\_maps[i][j]$ denotes the modifying information of memory page i collected in the j-th time, whose value is 0 or 1. 1 means the page is changed, and 0 means the page is not changed; $Weight_j$ that can be specified means the weight of dirty page information collected in the j-th time;

The weight of dirty pages is the sum of products of each modifying information and each page weight of each collecting time. We can know from the equation (1) that setting the weight of dirty pages in each collection time not only influences the weight of the whole dirty pages mostly, but also influences the performance of weight based Pre-copy algorithm directly. We can know from the discussion above, the weight of pages collected latest should be bigger than the earlier ones, which may measure the WWS accurately. We can set weights with different systems, such as binary system, $2^0, 2^1, \cdots, 2^i, \cdots$ and quaternary system, $4^0, 4^1, 4^2, \cdots, 4^i$, etc.. In order to make the weights of pages smaller for the convenient calculation, we take the binary system as the weight of pages. We set the weights $weight_1, weight_2, \cdots, weight_{ct}$ of pages that collected in first time, second time, $\cdots$, $collect\_times$ time as $2^0, 2^1, \cdots, 2^{ct-1}$. This way not only satisfies the need of the dirty page weight of each collection time is different, and the weight of latest col-lection is higher in one magnitude than that of last time. The Fig. 2 is an example of calculating page weights, where CT is 4; the weights of collecting 4 times and the weights calculated of ten dirty pages are shown in the figure.

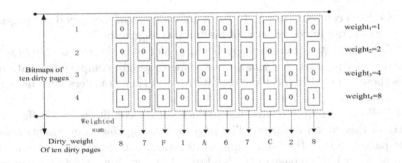

Fig. 2. An example of calculating page weights

4.4   Marking Memory Pages

When calculating the page weight, it needs to compare it with the predefined thresh-old to decide whether to send the page this round of iterative copy. Its important to set a proper value of the threshold, if too big it can make some frequently changed pages to be transferred repeatedly, which increases the network loads and total migration time; if too small it can lead some not frequently changed pages are mistaken as frequently changed pages to be sent at the last, which increases the pages transferred in the final round of iteration and prolongs the downtime of that machine. So the threshold must have a moderate value. There will be a threshold setting the highest number of weight of the collection times, which is $2^{(ct-1)}$. So we can mark the memory pages into three categories according to the threshold: (1) the pages that their *dirty_weight* values are equal to zero have never been modified and will be sent to the destination host in the first round of iteration; (2) the pages that the weights are greater than zero but less than the threshold can be thought as not frequently modified pages and will be sent at this round of iteration; (3) the pages that their weights are greater than the threshold are looked as frequently updated pages and will be updated recently, and will be skipped to transfer in this round of iteration. This can improve the efficiency of page transferring, reduce the times of iteration, and shorten the total migration time.

4.5   Weight Based Pre-copy Algorithm

In this paper, the process flow of weight based migration algorithm (WBMA) is generally the same with that of original xen pre-copy algorithm migration, while the difference lies in the memory migration. In WBMA, the measuring of WWS is not a simply comparison of the bitmap *to_send* and *to_skip* to decide whether to transfer a memory page, but introducing the weight calculation of dirty pages to determine the memory pages transferring. The weight based pre-copy algorithm is as following steps:

(1) Collects *collect_times* (CT) times information of memory dirty pages into *dirty_maps* array in the process of preliminary migration.

(2) When the iteration pre-copy begins, calculates the weight *Dirty_weight* of the memory pages in *dirty_maps* according to weight computing equation and marks those pages that meet the conditions, and then transfers into *mem_page_send* array.

(3) Collects M requirements pages which satisfy condition into buffer, as the objects of this round iteration. The pages satisfying the requirements refer to: a) the page is not in the final round of iteration, and its *mem_page_send* label not to be 1; Or b) The page of the final round of iteration, and its bitmap *to_fix* corresponding label to be 1; Or c) The page of the final round of iteration, and its bitmap *to_send* corresponding label to be 1, that is, the last dirty page of VM. Here the bitmap *to_fix* is the same with the original pre-copy algorithm, but the bitmap *to_send* here marks the final dirty page of VM, which is already not the same with the original algorithm.

(4) Transfer the memory pages in the buffer, repeat the operations in steps (3), (4) until all the memory pages of the VM are scanned.

(5) When transferring memory pages of a round, determine whether it would be the final round of iteration If not, repeat the operation of collecting dirty page messages in step (1), otherwise, copy the dirty messages into *to_send* directly.

(6)Repeat step (2), (3), (4), (5) until meeting the exit conditions, then transfer the last memory pages. The exit conditions are the same with original pre-copy algorithm.

(7)Suspends VM, and directly copies dirty page information into *to_send* bitmap, and then transfers the related memory dirty pages which are corresponding to the *to_send* bitmap. Due to limited space, the detail description of WBMA algorithm is omitted.

Table 1. The comparison of downtime (ms) with load

	pre-copy	ct=2	ct=3	ct=4	ct=5	ct=6	ct=7	ct=8
Mem intensive	22926	22568	22875	22922	22987	22990	23014	23425
I/O intensive	683	650	685	690	710	725	785	810
CPU intensive	732	689	715	730	745	763	801	832

5 Performance Evaluation

To evaluate the performance of the improved algorithm, we setup the corresponding experiment environment and make a large number of experiments; the comparison between original Xen pre-copy algorithm and the proposed algorithm are given in detail.

5.1 Experimental Environment

The environment consists of 3 PC (Intel Core 2 Quad Q8400 2.66 GHz CPU, 4G Memory, 1T Disk), among them there are 2 physical nodes, on which Centos5.6, Xen3.4.3, migration module and related resource monitoring modules are installed. The third node is used as a management server and NFS storage server. All nodes are connected with 1000M Ethernet.

5.2 Experimental Results

On the designed experiment platform, we create different full virtualization machine (FVM) and Para virtualization machine (PVM) with 128M, 256M, 512M, 1024M memory. Every virtual machine (VM) is installed with CPU intensive, memory intensive and I/O intensive applications respectively. We make large amount of experiments and analysis the performance of the weight based migration algorithm(WBMA) on the effect of collecting times, total migrate time, transferred memory pages and downtime.

(1) Effect of collecting times. To test the effect of dirty page collecting times (CT), we create one PVM with a VCPU, 512M memory, and make experiments with I/O intensive, CPU intensive, memory intensive applications. Fig. 3(a) and Fig. 3(b) describe the total migrate time and transferred memory pages with different collecting times. We learn from the figures that as the collecting times increase, the total migrate time and transferred memory pages decrease. When CT is 4, the total migrate time decrease by 15%, and the transferred memory pages decrease by 20%. When CT is greater than 5, the decreasing tread becomes weak. From the downtime of Table 1, when CT is 4 or 5, the downtime is close to the old pre-copy algorithm. When CT is greater than 5, the downtime increases. Because the more the collecting times is, the more accurate the WWS is. This makes the frequently modified memory pages are transferred at the final time iteration, and leads to the increasing of VM downtime.

Overall consideration of the effect of collecting times on total migrate time, amount of memory transferred and downtime, we advise the collecting times should be 4 or 5.

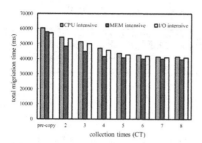

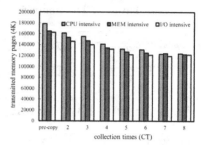

(a) Varying of total migration time   (b) Varying of total pages transferred

Fig. 3. The varying of total migrate time and transferred memory pages with different collecting times

(2) The total migration time. The total migration time is an important indicator for measuring migration algorithm, the less the total migration time is, the higher the performance of the algorithm gains. When running certain load applications and the CT value of WBMA algorithm is 4, the varying of the total migration time with different memory size of the virtual machines is shown as Fig. 4(a), we can see from the figure, the total migration time in-creased as memory increases. For the same algorithm, the total migration time of FVM is greater than that of PVM. Compared with the original pre-copy migration algorithm, the total migration time of the WBMA algorithm can be reduced by 15%, it shows that WBMA algorithm has higher performance.

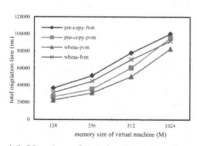

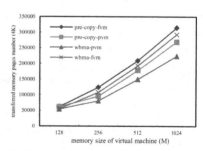

(a) Varying of total migration time   (b) Varying of total pages transferred

Fig. 4. The performance comparison of two algorithms with different memory size

(3) The total memory pages transferred. The total memory pages transferred is another important indicator to evaluate the performance of VM migration algorithms, the smaller the total memory pages transferred, the higher the performance of the algorithm. Under the same conditions as Fig. 4(a), to perform the two migration algorithm, Fig. 4(b) shows the change of total pages transferred with the different memory size. It can be seen that the total migration

Table 2. The comparison of downtime (ms) with memory-intensive workload

	8M	16M	32M	64M	128M	256M
Pre-copy-fvm-wirte	1166	2003	3877	6560	12897	28041
Pre-copy-pvm-wirte	793	1491	2969	5757	11554	22926
Pre-copy-fvm-read	328	323	322	316	322	329
Pre-copy-pvm-read	40	46	45	45	40	39
Wbma-fvm-wirte	1160	2000	3800	6550	12900	28045
Wbma-pvm-wirte	790	1500	3030	5772	11790	23390
Wbma-fvm-read	330	323	329	322	333	330
Wbma-pvm-read	42	45	50	51	50	55

pages increase as the VM memory size increases. Compared with the original Pre-copy algorithm, the proposed WBMA algorithm reduces total transferred memory pages by 20%. This is because that the dirty page rate increases along with the increasing of WM memory size, WBMA algorithm can accurately determinate the WWS, thus reduces the memory pages to be transferred and the number of iterations, in addition reduces the total migration time.

(4) Downtime. Downtime is a very important metrics in live migration ·of VMs. Long downtime will make the live migration lose its meaning, so good algorithm must be guaranteed within a certain time period to complete the live migration. Table 2 presents the comparison of downtime between the two algorithms with different WWS sizes. When a 512M memory virtual machine executes live migration, read and write operations at the same time, the WWS sizes are 8M, 16M, 32M, 64M, 128M, 256M respectively. It can be seen from the Table 2, when writing memory and executing migration, the downtime increases proportionally as the WWS increases. This is because the larger the WWS, the more the memory pages modified frequently, and those memory pages will be transferred only after the virtual machine is suspended, and this prolongs the downtime. For read memory operations, the downtime is considerable less than that of the write operations. This is because the read operations do not change the contents of the memory pages, so the memory pages modified frequently are relative few, and there is little pages need to transfer at the final stage. However, compared with the original pre-copy algorithm, the weight based pre-copy migration algorithm does not increase downtime of VM significantly.

From the comparison of the above three aspects, we can draw a conclusion that when the collection times is 4, the proposed weight based pre-copy algorithm is able to obtain a good balance between the total migration time and downtime. It can reduce the total migration time and the dirty pages transferred, and not increase the downtime significantly. It is a better optimization of WM live migration algorithm.

6   Conclusions

In this paper, we improve the WWS measurement method of original Xen pre-copy algorithm on the basis of the research and analysis on the existing live migration algorithms of virtual machines and the program locality principle. We change the two times dirty page information collection into multiple times collection, and weight the dirty pages collected to determine the WWS, the method can reduce the number of actual memory pages to be transferred. The experiment results show that the proposed algorithm can reduce the total migration time, at the same time it does not increase the downtime significantly, and has better migration efficiency. Next step we will consider other factors that affect the performance of the live migration, such as network bandwidth and etc., and improve the migration algorithm performance further.

Acknowledgments. This research was supported by the National Natural Science Foundation of China (No. 61073063, 61173029, 61100028, 61272182 and 61173030) and the Public Science and Technology Research Funds Projects of Ocean (No. 201105033).

References

1. Xen Hypervisor, http://www.xen.org/products/xenhyp.html
2. Sapuntzakis, C.P., Chandra, R., Pfaff, B., et al.: Optimizing the migration of virtual computers. SIGOPS Oper. Syst. Rev. 36(SI), 377–390 (2002)
3. Clark, C., Fraser, K., Hand, S., Hansen, J.G., Jul, E., Limpach, C., Pratt, I., Warfield, A.: Live migration of virtual machines. In: Proceedings of the Second Symposium on Networked Systems Design and Implementation (NSDI 2005), pp. 273–286 (2005)
4. Hines, M.R., Gopalan, K.: Post-copy based live virtual machine migration using adaptive pre-paging and dynamic self-ballooning. In: Proceedings of the ACM/Usenix International Conference on Virtual Execution Environments (VEE 2009), pp. 51–60 (2009)
5. Liu, H., Jin, H., Liao, X., Hu, L., Yu, C.: Live migration of virtual machine based on full system trace and replay. In: Proceedings of the 18th International Symposium on High Performance Distributed Computing (HPDC 2009), pp. 101–110 (2009)
6. Jin, H., Deng, L., Wu, S., Shi, X., Pan, X.: Live virtual machine migration with adaptive memory compression. In: Proceedings of the 2009 IEEE International Conference on Cluster Computing, Cluster 2009 (2009)
7. Ma, F., Liu, F., Liu, Z.: Live virtual machine migration based on improved pre-copy approach. In: 2010 IEEE International Conference Software Engineering and Service Sciences (ICSESS), pp. 230–233 (2010)
8. Liu, Z., Qu, W., Yan, T., Li, H., Li, K.: Hierarchical Copy Algorithm for Xen Live Migration. In: 2010 International Conference on Cyber-Enabled Distributed Computing and Knowledge Discovery, pp. 361–364 (2010)
9. Liu, Z., Qu, W., Liu, W., Li, K.: Xen Live Migration with Slowdown Scheduling Algorithm. In: The 11th International Conference on Parallel and Distributed Computing, Applications and Technologies, pp. 215–221 (2010)
10. Du, Y., Yu, H., Shi, G., Chen, J., Zheng, W.: Microwiper:Efficient Memory Propagation in Live Migration of Virtual Machines. In: 39th International Conference on Parallel Processing, pp. 142–149 (2010)
11. Sun, Y.: Researches on Xen virtual machine and live migration techniques. Shanghai University (2009)

Author Index